Penguin Books
Our Bodies Ourselves

Angela Phillips is a freelance journalist and
photographer specializing in subjects to do with
women and health. Jill Rakusen is a journalist,
specializing also in women's health issues.
Both writers have been actively involved in the
women's liberation movement for many years.

Our Bodies Ourselves

A health book by and for women

Boston Women's Health Book Collective

British edition by Angela Phillips and Jill Rakusen

Penguin Books

Penguin Books Ltd, Harmondsworth,
Middlesex, England
Penguin Books, 625 Madison Avenue,
New York, New York 10022, USA
Penguin Books Australia Ltd, Ringwood,
Victoria, Australia
Penguin Books Canada Ltd, 2801 John Street,
Markham, Ontario, Canada L3R 1B4
Penguin Books (NZ) Ltd, 182–190 Wairau Road,
Auckland 10, New Zealand

First published in the USA 1971
Published simultaneously in Penguin Books and Allen Lane 1978
Reprinted in Penguin Books 1979

Designed by Paul Bowden
Made and printed in Great Britain by
G. A. Pindar & Son Ltd, Scarborough, England

Set in 'Monophoto' Photina by Filmtype Services Limited, Scarborough

Contents

Photograph Acknowledgements

P. 8 Phyllis Ewen; p. 15 and 407 bottom right Jean Raisler;
p. 31 Ann Popkin; p. 33 Gregers Nielsen; p. 55 Mark Rusher;
pp. 70, 106, 113, 116, 127, 220, 232, 297, 340, 377, 463, 517,
532, 560, 565 and 569 Angela Phillips; p. 79 Andrea Black;
p. 97 Norma Pitfield; p. 228 Michael Ann Mullen; p. 316 Mark
Feldberg; p. 406 top Ed Pincus; pp. 406 middle and bottom, 407
top and bottom left and 549 Miriam Weinstein; p. 456
Elizabeth Cole; pp. 474–5 Marcia Kasabian.

Authors of the American edition listed
according to the chapters in that edition:

Preface, Wilma Vilunya Diskin, Wendy Coppedge Sanford; *Our Changing Sense of Self*, Joan Sheingold Ditzion; *The Anatomy and Physiology of Sexuality and Reproduction*, Esther R. Rome, Jill Wolhandler, Abby Schwarz; *Sexuality*, Nancy Press Hawley, Elizabeth A. McGee, Wendy Coppedge Sanford; *Living with Ourselves and Others — Our Sexual Relationships*, Paula Brown Doress, Nancy Press Hawley, Joan Sheingold Ditzion, Judy Norsigian; *In Amerika They Call Us Dykes*, a Boston gay collective; *Taking Care of Ourselves*, Judy Norsigian, Janet Jones, Carol McEldowney, Norma Meras Swenson; *Rape*, Judy Norsigian, with help from Boston Area Rape Crisis Center and Washington, D.C., Rape Crisis Center; *Self-defense*, Janet Jones, Carol McEldowney; *Venereal Disease*, Esther R. Rome, based on work by Fran Ansley, with help from Abby Schwarz; *Birth Control*, Wendy Coppedge Sanford, Barbara Bridgman Perkins, based on work by Pamela Chernoff Berger, with help from Kelly Mayo, Elizabeth A. McGee, Abby Schwarz; *Abortion*, Wendy Coppedge Sanford, Elizabeth McCord, Elizabeth A. McGee; *Considering Parenthood*, Joan Sheingold Ditzion, Ruth Davidson Bell, Wilma Vilunya Diskin, Paula Brown Doress, Nancy Press Hawley, Jane Kates Pincus, Wendy Coppedge Sanford; *Childbearing Unit*, Jane Kates Pincus, Robbie Pfeufer; *Pregnancy*, Jane Kates Pincus, Ruth Davidson Bell, Norma Meras Swenson; *Preparation for Childbirth*, Ruth Davidson Bell, Jane Kates Pincus, Norma Meras Swenson, Wendy Coppedge Sanford, Robbie Pfeufer, Barbara Cane; *Postpartum — After the Baby is Born*, Wilma Vilunya Diskin, Paula Brown Doress, Ruth Davidson Bell, Norma Meras Swenson; *Some Exceptions to the Normal Childbearing Experience*, Jane Kates Pincus, Barbara Eck Menning, Susan Siroty, Ellen Bresnick; *Menopause*, Pamela Chernoff Berger, Judy Norsigian, Marcia Kasabian, Wendy Coppedge Sanford; *Women and Health Care*, Mary Rollston Stern, Norma Meras Swenson, Jane Kates Pincus, Judy Norsigian, the section on The American Health Care System based on work by Barbara Bridgman Perkins, Lucy Candib, Nancy Todd.

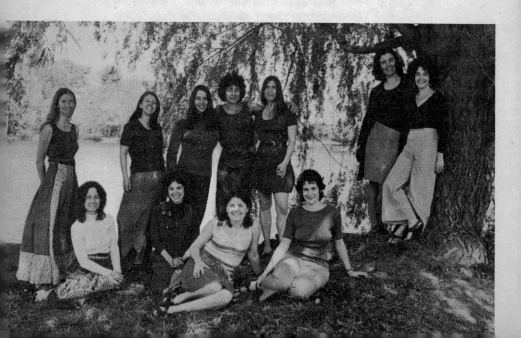

Preface to the UK edition

When we were approached by Penguin to produce this edition of *Our Bodies Ourselves*, we were delighted. As feminists, we had both been involved in health issues for some time: writing for the collective production of *Women's Report* and other publications, working in health groups, in campaigns around such issues as abortion, and/or in psychiatry groups, self-help groups or in health care courses. *Our Bodies Ourselves* was a book which had helped us in our lives and we wanted to make it more available and appropriate to women in this country.

The preparation of this edition has involved both up-dating and extensive adaptation. Since new information comes to light virtually every day, it is unavoidable that some of the text will be out of date by the time you read this. However, any significant changes in the law or in health policies will have been incorporated into the text up to January 1978.

In adapting the text, we have had to bear several points in mind. Firstly, our health care system is very different from that in the USA. This had particular implications for the chapters on Abortion, Childbirth, and of course on the final chapter — Women and Health Care. Much in these chapters has therefore been rewritten. Secondly, treatments and medical practices can also differ greatly (a reminder of how much medical treatment is still at the theory stage); thus in some places we have altered the original text considerably. For example, in the Menopause chapter, we have tried to provide a balanced, feminist view of the subject in the light of the fact that in this country, unlike the USA, doctors are loath to prescribe anything other than tranquillizers. The treatment of breast cancer also differs significantly from the more radical procedures commonly meted out to women in the USA: the text has been adapted accordingly.

We have kept to the spirit of the original book throughout, and, wherever possible, to the letter, diverging in instances like the above, or where we thought that more detail was necessary (as in the case of post-operative care of women undergoing mastectomy). Like the Boston women, we could have produced a book twice this size, but neither we nor our editor wanted the book to be prohibitively expensive. We have therefore had to shorten the original text – at times an extremely difficult job – in order to make way for new material specifically relevant to this country. We have also included new material on 'alternative medicine' where possible.

Inevitably, our own politics have coloured the content of the book. We decided to continue using the pronoun 'we' throughout but, as the Boston women explain in their preface, this does not mean that we all agree with everything that has been written. 'We', therefore, unless it is specifically stated otherwise, refers to the collective experience of all the women who have worked on this book. We believe that what we have written is in the spirit of a world-wide feminist movement, and although it was geographically impossible to work with the original collective we hope they will accept our changes as another contribution to the discussion of health care politics and feminism.

Many people have been involved in this book. We would first like to thank the Boston Women's Health Book Collective for producing it in the first place, and secondly, Julia Vellacott, who has acted more as a third member of a collective than as our editor. In expressing our thanks to the following groups and individuals who have helped and supported us in our work, and/or freely shared their experience and their knowledge, we are expressing our indebtedness, not only to them, but to the women's liberation movement as a whole. This book would never have been written without the existence of the women's liberation movement: the inspiration and ideas behind it are a product of the movement as a whole.

Thank you to: Lynn Alderson, Anne Anderson, Judy and John Bancroft, Sue Barlow, Berry Beaumont, Christine Beels, Valerie Beral, Lorna Carmichael, Children's Rights Workshop, Sam Collett, Anna Coote, Sarita Cordell, Kathy Engleman, everyone at the Manchester Women and Health Conference, Carragh Fiddian, Bobby Freeman, Gillian Frost, Lyn Gambles, Romola Guiton, Jeanne and Aksel Haahr, Mary Hemming, Annaliese Hennessey, Judy Hodgkin, Peter Huntingford, Barbara Jacobs, Lidwin Jury, Caroline Langridge, Lin Layram, Annie Lee, Isobel McGilvray, Nancy MacKeith, Dawn Marler, Carol Marshall, Elspeth Moir, Sylvia Morrison, National Childbirth Trust, Jenny Oswald, Di Palmer, Ruth Petrie, Griselda Pollock, Martin Richards, Maureen Roberts, Ann Satin, Scottish Lesbian Feminists, Marianne Scruggs, Joyce Sherlock, Margaret Stacey, Doreen Stewart, Penny Stock, Cathie Thomson, Women and Science Collective.

Angela Phillips
Jill Rakusen
1977

1 A Good Story

The history of this book is lengthy and satisfying. It began in 1969 in a small discussion group called 'Women and Their Bodies' at a Boston Women's Conference. For many of us, talking to women in this way was a totally new experience and we decided to go on meeting as a group to continue the discussion.

We had all experienced frustration and anger towards specific doctors and the medical maze in general, and initially we wanted to do something about this. As we talked we began to realize how little we knew about our own bodies, so we decided to do further research, to prepare papers in groups and then to discuss our findings together. We learned both from professional sources (medical textbooks, journals, doctors, nurses) and from our own experience.

For instance, many of us had 'learned' about the menstrual cycle in science or biology classes. But most of us did not remember much of what we had learned. This time when we read in a text that the onset of menstruation is a normal and universal occurrence in young girls, we started to talk about our first menstrual periods. We found that, for many of us, beginning to menstruate had not felt normal at all, but scary, embarrassing, mysterious. We realized that what we had been told about menstruation and what we had not been told – even the tone of voice it had been told in – had all had an effect on our feelings about being female.

The results of our findings were used to present courses for other women. We would meet in any available free space, in schools, nurseries, church halls, in our own homes. As we taught, we learned from other women, and as they learned, they went on to give courses to others. We saw it as a never-ending process always involving more and more women.

Some people have asked us why the book is only about women. As women we do not consider ourselves experts on men (as men through the centuries have considered themselves experts on us). We feel that it would be best for men to do what we have done for themselves.

After teaching the first course we decided to duplicate our papers for other women to use. This led to the first inexpensive edition of the book, which was published by the New England Free Press. There was so much demand for the book that in time it seemed logical to publish commercially to reach even more women. Over time we have revised and updated the material several times, using the royalties from sales to support health education work.

The material in this book comes not only from us but from other women living in or passing through the area who have read, discussed and added their own ideas. We in the collective do not agree with everything that has been written. Some of us are uncomfortable with part of the material. We have included it anyway because we give more weight to accepting that we differ than to our uneasiness.

Knowledge has freed us to an extent. It has freed us, for example, from playing the role of mother if it is not a role that fits us. It has given us room to discover the energy and talents that are in us. We want to help make this freedom available to every woman. This is why people in the women's movement have been so active in fighting legal restrictions, the imperfections of available contraceptives, poor sex education, and poorly administered health care that keep too many women from having this crucial control over their bodies.

For us, body education is core education. Our bodies are the physical bases from which we move out into the world; ignorance, uncertainty — even, at worst, shame — about our physical selves create in us an alienation from ourselves that keeps us from being the whole people that we should be.

We still work as a group; our current collective has been together for seven years. We are all white, middle-class, and our ages range from twenty-nine to forty-five. Some of us are married, some of us are single, some have children and some do not; we are all working, or have worked, outside our homes. In short, we are both a very ordinary and a very special group, as women everywhere. We realize that poor and non-white women have greater difficulty in getting accurate information and adequate health care, and are most often mistreated in the ways we describe in this book. Learning about our womanhood from the inside out has allowed us to cross over some of the barriers of race, colour, income and class, and to feel a sense of identity with all women in the experience of being female.

How the Experience Changed Us

We formed our group as individual women meeting together because we wanted to. Since most of us had patterned our lives around men, working together was a liberating experience. Like most women's groups we talked to each other about how it felt growing up female; this gave us a basis to discuss what we thought and felt about ourselves and how we wanted to change. At first it was rather scary admitting that we were not completely satisfied with our lives, standing back and taking a hard look at ourselves. Some of us were afraid that commitment to the women's movement and to the group would weaken our ties with men, children, jobs, life-styles; that we might lose control of our lives. We came to realize that this fear was unrealistic. No one could take from us what we did not want to give up.

Probably the most valuable thing we learned was to speak for ourselves and be ourselves. Many of us feared discussing personal details of our lives and relationships, we feared being ridiculed by others, but we soon learned that we had a lot in common. By facing up to our ambivalent feelings and being honest and open, we were able to build up more trusting relationships.

We discovered four cultural notions of femininity which we have in some sense shared: woman as inferior, passive, beautiful object, wife and mother. We realized how severely these notions had constricted us, how humanly limited we felt at being passive dependent creatures with no identities of our own. Gradually, with each others' support, we began to rediscover ourselves.

Rediscovering Anger

As we were changing we found we were frequently feeling angry. This surprised us and embarrassed us. We had grown up feeling that we needed to love everyone and be loved by everyone. If we got angry with someone or they with us, we felt in some sense that we were failures.

We shared memories of our pasts. Nearly all of us had had a hard time expressing anger verbally or physically.

I have very few memories of fighting. Each time I did I felt guilty and embarrassed.

We did fight a lot at home, but I never made a public display of any anger or aggression. That was unladylike.

My husband has this habit of not listening to me when I talk. I get angry at him, but I don't tell him.

I seem to put up with a lot of nonsense from people. It is as if I am always being the accepting, forgiving and accommodating person.

We began to admit that we had felt angry during our lives but that we had been using the anger against ourselves in hating ourselves. There were many ways we had learned to cover up our anger. It had built up for so long inside us that we were afraid we would explode if we let it out. We realized that there are many aspects of our lives that make us angry. Until we know and feel our own oppression we are not motivated to try to create constructive alternative ways of being and living. Many have accused us of being shrill. Our mood is far more complex. Our critics hear only the anger, and anger separated from real issues is a distortion. The anger that is in us is a starting point for creative change and growth.

Learning to Value Ourselves

When we started talking to each other we realized how deeply ingrained was our sense of being less valuable than men. In school we had learned that though we were expected to do well our real vocation was to be wife and mother. Boys were being trained for the important work in society. We learned that what our culture labelled work was not for us, and what we did was not seen as important. The few of us who did *not* stay out of 'male' work suffered the consequences.

For me the evidence of my mental competence was unavoidable, and I never had any trouble defending or voicing my opinions with men, because I beat them in all the tests. Consequently none of them would come near me in my first seventeen years of life.

It was as if to be considered women we had to keep our inferior place. If we challenged this we were treated badly and came to think of ourselves in negative ways. Our learned sense of inferiority affected the way we thought about our bodies – our physical selves.

We had lived our lives as though we were inferior but we learned that this personal sense of inferiority was in fact shared and that it was merely a reflection of the way power is distributed in society. While men continue to hold on to this power, women will continue to be denigrated. When we looked at our own lives we realized that we were partly responsible for the problem. We did not sufficiently respect ourselves or our needs and we did not sufficiently respect each other. By accepting society's view of us we were perpetuating it.

We all went through a time when we rejected our old selves and took on new qualities exclusively. For a while we became distortions, angry all the time or fiercely independent. It was as though we had partly new selves, and we had to find out what they were like. But ultimately we realized that rejecting our 'feminine qualities' was simply another way of accepting our culture's sexist values.

We began to reassess what we had felt were our weaknesses and to see them as strengths. As women we had been brought up to be sensitive to the problems of others and to take care of their emotional and physical needs. In the past we had lived mainly for others; we now recognized the need to live also for ourselves. We looked again at our passivity and dependence and recognized the value of being able to sit back when we need to, and we realized that dependence is an integral part of any inter-dependent, intimate relationship. We learned to incorporate the tradi-tional 'female' characteristics so that we could use them instead of *being* them. As we explore and change we discover things that we don't like about ourselves, but we realize that these things do not reflect our in-feriority, they are part of being human.

Although we learned to value the essentially servicing work that we do, we wanted also to incorporate more product-oriented work into our lives. This book falls into that category. It has been exciting to collaborate on a tangible product, but throughout the process we have in no way sacrificed the quality of our relationships with one another as men often do when they work together. We have genuinely collaborated and devised new ways of working together within the social context that we created. Along with this new, task-oriented activity has come a new sense of wanting to succeed, to get recognition for what we do. As women we had been taught to want to fail or at least not to excel.

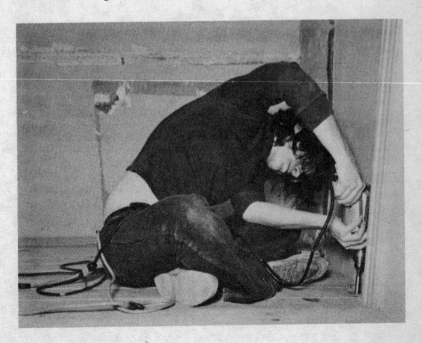

Our new confidence has led us to rediscover physical activity, climbing, canoeing, karate and car maintenance, and to take care of ourselves. We no longer feel the need for constant support from our families, particularly our men. We can choose to be alone and to seek support when we need it; we realize that we are no longer powerless, helpless children. Nevertheless we are forever fighting a constant inner struggle to give up and become weak, dependent and helpless again.

As we have come to feel separate, we have tried to change old relationships and/or enter new relationships in new ways. We now also feel positive about our needs to be dependent and to connect with others. We have come to value long-term commitments, which we find increasingly rare in such a changing society, just as we value our new separateness.

2 Anatomy and Physiology of Sexuality and Reproduction

Our Feelings

Our feelings about our bodies are often negative.

I remember coming home from school every day and going over my body from head to toe. My forehead was too high, my hair too straight, my body too short, my teeth too yellow, and so on.

We are always making some comparison, we're never okay the way we are. We feel ugly, inadequate. And it's no wonder! The ideal woman is something very specific. She may change over time (for instance, small breasts are 'in' these days, large ones 'out'), yet there is always something to measure up to. This ideal is not what *we* created. Yet we are encouraged to change in countless ways so we can fulfil this image. We are discouraged from appreciating our uniqueness.

We are encouraged to feel as though our bodies are not ours. Our 'figure' is for a (potential) mate to admire. Our breasts are for 'the man in our lives', for our babies to suckle, for our doctors to examine. The same kind of 'hands-off' message is even stronger for our vaginas. Sometimes it's hard to like our bodies because we feel so far away from our physical selves.

Having my first child was the first experience in my life in which I felt my physical being was as important as my mind. I related to my total body. I became very unselfconscious. I felt my body was fantastic!

Experiences in the women's movement have drastically changed our thinking and feelings about our bodies.

Recently, as I became more aware of my body, I realized I had pretended some parts didn't exist, while others now seemed made of smaller parts. I also discovered mental and physical processes working together. I realized that when my chest pulled down and felt collapsed I felt unhappy or depressed. When I felt sad my chest would start to tighten. When I became aware of some of the connections, I could start to change. Gradually I felt a new kind of unity, wholeness in me, as my mental and physical selves became one self.

Until we began to prepare this material, many of us didn't know the names of parts of our anatomy. Some of us had learned bits and pieces of information, but it was not permissible to find out too much. The taboos were strongest in the areas of reproduction and sex, which is why our book concentrates on them.

The first month I was at college some of my friends were twittering about a girl down the hall. She was having a painful time trying to learn to put in a tampon. Finally someone helped her and found she was trying to put it in her anus.

Finding Out about Ourselves

Knowing the facts about our anatomy and physiology has been very exciting for us. It's exhilarating to discover that the material is not as difficult as we once thought. Knowing the language of doctors makes them less mysterious and frightening. We now feel more confident when asking questions. Sometimes a doctor has been startled to find us speaking 'his' language. 'How do you know that? Are you a medical student?' we heard again and again. 'A pretty girl like you shouldn't be concerned about that.' Some doctors are very cooperative in response to our questions. Yet many others appear outwardly pleased while continuing

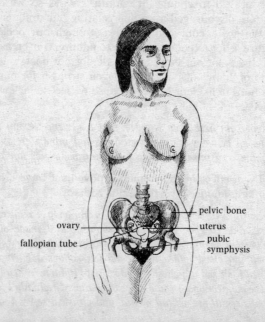

ovary

fallopian tube

pelvic bone

uterus

pubic symphysis

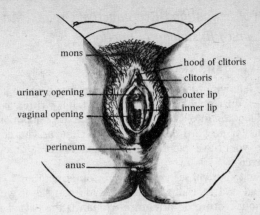

mons — hood of clitoris — clitoris
urinary opening — outer lip — inner lip
vaginal opening
perineum
anus

Vulva

to 'manage' us with new tactics.* From sharing our experiences and knowledge we develop an awareness of difference as well as similarity. We start to have confidence in our knowledge, and that confidence helps us change our feelings about ourselves.

I used to wonder if my body was abnormal even though I didn't have any reason to believe it was. I had nothing to compare it with until I started to talk with other women. I don't feel any more that I might be a freak and not know it.

Since doing a lot of talking about our sexual organs, we have been encouraged to look inside our vaginas by the women's self-help movement. (See 'Self-Examination', p. 135.) Some of us have taken a while to get over our inhibitions about seeing or touching our genitals.

When someone first said to me two years ago, 'You can feel the end of your own cervix with your finger,' I was interested but flustered. I had hardly ever put my finger in my vagina at all, and felt squeamish about touching myself there, in that place 'reserved' for lovers and doctors. It took me two months to get up my nerve to try it, and then one afternoon, pretty nervously, I squatted down in the bathroom and put my finger in deep, back into my vagina. There it was(!), feeling slippery and rounded, with an indentation at the centre through which, I realized, my menstrual flow came. It was both very exciting and beautifully ordinary at the same time. Last week I bought a plastic speculum so I can look at my cervix. Will it take as long this time?

We still have many bad feelings about ourselves that are hard to admit. We have not, of course, been able to erase decades of social influence in a few years. But we have learned to trust ourselves. We *can* take care of ourselves.

* Valerie Jorgensen, 'The Gynaecologist and the Sexually Liberated Woman'.

Description of Sexual and Reproductive Organs: Anatomy (Structure) and Physiology (Function)

PELVIC ORGANS

The following description will mean much more if you look at yourself with a mirror while you read the text. It is written as if you were squatting and looking into a hand mirror. If you are uncomfortable in that position sit as far forward on the edge of a chair as you comfortably can. Make sure you have plenty of light and enough time and privacy to feel relaxed.

First you will see your *vulva*, or outer genitals.* This includes all of the sexual and reproductive organs you can see in your crotch. The most obvious feature on a mature woman is the *pubic hair*. It grows from the soft fatty tissue called the *mons*. The mons area lies over the *pubic symphysis*. This is the joint of the pubic bones, which are part of the *pelvic bones*, or hip girdle. You can see that the hair continues between your legs and probably on around your *anus* (the opening of the *rectum*, or large intestine). The hair-covered area between your legs is also fatty, like the mons. This fatty area is called the *outer lips*. They surround some soft flaps of skin which are hairless. These are the *inner lips*. They are sensitive to touch. With sexual stimulation they swell and turn darker. The area between the inner lips and the anus is the *perineum*.

As you gently spread the inner lips apart, you can see that they protect a delicate area between them (the *vestibule*). Starting from the front, right below the mons area the inner lips join to form a soft fold of skin, or *hood*, over and connecting to the *glans*, or tip of the *clitoris* (klit'-or-is).† Gently pull the hood up to see the glans. This is the most sensitive spot in the entire genital area. It is made up of erectile tissue which swells during sexual arousal. Let the hood slide back over the glans. Extending from the hood up to the pubic symphysis, you can now feel a hardish, rubbery, movable cord right under the skin. It is sometimes sexually arousing if touched. This is the *shaft* of the clitoris. It is connected to the bone by a *suspensory ligament*. You cannot feel this ligament or the next few organs described, but they are all important in sexual arousal and orgasm. At the point where you can no longer feel the shaft of the clitoris it divides into two parts, spreading out wishbone fashion, but at a much wider angle, to form two *crura* (singular: *crus*), which attach to the pelvic bones. The crura are about three inches long. Along

* See Betty Dodson's 'Liberating Masturbation: A Meditation on Self Love' for beautiful drawings of vulvas.

† For a discussion of attitudes towards the clitoris read Ruth and Edward Brecher's excellent summary of the Masters and Johnson findings, *An Analysis of Human Sexual Response*. Also see Mary J. Sherfey's *The Nature and Evolution of Female Sexuality*.

the sides of the vestibule are two bundles of erectile tissue called the *bulbs of the vestibule*. These, along with the whole clitoris and an extensive system of connecting veins throughout the pelvis, become firm and filled with blood (pelvic congestion) during sexual arousal. Some pelvic congestion, giving a feeling of fullness or heaviness, can occur before your period comes. Both the crura of the clitoris and the bulbs of the vestibule are wrapped in muscle tissue. This muscle helps to provide tension during arousal and contracts during orgasm. The whole clitoris and vestibular bulbs are the only organs in the body solely for sexual sensation and arousal.

Vestibular or *Bartholin's glands* are two small rounded bodies on either side of the vaginal opening and to the rear of the vestibular bulbs. They are important only because they sometimes get infected and swell. You can feel them then.

You will notice that the inner lips attach to the underside of the clitoris. This is important for sexual stimulation. Right below this attachment is a small dot or slit. This is the *urinary opening*, the outer opening of a short (about an inch and a half), thin tube leading to your *bladder*. Below that is a larger opening, the *vaginal opening*. Because the urinary opening is so close to the vagina, it can become irritated from prolonged or vigorous intercourse and you may feel some discomfort while urinating.* If you have never had intercourse, you may be able to see the *hymen*. It is a thin membrane that surrounds the vaginal opening, partially blocking it and very occasionally covering the opening completely. Hymens come in widely varying sizes and shapes. The hymen can be stretched before intercourse by using a tampon, or simply by gentle finger pressure. (See Chapter 3, 'Sexuality'.) Even when stretched by intercourse, little folds of hymen tissue remain.

Now insert a finger or two into your *vagina*. Notice how the vaginal walls which were touching each other now spread around your fingers and hug them. Feel the soft folds of skin. These folds allow the vagina to mould itself around what is inside it, whether around fingers, a tampon, a penis, or a baby. The walls of the vagina may be almost dry to very wet, depending on whether you are in your reproductive years and, if you are, what stage you are at in your menstrual cycle and how sexually aroused you are. These continuous secretions provide lubrication, help keep the vagina clean, and maintain the acidity of the vagina to prevent infections from starting. The secretions taste salty. Only the outer third of the vagina is very sensitive. Now try to use the muscles around your vagina to pull it in around your finger. It might help if you imagine you are stopping the flow of urine. You are contracting the *pelvic floor muscles*. You can feel the contractions about one or two finger joints in

* See Chapter 7, p. 207, on urinary problems.

*Female pelvic organs
(side view)*

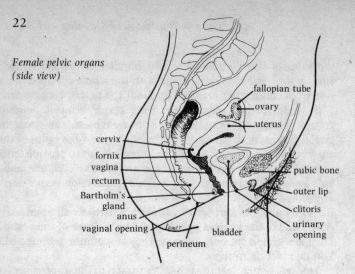

from the entrance of the vagina. These muscles hold the pelvic organs in place and provide support for your other organs all the way up to your diaphragm, which is stretched across the bottom of your rib cage. If these muscles are weak you may have trouble having an orgasm, controlling your urine (urinary incontinence), or your pelvic organs – particularly the bladder, lower intestine, or uterus – may sag and in extreme cases bulge out of the vaginal opening. These muscles are also important during pregnancy and childbirth. See Chapter 6, p. 137, for ways to strengthen these muscles.

There is only a thin wall of skin separating the vagina from the rectum, so you may be able to feel a bump in your vagina if you have some faeces in the rectum.

Now slide your middle finger as far back into your vagina as you can. Notice that your finger goes in towards the small of your back at an angle, not straight up the middle of your body. The end of your vagina is called the *fornix*. (If you are having any trouble reaching it, bring your knees and chest closer together so your finger can slide in farther.) A little before the end of the vagina you can feel your *cervix*. It feels like a nose with a small dimple in its centre. If you've had a baby the cervix may feel more like a chin. The cervix is the base of the *uterus*, or womb. It is sensitive to pressure but has no nerve endings on its surface. The uterus changes position during the menstrual cycle and during sexual excitement, so the place where you feel the cervix one day may be slightly different from where you feel it the next. Some days you can barely reach it. The dimple you felt is the *os*, or opening into the uterus. It is about the diameter of a very thin straw. No tampon, finger, or penis can go through it, although it is capable of expanding to allow a baby through.

You will not be able to feel the rest of the organs which are described. The non-pregnant uterus is about the size of a fist. This organ has thick walls made of one of the most powerful muscles in the body. It is located between the bladder and the rectum. The walls of the uterus touch each other unless pushed apart by a growing foetus or by an abnormal growth. The upper end of the uterus is called the *fundus*.

Extending outwards and back from the upper end of the uterus are the two *fallopian tubes* (or *oviducts*; literally, 'egg tubes'). They are approximately four inches long and look like ram's horns, facing backwards. The connecting opening from the uterus to the fallopian tube is so small that only a fine needle can penetrate it. The other end of the tube is fimbriated (fringed) and funnel-shaped. The wide end of the funnel wraps part way around the *ovary* but does not actually attach to it.

The ovaries are about the size and shape of unshelled almonds, located on either side and somewhat behind the uterus. They would be about four or five inches below your waist. They are held in place by connecting tissue and are protected by a surrounding mass of fat. They have a twofold function: to produce germ cells (eggs) and to produce female sex hormones (*oestrogen* and *progesterone*). The small gap between the ovary and the end of the corresponding tube allows the egg to float freely after it is released from the ovary. The finger-like ends of the fallopian tube move to set up currents which wave the egg into the tube. In rare cases when the egg is not 'caught' by the tube, it can be fertilized outside the tube, resulting in an abdominal pregnancy. See 'Ectopic (Misplaced) Pregnancy' in Chapter 10, p. 506, for more on this.

Development of Pelvic Organs

All female and male organs, including sexual and reproductive organs, are similar in origin, develop from the same embryonic tissue (homologous), and are similar in function (analogous). The following are examples of corresponding organs:

FEMALE	MALE
outer lips	scrotum
inner lips	bottom side of penis
glans of clitoris	glans of penis
shaft of clitoris	corpus cavernosum
ovaries	testes
bulb of the vestibule	bulb of the penis and corpus spongiosum
Bartholin's glands	Cowper's glands (bulbourethral glands)

Female and male foetuses appear identical during the first six weeks in the uterus.

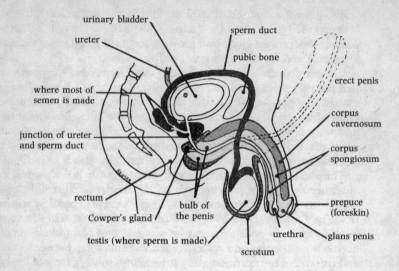

urinary bladder

ureter

sperm duct

pubic bone

erect penis

where most of
semen is made

corpus
cavernosum

junction of ureter
and sperm duct

corpus
spongiosum

rectum

prepuce
(foreskin)

Cowper's gland

bulb of
the penis

testis (where sperm is made)

urethra

glans penis

scrotum

Male pelvic organs (side view)

BREASTS

Breasts are made up of fat and a milk-producing or 'mammary' gland. Changing hormone levels affect the glandular tissue and hence the size of the breasts. Thus, the increase of sex hormones during adolescence accounts for the development of the breasts; changes of hormone levels at other times (e.g. during the menstrual cycle, pregnancy, or due to stopping or starting the Pill) can also affect breast size and shape. Most of the breast consists of fat around the gland, and this is what makes breast size vary from one woman to another. It also explains why breast size is not related to sexual responsiveness or capacity to produce milk.

In the middle of the *areola* (the darker part of the breast) lies the *nipple*. The nipple may stick out, it may not protrude at all, or it may sink into the areola. When exposed to cold or when sexually aroused, the nipple becomes more erect than usual. A slight secretion may collect periodically in the nipple. This is normal and comes from the ducts (small tubes of milk) inside the breast. You may see small bumps on the surface of the areola. These are glands which secrete a lubricant that protects the nipple during nursing. It is quite common for hairs to grow around the areola. They can be caused by hormonal changes due to pregnancy or changes in the use of the Pill. During pregnancy the areola often becomes darker and stays darker.

See Chapter 7 for breast disorders and how to examine your breasts, and Chapter 14 for breast-feeding.

Stages in the Reproductive Cycle

In childhood our bodies are immature. Then during puberty we make the transition from childhood to maturity. In women, puberty is character-ized by decreased bone growth; by growth of breasts, pubic and axillary (armpit) hair; starting of menstruation (menarche) and ovulation; and increase of sexual urges. The last stage of the cycle is when we are no longer able to reproduce. The climacteric is the transition between the reproductive and post-reproductive stages. Menstruation stops (meno-pause) and ovulation stops. (Although 'menopause' is commonly used to mean the whole transition period, technically this is incorrect.) For more on the climacteric see Chapter 16.

This entire reproductive cycle is regulated by hormones. Hormones function as chemical messengers and initiators in the body. Women have high levels of sex hormones (oestrogen and progesterone) during the reproductive period and low levels in childhood and after menopause. The signs and symptoms of the transitional periods are thought to be caused by the changing levels of hormones.

Within the reproductive stage there are hormone-caused cycles of approximately one month's duration; this is the menstrual cycle.

Ovulation

The ovaries at birth contain 300,000 to 400,000 *follicles*, which are balls of cells with an immature egg in the centre. Only about 300 to 500 of these will develop into mature eggs. The other follicles degenerate.

Each month during our reproductive years, one follicle (occasionally more than one) matures under the influence of hormones. One of the cell layers in the follicle secretes oestrogen. The follicle, with the maturing egg inside, moves towards the surface of the ovary. Ovulation is the process of the follicle and the ovarian surface disintegrating at a par-ticular point, allowing the egg to float out. For some women this can be felt as a cramp on either side of the lower abdomen or lower back, and there may be some discharge, possibly bloody, from the vagina. The cramp is occasionally painful enough to be confused with appendicitis. The phenomenon is called *mittelschmerz* (literally, 'middle pain'). If you look at your cervix with a speculum you may notice a drop of clear, stretchy mucus near the os. This happens within a day before and after ovulation.

Just before ovulation the same cell layer in the follicle starts secreting progesterone as well as oestrogen. After ovulation the follicle is called a *corpus luteum* ('yellow body', referring to the yellowish fat in it). If the woman becomes pregnant, the hormones produced by the corpus luteum help to maintain the pregnancy. If no pregnancy occurs, the follicle degenerates.

26

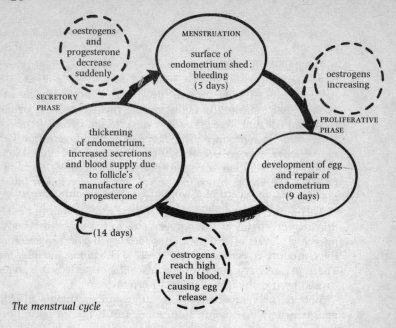

The menstrual cycle

After ovulation the fallopian tube carries the egg on its journey to the uterus. Fertilization, the union of an egg from a woman and sperm from a man, takes place in the outer third of the fallopian tube (nearest the ovaries). This is also called conception and usually occurs within one day of ovulation. The fertilized egg takes around 4 days to travel down the fallopian tubes to the uterus, where after 1½ to 2 days it implants in the uterine lining and develops through the next 9 months into a baby.

In rare cases the egg may implant in the tube instead of the uterus, or it may not be 'caught' by the tube at all. This results in a 'misplaced' pregnancy and requires surgery. See Chapter 15, p. 506, 'Ectopic (Misplaced) Pregnancy'. If the egg is not fertilized, it is sloughed off in the vaginal secretions. You won't notice it. This usually happens before menstruation.

Menstruation

Oestrogen, made by the maturing follicle, causes the uterine lining (*endometrium*) to proliferate (to grow, thicken, and form glands that will secrete embryo-nourishing substances). Progesterone, made by the ruptured follicle, causes the glands in the endometrium to begin secreting the nourishing substances and also increases the uterine blood supply. Thus, there are two linings: a proliferative lining and a secretory lining. A fertilized egg can implant only in a secretory lining.

The ruptured follicle will produce oestrogen and progesterone for only about 12 days, with the amount dwindling in the last few days, if conception has not occurred. As the hormone levels drop, the womb's lining is no longer nourished and most of it is shed during menstruation. (It is possible to menstruate without ovulating (anovulatory period), but this usually occurs only around the time of puberty or the climacteric.) Then a new follicle starts growing, starts secreting oestrogen; a new uterine lining grows; and the cycle begins again.

Menstruation starts generally at the age of eleven or twelve, though any time from nine to eighteen years is normal. See Chapter 16 for when it ceases.

There is no record of a woman with an absolutely regular menstrual cycle. The length of the cycle usually ranges from 20 to 36 days, the average being 28 days. (Menstruation is from the Latin *mensis*, for 'month'.) There are spontaneous small changes and there can be major ones when a woman is under a great deal of stress (such as a pregnancy scare). A normal period lasts 2 to 8 days, with 4 to 6 days being the average. The flow stops and starts, though this may not always be evident. A usual menstrual discharge is about 4 to 6 tablespoons, or 2 to 3 ounces. Each woman has her own cycle, which really is a more important guideline than the statistics. Many women feel an increased sexual urge during one part of the cycle. For some it comes around ovulation, for others it comes right before or during the period.

There is no need to stay in bed, avoid exercise, refrain from sexual intercourse, or observe any of the traditional taboos surrounding menstruation. If doing something makes you feel uncomfortable, it is only common sense to avoid doing it.

The Menstrual Fluid. The menstrual fluid contains mucous and endometrial particles as well as blood (sometimes clotted), but the content is not obvious since the blood stains everything red. This regular loss of blood can sometimes cause anaemia, although anaemia can often be caused by bad diet. (See Chapter 6 for 'Nutrition'.) The fluid does not smell until it makes contact with the bacteria in the air and starts to decompose.

Menstrual fluid can be absorbed in a variety of ways. The most common methods are sanitary towels and tampons which are needlessly expensive. In 1975 the Price Commission found that manufacturers had excessive profits and recommended that prices should be cut by at least 10%. We are still further penalized for being women by a levy of VAT on all such products (razor blades are free of VAT). Some women in the women's movement are campaigning that these products should be free (the Free Sanitary Protection Campaign can be contacted through WIRES, see addresses, p. 570).

In the meantime, we do not necessarily have to rely on expensive products. Some women have begun using a natural sponge often available at cosmetic counters. It can be washed and re-used. Others use diaphragms which can collect fluid too – and they are free! (See Chapter 9, Birth Control.) For many of us, tampons are of course very convenient. The packages give clear instructions on how to use them. If you have trouble inserting a tampon into your vagina, practise when you don't have a period. Use a mirror to help you find the entrance to your vagina; lubricating the tampon, for example, with KY Jelly (available from a chemist), may also help. Do not use vaseline, for it can cause irritation. You do not have to have had intercourse before you can use a tampon. Most of us are born with large enough openings in our hymens, but we can stretch them if necessary (see p. 38).

One other method of dealing with menstrual fluid is menstrual extraction. The Del'-Em menstrual extraction technique was invented and pioneered by feminists in the USA who have been using it for over two years with no complications. On or about the day they are due to menstruate, they extract their menstrual fluid by gentle suction, and are able to enjoy the convenience and comfort of a 5-minute as opposed to 5-day period. The same technique can be used for early abortions (see Chapter 10; and for more on the self-help movement, see Chapter 17).

Menstrual extraction cannot be used by a woman on herself. It is still at the experimental-research stage and has always been used in groups, by trained women who use it on each other. At no time is any woman allowed to experience discomfort. The technique differs from that employed by doctors, called 'Interception', 'Menstrual Aspiration' or 'Endometrial Aspiration', which is an inferior technique with a more powerful suction and which is known to cause unnecessary pain and bodily disturbance.* There is, however, no way of knowing yet whether there are any long-range effects on the uterus from regular menstrual extraction.

Menstrual extraction is probably not illegal under the Abortion Laws provided there is no intent to procure an abortion, but the legal situation is not at present clear.

Feelings about Menstruation. Many of us grew up with little or no knowledge about menstruation, so we were scared or even embarrassed when our periods started. Some of us thought we were dying when we first saw our menstrual blood. Some of us were terrified that a teacher or a boy would notice it. On the other hand, some of us felt inadequate if we didn't menstruate. We must tell both our sons and our daughters about menstruation so that they can be comfortable and open about it in a way that we were not.

---

* See, for example, *Women's Report*, Vol. 3, issue 5, 'Very Early Termination of Pregnancy'.

Menstrual Problems. Most of us experience menstrual problems at some time in our lives, and for many of us, pre-menstrual tension or painful periods are bad enough for us to seek medical help. For too long such problems have been ignored or ridiculed by the medical profession, but at last doctors are beginning to take them relatively seriously. We examine the various methods of treatment in Chapter 7, 'Common Medical and Health Problems'.

But do menstruation and the pre-menstrual syndrome affect our ability to function effectively and to hold positions of responsibility? During 'the last three Olympics . . . women won gold medals and established new world records during all phases of the menstrual cycle'. It is amazing that we are denied responsibility on the basis of menstrual cycles, while men, who are much more prone to seriously incapacitating diseases such as heart problems, continue in highly responsible positions even after these problems are discovered. There is also some evidence that men too have hormonal cycles. We are still allowed to work where we are 'needed' — at home, in factories, in offices — with no concessions in schedules or routines to take account of our cycles.

Bibliography

Crittenden Scott, Ann, 'Closing the Muscle Gap', *Ms* Magazine, September 1974.

Jorgensen, Valerie, 'The Gynaecologist and the Sexually Liberated Woman', *Obstetrics and Gynaecology*, Vol. 42, No. 4, October 1973.

Lennane, Jean and John, 'Alleged Psychogenic Disorders in Women, A Possible Manifestation of Sexual Prejudice', *New England Journal of Medicine*, Vol. 288, 1973, p. 288.

Llewellyn-Jones, Derek, *Fundamentals of Obstetrics* and *Gynaecology*, 2 vols., Faber, 1969–70. Quite a clear medical textbook with lots of explanatory pictures. This is about the best textbook we can recommend, although it is by no means perfect!

McKeith, Nancy (ed.). *The New Women's Health Handbook*, Virago, 1978.

Ramey, Estelle, 'Men's Cycles', *Ms* Magazine, Spring 1972.

Women's Report, 'Very Early Termination of Pregnancy', Vol. 3, issue 5, 1975.

3 Sexuality

The society we grow up in is sexually confused and repressive, particularly for women. On the one hand we are told by the state, the church and often our parents that sex is wrong unless sanctified by marriage and children. On the other we are encouraged by magazines, advertisements and the television to look sexy, to be available, and above all to enjoy it. These modern expectations can be as alienating and degrading as any Victorian puritanism.

Within this confusion it is not surprising that we are ignorant about our own sexuality. We learn that sex means intercourse and orgasm, that sex with other women is material for dirty jokes or guilt. We are ashamed if our experience doesn't live up to expectations. Instead of heeding our own rhythms and needs we try to mimic the responses we've seen at the cinema and we expect to be taught to feel by men who in fact share our ignorance.

Within the women's movement we are slowly learning about our own sexuality and sharing our experiences with each other. Our explorations have been helped by the research of Virginia Johnson and William Masters into the physiology of sex and by the growing volume of positive, creative work on sexuality, much of it written by women.

This chapter makes use of personal experience as well as research. Our greatest achievement has been in overcoming our inhibitions and learning to talk to one another. In sharing our knowledge we discover that we have problems and anxieties in common which our pooled experience can help to overcome. As our experience of learning from each other has been so valuable we would like to encourage other women to do the same.

Sexuality is much more than intercourse. It is a pleasure we want to give and to receive. It is a vital expression of attachment to other human beings. It is communication that is fun and playful, serious and passionate. We believe that as we accept ourselves and support each other, we can learn to express our sexual feelings in a way that strengthens our sense of self, deepens our pleasure and enhances the building and renewing of intimacy with others.

Sexual Feelings

We are our bodies. Our book celebrates this simple fact. Sexual feelings and responses are a central expression of our emotional, spiritual, physical selves. Sexual feelings involve our whole bodies.

When I'm feeling turned on, either alone or with someone I'm attracted to, my heart beats faster, my face gets red, my eyes feel bright. The lips of my vagina feel wet, and my whole genital area feels full. My breasts hum. If I'm standing up I feel a rush of weakness in my thighs. If I'm lying down I may feel like a big stretch, arching my back, feeling the sensations go out to my fingers and toes. These are special feelings whether I do anything to act on them or not.

We may have to learn to let our sexual feelings come without our judgement or control and to accept them as part of ourselves. They have a rhythm and flow of their own. They can't be forced, they come and go. Sensations and emotions simply are. However, when the feelings come we do have some choices — whether to act and how to act — and responsibility for the actions we choose. Though sexual feelings may be simple in themselves, they exist in the context of our society and feel complicated to us. For many of us sex has been confused with a special nurturing — with parental love, attention and acceptance that we needed as children but may never have had.

When I made love with Jack I felt he was feeding me. I felt full with his penis inside me. When I wasn't with him I would feel hungry again. Often I didn't have orgasms. I kept coming back to him, though it was an impossible relationship, because I needed to be fed. Later I realized he was mothering me, I was asking him to be my mother. That was a revelation!

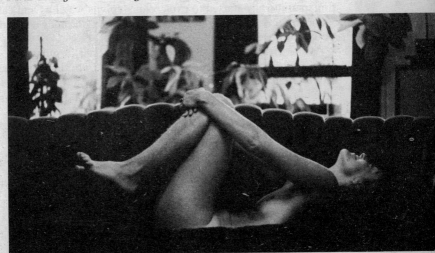

Sadly, some of our guilty, self-denying feelings about sex we have accepted for too long.

Our ambivalent feelings about our bodies and conflicted feelings about sex get in the way of sexual enjoyment. We can learn to let go of these feelings and at the same time to enhance the sexual feelings that give us a powerful sense of connection with other people and all of nature.

Growing Up

I watch my daughter. From morning to night her body is her home. She lives in it and with it. When she runs around the kitchen she uses all of herself. Every muscle in her body moves when she laughs, when she cries. When she rubs her vulva, there is no awkwardness, no feeling that what she is doing is wrong. She feels pleasure and expresses it without hesitation. She knows when she wants to be touched and when she wants to be left alone. She doesn't have to think about it — it's a very direct physical asking or responding to someone else. It's beautiful to be with her. I sometimes feel she is more a model for me than I am for her! Occasionally I feel jealous of the ease with which she lives inside her skin. I want to be a child again! It's so hard to get back that sense of body as home.

We are born loving our bodies.

Our sense of our own sexuality was shaped by numerous childhood experiences and memories. Sex was not talked about, not openly, in most of our families. We learned euphemistic terms for our genitals. From the embarrassed words, from the 'don'ts' that came as our fingers naturally started to explore our vulvas, vaginas and clitorises, we came to think of sex as dirty and *those* parts of our body as shameful, with power to harm us.

We learned as much from what wasn't said as what was. Perhaps a younger brother or sister appeared as 'a gift from the stork', with no real explanation of our mother's pregnancy. If our parents weren't openly affectionate with each other, if they were careful to keep us from seeing them naked, that taught us something.

When I was six years old I climbed up on the bathroom sink and looked at myself naked in the mirror. All of a sudden I realized I had three different holes. I was very excited about my discovery and ran down to the dinner table and announced it to everyone. 'I have three holes!' Silence. 'What are they for?' I asked. Silence even heavier than before. I sensed how uncomfortable everyone was and answered for myself. 'I guess one is for pee-pee, the other for doo-doo and the third for ca-ca.' A sigh of relief; no one had to answer my question. But I got the message — I wasn't supposed to ask 'such' questions, though I didn't fully realize what 'such' was about at that time.

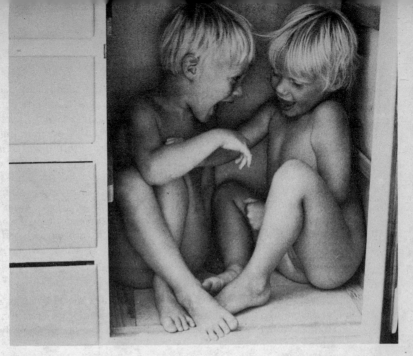

From the moment we were born we were treated differently from boys. We were programmed for domesticity, with dolls, toy sweepers and dresses which mustn't get dirty, while boys rolled in the mud and played with guns and building sets. As we grew older we learned that emotions are also sexually defined. We should be gentle and emotional, they must be aggressive and decisive. This division of characteristics deeply affects our sexuality — men lead, we follow.

As our bodies develop, we learn not about our own smells and shapes and rhythms, but about the commercial norm for beauty. We learn to compare ourselves to others and to images in the media. We learn to criticize our bodies for the apparent defects and we lose respect for our uniqueness. We learn to seek approval from everybody, friend or stranger, for evidence that we are winning the struggle. The constant comparing leads to competitiveness that separates us from each other.

At twelve I was among the first of my friends to begin to menstruate and to wear a bra. I felt a mixture of pride and embarrassment. For all of my life I had been a chubby, introspective child, but a growth spurt of a few inches, along with my developing breasts, transformed me one summer into a surprisingly slim and shapely child-woman. The funny thing was that on one level I had always known this would happen. Yet it was as if a fairy godmother had visited me. I felt turned on, but I was mostly turned on to myself and the narcissistic pleasure of finding I was attractive to boys.

Within a year or so, when we began to have mixed parties, we often played kissing games with no parents present. I didn't really like kissing whoever the bottle spun to or, later, necking with whoever took me out on a date.

Because multiple birth defects (cleft lip and palate, spina bifida) made my body different, my whole being is perceived and related to as different. My body creates feelings of denial, anger, guilt and rejection both within myself and within others. The only people who touched my body were medical personnel, with all their clinical coldness and detachment, and then it was to induce pain. I never thought my body could be itself pleasurable or be a source of pleasure.

In a disabled and disfigured body, I am 'desexed' by both society and myself. I was never aware of my sexuality until at twenty-two my emotional and social development put me into relationships where sexual attraction towards me occurred. A thirteen-year-old has greater knowledge, skill, and a sense of her sexuality than I did! I struggled to identify with and accept my 'womanness'. With no one there to help me, I was forced to go it alone. Always I've asked, 'Am I a person despite my physical handicaps?' Now I ask also, 'Am I a woman?'

Worst of all, we feel isolated — could anyone else be as ugly, dull, miserable as I? An ad for sanitary towels reinforces our aloneness and shame: 'When you have your period, you should be the only one who knows.'

Even if we were told that getting our first period was an exciting event (as well as 'the curse'), a signal that we were becoming *real* women, many of us could not celebrate this transition because we had not learned to accept our body processes as normal and desirable.

What did we really learn about sex in a positive way in our teens? We had to wait until our twenties, or thirties, to learn at last that we have the only uniquely non-reproductive human sexual organ, the clitoris. Almost none of us ever heard about that as we were growing up. In spite of all the experiences that taught us to repress our sexuality, we are learning to be proud of it.

As we remember the experiences of our own growing-up years, we want to help our children grow up differently, with healthier feelings about their bodies and their sexuality. We are trying to be more open with our words and affection, more positive when they explore their bodies, more ready with information when they ask for it. But we find it hard sometimes to move beyond our own upbringing. There are few good models, so we need each other's help.

The other day I was taking a bath with my almost-three-year-old daughter. I was lying down and she was sitting between my legs, which were spread apart. She said, 'Mommy, you don't have a penis.' I said, 'That's right, men have penises and women have clitorises.' All calm and fine — then, 'Mommy where is your clitoris?' Okay, now what was I going to do? I took a deep breath (for courage or something), tried not to blush, spread my vulva apart, and showed her my clitoris. It didn't feel so bad. 'Do you want to see yours?' I asked. 'Yes.' That was quite a trick to get her to look over her fat stomach and see hers, especially when she started laughing as I first put my finger and then hers on her clitoris.

At least I feel that I can have some greater ease and openness about sexuality with my daughter than my mother had with me.

It took us time to develop bad feelings about our sexuality, and we must allow ourselves more time to undo those feelings and develop new and healthier ones.

Sexual Language

The true language of sex is primarily non-verbal. Our words and images are poor imitations of the deep and complicated feelings within and between us. Unsure of touching as a way of sharing with another, we have let our fear and discomfort limit the rich possibilities for this non-verbal communication. Sexual expression has a power most of us are still just beginning to explore.

Sometimes when we want to talk or even think about sex we need words and we face the annoying dilemma — what words shall we use? For many of us there are no words that really feel right because of the attitudes and values they convey: the clinical, proper terms — vagina, penis and intercourse — seem cold, distant, tight; the street, slang terms — cunt, cock, fuck — seem degrading or coarse; euphemisms like 'making love' seem silly and inexact. So we use different words with our lovers, children, friends and doctors. We feel awkward, and this awkwardness convinces us that even if sex is a natural way of expressing ourselves, we have no natural way of talking about it.

But if we use those taboo street words in a loving way they lose their unpleasant connotations, and using words to describe how we feel not only helps us to communicate about sex, it's a turn on in its own right.

Sex in Our Imagination — Our Fantasies

For most of us it is difficult to acknowledge our sexual fantasies.

I never felt the freedom to explore parts of me that might come out in fantasy, dreams at night, daydreams, non-verbalized thinking. I was scared they would take me by surprise, tell me things about myself that I didn't know, especially bad things, and I was having enough trouble dealing with what came up without fantasizing. 'Let well enough alone' was my attitude.

I imagined I was sitting in a room. The walls were all white. There was nothing in it, and I was naked. There was a large window at one end, and

anyone who wanted to could look in and see me. There was no place to hide.
There was something arousing about being so exposed. I masturbated while
having this fantasy, and afterwards I felt very sad. I thought I must be so sick,
so distorted inside if this image of myself could give me such intense sexual
pleasure.

We feel we 'waste time' when we allow our minds to wander. We feel
our self-images are threatened when we think about sex as anything
except intercourse with a man. We feel we are disloyal when we fantasize
about someone other than the person we are with. Worse we feel we
might be losing our minds when we imagine ourselves doing something
we would never dare do in our real world, and then we worry that we
will do it.

Everyone has fantasies. They flash as fleeting images or evolve as
detailed stories. In talking with each other we have found that it is
common to have fantasies that scare or confuse us. It is true that, for a
few, fantasies can reflect deep emotional disturbances – if you truly fear
that your fantasies will lead to self-harm or hurt to others it may be a
good idea to check out those fears with a professional. For most of us,
however, fantasies simply reflect our needs, desires and dreams. Our
fantasies are depths in us wanting to be known and explored. In them
we can be whatever we imagine. Our fantasies are our treasures. They
enrich our sense of ourselves and the world.

Here are some of our fantasies.*

A fantasy before I made love to a plumber I know: I was entertaining myself
one night by imagining I was dancing with a stillson wrench (the most
enormous wrench I ever saw, very businesslike!), and it turned into the
plumber. He said, 'Well, men are still good for something!' We were fixing the
pipe while we were dancing, and the scene changed. We were swimming in a
sea of rubber doughnuts (the connector between the tank and the bottom part
of the toilet), and the doughnuts got stuck over our arms and legs. The scene
changed again, to the beach, where we fell asleep.

One time, just as I was climaxing with Steve, I suddenly saw and felt someone
else. I didn't realize until right then that that other person was on my mind.

I've had fantasies of having to drink urine from a man's penis while he was
peeing.

* Nancy Friday's *My Secret Garden* (Virago, London, 1976) is an exciting book full of
women's fantasies.

When I was a kid, every time I masturbated I imagined my parents spanking me as I climaxed. When I got older it changed to my parents making love, then to my being kissed by someone, then to my making love.

I used to have a recurring fantasy that I was a gym teacher and had a classful of girls standing in front of me, nude. I went up and down the rows feeling all their breasts and getting a lot of pleasure out of it. When I first had this fantasy at thirteen I was ashamed. I thought something was wrong with me. Now I can enjoy it because I feel it's okay to enjoy other women's bodies.

I had the fantasy of making love with two men at once. I pictured myself sandwiched between them. I acted on this one, with an old friend and a casual friend who both liked the idea. It was fun.

Virginity

What does virginity mean? It is in fact a physical state, but to most of us it is more a state of mind and traditionally it has also been a symbol of male domination. The hymen which partially blocks the vagina is the gift wrapping proving that the product is untouched when a father hands his daughter over to the care of her husband. She must keep her virginity because that is his prize for 'winning her hand in marriage'. For those of us who have been brought up in religious families, 'losing' our virginity before marriage is seen as a sin.

I confined my sexual involvement to heavy petting, since the Catholic Church makes intercourse seem like such a sin. The day I left the Church was the day I had an argument in the confessional with the priest about whether having intercourse with my fiancé was a sin. I maintained it wasn't; he said that I would never be a faithful wife if I had intercourse before marriage. He refused me absolution and I never went back.

Today, with the advent of the Pill and more relaxed attitudes towards sex outside matrimony, pressures are pulling in the opposite direction. We often feel obliged to have sex before we are ready and it is hard to explore our feelings under pressure.

Our first sexual experiences are important because they can affect our sex lives for a long time afterwards. For some of us though, virginity is just a hurdle to be jumped on the way to adulthood, an inhibition to overcome.

My first fuck was with a man I had just broken up with. I felt totally free and lacking in inhibition; in fact I had engineered the situation. Because the relationship was over I understood our feelings towards each other more clearly, that's why I felt I could do it. It was a very satisfying experience.

For others the first experience is something to be shared within a caring relationship. In this case it is important to share your feelings and your fears. Discuss birth control and try to decide on a method before-hand. It might help to read the relevant sections of this chapter together. Intercourse is only part of sexual experience; most of us will have learned a lot about each other's responses already. Don't be afraid to explore further and don't feel you are forced to have intercourse because your partner is aroused; he can control himself just as you can, so wait until it feels right for you.

Most of us look forward to our first experience of fucking with fear as well as expectation. Marriage manuals in common with pornography make much of the pain involved. For most women this first experience takes place with little or no pain at all; with care and gentleness there should be very little discomfort. If it is painful it is because the pliable membrane (hymen) which covers the entrance to the vagina has been difficult to break (see Chapter 2, 'Anatomy') or because the woman is not fully aroused. Test with your fingers to see if there will be room for penetration (two to three fingers' width). If you are tense it may be difficult to get any in at all, so choose a time when you feel relaxed. You can stretch the hymen with your fingers by gently moving them against the sides of your vagina; either of you can do this over a week or so before you attempt intercourse. Everyone is different: some hymens don't need stretching at all, and some of them completely cover the entrance to the vagina. (If intercourse seems impossible you could consult a doctor about surgical removal of the hymen.) Most of us feel some discomfort and bleed a little the first time, a few women bleed a lot, some of us feel nothing in particular. If you are highly aroused and wet it shouldn't be unpleasant.

Intercourse like many other things gets better with time and practice. Your first experience may not be all you had hoped for or expected – many of us felt disappointed the first time, but for most of us that has changed.

For lesbians the first experience of sex can be even more confusing; social attitudes and inhibitions combine with inexperience and often deep feelings of guilt.

After hanging around for about three months, one night we managed to get it together. We were sitting in front of the fire, seeming to get closer and closer, talking about anything but the situation we were in. She eventually took over and made love to me fully clothed. I didn't touch her at all – I couldn't, I was too caught up in my own feelings as to what was actually happening. (Red Herring, 2)

Homosexual Feelings

When we are born we instinctively do all we can to feel good. We need closeness, warmth and sensual pleasure, and we reach out towards those who offer them. Gradually we are taught to direct these sensuous — and increasingly explicitly sexual — feelings towards the opposite sex. Within each of us, however, the early sensual/sexual feelings we had for both sexes remain.

Society, through our parents, schools and churches, has told us that homosexual feelings are sinful and sick. For many of us these teachings have been very frightening. They have made it hard for us to acknowledge, let alone accept, the sexual feelings we may have for women. They have separated us, through fear, from women who openly act on sexual feelings for other women. Here is a friendship that suffered because exaggerated fears about homosexuality had been so well taught:

I had an intense friendship with Jan, a girl in my school. We wrote notes and went on walks and climbed trees, sharing dreams, reciting poems that we liked, and talking about coming back to the school in later years to teach together. We vowed lifelong love and friendship, but physically we could express the energy that was between us only by clowning around, bumping into each other — and once when she was asleep I kissed her hair. The intensity of my friendship with Jan made my family uneasy — I remember comments about seeing too much of one person. Their uneasiness got to me a little, because I was a bit uncomfortable with my strong pit-of-the-stomach feelings about her anyway. I remember being shy about undressing with her in the room, although I undressed with other friends without thinking about it. Then during the summer after we had graduated, having not seen Jan for several weeks, I was leafing through a psychology book and found a section that talked about the intense, bordering-on-homosexual friendships of young girls.

Before long I had labelled it as a silly, childishly intense friendship. I made no efforts to see her when we both went to college, for I decided we had nothing in common.

I think our feelings grew more intense as we tried to repress their sexual side. So I pulled away from Jan because I couldn't handle the natural sexual part of my feelings of affection for her.

Homosexual feelings need not be denied. In this chapter we have tried to provide information that will be of use to any woman, whoever she chooses as her sexual partner. However, in spite of changing attitudes towards lesbian relationships, those of us whose primary relationships are with women still face hostility from people who regard homosexuality with suspicion and fear. A group of lesbians in London have written more about their sexuality and how it affects their lives — both positively and negatively — in Chapter 5.

Female Sexual Response

Our sexual feelings can be affected by sounds, sights, smells and touch. We can be aroused by fantasies, a baby sucking at our breast, the smell of a familiar body, a picture of a bikini-clad model, anal stimulation, a dream, touching our own bodies, a lover's breathing in our ear, brushing against someone, or hearing the person we love say, 'I love you.' We can express our sexual feeling in an almost infinite variety of ways — writing a poem, rolling down a grassy hill in the sunshine, dancing to rock music, massaging a friend. We can also express them by masturbating or making love.

No matter how our sexual feelings are aroused or how they are expressed, physiologically our bodies follow a sequence of physical changes called the *sexual response cycle*, and culminating, if we are sufficiently aroused, in *orgasm*. Orgasm can be a mild experience like a ripple or a peaceful sigh; it can be a very sensuous experience where our bodies glow with warmth; it can be very intense with crying out and thrashing movements; it can even result in momentary loss of awareness. With continued stimulation, we can sometimes reach orgasm again and again. Afterwards our bodies return to their non-aroused state. Sexual tension can be released without orgasm, but the tension may produce an aching feeling in the genitals which may take hours to subside.

The knowledge that we are capable of having many orgasms has led many of us to feel that not only must we reach orgasm but that we must have several orgasms. If the old trap was ignorance, the new problem for women and men is increased expectation. So, whatever the manuals say, try to enjoy whatever feels best for you.

THE ROLE OF THE CLITORIS

It is arousing to stroke any part of our bodies, exciting to have our thighs caressed or our necks nibbled or our breasts sucked. However, the clitoris does play the central role in elevating our feelings of sexual arousal. It used to be thought that clitoral orgasms were 'immature' whereas vaginal orgasms were the expression of sexual maturity. We now know that all orgasms originate in the clitoris though they may be felt elsewhere. For a description of the clitoris see Chapter 2, p. 20. Here is a summary of how it works.

The clitoris has three parts: the glans, the shaft and the hood. The shaft of the clitoris is under the skin. The glans, which is the tip of the shaft, is covered by the hood. With sexual arousal, all of the clitoris fills with blood and swells. The hood becomes so swollen it balloons up, uncovering the glans. When sexual tension reaches a very high level, the glans retracts under its hood.

Stimulation of the clitoris helps produce the pelvic congestion and muscle contraction that are necessary for orgasm. When we are highly aroused, stimulation of the clitoris may bring on orgasm.

All stimulation of the pubic hair-covered mons area, the inner lips of the vulva and any parts of the clitoris itself is considered direct stimulation. (Since the clitoris is not in a rigidly fixed position, any stimulation in this area will move the clitoris and also may press and rub it up against the pubic bone.) The clitoral area is stimulated directly by touching with a hand, caressing with a tongue, applying a vibrator or pressing someone else's body close. Although some women say that they touch the glans to become aroused, the glans of the clitoris is so sensitive that touching it directly can hurt. Also, if stimulation is focused on the clitoris for a long time, we may lose the sensation and not feel excited any more.

Stroking the skin on the lower abdomen and inner thighs is another effective way to stimulate the clitoris (the tension of abdominal and thigh muscles pulls on the ligaments that attach the clitoris to the pubic bone).

At high levels of arousal, the clitoris retracts under its hood and can no longer be seen or felt. This occurs some time before orgasm, from one minute to perhaps thirty. Also, the clitoris can emerge and retract several times during a sexual experience. During orgasm the clitoris is always retracted; however, retraction doesn't guarantee orgasm, especially if stimulation doesn't continue and increase. To reach orgasm a woman needs continuous, effective stimulation of the clitoris — by penile thrusting, body pressure, or touching of the clitoral area with a hand or tongue. With direct stimulation, retraction will occur at lower levels of sexual excitement than with intercourse alone. With intercourse alone, very high levels of sexual arousal are reached before retraction occurs. This may explain why many of us have orgasm quicker through direct manipulation, and makes it clearer to us that intercourse is not better or worse than direct stimulation, it's just different.

In intercourse there is indirect stimulation of the clitoris. Penile movements and any movements in the vagina provide continual clitoral stimulation by moving the inner lips which, by their connection to the clitoral hood, move the hood back and forth over the glans. In addition, the inner lips become so swollen and firm they act as an extension of the vagina, hugging the penis as it moves back and forth. To reach orgasm during intercourse most of us need either direct or indirect clitoral stimulation before intercourse, and some of us need direct clitoral manipulation during intercourse.

SEXUAL RESPONSE

To help us understand how our bodies respond to sexual stimulation, Masters and Johnson separate the process of sexual response into four consecutive phases: excitement, plateau, orgasm and resolution. Together these phases make up the sexual response cycle.* They are for descriptive purposes only: we move from one phase to the next without any sense of demarcation. Although generally the first and last phases are the longest, we pass through the phases in differing amounts of time under different circumstances. The amount of stimulation needed or desired for orgasm varies from person to person and for each of us from time to time.

The two fundamental reactions of sexual arousal – vasocongestion (blood-engorged veins) and myotonia (muscle contraction) – lead to that feeling of fullness, warmth and arousal we experience as sexual excitement.

Here is what happens for us during a sexual response cycle (you may want to refer to the description of female anatomy in Chapter 2 while reading this).

Excitement – The Beginning Feelings of Arousal. The vagina becomes moist (lubricated) as the swelling blood vessels around it push fluid through the vaginal walls, making them 'sweat'. The vagina begins to expand and balloon and eventually the inner two-thirds double in diameter.

The inner lips swell and deepen in colour.

The clitoris swells, becomes erect, and is highly sensitive to touch. If there is clitoral stimulation during this time, orgasms of greater intensity are more likely.

The breasts enlarge, and become more sensitive. The nipples become erect.

The uterus enlarges and elevates within the pelvic cavity.

The heart rate increases; breathing becomes heavier and faster.

A flush or rash may appear on the skin.

The muscles begin to tighten, especially in the genital area.

Plateau – The Full Feelings of Arousal Necessary for Orgasm. While the inner two-thirds of the vagina continues to balloon, the outer third narrows by one-third to one-half of its diameter. This allows the vagina to hold the penis during intercourse. Some of us fear this narrowing means we are not sufficiently aroused for intercourse, and feel intercourse will be painful. In fact this constriction signals we are physically ready for intercourse. However, too many of us begin intercourse during the excitement phase, when we are only slightly aroused. Intercourse will be most pleasurable and most likely to include orgasm if we don't allow penetration until we are more completely aroused.

---

* Masters and Johnson's big contribution has been a scientific observation of people going through the sexual response cycle and measurement of their reactions. Wilhelm Reich did similar research thirty years ago.

Although the upper two-thirds of the vagina is relatively insensitive to touch, following sexual arousal the outer third is quite sensitive to pressure. For some of us, at times, the whole vagina feels responsive.

The entire genital area continues to swell, as do the breasts. (You may become increasingly aware of these areas of your body.)

The uterus elevates fully.

We breathe very rapidly; we may pant.

The muscles continue to contract.

During the plateau phase the clitoris retracts under its hood. Stimulation of the inner lips from manipulation or intercourse moves the hood of the clitoris back and forth over the glans.

Orgasm — The Release of Sexual Tension. For women, if sexual stimulation is interrupted, excitement may decline. This is especially true just before and during orgasm, when we need continuous stimulation. Then direct or indirect stimulation of the clitoris intensifies to orgasm.

Orgasm may start with a spastic muscle contraction of two to four seconds' duration. Orgasm is three to fifteen rhythmic contractions of the muscles around the outer third of the vagina at $0 \cdot 8$-second intervals, and orgasm is the time of our most intense sexual feeling. The uterus and rectum also contract (the contractions cause the release of the blood trapped in the pelvic veins). Just before orgasm some of us feel a sense of suspension, and after orgasm most of us feel a sense of release and warmth spreading throughout our bodies.

Resolution — Return to Non-aroused State. For a half hour or more after orgasm, if lovemaking doesn't continue, swelling decreases, the muscles relax, and the clitoris, vagina and uterus return to their usual positions. For those of us who reach plateau but not orgasm, this can take hours and can be uncomfortable. Orgasm speeds the release of pelvic congestion.

MALE SEXUAL RESPONSE

The male sexual response cycle is similar to ours, with the four phases following in sequence. The fundamental reactions of vasocongestion and myotonia are the components of sexual arousal in men as well as women. Our first reaction to arousal is vaginal lubrication, and a man's is penile erection. These things happen well before either partner is ready for intercourse (especially for those of us who want orgasm with intercourse). For both sexes the peak of sexual excitement is orgasm, which for a man includes ejaculation.

With men, the four phases of the sexual response cycle are less well defined. The first phase, excitement, is shorter, another way of saying we get aroused more slowly. After orgasm a man has a period of a few minutes or even hours (longer as he gets older) when he cannot have another erection. This is called the refractory period.

On p. 64 we talk about some problems that men may have with sex.

Sex with Ourselves — Masturbation

Tiny babies explore their own bodies with their fingers, enjoying the sensations and learning where the pleasure of their own body separates from their pleasure in others. As we grow older it is natural to continue that exploration and for most of us that pleasurable touching leads us to the discovery of masturbation. For some the discovery is made in the first years of life, for others it is part of an adolescent curiosity about our sexuality, others of us are not aware that we can masturbate until some chance article or discussion with a friend opens this new area for sexual discovery.

Whenever the realization of self-pleasuring occurs it is almost inevitably accompanied by guilt; children's hands are slapped away from their bodies by red-faced parents, teenagers indulge in elaborate fantasies of divine retribution for this 'sin', adults are ashamed that masturbation is a substitute for inadequate sex and indulge in it furtively, secretly or not at all. For some of us these feelings of guilt are now associated with sex in general, and often learning to masturbate and accepting it as a valid experience has opened up sex again.

Masturbation allows us the time and space to explore and experiment with our own bodies. We can learn what fantasies turn us on, what touches arouse and please us, at what tempo, and where. We can come to know our own patterns of sexual response. We don't need to worry about a partner's needs and opinions. Then, if and when we choose, we can share our knowledge by telling or showing our partner, by taking his or her hand and guiding it to touch the places we want touched.

Masturbation is a special way of enjoying ourselves. 'It is our sexual base. Everything we do beyond that is simply how we choose to socialize our sex life.'

Women have many ways of masturbating: some of us masturbate by moistening our fingers (with either saliva or juice from the vagina or a sterile lubricatory cream like KY Jelly) and rubbing them around and over the clitoris. We can gently rub or tweak the clitoris itself; we can rub the hood or a larger area around the clitoris. We can use one finger or many. We can rub up and down or around and around. Pressure and timing also vary. Some of us masturbate by crossing our legs and exerting steady and rhythmic pressure on the whole genital area. Some of us have learned to develop muscular tension throughout our bodies resembling the tensions developed in the motions of intercourse. Some of us get sexually excited during physical activity – climbing ropes or trees, riding horses. Still other ways of masturbating include using a pillow instead of our hands, a stream of water, or an electric vibrator.

It's exciting to make up sexual fantasies while masturbating or to masturbate when we feel those fantasies coming on. Some of us like to insert something into our vaginas while masturbating – anything will do provided it is clean and without any sharp edges. Some of us find our breasts or other parts of our bodies sensitive and rub them before or while rubbing the clitoris. Enjoying ourselves doesn't just mean our clitoris, vagina and breasts. We are learning to enjoy all parts of our bodies.

LEARNING TO MASTURBATE

You may feel self-conscious, awkward, even a bit scared or rather shocked at the thought of masturbating if you have never tried before, but learning about your own responses to sexual stimulation is part of getting to know your body. It is not unnatural to want to touch yourself; the fact that for many women there is one part of their bodies which is only ever touched by lovers or doctors is more shocking. Here are some suggestions for beginning to explore masturbation yourself.

Read over 'Female Sexual Response' and Chapter 2. Then choose a time when you will be totally undisturbed and a place where you feel comfortable and safe from intrusion. Indulge yourself, have a couple of drinks, look at your body full length in a mirror, feel its shapes and texture – your body is as capable of turning you on as anyone else. Settle down comfortably, let your mind flow freely into fantasy and relax. Stroke your body all over, with cream or body lotion if it feels good that way, vary the pressure and timing, close your eyes and move your fingers in and over the entire genital area.

Now focus your attention on the area around your clitoris, stroking or rubbing it gently. You might find that a vibrator will help (see p. 60 for information). As you get sexually aroused you will find that your vagina becomes moist and your muscles tighten in the whole pelvic area. Experiment with what you can do to increase your excitement, breathe faster, move your pelvis rhythmically, stroke the area faster or perhaps harder as the sensations dictate, do anything else that comes to mind and don't be afraid of making a noise.

For me the most pleasurable part is just before orgasm. I feel I am no longer consciously controlling my body. I know there is no way I will not reach orgasm now. I stop trying. I like to savour this rare moment of true letting go!

If you have never had an orgasm before you might find the build-up of sensation frighteningly intense, even uncomfortable. Don't give up –

if you allow the orgasm to come rather than blocking it you will learn in time to come more easily; and don't expect instant results — some of us will come to orgasm in 10 seconds with the help of a vibrator, for others it can take an hour. It's letting go that makes it happen. If you don't come the first time don't worry, many of us didn't either — just enjoy the sensations and try again some other time. If after a month or so you still can't reach orgasm, talk to someone you feel relaxed with and read the section at the end of this chapter on problems with orgasm.

Masturbating opens me to what is happening in my body and makes me feel good about myself. I like following the impulse of the moment. Sometimes I have many orgasms, sometimes I don't have any. The greatest source of pleasure is to be able to do whatever feels good to me at that particular time. I rarely have such complete freedom in other aspects of my life.

Sex in a Relationship

As we move into a relationship with another person, we carry our sexuality — our feelings, our fantasies, our masturbation experiences — with us as part of our whole selves. We can express our sexuality in relation to someone else both as a way of getting sexual pleasure and as a way of communicating loving feelings. Sexual sharing that is satisfying deepens our relationships in a way few other shared experiences can, and good relationships in turn improve our sexual pleasure.

Yet sex in a relationship is as complex as relationships themselves:

I enjoy sex with Mike more than I have with anyone. When we get turned on, we make the most beautiful music together! Still sex often feels difficult for me. When I feel good about myself and close to him and when the pressures of our children and my work and my friends are not demanding a lot of my energy, our sex is very fluid and strong. When I feel angry or sad or depressed or very childlike and needy, or any combination, or busy with other people in my life, I have a hard time being sexually open with Mike. We've talked about this, and he experiences a lot of the same ups and downs and distractions as I do.

Sex in relationships can vary in meaning and intensity for us.

Sometimes I make love to get care and cuddling. Sometimes I am so absorbed in the sensations of touch and taste and smell and sight and sound that I feel I've returned to that childhood time when feeling good was all that mattered. Sometimes I am the tom-girl as we tumble and tease. Sometimes sex is spiritual — high mass could not be more sacred. Sometimes I fuck to get away from the tightness and seriousness in myself. Sometimes I want to come and feel the ripples of orgasm through my body. Sometimes tears mix with come mix with sweat, and I am one with another. Sometimes sex is more powerful than getting high, and through it I unite with the stream of love that flows among us all. Sex can be anything and everything for me. How good that feels!

Sometimes a brief encounter can be intensely exciting and can free us to try things we wouldn't with someone we were in a certain pattern with. On the other hand, a brief encounter or an affair we know will end can be unsatisfactory if we don't know or trust our partner well enough to ask for what we want. In a long-term relationship there is an opportunity to learn about each other's bodies over time; to explore different sexual techniques, roles and fantasies; to express deeply our many and varied feelings through sex.

I couldn't bear the thought of getting really involved with someone so that I would have to give up faking [orgasms] and worst of all, really face up to the possibility of a less-than satisfactory sex life stretching ahead of me for years. One night stands became the norm. The excitement of a new encounter was enough in itself . . . eventually I realized that my inability to achieve orgasm was becoming a major issue in my life, I knew that everything would not suddenly 'come right' outside a totally trusting relationship.*

Yet some long-term couples get into sexual patterns that fail to satisfy either or both partners. Some of us have had short-term relationships and have been able to use what we've learned in them to get out of unsatisfying patterns with a long-term partner. (Some relationships can last through such changes, others cannot. See Chapter 4 for more detail.)

Others are trying to evolve new ways of creating trust and closeness outside pair relationships, perhaps by extending special friendships to include a sexual element. Such parallel relationships need a high degree of trust and openness from all those involved; jealousy can be very destructive and it is not always easy to control our emotions to conform with our theoretical desires for less possessive relationships. It is particularly hard for those of us in stable relationships who want to spread out and include others in our sexual lives, to be aware that the 'outsiders' are particularly vulnerable. We must beware of using other people to test out our own emotions.

Whatever kind of relationship we have, good sexual sharing requires trust, clear communication, appropriate technique, a sense of humour, time and privacy. We want relationships based on mutual respect and equality. We want relationships in which our commitment allows us to share our vulnerable places as well as our joyful places. We need to cry and laugh together. We want to spend many quiet, unhurried hours with each other, finding what pleases and excites us.

---

* From *Spare Rib*, issue 23.

COMMUNICATING ABOUT SEX

When we asked a group of male and female students, 'How do you let someone know that you want to go to bed with them?' they started to laugh. The laughter expressed, 'Well, you know the games, too, so why are you asking?' It was also saying, 'It's hard to think seriously and talk openly with each other about sexual feelings.'

We pressed on beyond the laughter. One woman responded, 'By the eyes – the way you look at each other, you know.' A man said, 'I ask her if she wants to come to my room and smoke a joint.' Others spoke of how they touched each other – squeeze on the hand, arm on the shoulder – to communicate a desire for sex. 'How are you sure that the other person gets the message you intended and wants to have sex too?' More laughter. A man spoke up. 'Well, it's obvious – she got into bed with me.' I continued, 'Was she aware of how she felt, and if she felt she didn't want sex now, could she have said no comfortably?'

One woman joined in and very clearly said, 'I've been in that situation and couldn't say no because even though I didn't want intercourse, I did want to be physically close to someone and be held and touched, and I felt they all go together.' Another woman added, 'This is the first time I've talked about things like this in a mixed group, and I have not always known what I felt, or if I have, haven't felt I could say it.'

A man continued, 'Frankly, there have been times I've felt so horny it didn't matter to me what the other person felt.' (Nods from both women and men to this.) 'There have been other times I didn't feel like sex – holding hands and a good-night kiss were fine, and yet I felt the girl expected it, and the men I live with expected it, so I had sex.'

This discussion illustrates some of the issues we all face in a sexual situation, whether it's with a date, long-time lover, or spouse: How do I feel at the moment? Do I want to be sexually close with this person now? In what ways? What if I don't know; can I say I'm confused? Then can I communicate clearly what I want, what I don't want? Do I feel comfortable saying it in words or letting him/her know some other way? What are the unspoken rules? Is there enough trust between us, enough caring, for this person to listen to my feelings and respect them if I feel differently from him/her?

These questions come up all the time, and there are no easy or permanent answers. We can try to be as fully aware as possible of our feelings at the moment, and to be honest with ourselves about them.

Communication about our sexual needs is a continuous process. One woman who had got up the courage to talk with her man about their sexual relationship said in frustration, 'I feel like I told him what I like *once*, so why doesn't he know now? Did he forget? Doesn't he care?' None of us is a mind reader. Sometimes we can sense what someone close to us wants or needs. Other times we can't. We are aware that our own sexual feelings are different at different times, yet we're not always comfortable telling our lover how we feel from time to time.

I felt passionate and intense last time we had sex. This time I'm feeling mellow and wanting to be physically close and don't care if I have an orgasm. While I'm clear about what I want, I have trouble saying it. The voices in my head say:
— I felt so physically, spiritually and emotionally close that I crave that peak experience again. Anything else is less than that.
— I fear he expects me to want intercourse and an orgasm and he'll feel bad if I don't.
The voices go on. I want to scream, to shut them off. The more I let them go on, the less I feel like any kind of sex.

Letting Tony know what I need at a certain point was not always so simple. I knew that he had grown up believing males are supposed to know more about sex. So even when he told me he wanted to know what made me feel good, I had this feeling that telling him would seem like criticism of what he was doing.

We were both really excited. He began rubbing my clitoris hard and it hurt. It took me a second to work out what to do. I was afraid that if I said something about it, I would spoil the excitement for both of us. Then I realized I could take his hand and very gently move it up a little higher to my pubic hair.

Communicating about sex is often awkward at first. Here are some of the barriers that we have felt:

We are afraid that being honest about what we want will threaten the other.
We are embarrassed by the words themselves.
We feel sex is supposed to come naturally and having to talk about it must mean there's a problem.
We aren't communicating well with our partner in other areas of our relationship.
We don't know what we want at a particular time, or we need to react to something our partner does. The barriers can be within us, not just between us and our partners.

How do we work on better communication in sex? We are discovering that talking about sex with our partner — the sharing of what we feel, of what we enjoy and don't enjoy in our lovemaking — is part of the whole experience. Sometimes it's helpful to talk while we are making love. This can create surprises and add to our excitement. At other times it feels better to wait until later to talk.

Either way, talking can add new dimensions to the experience and can make for a greater sense of closeness and intimacy. Talking about love-making can also be painful, because sometimes when our sex isn't as we want it to be, it is clearly reflecting our general inability to connect, and that's disappointing.

Making love is one of the special times when we have more than words to use to reach each other. Taking our partner's hand and putting it in a new place, making the noises that let him/her know we are feeling good, speeding up or slowing down our hip movements, a firm hand on the shoulder meaning 'let's go slow' — there are many ways we have of communicating, if we will use them.

We have so many ways of expressing affection, trust and pleasure — touching, hugging, kissing, communicating through words and gestures, teasing, laughing and crying.

I can so clearly remember moving in and around him and him in me, till it seemed in the whole world there was only us dancing together as we moved together as we loved together as we came together. Sometimes at these times I laugh or cry and they are the same strong emotions coming from a deep protected part of me that is freer now for loving him.

With all our old stereotypes about who does what in sex, these kinds of communication don't happen overnight — we move gradually away from the old myth that men know all about sex, women just have it done to them, and no one talks about it. However, more and more of us are finding that telling or showing each other what feels good is not complaining or demanding; it's a profound kind of honesty.

THERE'S MORE THAN INTERCOURSE

The pleasures of sex include a wide variety of feelings and experiences. The categories we learned — foreplay, intercourse, orgasm — confine us. They imply that all sex is a prelude to, culmination of or substitute for vaginal intercourse.

We have many ways of getting and giving pleasure. We can touch, stroke and caress each other, spend time finding the ways in which we can turn each other on. We can find out about the sensations we feel all over our bodies; sometimes we build up more excitement by avoiding the 'erogenous' zones of breasts and genitals until we both feel really aroused. Then there are many different ways of coming to orgasm. We can do it by 'mutual masturbation', stimulating each other with our hands, or with our mouths or tongues (this is called cunnilingus if done to a woman or fellatio if done to a man).

The anus can be stimulated with fingers, tongue, penis or a slender object. The anus is highly sensitive to erotic stimulation, however it is not as elastic as the vagina. Be gentle, careful and use a lubricant (KY Jelly, saliva, etc.).

All these techniques can be used as a prelude to intercourse, *but don't put anything into your vagina which has been in your anus without washing it first. The bacteria in the anus can cause vaginal infections.* The possibilities for arousing each other are endless, so use your imagination. For further suggestions see *Loving Women* – written by women – or *The Joy of Sex* and *More Joy* by Alex Comfort – a man (see Bibliography).

SEX WITH INTERCOURSE

Sex with intercourse includes what is traditionally called foreplay. Giving more importance to intercourse is unnecessary: all sexual pleasures are equal.

Unfortunately, the 'norm' for female sexual response has been defined by all experts as orgasm during vaginal/penile intercourse. Women who *don't* have this experience are still labelled 'sexually dysfunctional' even if most can achieve orgasm quickly and easily through masturbation.*

Most of the time we want intercourse to lead to orgasm because it feels so good for us and our partner. There are many ways to enjoy ourselves and to come to orgasm; there is no one right way. Sometimes we feel like having intercourse and having an orgasm is not important to us. Then it is a different experience from intercourse with orgasm, not a lesser one.

Here is one experience of sexual intercourse with a man:

We got home late in the evening after a long visit with friends. Bryan and I went straight to bed, both of us feeling very sleepy. After a few minutes of cuddling and good-nights, I began to feel somewhat sexually aroused; but thinking I was too tired to enjoy making love, I rolled over to go to sleep. Bryan, also feeling aroused, reached around me and began to stroke my body. As I felt his hand on my breast and then on my stomach, I smiled to myself and rolled back towards him. At this point I knew I wanted to make love and was amazed at how quickly my moods could change.

We moved our bodies against one another gently. Neither Bryan nor I was very energetic or passionate, but we were both feeling aroused. I kissed his chest and then slid my cheek along his stomach and thighs. I stroked and held his penis, which had been erect for several minutes, and lay quietly upon his stomach. We touched and kissed each other affectionately, sometimes laughing and biting playfully, sometimes looking into one another's eyes with that very special non-verbal expression of our love.

When I felt ready, I lay on top of Bryan and guided his penis into my vagina. I moved my pelvis slowly back and forth enjoying the familiar, warm sense of fullness of feeling Bryan inside me. The muscles in my vagina began to contract and release rhythmically. At the same time, I began to fantasize about being by the ocean, with the rhythmic sound of waves breaking on the shore. Then

* See Shere Hite, *The Hite Report*.

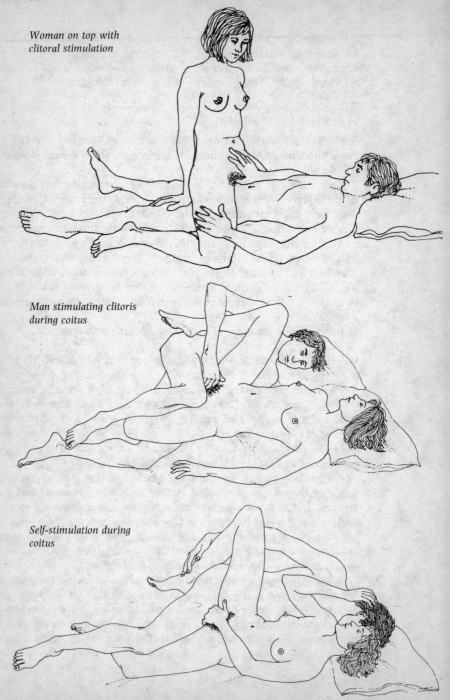

*Woman on top with
clitoral stimulation*

*Man stimulating clitoris
during coitus*

*Self-stimulation during
coitus*

Bryan put his hands on my hips and asked me to stop moving for a while — he was close to the point of orgasm and didn't want to come yet.

We lay still for several minutes and talked about the evening with our friends as well as plans we'd made for the following day. I began to move my pelvis again and felt that I wanted to have an orgasm. Though I had nice sensations all over my body, I sensed that I needed to change positions, that my clitoris needed a lot of stimulation before I could have an orgasm. We both knew from experience that at times like this I felt best if Bryan penetrated me from behind and reached around me with his hand to rub my clitoris. Sometimes I liked to do this while lying on my stomach with him on top of me, but this time it felt better to lie with my back to his stomach. Bryan knew from my movements and my breathing when to increase the pressure on my clitoris and when to move his fingers more rapidly. I communicated this non-verbally by rubbing my hands against his thighs: he knew how to match the movement of his fingers with the movement of my hands.

I soon became very excited, experienced tingling sensations all over, and then felt the intense pleasure of those moments just before orgasm, when I seemed to be soaring over the top of a waterfall. My orgasm was a rush of wonderful feelings.

I moved rhythmically for several minutes, enjoying the sense of release and looseness after my orgasm. Bryan said how much he had enjoyed tuning in to my orgasm. (He often likes to hold back from coming himself so that he can share in my orgasm more fully.) He then started to thrust inside me, moving more and more forcefully and rapidly. As he approached orgasm, I became aroused again and started to rub my clitoris. When he came, he moaned softly and kissed the back of my neck (one of my most erotic places). His orgasm was especially arousing for me and I came soon after him. We both felt a warm glow and snuggled against each other for a while.

For most of us it is quicker, physiologically, to reach orgasm with direct clitoral stimulation by hand or mouth or vibrator than solely with the indirect stimulation of intercourse. Yet many of us also feel that orgasm with a penis in our vagina is pleasurable and emotionally satisfying. Since many of us find it difficult to get sufficient stimulation with a penis in our vagina but want orgasms through intercourse, we have included some suggestions that have helped us reach orgasm with intercourse. (There may also be other reasons for difficulty in reaching orgasm — see 'Problems with Orgasm', p. 59.)

Take the penis into your vagina only when you are very aroused (see 'Masturbation' and 'Female Sexual Response' sections, pp. 44 and 40). Over time you will learn to know when you are ready to begin intercourse without giving it much thought.

Sometimes when you make love you may be eager for penetration without clitoral caresses, but more often most of us need clitoral stimulation manually or orally for some time before intercourse.

If you are highly aroused when actual intercourse begins, the minor lips around the entrance to your vagina will be swollen and will stimulate your clitoris (see 'Female Sexual Response', p. 40). You may want additional manual stimulation of the clitoris during intercourse. You or your partner can do this easily if you are sitting on top (female superior position) or the two of you are lying side by side (lateral coital position) – see figures, p. 52. For many women the female superior position is the easiest and sometimes the only way to achieve orgasm with intercourse. It is also easier to get breast stimulation in this position. The man on top is not a more 'natural' position for intercourse. You can both sit up with your legs over his and his penis in you. Or your man can enter you from behind and use his hands to reach around and stimulate your clitoris. We are all different shapes and need to find the positions that suit us. We can gain a lot of pleasure by trying different positions.

If you are not ready for orgasm and your man is highly aroused when you begin intercourse, you might bring him to orgasm too soon for you if he engages in vigorous penile thrusting and you move your pelvis against his quickly. You can both slow your movements down until you are more excited.

With these subtle movements you can hover at the edge of orgasm for a long time, which is exquisitely exciting. Also, you are more likely to both reach orgasm and to do so within minutes of each other. (Simultaneous orgasms are not important – or frequent.) These experiments with moving slowly can help men learn to delay ejaculation, which can make intercourse more pleasurable for both of you.

The first few years we had a great sex life. We were very attracted to each other and I loved sex with Ralph. I didn't have orgasms and I didn't even know what an orgasm was. Then I learned about orgasms, partly by reading some of the new books and articles, and partly by having one while masturbating. It felt so good that I wanted to have it with Ralph. The next two years were awful in bed. We had this goal – my orgasm – and it was like we'd look at our watches and say, 'One, two, three, go,' and work at it until we succeeded. Now, finally, we're back on an even keel. Usually I come, sometimes I don't. I let Ralph know which way I'm feeling. We can forget that goal and just do what feels good. But I wish I'd known everything I know now back when our feelings were so intense.

We owe it to ourselves and each other to make the time and space we need to enjoy sex, to learn about each other to discover what feels good and what feels better. For many of us, work schedules, crowded homes and exhaustion make privacy and time seem like unattainable luxuries. Our lives are organized for others, not ourselves, but even within the narrow limits that society allows us we can help each other to find that time. When we fight for socialized child care, for part-time work, for good homes, we are fighting also for time — for ourselves, for our children, for each other.

A LIFETIME OF SEX

Our powers to express ourselves sexually are powers that last a lifetime — from birth to death. For some of us that may be a new notion. Certainly many of us don't see our parents as sexual beings; they are our parents, and many older people haven't felt comfortable sharing that part of themselves with us.

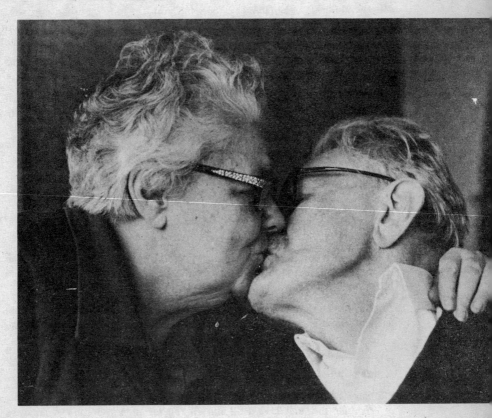

When he was drinking, an old family friend (he's in his late sixties) said to me, 'Your generation doesn't believe we had sex before marriage. Well, my wife and I were sleeping together for three years before we got married, and we are still enjoying it!' I drew back for some moments. My response was one of surprise and I said, 'Well, how could we know, you never talked about it.'

As we start to be more open about sex with the older people in our lives, and they with us, we discover, happily, that there is no age limit.*

Recently I heard this story: The seventy-five-year-old mother of a friend told her daughter that an eighty-year-old man she knew had propositioned her. She was delighted and said, 'Walter you really want to make love with me and I accept!' I was surprised and also excited that sexual loving doesn't end at sixty!

Over our lifetime we can have many changing feelings about our sexuality – how we want to explore it, with whom, etc. Sometimes these changes take us by surprise.

I have trouble talking about sex right now because there isn't much. I feel closeness and deep connection with my husband and still I'm disturbed. We used to always count on being able to make love, no matter what else was wrong. And that just isn't true any more. I feel uneasy.

If we're not having a sexual relationship or not getting what we want in the one or ones we're in, it's hard to accept that sex isn't everything we always thought it would be. We can begin to feel deprived, discouraged, less a woman. But we *can* take these changes quite easily.

I'm feeling this is a space in my life for myself, to explore certain issues I've never allowed myself to explore before. I want male companionship from time to time. Yet I don't want an intense, continuous relationship. That means I have sporadic and spontaneous encounters with men (some sexual, some not) – momentary intimacies. This is a new experience for me, and the newness of it sometimes makes me feel shaky. Most of the time I feel okay.

It helps us feel easier with fluctuation in sexual feelings when we see that while our sexual feelings can go just as they can come, they can also come back again.

I've been so angry that I could easier kill him than sleep with him. At first these feelings scared me. Now I know they pass and change and I feel loving again.

There are times in our lives when sex is in the background of a relationship. We go on a business trip for a month, we visit a sick relative and stay awhile, we spend time with a friend.

I'm absorbed right now in sorting out what work I want to do. This is a time of crisis for me, and I need all my energy for myself. I can't relate very intimately to the man I live with. We've been together for several years and I trust this is what is happening right now and will change.

It felt so good to talk to Anne. We've been married about the same time, ten years. I was feeling there was something wrong in my relationship with

* For more information see 'The Effects of Age on Sexuality', in Helen Kaplan, *The New Sex Therapy.*

Steven — we haven't had sex for a month. I was feeling, 'What's wrong with us? I need to create some excitement, perhaps have an affair, do something different to keep the sexual fires burning.' She was very reassuring. She said she'd had a similar experience and felt the same way at the time. She said that after that time they began having sex regularly again.

People who have lived together for a long time may feel less energy or urgency for sex.

We have been married for fifteen years. For several years we were passionate lovers, there was a lot of romance in our lives. Now there is less romance and very deep love and friendship. Sex is no longer the most important thing in our lives. We have sex less frequently and yet our lovemaking feels good in different ways than in those early years. We feel very warm, intimate and deeply trusting of each other.

IN BED

Discontinuous we lie
with an old cat asleep
between our backs

where jealous children
used to squirm
wedged in between us.

We grow old, you and I,
to be so equable, lying
back to cat and cat to back.

(ALICE RYERSON)

For many couples, sex becomes more meaningful over time:

I didn't marry for love or sexual passion. Sex was something I didn't know much about and neither did my husband. Just in the last two years — after fourteen years of marriage — we've been able to talk to each other about sex. That's mainly because we're not playing games, we're not criticizing and tearing each other apart. We are each more responsible for who we are as individuals. We are not expecting the other to live up to our expectations, to live out prescribed roles. So when we were making love the other night I felt clearest that I was making love as an adult, not a child. We didn't talk at the time — it wasn't necessary. Next morning we both felt the same thing. What I mean by adult is a deep kind of un-crazy passion. When you are in love it's crazy passion — you want to swallow each other up and be swallowed. This, in contrast, is a relaxed openness, anything goes, no hurry, free of guilt. We are more sexually connected than we've ever been in our lives and able just to be with each other.

We look forward to a lifetime of ups and downs and growth and change in how we live our sexuality. We will be fascinated to see how our daughters revise this chapter!

Problems with Sex

At one time or another all of us have problems with sex. We should not be afraid or ashamed to find out more about our difficulties and seek help, from friends, through reading or sex therapy. Two useful books are Helen Kaplan's *The New Sex Therapy* and Masters and Johnson's *Human Sexual Inadequacy* — both are listed in the bibliography to this chapter.

Many sexual problems arise through ignorance of how our bodies work or, for example, about the existence and whereabouts of the clitoris, and through lack of communication. These problems are increased by male and female role expectations, lack of trust, or unresolved conflicts. Sexual problems within a relationship involve both partners, and they cannot be solved without admission that they exist and discussion and exploration of our feelings and reactions to each other.

Some of the difficulties may not be easy to recognize. Here are some possibilities:

We are so concerned with sexual images and goals that we cannot think of sex outside the context of success/failure.

We grew up feeling that sex was bad and dirty and deep down we still feel that way.

We fear becoming pregnant.

We are afraid to follow our own feelings — we may not even be sure what they are.

We are ignorant of facts that would help us.

We are too shy and embarrassed to ask for the touching or other sorts of sexual stimulation we would like.

We fear if we ask for something different we will embarrass or threaten our lover, and our lover might leave.

We sleep with someone we are attracted to but do not feel comfortable with.

We always have sex at the end of the day when we are tired.

We make love with someone with whom we are angry.

We have been with one partner for many years and we are stuck in patterns that no longer excite us.

We expect to be instantly free and at ease with people we don't know well or feel very close to.

We don't have any friends with whom we talk about our experiences, feelings and concerns.

We don't have anyone we want to sleep with.

There are some problems which do not stem directly from a particular relationship. They may come from deeply hidden fears and inhibitions. If the problems come from our own minds we cannot expect another person, however loving, to solve them; at best he or she can give patient support. We must learn about ourselves before we can teach others to please us. How we think and feel about ourselves powerfully affects how our bodies respond. Our problems can take many forms, which we will discuss below. If we have any problem we owe it to ourselves to explore further. We need not be in agony or a freak to seek help. Sexual problems are common.

PROBLEMS WITH ORGASM

Many of us experience difficulties reaching orgasm – either by ourselves or with a lover. Shame about exploring and touching ourselves keeps us from learning to bring ourselves to orgasm through masturbation. A variety of problems keeps us from having orgasms with another. Here are some of the reasons why:

We don't notice or else we misunderstand what's happening in our bodies as we get aroused. We're too busy thinking about abstractions – how to do it right, why it doesn't go well for us, what our lover thinks of us, whether our lover is impatient, whether our lover can last – when we might better be concentrating on sensations, not thoughts.

We feel ourselves becoming aroused, but we are afraid we won't have an orgasm, and we don't want to get into the hassle of trying, so we just repress sexual response.

We hold our breath the more excited we get and cut off the feelings of our own orgasms.*

We don't know how to coordinate our breathing with the movements of our pelvis.*

We can't tolerate too much pleasure and our orgasms – if we have them – are less satisfying and intense than they could be.*

We are afraid of asking too much and seeming too demanding.

Although we really want to cuddle, we feel we must have intercourse, since our partner has an erection. We fear it is physically painful for him not to come, although becoming aroused and not having an orgasm is no more uncomfortable for him than for us.

We haven't learned, and often neither has he, that the getting to orgasm is as pleasurable, if not more pleasurable, than orgasm itself.

We find it takes longer for us to get aroused, and we are anxious our partner will become impatient. That anxiety assures our not getting aroused.

* For more detail on these points see *Total Orgasm*, by Jack Rosenberg, and also *For Yourself*, by Lonnie Barbach.

We let him enter before we really want him inside us. We rush into it —
or let our partners rush us into it. We end up fucking with great intensity —
swept off our feet like in the films and swept under the rug when it comes
to climaxes.

*I really love to stroke and kiss and lick Ned! Why can't I trust that he likes to
do the same for me, when I know he does? Maybe it's just too good for me to
feel it could be true!*

We are afraid that if our partner concentrates on our pleasure we will
feel such pressure to come that we won't be able to — and then we don't.

We are trying to have a simultaneous orgasm — which seldom occurs
for most of us. It is just as pleasurable if we come separately.

We have conflicts about, and are often angry with, the person we are
sleeping with. Unconsciously we withhold orgasm as a way of withholding ourselves.

We feel guilty about having intercourse and so cannot let ourselves
really enjoy it.

We don't want to make love in the first place.

An orgasm is a physical response like sneezing which can be triggered
off by the right stimulus. You can learn what the stimulus is for you and
once learned it will never be forgotten. Certainly some people 'come'
more easily than others; you may simply need much longer stimulation
than you have ever allowed yourself or been allowed. The average time
can vary from a few minutes to an hour and the amount of concentration
needed varies as well. For some of us, total concentration is required. It
can be shattered by a sudden noise, or even a change in tempo; almost
anyone can be put off by a flatmate walking into the room! If you are
concentrating on your partner's pleasure instead of your own you may
never make it. Concentrate on enjoying yourself; your pleasure will
certainly be more stimulating to your partner than solicitous attention
would be.

If you have never had an orgasm in spite of a longstanding relationship
and many attempts, try masturbating on your own (see p. 44). It may
well take a long time, so make sure you will be undisturbed. Invest in a
vibrator which will take the strain off your fingers. Plenty of lubrication
(saliva, or KY Jelly) massaged around the clitoris improves the sensations
and protects it. A drink or two beforehand will help you relax, and don't
try too hard the first time, anxiety about failure is a real killer. Vibrators
are often called Personal Massagers. They are sold in most chemists and
sex shops or by mail order. Some of us tried little plastic ones and only
got a tickle for our trouble, the heavier ones seem to work better and we
would recommend the Personal Massager from Pellen Personal Products,
5 The Campsbourne, London N8. Vibrators can cost between £1.00 and
£5.00 (probably much more by the time you read this). It sounds
expensive — but it's cheap if it works!

In a fit of rather panicky depression I brought up the orgasm problem with a friend. She not only suggested a vibrator but provided me with one. Luckily I was feeling reasonably optimistic, nobody knew, nobody was listening and nobody was awaiting results. I lay back and searched out the most sensitive area. After a while I began to feel sensations which I recognized from previous attempts at masturbating. They were uncomfortable, almost painful and I'd always stopped when they started. This time I didn't stop and sure enough my body was jerked with a series of frightening contractions. I'd had an orgasm at last. Looking back I realized that I'd developed a kind of stalling mechanism. As I came near to orgasm my muscles would tense and actually resist. The sensations became unbearable and that is why I'd always stopped.

Some of us find that we cannot work things out on our own. In response to this need, pre-orgasmic groups have been started. (See Addresses at the end of this chapter.)

LACK OF INTEREST IN SEX — SEXUAL AVERSION (LACK OF LIBIDO)

Sometimes we feel that we have no interest in sex at a particular time. For most of us this is a passing phase: we are angry, depressed, too involved in other interests or preoccupied with worries. When the problem passes our sexual interest returns. But sometimes the phase seems to be going on for ever, causing anxiety and tension in a relationship. In this case it is important to find out what is bothering you.

It may simply be that after the initial excitement you are not as interested as you used to be. As long as you are both happy with this arrangement it isn't a problem, though it is important to discuss it. You might find that you are both misinterpreting each other's needs. Sexual appetites are as varied as appetites for food.

Sometimes it is hard to accept that sex doesn't always have to be electrifying; it can be gentle, the sensations quite mild. Learn to allow your body to respond to even mild feelings; they will probably build up after a while, and even if they don't you can enjoy the pleasure of physical closeness.

However, lack of interest may be concealing other profounder problems within a relationship and it shouldn't be ignored. It could be covering unresolved conflicts which you may or may not be aware of; it might herald the end of an unsatisfactory relationship. Whatever the reason, it is important to be open about how you feel. It may be difficult to remember that your partner is suffering too.

If you hide the problems and 'submit' to sex when you are unhappy about it you may be building up bigger problems, completely covering your own needs and learning to fear sex. Talking and re-learning about each other's bodies and responses may help to resolve the conflict, strengthen your relationship and improve your sex life as well.

Masters and Johnson use a technique for re-kindling sexual interest —
though no technique will be completely successful if you haven't
resolved the deeper problems as well. It is called 'sensate focus'. Each
partner must take turns at pleasuring the other without touching
genitals or breasts. The passive partner of the moment gives feedback on
how it feels. On the second or third days you can move to the genitals but
must make no attempt at intercourse and/or orgasm until both partners
feel absolutely ready for it.

Some of us have conflicts about sex which go so deep that we never
have any interest in it. We may feel unpleasant sensitivity to touch, or
so ticklish we can't relax. If our problems are deep inside our own minds
we may need help to unlock and resolve them through some kind of
psychotherapy.

PAINFUL INTERCOURSE (DISPAREUNIA)

You may experience discomfort, even pain, with intercourse for physical
rather than emotional reasons:

Local Infection.   Some vaginal infections — monilia or trichomonas, for
example — can be present in a non-acute, visually unnoticeable form. The
friction of a penis moving in the vagina might cause the infection to
flare up, making us sting and itch. (See Chapter 6, for more details.)

Local Irritation.   The vagina may be irritated by the birth-control foam,
cream, or jelly you are using. If so, try a different brand. Some of us react
to the rubber in a condom or diaphragm. Many of the vaginal deodorant
sprays can irritate the lips of the vagina; if sprayed inside, they can
irritate the inside too. If you've been using one of these and intercourse
makes you itch, don't switch brands, just stop using any.

Insufficient Lubrication.   The wall of the vagina responds to sexy
feelings by 'sweating', giving off a liquid that wets the vagina and the
entrance to it, which makes the entry of the penis easier. Sometimes there
isn't enough of this liquid. Some reasons: (a) you may be trying to let
the penis in (or the man might be putting/forcing it in) too soon, before
there has been enough foreplay to excite you and set the sweating action
going; (b) you may be nervous or tense about making love (e.g., it's the
first time, or you're worried about getting pregnant), so there isn't
enough liquid; (c) if the man is using a condom you may need to add
lubrication. Be sure to give the vagina time to get wet. If you still feel dry
you can use saliva, lubricating jelly (e.g., KY) or a birth-control foam,
cream or jelly. (Never use vaseline to lubricate a condom or diaphragm.
It will deteriorate the rubber.) Occasionally, insufficient lubrication is

caused by a hormone deficiency. After childbirth (particularly if you are nursing your baby or if your stitches hurt) and after menopause are the two times when a lack of oestrogen can affect the vaginal walls in such a way that less liquid is produced. A doctor can give you vaginal suppositories or some kind of hormone therapy. Meanwhile try the lubricants suggested above.

Tightness in the Vaginal Entrance. The first few times we have intercourse, an unstretched hymen (if we have one) can cause pain. Anyway for a penis to get in easily, our vagina and its entrance have to be relaxed as well as wet. If we are tense and preoccupied the vaginal entrance is not likely to loosen up, and getting the penis in might hurt. Even if we feel relaxed and sexy, timing is important. The vagina gets wet well before the clitoris, vaginal lips and the outer third of the vagina are fully sensitized and ready for orgasm. If we try to get the penis in before we are fully aroused, we might still be too tight though we are wet enough. So don't rush, and don't let yourself be rushed.

Pain Deep in the Pelvis. Sometimes the thrust of the man's penis hurts inside. Masters and Johnson say this pain can be caused by: (a) tears in the ligaments that support the uterus (caused by obstetrical mismanagement during childbirth, a botched-up abortion, gang rape); (b) infections of the cervix, uterus and tubes (such as pelvic inflammatory disease – the end result of untreated gonorrhoea in many women); (c) endometriosis (see 'Common Medical and Health Problems', Chapter 7); (d) cysts or tumours on the ovaries. These can all be treated successfully. Also, if the penis hits the cervix we feel pain. That pain can be relieved by having the man not go in so deeply or by being more fully aroused (which moves the cervix away) before penetration.

Clitoral Pain. The clitoris is exquisitely sensitive, and for most of us direct touching or rubbing of the clitoris is painful (many men don't know this until we tell them). Also, genital secretions can collect under the hood, so when we wash we need to pull back the hood of our clitoris and clean it gently.

PAINFUL PENETRATION (VAGINISMUS)

For a few of us, intercourse is painful and sometimes impossible. While there are physical reasons why we experience this pain (see 'Tightness in the Vaginal Entrance', above) we most often experience vaginismus because of strong conflicts and fears about sex, which we express, often unconsciously, by making it difficult for us to have or enjoy intercourse.

If you have vaginismus you experience a strong, involuntary tighten-ing of your vaginal muscles, a spasm of the outer third of your vagina, which makes entrance by the penis acutely painful.

Vaginismus can be your body's defence against a sexual situation you can't handle or don't want to be in. It can also be the result of bad experiences, such as rape. If you think you are suffering from vaginismus, read about it in *The New Sex Therapy*. There is a physical treatment for vaginismus which you can learn to do. For some of us, good psycho-therapy can also help change unhappy sexual patterns.

Whatever the cause, if intercourse is at all painful, don't put up with the pain! Find out what is causing it and do something about it. Until the problem is solved, work out other ways to make love. The power that each of us has, and the power that we have together, to make our lives more satisfying is enormous.

A WORD ABOUT MEN

If we are having sex with a man and he's having sexual difficulties, it is hard to share the kind of pleasure both partners would like. Further, his difficulties may complicate our own problems – even create some for us. (For example, if our partner ejaculates prematurely, we will probably not have an orgasm. It is difficult for us to climax with stimulation from penetration alone if he lasts just a few minutes once inside the vagina.) We need to give him the kind of patience and encouragement we want from him if the two of us are to overcome anxieties and establish a satisfying sexual relationship.

Men can suffer problems similar to ours, and for many of the same reasons. The common male sexual problems are: (1) premature ejacula-tion – the inability to control the ejaculatory reflex; (2) impotence – the inability to maintain, or even be aroused to, an erection; (3) dispareunia – pain with intercourse; and (4) sexual aversion – lack of interest in sex altogether.

Some sexual problems can be worked through with a little knowledge and a caring partner, while others might call for professional help.

It is important to recognize that a sexual problem that develops within a relationship is a shared problem. Too often women are made to feel guilty about their partner's difficulties as well as their own. Myths about independent women 'castrating' their husbands psychologically should be ignored. Of course changing roles between men and women can create insecurity for both partners and this can be expresssed through sexual difficulties. The answer is to be open about your feelings and try to work out tensions as they come up.

Men are more reluctant even than we are to discuss their sexual anxieties with friends, so we often find we are carrying much of the psychological load in supporting them. Books referred to in the bibliography will be of help to them as well as us.

GETTING HELP

If you are feeling pain in your pelvic, genital or vaginal area, go to a doctor and insist on being examined. Many doctors, if they cannot find an obvious cause, will just dismiss you and say, 'It's all in your head dear.' Few gynaecologists are equipped to help with sexual problems, and at the very least they should make sure they have carefully checked out the physical ones. We know of one woman who had an exploratory operation in a London hospital; she was sewn up again and told that her problem was depression. On a subsequent examination from another doctor she was diagnosed as having endometriosis (see Chapter 7).

Despite our knowledge about sex, despite the support of friends and partners, sometimes we cannot work through our difficulties. Psychosexual counselling is not as widely available in this country as it is in the USA and there may be waiting lists at the better places. The two bodies which are mainly responsible for running psycho-sex clinics are the Family Planning Association and the Marriage Guidance Council. Between these two agencies it should be possible to get some kind of help almost anywhere in the country but the quality of that help is a different matter.

The most popular training method for GPs and family planning doctors and nurses is that provided by the Institute for Psycho-Sexual Medicine. Most of its members are women and they mainly treat women, but their methods are based on psychoanalytic techniques and a very reactionary view of women. In her book *Contraception and Sexual Life*, the secretary of the Institute, Dr Prudence Tunnadine, seems to describe success in treating patients in terms of their acceptance of the traditional feminine role. They make little use of the more practical Masters and Johnson techniques, so it is probably not surprising that the success rate in a London FPA clinic was only about 30%, with orgasmic problems (referred to as 'frigidity') proving most difficult to treat. In clinics using M. & J. methods the 'success' rate is usually much higher. We feel that most women, if they are taught to bring themselves to orgasm through masturbation, will be more successful than if they are encouraged only to discuss the problem with a therapist and their own partner, in the end leaving him in charge of the practical aspects. The institute 'line' seems to be very much in favour of male sexual domination.

In spite of these very real drawbacks, individual doctors might be different in their approach, and as the FPA is for many people the only available source of help it might be worth a try.

The Marriage Guidance Council has a different approach. It uses lay counsellors for a start, not doctors, and the technique is based on

Masters and Johnson. The results of the first year of operation were considered 'very encouraging'. They work in couples and only treat couples (a restriction for some of us). There are only six of these centres but the treatment is free and they sound quite useful.

There are about forty NHS hospitals which run psycho-sexual clinics. They are usually attached to psychiatric departments but may also be found in gynaecology departments. Few of them use Masters and Johnson; those which do are listed at the end of this section.

The opening of the Women's Therapy Centre in North London is a welcome alternative to the existing institutions. It is not free, and can provide for only a small number of women; however it does provide a model for others to take up. There is no pressure here to be part of a heterosexual couple; much of the work is done in groups where women are encouraged to help each other. For the rest of us, if we do not conform to the heterosexual, monogamous couple norm that society expects of us, we will have difficulty getting help. Some of the places listed will help single people; most of them prefer not to and few of them are likely to approach the problems of sexual difficulties among lesbians.

LEARNING TO TALK TOGETHER ABOUT SEX

In a group we can discuss factual information, talk out problems, learn to communicate verbally and non-verbally, and learn alternative ways to get what we want sexually. Some women's groups have decided to spend a month or so discussing sex, other women have come together specifically to talk about it. Here are some suggestions for organizing discussion.

At the first meeting draw up a list of topics. Get different members of the group to research on practical aspects and suggest material for other group members to read. Some topics which you might like to discuss are: childhood and adolescent memories of sexuality; your feelings about your body; differences in male and female socialization; masturbation; fantasies; virginity; homosexuality; aspects of love-making; your relationships with women and men; sexual problems.

This is one way of starting discussion; after the first or second meeting two of you can draw up a list of questions about different aspects of sexual experience, starting with questions about childhood memories (what did you enjoy touching), sex play (doctor games, etc.), through to recent experiences. The rest of the group lie down with eyes closed while the questioners go through the list they have drawn up, asking questions to each other member, slowly, giving time for thought. When all the questions have been asked, the entire group then discuss their reactions and new thoughts that have occurred. When discussing aspects of our lives that we have always kept hidden and private it is important to build up trust in each other. It might help to make it a rule at the start not to discuss anything that happens within the group outside meetings even with other group members. The simple experience of expressing deeply hidden worries about sex can be enormously liberating in itself.

Bibliography and Resources

Barbach, L. G., *For Yourself – The Fulfilment of Female Sexuality*, Doubleday, New York, 1975. Not yet published here – a guide written for 'pre-orgasmic women' but an excellent guide for all of us. Try Compendium Books. 240 Camden High Street, London NW1.

Belleveau, Fred, and Richter, Lin, *Understanding Human Sexual Inadequacy*, Hodder, 1971. A shortened version of the Masters and Johnson research. Very useful.

Brecher, Ruth and Edward, *An Analysis of Human Sexual Response*, Panther, 1971. A very readable version of the first Masters and Johnson study.

Chartham, Robert, *Sex and the Over Fifties*, Frewin, 1970.

Comfort, Alex, *The Joy of Sex*, Quartet, 1974, and Comfort, Alex, *More Joy of Sex*, Quartet, 1977. Both give encouragement and helpful suggestions though some people find the cookbook style offensive.

Dodson, Betty, *Liberating Masturbation: A Meditation on Self Love*, 1974. Available from Compendium. Published by Bodysex Designs, PO Box 1933, New York, NY 10001. Highly recommended.

Ejlersen, Mette, *I Accuse*, Tandem, 1969. A supportive book on female sexuality, particularly clitoral orgasm.

Falk, Ruth, *Women Loving*, Random House, 1975.

Freud, Sigmund, *On Sexuality*, Penguin, 1977. An outline of Freud's basic ideas on female sexuality. We don't agree with some of his theories, but as his texts are slavishly followed by many people we should know what he said.

Friday, Nancy, *My Secret Garden*, Virago, 1976. A book of women's sexual fantasies.

Hegler, Inge and Sten, *An ABZ of Love*, Spearman, 1969. Honest, open view of female sexuality with respect for women.

Hite, Shere, *The Hite Report*, Summit (Hamlyn), 1977, and *Sexual Honesty*, Warner Books, 1974. Research on female sexuality compiled by a feminist. Very important.

Kaplan, Helen S., *The New Sex Therapy*, Penguin, 1977. Readable discussion of male and female sexual dysfunction and their treatment. Pictures particularly good.

Loving Women, Nomadic Sisters (USA), 1975. (Compendium.)

Masters, William H., and Johnson, Virginia, *Human Sexual Response*, Churchill, 1966. A revolutionary research study, important though hard to read.

Masters, William H., and Johnson, Virginia, *Human Sexual Inadequacy*, Churchill, 1970. More research and treatment of sexual dysfunction.

Mead, Margaret, *Male and Female*, Penguin, 1970.

Mitchell, Juliet, *Psychoanalysis and Feminism*, Penguin, 1974. Hard going, a reassessment of Freud's view of female sexuality.

Reich, Wilhelm, *The Function of the Orgasm*, Panther, 1968.

Reich, Wilhelm, *The Sexual Revolution*, Vision Press, 1972. Important work on human sexuality which predates Masters & Johnson.

Reich, Wilhelm, *The Invasion of Compulsory Sex-Morality*, Penguin, 1975.

Rush, Anne Kent, *Getting Clear: Body Work for Women*, Wildwood House, 1974. Book of exercises, experiences, etc. to help us get in touch with our bodies.

Rosenberg, Jack Lee, *Total Orgasm*, Wildwood House, 1974. Suggests exercises to help us enjoy sex together.

Sherfey, Mary Jane. *The Nature and Evolution of Female Sexuality*. Random House, New York, 1972.

Spare Rib (see p. 570) has published a number of articles on female sexuality – particularly good on difficulties with orgasm:

Machin, Alison, 'Good Vibrations', *Spare Rib*, issue 23.

Pre-Orgasmic Therapy Group, 'Earthly Delights', *Spare Rib*, issue 52.

Stephens, Eleanor, 'The Moon Within Your Reach', *Spare Rib*, issue 42.

Stephens, Eleanor, 'Unlearning Not to Have Orgasms', *Spare Rib*, issue 44.

Stephens, Eleanor, 'Making Changes Making Love', *Spare Rib*, issue 48.

FOR CHILDREN AND YOUNG TEENAGERS

Claesson, Bent, *Boy Girl Man Woman*, Calder & Boyars, 1971. Needs updating and is not as good as it should be on female sexuality, but it is straightforward and unpatronizing, discussing sexual technique, sex problems and contraception, etc. New Penguin edition due Spring 1979.

Knudsen, Per Holm, *How a Baby is Made*, Piccolo, 1975. For very young children.

Sheffield, Margaret, *Where Do Babies Come From*, Cape, 1973. Simple, for young children.

ADDRESSES

London Pre-orgasmic Workshop, 58 The Pryors, East Heath Road, London NW3.

The Women's Therapy Centre, 19a Hartham Road, London N7 (01 607 2864). Run by feminists.

The Family Planning Association, Margaret Pyke House, 27–35 Mortimer Street, London W1. Costs about £6.00 per session or free where NHS-controlled. Lists of clinics available from the above address.

The Institute of Psycho-sexual Medicine. Contact Dr Margaret Blair, Department of Obstetrics and Gynaecology, Charing Cross Hospital, London W6, for lists of private therapists available.

The National Marriage Guidance Council, Herbert Gray College, Little Church Street, Rugby, Warwicks (Rugby 73241). No charge; six clinics, mostly in the Midlands.

The following hospitals provide Masters and Johnson therapy on the NHS:

Carlton Hayes Hospital, Leicester

Claybury Hospital, Woodford, Essex

Doncaster Royal Infirmary
Guy's Hospital, London
Knowle Hospital, Fareham, Hants
Rochford General Hospital, Essex
St George's Hospital, Hyde Park Corner, London
Whitely Wood Clinic, University of Sheffield
Withington Hospital, Manchester

The following places give counselling with or without further referral at reasonably short notice:

British Pregnancy Advisory Service, 2nd Floor, 58 Petty France, Victoria, London SW1 (01 222 0985).

The Brook Advisory Centre for Young People, central address: 233 Tottenham Court Road, London W1 (01 580 2991).

The Forum Clinic, 2 Bramber Road, London W1 (01 385 6181). This has the singular disadvantage of being attached to *Penthouse* magazine, but the people who run the clinic are serious and helpful, and sessions are modestly priced.

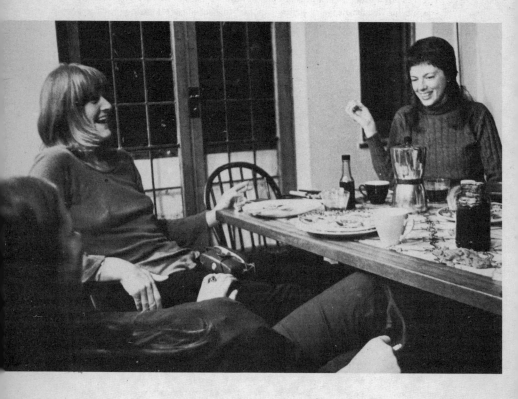

4 Living with Ourselves and Others – Our Sexual Relationships

Some Different Life-Styles

In this section we present the experiences of a lot of different women. These experiences are not meant to be models. We hope that no woman reading this chapter will feel that these are goals she has to get to someday. We want to share our confusions and regrets as well as the joy and growth we've experienced, so that every woman can be more aware of what her own choices are. We have chosen to use poetry, narratives and conversations from the lives of several women who have passed in and out of one or a number of these options on their way to finding what's best for them.

We have found for ourselves that broadening the scope of our close relationships has been very difficult and has taken a lot of time and energy. The support of other women has allowed us the space to grow in many directions.

THE EXPERIENCE OF BEING SINGLE

Many Voices: Excerpts from Taped Conversations Among a Group of Single Women in Boston, USA

It is an old belief that heterosexual couples are the only natural and necessary form of existence. Think of Noah's ark. Everything leads up to finding a mate – for love, for intimacy, for economic security, for survival of self, and for the survival of the species. Any other form of adult life is an exception to be pitied (old maid, widow), maligned (homosexual), or possibly tolerated (playboy bachelor, eccentric artist).

We all grew up with these assumptions. People outside our families were defined as 'outsiders'. We expected to be inside a couple and inside our own families when we grew up. We might be single women and do exciting things for a while, but that would be just a breathing space before marriage.

It didn't work out that way for us. For the past few years we have all been deeply, personally involved in the women's liberation movement, and our lives have changed drastically. All of us have varying degrees of intimacy with people now, primarily with women. None of us has a primary relationship that defines who we are. Together we are trying to explore our independence and find positive identities for ourselves – not in isolation from other people, but outside relationships that feel limiting or defining.

We have different fantasies for the future. Some of us want more intimate relationships. But in our lives outside of couples we've felt a lot of strength and joy – alone and as part of a group. What we've learned from being single is much more than the skills of survival in a 'transitional' state. And we look forward to new options for women in the future.

ELAINE. As a child I was often told it was impossible for a woman to take care of herself alone in the world, that she needed a man to manage things for her. No one took a woman seriously. I knew a repairman would come immediately if my father called, but it would take my mother many phone calls before he'd finally come around.

JUDITH. I was brought up with the idea that not getting married was the worst thing that could happen to you. If you didn't get married, your life was doomed to loneliness.

DEBORAH. I'll always remember the day I was supposed to go to a film with my friend Darlene. She called me at the last minute and told me that a boy she knew had called her up and they were going to go somewhere instead. I got really upset. I hung up the phone and said I didn't understand why she had cancelled her date with me. I really didn't understand it – I hadn't learned yet. My older sister and my mother said that I shouldn't get upset, because that's what girls do. It's more important for them to be with boys, and I just had to start getting used to it.

In high school I decided it was silly that boys should pay for girls. So I remember saying to my family that I should pay for myself, and my father started ranting and screaming at me, 'If you have that attitude, Deborah, boys will never like you and no one will ever take you out and you'll never get married!'

SUSANNE. In high school I found it harder to be without a boyfriend than it is now at twenty-three. All of us were expected to have a rocky time in adolescence, but those of us who didn't go on to get boyfriends and husbands still have a rocky time.

JUDITH. I would talk with many of my women friends about careers, but by the time of my last year at college I was the only one in my group who wasn't getting married. When I thought about doing a post-graduate degree, a male professor told me not to go – that I would become too much like a man and never get married.

Like many other single women I spent months looking for an 'exciting' job to meet 'exciting' people. Of course I didn't get the ideal job but finally settled for enough to live on.

I came home after the battle in rush hour to eat dinner with my flat-mates and talk about meeting men. The evening was spent waiting for someone to call for a date or trying to find someone to do something with.

I went to parties dressed in my new and most sophisticated attire. I tried to learn the art of cocktail chatter, taking subtle initiatives, looking confident and above it all. Going out on dates was another ordeal. Coolness and dishonesty seemed like the only qualities of the early parts of relationships. Informal socializing over real interests was almost impossible. Then, of course, there were the sex hassles — will you or won't you? I knew that I wasn't ready to get married. There were still so many things I wanted to do — travel, meet people, find exciting work. But I didn't know how long I could last; marriage seemed the only way out. For me the horror of being single was the loneliness, the lack of intimacy and honesty, as well as the lack of commitment between women.

As a single woman I felt a lot of anger and pain in my life. There was no outlet for the feelings, no focus for my anger and disappointment. I wanted freedom and independence, but I also wanted to be loved. Getting both seemed impossible. In retrospect I realize that I chose to be single. I wanted independence and excitement more than marriage. But at that time, I couldn't see it as a choice. It seemed impossible to share my feelings with other women. Everything made me feel ashamed; it must be my fault, there must be something wrong with me if I didn't have a permanent and lasting relationship with a man.

CAROLYN. When I tried to 'make it', become successful in my own right, I became aware of the incredible social stigma put on independent women. It became clear that one could not be seen as womanly and at the same time be successful in the 'active work world of men'.

RACHEL. When I got out of college I lived with several men, one after another. I got a lot out of those relationships — love and security and understanding and support. I thought I had what I'd always wanted. But underneath I was terrified. I was very dependent on my sexual relationships, and that frightened me.

Being out of a couple for several years has let me grow up and learn to function independently in the world. I really feel as if I can rely on myself now. And I feel I want more intimacy and am ready for it, but I don't know if I'll ever want to be part of a couple that develops a lot of dependency.

As a group of women we felt free to talk about our problems and begin to act on our feelings; we began to look at each other differently. We rediscovered a common bond that allowed us to stop judging ourselves and other women by men's standards. We tried to stop competing with one another. We worked to respect our emotions and to support each other's strengths. We learned to take each other seriously.

We joined women's consciousness-raising collectives and worked on various women's projects and organizations. We moved into houses with other women and began to acknowledge our feelings of love towards women. We changed our lives — our expectations, our environments, our definitions of meeting our needs.

Within the women's movement we have found that our interests and our needs sometimes differ from those of married women. At times we have felt excited that single women seemed freest to change their lives. At other times we have felt burdened and saddened by the insecurity of being single. We want to find new ways of relating to men, but we have no models. The possibility of gay relationships has opened new options for us, but being gay does not resolve the conflicts we feel about couple relationships.

When we tried to summarize the differences that the women's movement has made in our lives, we ended up with a lot of confusion. There is still fear, but also joy and relief about the roles we have grown out of and the possibilities we see ahead of us.

ELAINE. Now at most parties I go to, people function independently whether they're in couples or not. There's some sense of community. Your goal at a party is not necessarily to meet someone.

JUDITH. When I felt there was a clear community of women that was autonomous, I think I stopped thinking about myself primarily as a 'single' woman and started to think of myself more as a woman.

KATHY. I think there has been a growing respect for women who are more aggressive. A woman who is single is now given a certain amount of respect for having the strength to go out on her own. I always liked doing things that were thought of as boys' things, and in the women's movement these have become acceptable for women for the first time. Learning car mechanics and feeling that people respected me for it has been very important to me.

SUSANNE. Now I really count on other women as being prominent in my life. I no longer feel that I just happen to be there with other women who happen to be there because they aren't married or aren't with men.

KATHY. I still look towards the future with a lot of dread. I'm really scared that it's all going to collapse and I'll still be left alone. I have an absolute fear of what it means to be forty — I mean for me. The fact that many women are going back into couples — some with men and others with women — is what brought that fear back, since I've never related primarily as part of a couple.

DEBORAH. The women's movement opened up to me for the first time the option of not getting married. That's frightening, because it means that I have to create something new; there aren't the old forms of security. On the other hand, I feel better, since those old forms never really seemed quite so secure or didn't really give me the kind of happiness they were supposed to.

In giving up the idea of getting married I gave up one sense of the future. Now it feels as though I'll be making certain decisions for a few years at a time, but I don't have any sense of where my future is headed. Some of that's really good. It allows me to live from day to day and to express my needs for the present. On the other hand, I do need a greater sense of continuity.

I still want some kind of permanent relationship, to feel security and love. I want to have children of my own or share ongoing responsibility for friends' children. Now both those possibilities seem so hard to achieve; I have no models for what I want.

Stephanie: Communal Living

Living with others has been mostly a good experience. I've learned much about myself — about my strengths and weaknesses, about my needs for both intimacy and aloneness, and about the things I like and don't like.

When I first lived collectively, I had little understanding of how much time, energy and commitment it would take to create trusting, loving and caring relationships. I thought that simply our desire for a warm, loving home was enough — that working out conflicts and differences would all happen in time, without too much hassle. We certainly did hassle and struggle, but it took many months of living together for us to realize that we could not work through our conflicts. I learned a lot from that first communal experience. I realized how emotionally draining it could be for me to be close to four or five other people at the same time. I learned that I had important needs for space and time spent alone, needs which I often failed to recognize until I was already feeling very fragmented and pulled away from my 'centre'. It was particularly hard for me to know my own feelings and to find my own pace, since I was so easily sucked into my environment: if others were cheery and playful, then I would be, too; if others were depressed, then I'd feel sad. The people I lived with helped me to become more aware of my feelings — it's now much easier to be around others and to still be in touch with the 'me inside'.

One of my most intense and growthful experiences was a year of communal living on a farm. We started out as eight adults and two children who had met regularly for almost six months before actually living together. We felt a strong sense of family during the first few months of living together. At times, I would imagine that we might all be together for years, though that fantasy came more from my need to create lasting bonds and deep commitments rather than from any realistic perception of the potential of our staying together.

So much happened so fast it's still hard for me to believe that we were on the farm less than a year and a half. Most of us wanted to share an intense process of day-to-day encounter – a commitment to 'dealing with feelings' first and foremost. This frequently drained our energies. It was also a process that often conflicted with some of our most basic needs for space and time alone.

Though we started out as four couples, most of us were interested in moving away from 'coupledom'. Some of us became sexually involved with others both in and out of the commune; others felt very threatened by any sexual sharing at all. Sometimes we felt excitement and joy in being sexually intimate with more than one person; other times we felt pain and fear and sadness. Some of us experimented with making love in threes or fours (though we did not consider it an experiment at the time; it feels that way looking back). On a hot summer afternoon, three of us along with a friend (all women) had our first homosexual experience together. It was loving, playful and sexually arousing in a newly titillating, exciting sense.

We talked about all these experiences, shared our feelings and responses, and became more comfortable with and accepting of our sexuality. We had the most trouble in working out our sexual relationships with each other within the commune, and sometimes we couldn't: one woman left largely because she wanted a monogamous relationship with a man who didn't. Sometimes I think we fooled ourselves into thinking we were more open to and accepting of multiple sexual involvements than we really were (both for ourselves and one another). Given our socialization and the incredible importance that's always been attached to 'the sexual relationship', it's no wonder that we had trouble radically changing our gut feelings about sexual intimacy. A few of us often did feel comfortable with sexual sharing. I most often felt good about my mate's being involved sexually with another person, though my being sexually intimate with another man usually threatened him, but we almost always worked it out in a good way. We knew that we were taking risks and needed to be especially sensitive to one another. What was important to us was that our risk-taking be a mutual decision.

For most people in the commune multiple sexual relationships were painful (and probably somewhat destructive for a few of us). We weren't going to change any faster or make our guts react any differently just because we wanted to. This is an area where change comes much more slowly and with more difficulty than I think we had realized.

The story of our breaking apart is long and complicated. Our inability to resolve our sexual relationships in a good way is only a part of this story, though I'm not quite sure how big a part. It took almost a year for us to break up; though I would often have a glimpse of this inevitability, I refused to accept it. In my diary at one point I wrote, 'Somehow I feel that our love for one another should go beyond our differences, beyond how we'd like each other to be different.' Today I'd never write that. There are some things I don't think I'd ever be able to accept in another person, however much love I felt.

During the past few years my sexual relationships have become more fulfilling and more intense, both physically and emotionally. Maybe because of this I've wanted fewer sexual relationships and only with those I could potentially live with. My relationships with women, whether sexual or not, have also taken on a special importance for me. In part this is because I've found exciting, meaningful work and have a wonderful sense of integrating my personal life and political involvements. Because of a unique understanding I've felt with women, and only with women, I know I'll probably never live alone with a man.

I still want very much to create a home with several people that I love and feel committed to. I want to build the deep bonds that can come only with time, to have a family including children, and to feel rooted in land I love. All this now seems to be happening in a beautiful way with three of the people (a woman, a man and a child) that I lived with communally on the farm. Possibly another man who has become very important to me will be included. The two of us have a very fine relationship, and I hope we will eventually feel the same long-term commitment that I feel with the others.

We've all become more patient, accepting and realistic. We've learned to respect our individual needs for space and our different natural paces. We understand that we need to nourish both our relationships with one another and ourselves as individuals. Sometimes this is hard to do and we won't always succeed, but that's okay, too. Whatever happens, I feel like I'm moving in the right direction.

Margaret: A Middle-aged Single Woman

I've always wanted to have a family, but I wasn't going to get married just to have children. I've never met a man who was a good friend and a good lover, as well as someone who loved to be with children. So now I'm fifty and I'm still single with no children of my own. I feel sad about this sometimes, but since my work has been so fulfilling and involves working with children — I'm a teacher — I still feel that my life has been rich and complete.

Hannah: An Older Single Woman

I am eighty-eight years old. I have never been married, nor have I had sexual relations. I have all my life had fine relationships with men as fellow students, as warm friends, and as co-workers in various causes. I would like to have had a devoted marriage, but I never considered marrying just for the sake of being married, and I have never met a man whom I loved enough to marry. My philosophy about sex has been that the only justification for sex relations is total mutual devotion, and that it should be a permanent relation, not a mere temporary physical attraction. I believe this mutual love is what constitutes a marriage even if there is no wedding ceremony and that a couple who go through that ceremony merely for other material reasons are really not married.

In my school and early college years there was a neighbourhood group of boys and girls who regularly played together, went on picnics, etc. One of these boy friends was a particular pal of mine. After he graduated from college he got a job in the Midwest. For seven years he wrote to me twice a week, and in every letter he asked me to marry him. Unfortunately I felt a very warm friendship for him, but not the love to warrant marriage.

I have no living relative and, as I have learned from experience, living in an apartment all by yourself is a very inhuman existence. I have tried it. So for about twenty-five years I have been a member of one or another commune, having anywhere from five to fifteen members, all but one of them including both sexes. I was always the only old member, the others usually being in their twenties or early thirties. It was an approximation of family living – we ate together, shared all the household tasks and expenses, swapped news and views, and often members would go out together to meetings or social gatherings.

The members of these communes were inclined to leftist opinions, and whenever a vacancy occurred we took care that the new member would have congenial views. So I felt that I had a satisfying substitute for the family relationships that circumstances denied me.

I carried on my soul-satisfying activities in many vital social movements – the women's movement and many civil liberties battles. In the last few years I have filled over 150 speaking engagements. So life for me is still interesting and worthwhile.

THE EXPERIENCE OF BEING MARRIED

We learn from our culture that the relationship of a married woman with her husband is the most intimate and lasting relationship a woman has, and that a woman is always expected to put this relationship before everyone and everything else in her life. We want to counteract this misleading and confining message. We want to open the definition of marriage and to explore intimate relationships in addition to marriage.

Although in this society the monogamous, nuclear family is seen as the ideal living situation, there are, in fact, other choices we can make about how and with whom we live..

We have no one opinion about monogamous or non-monogamous relationships. We want to express both our good and bad experiences. We want to begin to separate the good reasons for staying in monogamous relationships from the good reasons for leaving. (And remember, monogamy is not limited to just heterosexual relationships.) We want to explore the possibilities of getting love and support from several people, rather than having one primary intimate relationship that is supposed to satisfy all needs. For those of us who decide that marriage *is* a very deep and important relationship for us, our marriage will be far better if we feel that it is our clear choice rather than our only alternative or our life-defining duty.

Mathilde: A Deepening Relationship

Julien and I met when we were very young, eighteen and nineteen years old. We had a fiery, emotional, story-book love affair — read poetry to each other, took long walks in the country, went skiing. We spent whole afternoons, days, weekends in bed, holding and touching each other,

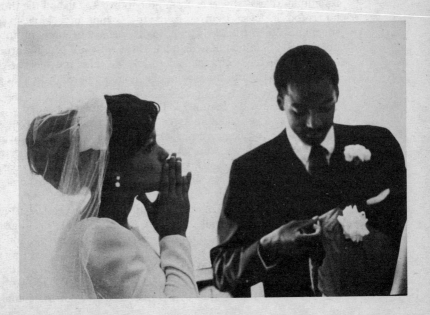

bringing each other to orgasm many times, even though we didn't actually have intercourse with each other for over a year. After a couple of years we got married.

The years before we had kids we spent a lot of time together, building up a reservoir of experiences we shared and talked about. They have become a part of us both, have somehow made us part of each other.

Over the past ten years we've had plenty of fights and disagreements, but I've had only one huge trauma. In our third or fourth year of marriage we had a fight over something – I don't remember what – and he wouldn't talk to me for over a week no matter how much I cried. I hated that coldness more than anything else in my life.

When we were first married and had got over the first high excitement of early lovemaking, we started talking about how we would handle it if either of us wanted to have an affair. Well, we blissfully thought, that would be easy! We would simply bring the third person into our relationship and all make love together! It actually almost happened once.

We also talked about having sexual relationships with other couples. Both of us had had very little sexual experience before we met each other and wanted to 'broaden our love relationships' (though we didn't want to betray each other). I realize now that those things could not possibly have happened the rational way we planned.

The women's movement coincided with my very little babies and with Julién's getting a job for the first time. Before the movement we played traditional roles – I worked from nine to five and did all the things in the house too. It never occurred to me to ask him to cook, clean, or do the shopping. When the kids came, there was a lot more stuff to do in the house, and I didn't want to do it all. There were lots of fights around those things, but he really changed a lot. Now we share much of the child care. But still, he has a full-time job, while I stay home with the kids and work part-time.

Julien has always been a good lover, has always wanted to do what I liked. It was a couple of years before I had orgasms during intercourse, but I was never left unsatisfied. Our love affair remained a love affair for a long time after we were married. Then, inevitably, it became more tranquil. But our relationship never lost the closeness, the basic understanding we have of each other: we love each other very much and we tell each other so, often.

That wild sexual excitement of our early lives has been gone for a long time, along with all those wild positions, antics, lotions, honeys. But then we're now much more proficient at lovemaking, and when we do it we do it very well.

We have both made compromises in our lives for each other, for our kids. We have both changed a good deal over the years we have been together. I often think that it was just luck that our individual changes did not make us grow apart but allowed us to draw together. I'm very glad they did.

Laura: Family, Marriage and Separation

Okay. So I am twenty-nine years old now. Following the only model I knew, I lived with and then was married to my husband for ten years. We had two children together. I separated from him six months ago.

I got married at nineteen. We were both in college, both young, scared and alone. We got together. It was a way to break ties with our parents, to be on our own in a comforting, secure way. For many years we grew alongside each other as friends and as lovers.

As we grew up we felt our differences more too. But we found it hard to see those differences as legitimate, since all our expectations told us that we were a special 'unit'. If I wanted to spend time with him and he wanted to read, I felt hurt. If I wanted to visit my friends and he needed to be with me at that time, he felt hurt. If one of us didn't want to make love and the other did, the hurt was worse. At times the hurt turned to anger and resentment.

Being intimate with only one person did not seem to be enough to meet our needs. But it was hard to go outside the marriage for intimacy, since that would break the 'contract'. Friendship with others was okay, but sexual intimacy was another matter.

At the point that we both reached out for other intimate relationships we were reaching out for ourselves. Friends still referred to us as the Greenways rather than as Laura and Joe. But the need for each of us to feel whole, distinct, separate and centred in ourselves was pressing; it took priority over the marriage.

How do you know when you reach the point when you no longer can change together? When is separation a cop-out? When is it a positive moving forward? These are crucial questions with no easy answers. Many, many couples get to this point, sometimes over and over again. There are different ways of dealing with the impasse — keeping up a marriage of convenience, splitting up angry, splitting up when the kids are less dependent. For me it was very difficult and painful to think about separation and finally separating. Breaking up doesn't have to mean the whole relationship was bad, but deep down the myth is that marriage should be 'for always' and we are failures if our marriages come to an end. I still feel the pain of losing the closeness and intimacy that we had built up over ten years. It was hard to give up even when the marriage lacked joy and things between us were clearly sour.

Ungluing our marriage took at least two years. It began with the women's movement, which gave me support to move out on my own, to develop new skills and new relationships. I still felt in contact with my husband on some levels. I was involved in two different relationships during that time – one with a woman, one with a man. They were each long-term friendships that grew more intimate – emotionally and sexually.

During this time my husband and kids and I were living with a group of people. With other people around, we thought we could perhaps be more independent and still live together. It didn't work. For us, more people meant more conflict and tension as well as more resources.

I split for a while. I left the house to sort out my feelings, though I still wanted to live with my husband and kids. I wound up staying away for several months, and finally left for good. The decision to leave was especially painful because I was breaking up a family as well as a marriage.

So where am I now? I feel in many ways I've exchanged one set of problems for another. I live by myself half-time and with my kids half-time. (Relative to other women, I'm fortunate that my husband and the people he lives with are willing and able to care for the children half-time.) I feel much more centred in me than when I was married. Sometimes my centre feels warm and strong, other times cold and lonely. My kids are very important to me, especially now. They are a stable, loving element in my life.

And my friends – I couldn't be living alone without support from them. Some of them have lived or do live alone. They tell me, 'Keep going, it's good for a time.' It's the first time in my life I've had space to focus on me, to love myself more, so that I can deeply love others, whether men or women.

Alice: The Experience of Being Widowed after Twenty-Six Years of Marriage

I never liked being married, but in spite of my reluctance I was competent as a wife and mother. I never had sexual satisfaction in my marriage, but this wasn't such a problem since I couldn't miss what I had never experienced. Besides, I was always too busy and too tired and ready for sleep even before I collapsed into bed. I felt overburdened with the responsibilities of raising five children and keeping house for seven people, but my husband felt that his contribution of eight hours a day at the office was sufficient. I guess my resentment about this was one of the hardest things to live with, especially since there was no support from anyone then for changing this situation. We sometimes talked about divorce, but my husband felt that we couldn't afford it. After he died I grieved for him and suddenly realized that I had in fact loved him. In retrospect, I think that our marriage might have been salvaged if we had arranged for a lengthy separation, for at least a year. I had so much to settle with myself, by myself, that I could not cope with the way we were married. In many ways the state of marriage just goes against the grain. We might have been better mates under different circumstances, but time ran out. Four years ago when my husband died I cried for his life — not for ours together.

Now I like not having to account to a rigid mate, not having to do things and be someone that I'm not. I like to travel, practise yoga, go to concerts and lectures, and read. These are things I could never find time to do before. Though relatives are often critical of my current interests and activities, my children are wonderfully supportive. In return, I can support them in pursuing unconventional life-styles without nagging from me. It's good that my children are near me, since we get along so well now.

I can see many advantages to a compatible mate, though I think such a person is hard to find. Fortunately life is full of adventures that don't have to be shared with just one special mate. As for exploring my sexuality with another person, I've never felt much sex drive, so sex hasn't been important to me. Though my sexual experiences both during and after my marriage have not been very good, there has been one exception, a good friend and lover whom I see once a week. However, even though I enjoy sex with him, I don't feel much sexual energy at other times.

I still feel that I would like to be really alone sometimes for a long period. That's something I've never tried out. Unfortunately I still have difficulty making time for myself — I so often feel that I ought to do things for other people, whether or not they actually ask for help. So I find myself making dinners for my sons and their friends or listening to other people's problems or driving someone to an appointment or working part-time, whether or not that's what I really want to do. It's very hard to change this tendency in me and to begin to think more about some of my own needs too.

Declaration

For years I charted my independence
in miles traveled away from you.
You were New York and I a car
fleeing in every artery.
That I made you the center, there is no question.
No question I could rule on
without your opposition. No adventure unless
it wasn't yours. Today I think of Concord grapes,
those little pyramids, depending;
of the bay's water angrily repeating
its leap up the beach. One man's
violent need becomes a woman's service job.
But I don't work for you.
I'm crazy now.

MIRIAM GOODMAN

The Edge

Time and again, time and again I tie
My heart to that headboard
While my quilted cries
Harden against his hand. He's bored —
I see it. Don't I lick his bribes, set his bouquets
In water? Over Mother's lace I watch him drive into the gored
Roasts, deal slivers in his mercy . . . I can feel his thighs
Against me for the children's sake. Reward?
Mornings, crippled with this house,
I see him toast his toast and test
His coffee, hedgingly. The waste's my breakfast.

LOUISE GLUCK

THE EXPERIENCE OF CELIBACY: TIMES WHEN WE ARE NOT HAVING SEXUAL RELATIONS

The dictionary defines celibacy as a state of being unmarried, usually in connection with religious vows, but in general usage it has come to mean abstaining from genital sex in our relationships with others, even if temporarily.

Many of us enter periods of celibacy deliberately, feeling that we have a need for a time not to be in a sexual relationship of any kind. We may want to mobilize all our energy for our work, our children, our friends; we may want to explore our own sexuality without the distraction of another person; or perhaps we just don't feel 'sexy'.

Yet many of us have entered periods of celibacy with apprehension — we have feared the insecurity of being without a partner. Often this anxiety diminishes because being alone is a very positive experience. It has given us back our integrity, our privacy, our pride.

Of course there is a difference in how we feel when we choose celibacy and how we feel when being without a sexual partner is not our choice. But either way many of us have found that periods of celibacy — a month, a year, or even longer — can be freeing and growth-producing. We are freed to explore ourselves without the problems and power struggles of a sexual relationship. We can begin to define ourselves not just in terms of another person.

Not being in an intense, intimate relationship has been good for me. I've had space to learn more about me — my needs, my talents, my potentials, my own natural rhythms. I now feel much more capable of sustaining intimacy with another person in a way that could better meet both my own needs and those of the other person. It's important to me now that I don't 'lose' myself in an intimate relationship — some of the time I need to feel whole and complete as an individual, as the person I am apart from the relationship.

I have been celibate for over a year, since the beginning of my involvement with the women's movement, which gave me a lot of support. I work very hard and feel good about working. I have created my own physical environment, building a house, and have provided my own psychological space — a good combination. I masturbate a lot and enjoy it. I feel happy, independent and free to figure out my own expectations of me.

My first reaction to being without a man was frustration and anger. I thought, Well, here I am feeling pretty liberated sexually, and there's no one to sleep with. Over time, I thought less and less about being with a man. I had very relaxed times with my friends and never had to think twice about making plans with them for dinner. I was not asexual during this time. I was masturbating with much pleasure, having different kinds of orgasms — some long and slow and ripply, others short and jerky and tenser. I explored my sexuality in a way I had not with men. It was also easier to work at what I wanted to, because I was my only obligation.

Some of us come out of celibacy deliberately, feeling that we need a sexual relationship. Some of us, feeling isolated and outside the norms of society, give up and flee into the arms of the first person to come along. Some of us may find we feel better being more autonomous.

But for most of us, being celibate has not provided a long-term solution to the problems posed by sexual relationships. There are also some very real drawbacks to long periods of celibacy.

Most of us crave physical contact and physical affection. To be alone, or to receive physical affection only from our children or pets doesn't quite work. We can have fantasies about sleeping with them, but it doesn't feel right to act on them. We need other adult human beings to meet our deeper sexual/sensual needs.

Going without physical affection for long periods can be a kind of starvation. We won't die as we would without food or air, but the effects may still show in our bodies. We may get stiffer and out of touch with our sensuality. Many of us have found that being physically affectionate with family and friends can prevent this from happening during celibate periods.

When celibacy no longer feels good we want to change it — but that's easier said than done. And it feels harder the longer we have been celibate. Coming out of celibacy, we may feel awkward or defensive, or we may feel embarrassed by needs that seem insatiable. Sometimes it's easier to start a new relationship with someone else who is also coming out of celibacy.

One unresolved thought: Do we ever choose celibacy out of fear of any kind of physical intimacy? What does this mean?

It's hard to take on the loneliness, the bad parts of being alone as well as the good parts of getting in touch with ourselves. It's also difficult to explore fully what being celibate can mean to us, since society does not generally accept the idea of choosing to refrain from sexual activity.

The Influence Coming into Play:
The Seven of Pentacles

Under a sky the color of pea soup
she is looking at her work growing away there
actively, thickly like grapevines or pole beans
as things grow in the real world, slowly enough.

If you tend them properly, if you mulch, if you water,
if you provide birds that eat insects a home and winter food,
if the sun shines and you pick off catepillars,
if the praying mantis comes and the ladybugs and the bees,
then the plants flourish, but at their own internal clock.

Connections are made slowly, sometimes they grow underground.
You cannot tell always by looking what is happening.
More than half a tree is spread out in the soil under your feet.
Penetrate quietly as the earthworm that blows no trumpet.
Fight persistently as the creeper that brings down the tree.
Spread like the squash plant that overruns the garden.
Gnaw in the dark and use the sun to make sugar.

Weave real connections, create real nodes, build real houses.
Live a life you can endure: make love that is loving.
Keep tangling and interweaving and taking more in,
a thicket and bramble wilderness to the outside but to us
interconnected with rabbit runs and burrows and lairs.

Live as if you liked yourself, and it may happen:
reach out, keep reaching out, keep bringing in.
This is how we are going to live for a long time: not always,
for every gardener knows that after the digging, after the planting,
after the long season of tending and growth, the harvest comes.

MARGE PIERCY

5　Lesbian Perspectives

(by a group of socialist lesbians in London)

Introduction

Women's politics and the ideas of women's liberation are now part of everyday life. From the women's movement comes the idea that the personal is political. We need to work out our ideas by understanding the oppression we all experience. Women continue to be put down by our male-dominated society, and lesbians are no exception. Much of the open challenge and freer expression of lesbianism come directly from the women's movement. Although in the past aspects of the movement have been oppressive to lesbians struggling to raise this 'touchy' question in their groups, this is far less so now. The relationship between lesbians and the women's movement has become a close one. The sixth demand of women's liberation expresses this: 'We demand an end to discrimination against lesbians and the right of every woman to a self-defined sexuality.'

Sexual stereotyping is one of the most pervasive and limiting of the pressures put on us as women. As lesbians too we are role-defined, activity-defined, lifestyle-defined. We are supposed to be the 'women who can't get a man', 'the women who want to be men'. We are sick, perverted, 'a malignant cancer in the community', thoroughly unnatural! We are unfit to be mothers. Even some socialists say we will disappear under socialism because we are an expression of 'the decadent bourgeois system'. We are perceived as masculine, aggressive, hard; we 'drink too much', were born with 'hormone deficiencies', are the children of unhappy, unbalanced homes. The list is endless. Society permits no alternative. Heterosexuality is the only possible norm, and this is legally reinforced.

Yet, in the face of all this, we are declaring now that it isn't so. Challenging what has for so long been accepted is not easy, but we make this challenge every time we declare ourselves lesbians. Not all of us do it in the same way, but the more of us who do it, the stronger we all become.

Contrary to what some advocate, 'gay' is not automatically great. It isn't everything; sometimes it is not even good. For many of us the individual act of coming out (acknowledging our lesbianism) is the most we can manage. To throw off the conditioning of a lifetime is not easy. We recognize that it is not even easy to make the statement, 'I am gay', indeed often not possible. It is, however, easier today than ten years ago and, as our *combined* strength grows, we feel that lesbians do have to go further than this courageous individual statement. There is now a new lesbian consciousness which understands that just to say 'I am gay' has implications far beyond the personal and that, collectively made, it is beginning to generate a basis for radical change affecting the whole of sexist society.

Those responsible for writing this chapter are all socialist, lesbian feminists. For us, gay goes way beyond sex. Our sexuality doesn't just show itself in our sexual preferences and in our activities in bed. This is a male notion of lesbianism. We reject the notion that lesbians, like many men, see women as potential sex objects. We hope that the contents of this chapter will clarify how we actually see and live our lesbianism, recognizing it as a political force, and some of the ways in which we are attempting to make changes.

Black Lesbians: Some women reading this chapter may notice the absence of anything specifically about black lesbians, especially if they are themselves black, and also, as it must be obvious from the personal accounts that one of us is black. This is, therefore, an attempt by a black lesbian to explain this absence. It largely revolves around the fact that in no way did I want to come across as, or be put into the role of, a spokeswoman for all black lesbians, or as token black for the group writing this chapter. If this was to be avoided I felt, therefore, that the piece would have to be a theoretical perspective developed out of deep and lengthy discussions by a group of black lesbians committed to a socialist analysis of the complexity of their oppression as black lesbians. Given that there were neither time nor contacts to develop this theory, however, I attempted something on my own. Eventually, though, I found this unacceptable as it was too personal and, in a sense, just a re-hash of my personal account. I finally came to the conclusion that I would do most justice to other black lesbians by not writing anything, and hope that this brief explanation will be acceptable.

Coming Out – Three Women's Experiences

We have written this chapter collaboratively, but want to start with three personal accounts from women about discovering their lesbianism and coming out.

I was twenty-five before I seriously questioned my sexuality. As a younger woman I had been extremely active heterosexually, running at great speed from one relationship to another, very much (at least as I view it now) into power trips. Brought up in the fifties and sixties, I needed the affirmation of a man because my own sense of self was somehow confused, though I frequently felt myself 'better' than those men I was with. When I was twenty-two, and the veteran of a disastrous marriage, I met a man quite different from those I had previously known. He actually likes women — rare indeed! — and is an immensely sensitive and perceptive human being. I raced through my usual bag of tricks and attempts to shock, estrange, disgust, but quite failed to do so. He refused to do anything but understand my weird mixture of puritanism and promiscuity. My emotional life was in a turmoil. Should I actually trust this man? And then who would have the power? We didn't live together. He chose to study away. I immediately fell into having other affairs. His style was not to criticize, but to question. It was very seductive and gradually I was asking myself more searching questions too. My sexual expression was very tough, nearly violent. But it was spontaneous; was it saying what I really felt? There was a desperation about it which indicated that it sprang not from love or good old-fashioned lust — though they were not absent — but from an unease with sex, with myself as a sexual person, despite the 'sexy' role I had cast for myself. We probed these questions from this direction and that for two or three years, then tried a new perspective. Would I feel more at ease with myself, as a woman, if I learned sexually to love another woman? He was more in touch with the lesbian life-style than I was (I wasn't in touch at all!), as the lover he was with before me had been bisexual and they had both felt very relaxed and unthreatened by her relationships with women. (When I met her for the first time, my first 'real' lesbian, it was with great delight that I discovered I wasn't shocked, so my expectations must have been heavily biased.)

Having tuned in to the idea of making love with a woman, I became quite obsessed with the idea. I also began, for almost the first time I think, to have sexual dreams. These were about women. I made a decision to begin to masturbate, which I had always resisted as I had felt that the intense closeness of intercourse was enough and that I had no need for clitoral stimulation. But in a rather calculated if hazy way I thought I should prepare myself for this future encounter by practising what I imagined (correctly) would be part of lovemaking between women: clitoral stimulation. Like most women who learn to masturbate later, I discovered I liked it very much indeed, and it certainly made gradual but quite perceptible changes in my attitude to love-making as it increased my sense of independence which, at the time as well as subsequently, was being reinforced by work success and more comfortable financial independence. My lover was very happy that I had made this step towards freeing myself from a sexual taboo (touching myself) and we both felt that an extra dimension had been added to our relationship. Unfortunately, this proved to be only partly true as from that time it slowly became more difficult for me to enjoy 'ordinary' intercourse, so there was some subtraction as well as growth.

As a feminist it is sad to have to say that I didn't at this stage meet a woman and, in a mood of mutual liking and trust, have my first lesbian affair. The situation was very different. I believe now it would have been much more comfortable had I been active in the women's movement, but my career was running my life . . . and there was shyness/diffidence/ignorance. In a very sexual, even sexist way, I saw a very pretty woman in a club, took boldness by the hand, and approached her. We arranged to meet and, after a couple of rather tense meetings, went to bed. Out of that kind of tension comes more tension, and that is what I got. I was extremely nervous, embarrassed and fairly convinced that lesbian relationships were not for me. But the dreams continued, the fantasies continued. I spoke about lesbianism only to my lover, and felt emotionally and socially quite distanced from my sexual upheaval. I continued to have affairs outside my relationship, though these were with men and in a sense more important socially than sexually. I liked them better than I liked going to bed with them, and on the whole we have remained good friends.

About a year after that first experience I met a woman to whom I was immediately and quite violently attracted. This was extremely unsettling. I did not feel that we had a great deal in common and was frequently distressed by her, but she made a profound impression in that the effect she had on me forced me to question how important or potentially important lesbianism was in my life. She was involved with someone else so there was very little emotional space left in her life and that was, in a sense, a selfish bonus as I was able to acknowledge the intensity of feeling and deal with its effect, but without commitment to her. Adversely though, I had very little support from her. She did, however, involve me in the lesbian social world (or a part of it at least) which I hadn't previously had any but the most peripheral knowledge of. I was really enchanted, fascinated, horrified. I believe now, as then when it was fresh, that there are few experiences lovelier than being with a group of women who really feel close and take pride in being together. At its best, that is comradeliness, tenderness and sexuality mixed perfectly. I did, however, sometimes fear that the strongest link that I had with many of the women was my sexuality, and that politically and emotionally we were far apart. I was also barraged with criticism about my 'straight' relationship, made to feel that I would get the key to the magic gate of belonging only when I had cast him off, despite my repeated insistence of how supportive he was being during this time which was so difficult for us both. My sexual interest in men had virtually disappeared, so my lover and I were forced to question most closely why we should or how we could continue to stay together when my general sexual orientation was now clearly towards women, and when politically I preferred to be active in women's politics rather than a mixed left group. Gradually I spread this discussion wider and told friends about my lesbianism. This was accepted without surprise (usually), though there was natural concern about my lover and about our relationship which friends had always felt close to.

My split life continues. I am very involved with a number of women socially and increasingly politically. I have sexual relationships which seem usually to be brief and vaguely unsatisfactory but that may be understandable in the context of intense self-questioning which inevitably continues and probably makes me very difficult to be with, or get close to. I would probably enjoy a longer-term relationship with a woman but am aware that my ideas about it are so complicated that it may remain an ideal. I value my gay friends enormously, though feel fleetingly sad that I am so involved with them that there is very little time left for heterosexual friends . . . I still feel very much in touch with what attracted me to women: the tenderness, the intensity, the mutual striving, the sheer womanliness. I am very comfortable with the tie between loving women and the political strivings of a feminist, but am uncomfortable with the seductive exclusivity of this. I attempt (and often fail) to resist social labels and definitions, and though sorely tempted sometimes to embrace exclusivity feel that this would, for me, be a defeat. My lover continues to be my lover, and my comrade. We have many difficulties and don't always feel we have the means to cope with them, but emancipation doesn't come from retreat and perhaps the question of emancipation is what I am struggling with: have I moved away from the limits of heterosexuality to shut doors, or to open them?

*

It is significant that in our society discovering one's homosexual potential and 'coming out' are two different processes, and whilst many individuals do not discover the first, an even smaller proportion achieve the second. For several years I had indications of my sexuality whilst at the same time denying them, even to myself. I saw gayness as a particularly nasty slur on one's entire personality, and even when I became conscious that I was also capable of emotional and sexual feelings towards other women, felt that it was a facet of my feelings which I in no way wanted to realize or confront. What stopped me from defining myself as a lesbian, even to myself, was nothing to do with my feelings or any sense of disgust at the idea of touching other women's bodies, but the absolute horror I felt at the idea of being, as I then saw it, socially disgusting and of provoking scorn and disgust.

Ironically, I was, in fact, imposing a form of social alienation on myself through the techniques of evasion which I was employing to avoid it. Because I felt that on a certain level I had something unsavoury lurking in my consciousness, I could never allow myself direct expression. Actions, emotions and thoughts had to be filtered through an exaggeratedly rigid mesh of stereotypical social acceptance which I had internalized.

When I finally did confront my lesbianism I found it an incredibly emotional experience, since I felt that for the first time in many years, probably since I had first acted on internalized heterosexual values as an adolescent, I was in touch with emotional roots in myself and that my experience was drawing directly on my emotions.

In common with what I would imagine still to be the majority of lesbians' experience, I unquestioningly assumed that I wanted to experience myself through relating to men. My first sexual experience with a man was much better than subsequent ones. Firstly, we were both virgins, and although our sexual encounters obviously did not occur within a social vacuum, and we both adhered to quite stereotypical roles and role expectations of each other, I think that our common sexual naivety allowed me more say in the sexual direction of the relationship. Secondly, my emotional feelings towards him, which were totally obsessive and dependent, were an almost total transference of the emotional dependency engendered by the family for which, through particularly bad familial relations, I felt no outlet for in their originating context. My family had been quite obsessive about my chastity. I therefore took a particular delight at fourteen in being a 'bad girl'; adolescent sexual experience with all of its clandestine undertones became a source of personal identity and an affirmation of my autonomy. Significantly, when, after dragging on and off for well over two years, this relationship finally ended, I developed anorexia nervosa, an illness traditionally associated with lack of self-value and the unaccomplished need to break away from the family.

During this period of my life I also experienced sexual and emotional feelings towards other girls. I found them so unacceptable that on one occasion, after having had an explicitly sexual dream about a close friend, I went into school the next day and told her that I had dreamt of murdering her!

The rest of my heterosexual relationships were tales of ever-increasing alienation which led me to decide eventually that since I was not attracted to men, bored in bed, and emotionally dead towards them, I must be asexual. At this particular point I feel that society's lack of recognition of lesbianism and the more general suppression of women's sexuality are politically fused. Through agents of sexual repression, capitalism defines women's sexuality as a negative rather than a positive force. Because one is taught to view one's sexuality as latent, and men as the catalysts which bring female sexuality into existence, it is not surprising that a failure to respond to men sexually can be interpreted as a failure to be sexual at all. However, whilst being a comfortable self-definition theoretically, in practice it was boring in the extreme and no long-term solution to avoiding confronting my lesbianism. My attraction towards other women would periodically seep through the bland exterior. As my feelings towards other women became more conscious, my confusion increased. I had one final disastrous attempt at a heterosexual relationship, which was accompanied by my having enormously strong romantic feelings towards various unapproachable women (surely a symptom of incredible sexual repression at work — and perhaps romanticism as a whole is one of the strongest ideological weapons which militate against women's discovery of their own strength). In addition to this I slept with a couple of women friends of mine. This was also entirely unsatisfactory since I don't think that they were consciously sexually attracted to me, and the sexual dimension of our *friendship never seemed to have any momentum as neither of us could properly relax in the situation, since we did not experience lesbian sexuality as a valid and confirming thing to feel.*

Eventually this situation was brought to a crisis by my becoming pregnant on one of the rare occasions on which I slept with the man I was relating to. For months prior to the pregnancy I had been sexually frigid, and if anything entered my vagina it would become immediately de-sensitized and any possibility of my achieving orgasm ended abruptly. The four months from the beginning of my pregnancy to its termination forced me to look at the total bankruptcy of my life-style. I had frequent nightmares — many of which were concerned with other people's discovery of my lesbianism coupled with the sense of panic and violation which my pregnancy engendered.

After the abortion I started going around with a group of gay men and getting very heavily into drink. Gay men were less sexually threatening and had the possibility of leading me to places where I could meet other lesbians. Usually this was not the case, as the clubs and bars which we frequented were ghettoized and yet another facet of male-dominated culture both in form and attitude. Everyone rushed frantically to them at the end of a tiring week posing as straight, and drew no political lessons about the 'double life' they were being forced to lead. Therefore their gayness posed no threat to the dominant ideology by taking a political direction. So the rip-off merchants who ran these clubs continued to profit from the creation of a little pocket within society where we could all pretend that the world was gay for a few hours. I, for instance, was threatened with being chucked out of one disco for trying to collect signatures for an anti-fascist petition.

Gradually, however, I got to know other lesbians and began to see lesbianism as a possibility for caring relationships with women with whom I was involved in the same personal and political struggles. (Until this time my identity as a lesbian and my involvement in the women's movement had, to a large extent, been separate entities.) I began to know other women whom I could relate to politically, socially, emotionally and sexually, and for the first time felt confirmed and 'natural' about my gayness and began to experience my sexuality as an integral part of my identity and practical political struggle.

*

Any retrospective discussion about the discovery of one's lesbianism is bound to be extremely difficult and cause many conflicts in the individual concerned, especially if it is to be couched in a political framework. I think this is inevitable when we become more politically aware, and begin to relate our experience to the political structure in which capitalist social relations are formed. In trying to make this link we may be liable to make deductions which may or may not be valid or true. For example, I can now think that one reason for the suppression of my lesbianism until a fairly late age was related to my having to find my pride and identity as a black woman in a racist society. That is, my identity as a black woman and the way this influenced my relationship (and all black people's) to the class struggle presented itself as a more urgent need.

No lesbian can isolate herself from the social environment, and because of our internalization of society's view towards lesbianism, there appears to be an inbuilt mechanism to deny this 'deviance' in ourselves. This was certainly the case for me. Indeed, this internalization was so complete that even in the face of what are now obvious 'lesbian tendencies' any surfacing of these was completely obliterated. This led to a tremendous contradiction between my emotional and intellectual life. Whilst I felt deep emotional attachments to women in my school years and after, I never consciously associated these with lesbianism. On an emotional level they felt natural and right; however, any attempt at analysis of what they were and therefore of naming or labelling them immediately turned them into disgusting, shameful feelings since the words 'lesbian', 'queer', 'pervert' naturally arose. Now I can see that this was due to the relationship between the existing ideology and language, i.e. the way in which society's views of good/bad, moral/immoral, etc. are reflected in the language of that society. As a result of this, and rather than having to deal with this disgust of myself and the fear of rejection by family, friends and society generally, I simply ceased (with only a degree of success) to equate my emotional attachments to women with lesbianism. One factor which enabled me to do this was that despite my absorption of social attitudes, these never quite managed to destroy the feeling of 'rightness'.

When I was five, six, seven years old, my sexual experimentation with other children involved both girls and boys. This I found difficult to admit to until fairly recently because it seemed to point to confirmation of the 'born that way' arguments, especially because I didn't know, until I had actually talked with others about it, that lots of girls only experiment with other girls. An instructive point in itself. Anyway, anything that pointed to confirmation of this biological argument was a tremendous pressure for me since it implied I was a genetic fuck-up. On the other hand, there are certain experiences in my childhood which could equally validate the psychologically created argument, for example, bad or non-existent relationship with father or mother. Both arguments are equally unpalatable because of the way in which they are used to invalidate lesbianism as a viable alternative to heterosexuality. I myself believe in social determinism, which means acknowledging the way in which our psychological make-up is formed by the interaction of various social forces within our culture.

Important factors in helping me to accept my lesbianism after the long period of its discovery and metamorphosis were (a) that my political consciousness had further developed to see the fundamental importance of feminism, which in turn led me to the importance of self-definition, and (b) that this led me into the women's movement which itself was just undergoing an acceptance and recognition of lesbianism and therefore was an area of my life in which it was comparatively easy to 'come out'. Certainly I am aware that the positive effect of the movement on my acceptance of my lesbianism will not hold true for lots of women, especially those who have not been involved with the movement at all or who became involved at its inception and infancy. Nevertheless, I gained the support needed but feel this needs to be put into perspective, since to a large extent I had already reached the stage of acceptance and just needed support for it to be on-going.

In a sense the hardest area of my life in which to 'come out' was to my family. There are two main reasons for this. Firstly, because I'm very close to Mum and Nan, the two most important people to me in my family. All the feelings of guilt, etc., and the idea that their happiness was of greater importance than mine, kept stopping me from telling them, despite the fact that I was losing all sense of self. This is of course a manifestation of one of the ways in which lesbianism is kept invisible, what Abbott and Love (in Sappho was a Right-On Woman) call 'the parent within'. By denying yourself the quite liberating experience of declaring your sexuality you collaborate with your oppressors in lying about your existence. The second reason why telling my family presented itself as the most painful area is related to the fact that I am married and still living with my husband, even though there is no sexual relationship. This fact seemed to add a double edge to my fears of hurting them because it seemed to me that I would not only destroy what I thought their image of me was, but also shatter any hopes they might have of my only going through a phase'. I finally came to the conclusion, however, that I must tell them because not doing so was affecting the way in which I related to them in general. I suppose I did this over a period of time, not wishing to face an 'I've got something to tell you' situation. But basically it amounted to my just telling them that I felt a strong emotional and physical attachment to a particular woman and that I felt completely at ease and comfortable in the relationship. I then went on to try and explain to them that lesbian relationships were completely valid and that they themselves had had strong emotional feelings towards friends that might well be termed 'lesbian'. I suppose I was able to discuss it with them in this way because of the closeness of our relationship and because they seem to be willing to consider my ideas and experiences. Nevertheless this is still an extremely difficult dilemma for me because whilst I continue to have an emotional relationship with my husband, I also feel I must continue to push my lesbianism on my family lest they interpret this wrongly. Since the best way to do this would be to sever completely my marital relationship, and as I haven't done this, I am in effect giving in to the pressure applied by parents to keep a marriage together despite any degree of breakdown in the relationship which might have occurred.

P.S. It is two months since I wrote the above and during that time, and partly as a result of the support and strength gained in doing this work, I have

*made the final break with my husband by moving out. This represents for me
a strong commitment to 'staying out', that is, refusing to be re-absorbed into a
heterosexist society whose norms I reject. Staying out means aligning theory
and practice, despite the struggle involved.*

Coming Out: A Collective Summary

During our development as lesbians we were continually confronted with
heterosexuals' explanations of our sexuality. Traditional ideas of lesbianism imposed upon us a sense of 'unnaturalness' and 'perversion',
along with an image of the lesbian as someone singled out from other
women. Viewing sexuality as biologically determined, rather than
socially conditioned, leads to a static interpretation of sexual potential
and expression, and ignores the political significance of being gay in a
heterosexist society. If sexuality in all forms is social in origin, then the
denial of gayness in any society as a valid way of loving and relating to
others is a political factor and must lead us to begin to hold society up to
the light for analysis, rather than delving into our genetic or psychic
make-up for evidence of dysfunction. In this way, while we have early
recollections of sexual feelings towards other women, we do not regard
ourselves as having been 'born that way', but rather see our lesbianism
as a result of a particular process of social interaction. Biological
determinist interpretations of homosexuality lead only to limited pleas
for reform based on tolerance. 'Really, they can't help it . . .'
  We believe that we pose a radical alternative to heterosexual society.
Because of this, we do not feel that coming out is in itself enough. We also
plan to stay out, resisting the liberal view that what we do is our own
affair. Oppressed groups have constantly to make sure that their oppressors move beyond a position of mere tolerance. Lesbians who repeat the
heterosexual pattern of living in monogamous couples are more easily
tolerated by society. Indeed, many lesbians who made a strong coming-
out statement as a couple, when such matters were not easily made
public, may now feel a new sense of oppression as they struggle to
explore alternatives to the restrictions of this normative pattern.
Lesbians are currently in a very advantageous position to challenge
the implicit moral assumptions of monogamy, for instance concepts
such as possession and unfaithfulness, and can show how it is fundamental to the maintenance of a male-dominated society. By staying out
we mean channelling our lesbian commitment towards changing the
bases of contemporary sexist society which tries so constantly to
assimilate us, and thus to submerge our revolutionary potential.

Life-style

How we live our lives will depend on our age, class, race, work and politics, and these factors are, of course, intricately related.

Work and leisure time in our society is normally strictly compartmentalized. For some of us the split is even more pronounced because we will probably be 'passing' as straight (heterosexual) at work and having to spend our leisure time at specific places where we can openly be lesbians. Even if a lesbian does not wish to pass as straight at work or in public generally, she will nearly always be *assumed* to be straight. This daily denial of our sexual identity sometimes forces us to go to clubs, discos and meeting places where our lesbianism can be made comfortably public for a short time. We want to spend time together, even though we know that some of the places in which we meet feed off those very definitions of us which we wish to resist. Discos for women only, organized by lesbians, are relatively free of any commercial exploitation or 'ghetto tension'. (Details of those held in the UK are obtainable where there are women's centres. See p. 570.)

It is usually difficult, sometimes even impossible, to come out in the working situation, though obviously it is easier for some. We think, for

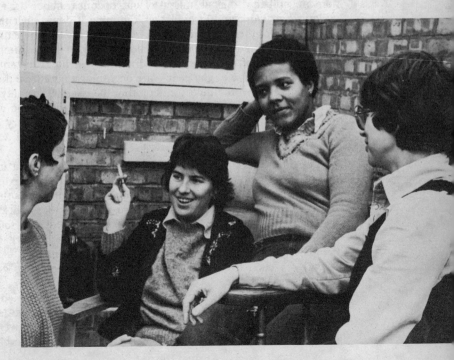

example, that the arts and related professions have a tradition of accepting 'eccentrics' and even capitalizing on them. But even here it is easier for male homosexuals than for lesbians. If there is less disapproval anywhere, it tends to be where middle-class liberals work, though even this is not a reliably supportive milieu. Teaching, nursing and some areas of social work contain their own special prejudices against gays who might 'contaminate' children or dependent people. However teachers and, even more actively, social workers are in the vanguard of those organizing to make sexuality a political issue in the work place.

For the working-class lesbian the situation is usually especially difficult. On the factory floor or in the normal office situation the conversation is predominantly about heterosexual relationships, and any references to homosexuality will almost invariably be in the form of 'jokes' or derogatory jibes. Overall, we don't think that there is any type of work where being a lesbian can be easily and openly evident without at best, a painful period of 'explanation' and 'acceptance'.

Gays were once moderately content to restrict their expression of homosexuality to their leisure time, perhaps because they assumed that heterosexuals expressed *their* sexuality only in their 'own' time. But we have come to realize that heterosexuals express their sexuality at every moment, and that their dismissal of our openness about declaring our lesbianism at work and in public as 'ramming it down their throats' is quite unjust, for their sexuality confronts us at every turn, whether or not they are acting in a specifically sexual way. The endless assumptions by heterosexuals that they are the 'normal' people has constantly to be challenged. This is why gay people are beginning to organize themselves in their places of work, understanding that the issue of sexuality must be raised in and through their unions. Otherwise aggression and victimization of gays will continue explicitly and implicitly in every working situation. Lesbianism is not a spare-time private activity that waits until the lights are low.

Nevertheless leisure-time clubs and organizations do exist in Britain to support lesbians who want to contact each other and extend their group of friends. CHE (Campaign for Homosexual Equality) is the largest national network in England. In Scotland it is SMG (Scottish Minorities Group). Many lesbians who want to come out discreetly and safely go at first to their meetings. They are run by male gays, and the organizations mainly reflect their concerns in the area of law reform and so on. Recently, women from CHE have formed a separate group called the National Organization of Lesbians (NOOL).

There are groups, like Sappho, exclusively for women, which run discussion and social evenings, and are not generally involved in lesbian or women's movement campaigns. There are also many less well-defined groups, sometimes based on 'women's houses' where lesbians live communally, working out their life-style and politics in a way distinctive to that group. These women do not restrict their lesbianism to their leisure time, but live it out in all aspects of their lives. This total commitment is not, however, possible for everyone, though certainly the principle that 'the more there are, the easier it is' does apply.

Women from all or any of these groups may go to the same discos or meeting places, but tend to identify within their own groups. Usually lesbians choose the life-style best suited to the level of their political commitment to lesbianism. Obviously we as a group identify with lesbians who are socialist and feminist, also attempting to work in jobs where expression of our position is possible, and spending a lot of time working politically.

Ageism within lesbian groupings still reflects the general pattern of our society. Unlike much of the male gay scene, sexual attractiveness is not thought by lesbians to be found only among the very young. However, there is a definite age prejudice which is felt by middle-aged lesbians. Many of these lesbians also feel excluded from the women's movement. It isn't that older lesbians necessarily see themselves as less sexually attractive, but less socially and politically acceptable. The fact that they came out before the women's movement was established, and before women's politics really gained momentum, tends to make them feel cut off from the issues which occupy younger lesbians in the movement. And the meeting places which lesbians can go to are often geared to younger women's interests.

Adolescent lesbians have an impossible time if they want to come out at school. They have to resist constant propaganda that they are just 'going through a phase'. The pressures on every adolescent girl to become the object of a boy's desire are tremendous. The idea that a relationship with a woman can be mutually beneficial and supportive is never advanced, so that the young lesbian may have to wait several years to find the support she needs to establish her identity.

Do lesbians choose a particular life-style? There is no such thing as real choice when the material conditions of our lives will inevitably restrict, constrain and determine our activities. Probably working-class women have considerably less room to express their lesbianism than those lesbians who are freer in their time or more powerful in their position (students, lecturers, writers and so on). A lesbian who has at all costs to keep her job (for example, an unsupported mother) can hardly choose to lead a life which seems sure to threaten her source of income.

Isolation

Sexuality is such an integral part of one's whole personality that the experience of being isolated as a lesbian cannot be compared with other forms of isolation which only pertain to certain more superficial interests. In a society which only subscribes overtly to one form of sexual expression, all lesbians are bound to feel isolated in a general sense through a daily confrontation with the dominant heterosexual ideal. This is further complicated by the fact that, although finding other lesbians after a period of complete isolation may initially feel euphoric, having only your sexual orientation in common with other women can quite quickly prove not to be as personally satisfactory as one had originally hoped. As a group, we have found that a common basis of politics and values has meant much more to us and has combated our sense of isolation much more effectively.

Appearance and 'Fancying'

Some of us demonstrate our opposition to what is considered the 'ideal' female appearance by wearing clothes and hairstyles which are deliberate attempts to show men we are not interested in them. This is not because we want to appear masculine, but because we reject the consumerism of fashion pressures and the artificiality and constraint imposed by commercially propagandized notions of beauty. There are no 'rules' about lesbian dress and we cannot necessarily recognize other lesbians by their appearance or mannerisms, nor do we want to. We aspire to find our identity and solidarity through our politics, not through physical features. That is a significant difference between ourselves and the majority of homosexual men.

We, as a group, are trying to rid ourselves of the whole idea of 'fancying', and the all-too-familiar process of choosing lovers which goes along with it. As a group, we are making a conscious and concerted effort to liberate our sexual feelings from the tyrannical implications of having to compete in sexual attractiveness. This is an aspect of heterosexist behaviour which some homosexual men and women also act out. We are struggling to understand how the concept of sexual attraction serves a society which is based upon individualized identities and the amassing of personally owned commodities. We want to understand the anxiety we have all felt about gaining, and sustaining, the sexual interest of other women, and with that we want to re-examine the concepts of passion, intensity and romance. We believe that the particular pains we suffer from having to emphasize such emotions will, with gradually changed experiences, become less absorbing and that they are not a 'natural' and permanent part of our lives.

Lesbian Mothers

Most people now know that lesbianism is not against the law. But this does not mean that the law smiles benignly upon us, or even turns a constantly blind eye. A current area of publicity and debate is the plight of lesbian (previously 'heterosexual') mothers whose ex-husbands want custody of the children. At last one or two custody cases are being fought openly and with a modicum of success, but the judges still fulminate about the mother's sexuality, especially if she is also a feminist. Indeed, heterosexual, declared feminists can also have a rough time in the custody courts.

Nowhere is the public disgust at lesbianism more clearly seen than in the arena of child-rearing. Even liberals have been seen to retract their patronage when it comes to our contact with children, as teachers, social workers, and above all, as mothers. The current concept of childhood in our society contains the notion of children as asexual: children must not be tainted with adult sexuality. Information about how adults relate sexually, and the difficulties they have, is deliberately and consistently withheld from the children of our century. This has happened only recently, within the last 200 years or so, and is related to the rise of the 'ideal' family, universal marriage and nuclear family economics. Before that time children and adults were much less differentiated, and children were not seen as tender plants to be cultivated. While no one, we presume, would want to see a return of child poverty, mortality and economic exploitation, the present situation, where children are regarded as in need of years and years of delicate nurturing and censored educational input (no sex or politics), is distinctly nostalgic of how middle-class women were regarded until they began their concerted liberation movement. While we totally support the rights of lesbian mothers to keep their children, we also see the need to prepare a broad struggle against the whole concept of the 'ideal' nuclear family which oppresses children at least as much as it has oppressed women.

Many lesbians have children and a majority of these, for one reason or another, have not had to fight custody cases. Obviously the lesbian who hasn't been married can bring up her child without legal interference. But these mothers, and their children, are never ever free of the watchful, critical eyes of other parents, the children's friends and teachers. The children of a lesbian mother, especially if that woman is committed politically, do have a rough time, never being able to state categorically their mother's real views, or describe their mother's relationships honestly. Such children spend their days in classrooms where they constantly see and hear heterosexual norms propagandized. Even their gay teachers have to disguise themselves as straight. And such children, on return from school, see heterosexual images on TV till bedtime, hear model heterosexist relationships celebrated (or mourned) in every pop record. The heterosexual feminist mother also has a difficult time, in constant conflict with a world which propagandizes her loved child into heterosexist attitudes. For the lesbian mother, it is even worse. Never do our children see *one* image, hear *one* story that could reflect back to them that we are solid, real people.

'Action for Lesbian Parents' is struggling to prove to the judges that our children grow up just as 'normal' as others. This is the battle which we first have to win, before we can show that some of us don't *want* our children growing up in that so-called 'normal' way. We are still trapped in the vice of showing that we can be just as adequate as heterosexuals, whereas what we really want to get on with is studying and working out potent, viable alternative concepts of childhood so we can move towards different kinds of relationships in which we can live with our children. We do not want to pattern ourselves on the same family-life system which has caused so much distress to so many people, gay and straight, and which is a fundamental underpinning to the hierarchical structure of our society, a society which says it loves children but shuts them away from us daily into normalizing institutions and never gives them any real say in what is happening to them. The child of a lesbian mother shares in the mother's oppression, whether or not that woman has had to endure the terrible battle for custody. We fight for the right to custody and we fight in addition against the culture which bombards our children's ears every night on TV, and the next day in the playground with 'jokes' about 'poofs', 'homos' and 'lessies', reinforced by endless heterosexist propaganda about 'normal' family life.

Daughter (11 years old) of a Lesbian Mother

The world that my mother lives in is very frustrating for her. When anybody straight sees that she is gay they cut her off from their world as if she were alien. This also has upset me sometimes as I have many friends and sometimes they make jokes about homosexuals as if they were dirt. I am sure they have been given this impression by parents and adults. I think people had better start realizing that what lesbians do in bed is no more 'disgusting' than what heterosexuals do.

Lesbians and Therapy

Most psychoanalytic theories have little positive to say about lesbians. We tend to suffer in two ways at the hands of these 'experts'. We are women — and female psychology is generally much abused and misunderstood. In addition we are homosexuals and this is most often seen as deviant by therapists, whether it is diagnosed as due to 'biological' or 'environmental' problems. In general psychological theory, women are equated with men and not seen as separate in their own right. This extends to lesbianism where there is seldom any attempt to separate lesbianism from male homosexuality in cause, effect or 'treatment'. Homosexuals are usually portrayed as regressive, infantile, with mother/ father fixations and such like. Until recently, few psychologists were seriously interested in female psychosexuality. The male bias of the profession has weighed heavily on women. If there has been any separation on the question of homosexuality, it has been to see male homosexuality in a more favourable light. The tradition of male friendships is long and goes hand in hand with the concept that love of men for men is elevating and ennobling. Lesbians do not have the same historical advantage; like all women, we are part of the subordinate section of society. Lesbianism is still to so many merely a 'disease' to be treated and cured (if possible). There are those in the profession who do take a more 'liberal' view and still suggest that it is just limiting: 'After all, we are all bisexual.' Even then, homosexuality is seen as a less favourable option to heterosexuality. Many of these ideas come from Freud and his successors, but it would be foolish of us totally to reject Freud's views or influences, as those ideas are now part of our lives. Also, much that Freud wrote has been subsequently misquoted or distorted to fit the ideas of others.

When we lesbians are in therapy, we are generally unsure and struggling to come to terms with society's attitudes, as well as with ourselves. Consequently we are vulnerable. Our education about homosexuality has usually been negative or non-existent and we are subject to countless fears and myths. This is why so many will continue to seek help. But therapists, counsellors and advisers free from bias are few and far between. Most lesbians will never meet them because of the prohibitive costs. If we can afford it most lesbians will find that the psychiatric bias emphasizes the *personal* nature of lesbianism and the solution has to do with reorganizing aspects of your personality, generally along heterosexual lines. Often the local GP will be as far as we will get. Here we will usually be fobbed off with tranquillizers and other medicinal cures. The attitude of most general practitioners towards sexuality is far from enlightened. If we do encounter therapists and psychiatrists, they are likely to uphold any distorted views we have of ourselves. Most work with, and very often make money out of, those in society who believe they are 'sick'. They tend to believe in the existing norms, in which we as lesbians do not figure. It is important for all of us to realize that those from whom we seek help are part of that very structure which oppresses gay people and women everywhere. Yet, as long as our society exists in its current form, women will need and look for some 'therapy'. What then is available apart from the local GP, the psychiatric specialist, the expensive Harley Street analyst?

For many of us, consciousness-raising groups and women's self-help therapy groups within the women's movement will do far better than most therapists. In these *we* control content and analysis, not the therapist. The development of the growth movement has seen a proliferation of various alternative therapies, predominantly based on the group. The growth movement, or human potential movement, is popularized in such things as encounter groups, Gestalt, co-counselling, T-groups and sensitivity training. Lesbians are using these, and for personal growth some work extremely well, though the extent to which they can help an individual lesbian in crisis is doubtful. Lesbians also need to be aware that the original principles of some alternative therapies are not favourable to homosexuals, or to women.

For those of us who prefer individual therapy the choices are even more limited. If you can find a woman therapist she may be more helpful and sympathetic than a male therapist, but this is not automatically true because of the discipline in which she has been trained. A feminist therapist is even better, but is a rare find. (Contact the Women's Therapy Centre for details; see chapter on Sexuality, p. 68.) Co-counselling is another form of one-to-one counselling which can be less restrictive and oppressive (see Contacts, p. 110).

However, we have to face the fact that the forms of 'help' available to us are few, and all are, with minor exceptions, governed by forces beyond our control. Until women's position improves in relation to this control, we should approach all instruments of the patriarchal society with extreme caution.

What We Do In Bed

It is not surprising that women might feel apprehensive about going to bed with other women, given the repressive influences on women's sexuality in general and the taboo on lesbianism in particular. Here are some thoughts which we hope will dispel some of the myths about lesbian lovemaking.

There are, of course, no set patterns we follow; responsiveness is the key element. The interplay possible between two women is marvellously and almost limitlessly varied. Some of us erroneously assumed that sex with another woman would be as loaded with expectations as heterosexual sex, that foreplay would lead to manual and oral exploration, then to orgasm. Instead we found that orgasm was only a *part* of lovemaking and that it was not seen as a goal, an end or *the* end. Most women receive enormous pleasure from mutual, diffused sexual contact, perhaps so diffused — at least initially — that it should be described as *sensual* contact and seen as an extension of other shared activities.

Lesbians regard the whole body as an erogenous zone and we emphasize the pleasure of caressing, stroking gently, exploring the softness of another body mirroring our own, expressing our sexuality as a sharing of mutual pleasure. Kissing may be the most purely mutual of all acts; the giving and receiving of pleasure is merged in a way which is the theme of all lesbian lovemaking. We do not view kissing as a prologue to something 'more important'. We *add* activities to our initial talking, laughing, kissing and touching, but we don't replace them. When we want more specific genital/sexual arousal this will also be mutual, even when the emphasis may move from one woman to the other and back again. We use hands and mouths, and usually both. Individual preferences naturally vary. Some of us enjoy manual penetration, also finding excitement in being stroked inside. Others prefer all genital arousal to be clitoral. There seems to be no 'reason' for this, or predictable inferences to be drawn. Some women who have had quite satisfactory heterosexual relationships simply don't enjoy penetration. Other women who loathe the thought of a penis enjoy the sensitivity of their female lover's hand.

In lesbian relationships we try to reject 'roles'. The mutuality of lesbian lovemaking is its strength.

Sex: A Political Statement

As a group we do not see personal relationships as cordoned off from our political struggle, nor as a private sanctuary from an otherwise hostile world. We feel that the struggle in personal relationships is completely interrelated with the class struggle and the struggle against male dominance. Sexual relationships can reproduce class and sex divisions, and notions such as 'property' and 'dominance' have to be combated in our day-to-day contact with others, and in ourselves.

As women and as lesbians we have had our sexuality defined and distorted and have internalized false definitions of ourselves. Thus the first step is to re-define our sexuality and to destroy the idea of lesbianism as an inferior form of heterosexuality. We are disclaiming the need for male substitution in any form, whether by imitating oppressive heterosexual roles, or directly in our sexual activity by seeing lesbian sex as a form of deprivation, or of envy of the penis. We do not see penetration as the ultimate and inevitable climax to sexual activity, nor do we see sexual activity as being a gradual progression towards orgasm.

We are exploring ways of relating sexually which are uncompetitive

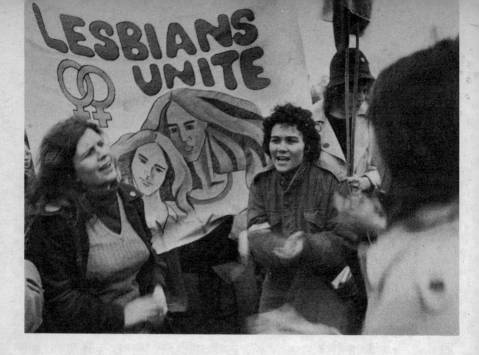

and which do not adhere to qualitative notions of performance, and trying to explore forms of reciprocity which we create together instead of having preconceived standards of something which amounts to 'satisfaction' and 'being good in bed'. We want to release our sexual responses and activities from the over-concern with orgasms as the test for the viability of a sexual experience.

We are rejecting the competitive basis of meeting each other with ideas of success and failure, and are looking for alternatives in which mutual freedom and communication are the basis, so that each sexual encounter can be experienced as a fresh recreation, rather than a habit or ritual.

Bisexuality

As bisexual women who take ourselves and our relationships seriously, we inevitably find ourselves in a particularly invidious position. We are generally viewed by the heterosexual world in purely sexual terms: a sensual receptor for come-what-may. Lesbians may also regard us as sexually predatory, feeding off their full-time commitment but unwilling to make it ourselves and free to 'choose' the safety of the straight world when necessary. In fact the question of a 'choice' may be, for us, the source of uncertainty. While struggling to understand our emotional needs, which may well have to find sexual expression, the isolation and hostility we feel, sandwiched between those belonging to the heterosexual and homosexual worlds, add powerful feelings of defensiveness to feelings of confusion. There are great temptations for everyone, no matter how strong their individualism, to adapt to the mores of the world which most matters to them. Increasingly the lesbian has her world, has an 'us' to be against 'them'. The bisexual has no such world and it may be that we should get together and begin to examine our position and work towards self-definition and shared strength in the way that lesbians have done and are doing. But the very nature of bisexuality means that it is not easily defined, that we are not easily 'grouped'. It may be a matter of transition for some, self-deception or fear for others, a positive choice for a few. So for some time yet many of us will choose to align ourselves with lesbians. We may not easily be understood, frequently we don't understand ourselves, but our freedom to see our sexuality positively will be enhanced when pressure from gay women at least subsides, when we are viewed not with suspicion but as sisters joining in the struggle against sexism, and perhaps against sexual definition too.

Conclusion

It is difficult for us to talk about our role in the women's liberation movement, as that would be to presuppose some artificial separation from the rest of the movement, which we do not feel. We see our oppression as lesbians as part of the general oppression of women, and as socialists feel the need for a class analysis, whilst considering struggles around the particular oppression of race and sexuality as central revolutionary issues rather than as subordinate to the class struggle.

In this way, we need to organize separately as lesbians in order to understand our specific oppression and how it is linked to capitalism, and to gain support from our common experience of this. We do not, however, believe that the fact of our lesbianism pre-empts the need for our involvement with the struggles of other women. We no more see the National Abortion Campaign as the domain of heterosexual women than we see the issue of sexuality as relating solely to lesbians.

Whilst we support single issue women's campaigns and demands such as the Working Women's Charter, Women's Aid, Nursery Campaign, National Abortion Campaign, etc., the interrelated nature of women's oppression demands an overall feminist perspective if these demands are to be carried beyond reform. This is crucial for us as lesbians if we are to challenge the view which sees our struggle as best contained within the particular issue of sexual preference and civil law reform. Lesbians in the women's movement cannot avoid confronting the issue of sexuality, but we need to work with all women in the movement in order to develop an analysis of sexual oppression. Without this, lesbianism will remain an issue of who one goes to bed with, and feminism will face considerable difficulty in moving beyond individual rights and a series of demands for equality. Unless we work together as women to develop this analysis we will never be able to challenge economist positions of the left which see revolution as the transference of power to the working class, after which all other forms of oppression will disappear, e.g. women's oppression. Women know from bitter experience that this is not the case, and while we cannot conceive of women's liberation as being achieved under capitalism, neither can we see much hope for a revolution which does not have women's liberation as one of its central goals. Women are building such a revolution.

Bibliography and Resources

The following books and pamphlets contain ideas and information about lesbians and the lesbian struggle. They are all obtainable from Compendium Books, 240 Camden High Street, London NW1 (who do mail order), and will also often be on sale in good book shops local to you; for a list see p. 573.

Abbott, Sidney, and Love, Barbara, *Sappho was a Right-on Woman*, Stein & Day, 1973. Descriptions of various life-styles and personal histories, in the context of gay liberation, and a section on how the growing lesbian struggle influenced the American women's movement.

Altman, Denis, *Homosexual — Oppression and Liberation*, Allen Lane, 1974. An account of oppression as experienced by gays in the context of the growing liberation movement. Mostly about men.

Birkby, P., *et al.*, *Amazon Expedition*, Times Change Press, 1973. Lesbian feminist anthology.

Cassidy, Jules, and Stewart-Park, Angela, *We're Here: Conversations with Lesbian Women*, Quartet, 1977.

Conditions of Illusion, Feminist Books, 1974. Collection of writings on feminist issues, some emphasizing lesbianism in a feminist context.

Gay Left, Gay Left Collective. Male collective magazine considering the relationship between homosexuality and socialist commitment. Published two or three times each year.

Johnston, Jill, *Lesbian Nation*, Simon & Schuster, New York, 1973. American radical feminist's writing, advocating separatism.

Klaich, Dolores, *Woman Plus Woman — Attitudes towards lesbianism*, Morrow, 1974. Personal psychological and historical perspectives on lesbianism.

Loving Women, Nomadic Sisters (USA), 1975. A sex manual by women for lesbians, bisexual and heterosexual women.

Martin, Del, and Lyon, Phyllis, *Lesbian/Woman*, Bantam, New York, 1972. Personal account by a lesbian couple who founded first lesbian movement in USA. Enlightening account of how older lesbians have struggled to get lesbianism incorporated into the women's movement, with other case histories.

Milligan, Don, *The Politics of Homosexuality*, Pluto Press (London) pamphlet, 1973.

Move. Lesbian feminist magazine from Bristol Women's Group (see bookshops, p. 573).

Myron, N., and Bunch, C., *Lesbianism and the Women's Movement*, Diana Press, 1975.

Red Herring. An excellent magazine from the Scottish Lesbian Feminists. No longer produced, but back copies available from Glasgow and Edinburgh women's groups (contact WIRES, p. 570) and some bookshops (see p. 573).

Rule, Jane, *Lesbian Images*, Peter Davies, 1976. Studies of lesbian images in fiction with special references to lesbian writers.

With Downcast Gays. Pamphlet about self-oppression, by A. Hodges and D. Huttet, Pomegranate Press, London, 1974.

PSYCHOLOGY, PSYCHOTHERAPY AND LESBIANS

Baker Miller, Jean (ed.), *Psychoanalysis and Women*, Penguin, 1974. Essays which attempt to dispel current and longstanding myths about 'female' psychology (e.g. penis envy).

Chesler, Phyllis, *Women and Madness*, Allen Lane, 1974. Again explaining how and why women have often been labelled 'mad', 'hysterical', etc.

Rough Times: A Journal of Radical Therapy, December 1974, November 1975. Articles on women/lesbians and therapy.

Psychiatry and the Homosexual, Gay Liberation Pamphlet 1. Shows attitudes of psychiatrists to homosexuality as 'deviance' which makes people 'ill' and criticizes these.

The Radical Therapist, Penguin, 1974. Collection of papers by therapists who disagree with 'deviance' concept and other psychoanalytical myths.

Issues in Radical Therapy, summer 1975, winter 1975. Articles on women/lesbians and therapy.

Szasz, Thomas, *The Manufacture of Madness*, Paladin, 1973. Traces links between religious persecution of heretics and witches and society's use of homosexuals as scapegoats — labels of 'madness' and 'eccentricity' seen as control instruments of the dominant ideology.

Wolff, Charlotte, *Love Between Women*, Duckworth, 1971. Lesbian psychoanalyst's accounts of lesbians and lesbian relationships, using a case history approach.

NOVELS AND NARRATIVE MATERIAL ABOUT LESBIANS

Bedford, Sybille, *A Favourite of the Gods*, Collins, 1963, and *A Compass Error*, Collins, 1968. Two linked novels describing an intense relationship between mother and daughter and subsequently between daughter and lover.

Brown, Rita Mae, *Rubyfruit Jungle*, Daughters Inc., 1973. Loosely autobiographical American working-class teenage girl in lively development as a lesbian. Has written several books — novels and poetry.

Falk, Ruth, *Women Loving*, Random House, New York, 1975. Autobiographical account of one woman's search for her identity through her relationships with other women.

Hall, Radclyffe, *The Well of Loneliness*, Corgi, 1968 (first published 1928).

Mavor, Elizabeth, *The Green Equinox*, Wildwood House, 1974.

Mavor, Elizabeth, *The Ladies of Llangollen: A Study of a Romantic Friendship*, Penguin, 1973. Historical biography of two lesbians.

Miller, Isabel, *Patience and Sarah*, Fawcett Crest, 1973. Out of print in the UK. Available from *Gay News* mail order. Based on fact, this is the story of two lesbians who set up a farm together in early nineteenth-century Connecticut.

Millett, Kate, *Flying*, Paladin, 1976. An autobiographical account by an American feminist of the growing strength of her lesbian feminism, through a description of her work and relationships over a period of a year.

Nicolson, Nigel, *Portrait of a Marriage*, Weidenfeld & Nicolson, 1973. Story of a marriage in which both partners had relationships with members of their own sex, based on the personal papers of Vita Sackville-West.

Riley, Elisabeth, *All that False Instruction*, Angus & Robertson, 1975. An Australian lesbian describes her life, her relationships and her conflicts in a society where female independence is seen as particularly suspect.

Russ, Joanna, *The Female Man*, Bantam, 1975. Science-fiction account of female societies.

Sappho of Lesbos, *Works*, University of California Press, 1958.

Wolff, Charlotte, *An Older Love*, Quartet, 1976. Novel about lesbian relationships involving older women.

Woolf, Virginia, *Orlando*, first published 1928. Triad/Panther, 1977. Novel in which the author explores the constrictions of socially imposed sex roles – the central character lives through four centuries, and in both sexes.

CONTACTS (see also general section, p. 568)

Action for Lesbian Parents, c/o 57 Maids Causeway, Cambridge CB5 8DE.

Campaign for Homosexual Equality, POBox 427, 33 King Street, Manchester M60 2EL (061 228 1985).

Anne Dickson, 83 Fordwych Road, London NW2 (01 452 9261). For co-counselling.

Friend. National network advice and counselling service. London number (01 359 7371) will advise you on your nearest service. See *Gay News* and *Time Out* for other supportive services.

Gay News. A fortnightly newspaper on sale nationally. It is mainly by (liberal) men for men, although it is always saying it is for women, too. But it publishes a comprehensive guide to gay pubs, discos and so on, on a national scale, and runs small ads section.

Gay Switchboard, 01 837 7324. They will tell you whether there is a switchboard nearer your area if you do not live near London. This is a free, 24-hour service: what's on, flats, flatshares and information about women's groups, advice centres and so on.

Lesbian Line, telephone advice, contact service available on Monday and Friday afternoon and evenings, 01 837 8602.

National Organization of Lesbians, contact through Sappho.

Sappho, Basement, 20 Dorset Square, London NW1 (01 724 3636); they also publish a magazine of the same name.

Scottish Minorities Group, 60 Broughton Street, Edinburgh EH1 35A (031 556 9473).

Time Out. A weekly magazine. A guide to cinema, theatre and events in London; contains an Agitprop page which sets out any leftist/feminist meetings, discos and other activities which are taking place, along with specific lesbian events. *Time Out* also runs small ads which include information about advice services, flatshares, and general contact information.

Information about specific lesbian groups is best found out by going through one of the above channels, which will give you the up-to-date information you need. (Anyone who feels they are in a state of emergency should note that the London **Gay Switchboard** is a 24-hour service and you can ring them wherever you live, if you have not got your more local number which they will give you if you want it.)

6 Taking Care of Ourselves

Do we really take care of ourselves? Most of us just drive ourselves to the limit and then go to the doctor to have our minds and bodies repaired with pills. We know that doctors cannot provide a cure for overwork, sandwich lunches, late nights, unhappy marriages and lack of exercise, but we go along after the damage is done, hoping for a panacea. Our lack of care is partly ignorance, and partly apathy; we feel that the medical profession knows best and will take care of us.

Most doctors treat symptoms, not causes. They look at the bit that hurts and ignore the rest. It is rare for a traditional doctor to ask questions about our diet and life-style, and too often they don't listen to our attempts to give them relevant information or dismiss it as attempted self-diagnosis which they see as dangerous.

Socially there is a lot working against good health: firm muscular bodies and rosy cheeks are not fashionable. Here are ten reasons why many of us see good eating and exercise as a drag:
(1) Health food is sold at rip-off prices; (2) food faddism labels you as a nut; (3) my ulcer proves what an important job I'm holding down; (4) nutrition is so complicated it takes a lifetime's study to understand it; (5) and even then the experts disagree; (6) why get fit like an athlete when all I ever do is ride on buses and sit in an office; (7) exercising at home is sterile and boring; (8) and anyway Charles Atlas is muscle-bound; (9) delicious things to eat are supposed to be bad for you; and (10) as if all that were not enough, I feel all right anyway, thank you very much.

Tip-top health probably afflicts one in 1,000 people, but no one ever bothered to measure good health. It is sold to us as being the opposite of being sick, so if you are not actually seeing your doctor, or recovering from an infection, or dying in hospital, you are supposed to be well. But health is a spectrum and really good health — the golden radiance plus bounce sort — is probably as rare as rabies. Here's how one woman learned what good health feels like.

I used to think I felt fit, until I returned from a short spell in the country to the city where I was greeted with a chorus of 'But you look so well.' And as these whey-faced city dwellers peered earnestly into my face trying to fathom the mystery of my new condition I realized that there had been a change. I hadn't exactly looked pinched and peaky before, but if you are not actually ill, then it seems to be almost impossible to remember what it felt like to be in peak condition.

On top of this there are political, economic and cultural reasons which combine with these other factors to load the dice against the achievement of good health. Food production is big business, it is dominated by the monopoly companies who rake in huge profits from convenience foods. Governments also make money from unhealthy products through taxation; in spite of a public anti-smoking campaign only 6p of every £100 gathered in taxing cigarettes is used for anti-smoking propaganda in Britain. Culturally, pill-popping and surgery have become the backbone of recognized medicine. Public attitudes to homeopathy, acupuncture, and a hundred other practices illustrate the confines of our understanding of healing. The drug companies have a lot to answer for here. The very pattern of work – cerebral work, office work, automation and the division of labour – mitigates against health.

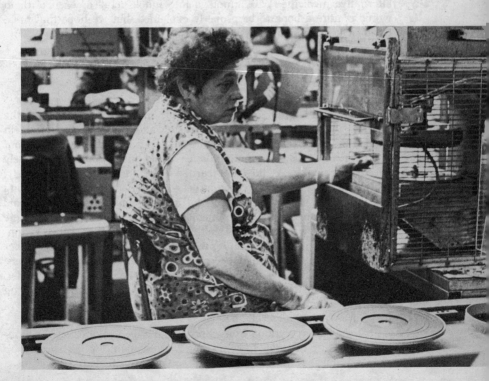

Nonetheless, we can do more to help ourselves. Nobody is going to help us stop limping around this planet at half steam. No one has to obtain a licence or pass a test to be in charge of a body. Health is our own responsibility.

What We Can Do and Why

Many of the fatal diseases of middle life like heart disease, strokes, ulcers, diabetes, are a direct result of our ill-treatment of our bodies. We are all equipped with a variety of built-in checks and filters which under normal conditions fight disease and expel unwanted or poisonous foods from our bodies. But if we continually consume food with the wrong balance of nutrients, if we overload our bodies with 'fat', if we neglect the exercise that our system is built for and if we insist on inhaling hot smoke which damages the delicate tissue of our lungs, we are asking for trouble in the end. But many of us do not know what normal conditions should be. This chapter is divided into three sections on nutrition, exercise, and alternative medicine. We cannot go into much detail as each of them would require a book to be properly explained, but we hope that these basic facts will encourage people to explore further.

Nutrition

This century has seen a massive change in the eating habits of the affluent nations. Fewer people die of starvation, but the revolution in food production has been a mixed blessing — our lack of knowledge about nutrition combined with an abundance of bad quality food has adversely affected our health. We have not learned to use our food resources wisely.

During the war years, rationing distributed food fairly evenly among the population of Britain, probably for the first time. Attention was paid to the balance of nutrients, and people were advised on how to get the best from what was available. Health improved as a result. When rationing stopped, like a nation of fatties released from a diet, we filled ourselves with all the things we had been denied: sugar, white bread, sweets, chocolate, coffee, butter and larger quantities of meat if we could afford it. These bad habits have been passed on to our children and are being passed on to our grandchildren. Britain now has the highest incidence of heart disease in the world.

How has the revolution in food production affected our diet? Technological farming methods have increased production, but the speeded-up growing times retard the growth of some vital nutrients. Pesticides used to protect crops, and chemicals for fattening livestock may in the long run do us harm. New methods of transport have given us a wider variety of food, but by the time we get them vegetables may be weeks old and vitamins may be lost. Food preservation has protected us from the ravages of food poisoning and allowed us to feed our urban populations safely. However, bread which stays fresh for days has been stripped of the live wheat germ containing many vital nutrients, only a few of which are replaced. In canning, food is heated to very high temperatures which destroy much of the vitamin content. In addition, it is usually preserved in sugar or salt, both of which we eat in dangerously high quantities.

Perhaps the greater availability of food outweighs the disadvantages of technology. Certainly if food was distributed evenly throughout the world higher yields would ensure that nobody starved. But we are faced with an additional problem, the profit motive. The agricultural lobby in most developed countries is strong enough to ensure government protection of price levels. When yields climb too high, the excess is often destroyed to preserve prices. On the manufacturing side a relatively small number of companies are making huge profits from food, some of it totally synthetic and much of it produced to appeal to our sugar addiction rather than our food requirements, or processed for our convenience at the expense of our health. Even farming is heavily controlled by the manufacturers. Many farmers sell their entire crops to the companies long before harvesting and this obviously affects the kind of food that they grow as well as the final market price of all foods. Most farmers find it uneconomic to use non-technological farming methods or to sell direct to the consumer.

Increasingly, multinational corporations like Unilever are taking over all aspects of food production, from farming to retail selling in the supermarkets. Such monopolies make it more and more difficult for us to improve the quality and reduce the cost of our food. Unilever will continue to spend 30% of its income from product sales on advertising, so that little Susie will continue to demand her marshmallows and synthetic food instead of carrots and brown rice.

What can we do about this control over our lives? Well, for a start we can find out what food we should eat to keep healthy and how to prepare it simply. Few of us have the time or inclination to spend hours over a hot stove every day, but eating out of a tin is not the only alternative.

BALANCED EATING

All fresh untreated foods contain one or more of the three basic nutrients: protein, fat and carbohydrate, in varying amounts and some of the vitamins and minerals which are also vital to health. If we eat a diet of mixed fresh foods containing all three basic nutrients the combination

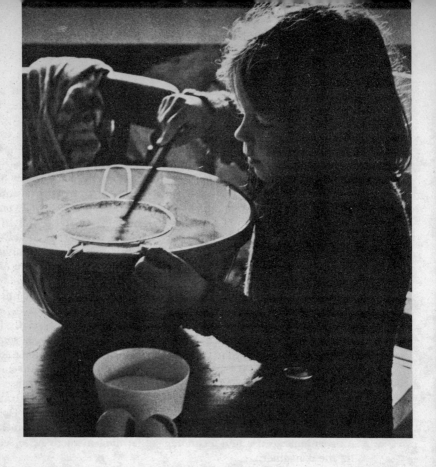

should ensure that we are not deficient in anything. That combination is important because the nutrients work together in the short term as well as the long term and an imbalance will probably cause sluggishness and apathy.

Protein is the body building food. It is responsible for running repairs and growth and for keeping up the supply of chemicals which control body processes, fight disease and aid digestion. We don't need a vast amount of protein to keep us in trim; official estimates vary from 55–75 grams (2–2¾ oz) per day but it could be less than that; our protein needs are largely defined by our size and weight and rate of activity. Good protein sources are: milk foods, eggs, fish, soya beans and wheat germ. (You will need about 12 oz of a combination of these foods to provide 2–2¾ oz of protein). Meat is of course also a good source but it is expensive; it takes only half an acre to feed a vegetarian and 1·63 acres to feed a meat-eater. In addition, meat-eating causes a build-up of potentially harmful substances which have to be eliminated by the kidneys and liver. They manage well with a small amount but if we overload them they could stop functioning properly.

Beans and brown rice contain incomplete protein, but if they are eaten together they provide a good and economical source of complete protein. In the same way, whole wheat bread eaten with cheese or lentils provides complete protein.

Fats are a concentrated and long-lasting form of energy because they are slowly digested. They divide into two categories: saturated and unsaturated fats.

Saturated fats: most animal fats (e.g. beef fat and butter) and solid vegetable shortenings (Spry, Cookeen, etc.) are saturated fats. Too much of these fats can contribute to heart disease. This is thought to be because of a waxy substance called cholesterol which is found in all animal fats (including our own). Cholesterol in small doses is essential to the body's chemical processes. However, if cholesterol deposits build up on the artery walls they can block the artery and cause a heart attack.

Although cholesterol is not found in vegetable fat, too much saturated vegetable fat has the same effect as too much animal fat. Therefore, we need to cut back on all saturated fats to guard against cholesterol deposits.

Unsaturated (or polyunsaturated) fats are almost always oils which are both liquid at room temperature and of vegetable origin. They help to build cell membrane, arteries, nerves and brain. There is increasing evidence that a high ratio of unsaturated fats to saturated fats is what really matters. That is, to keep a low cholesterol level, more of the fat we eat should be unsaturated and less of it should be saturated. One way of doing this is to substitute polyunsaturated margarine for butter (beware, not all margarines are polyunsaturated; when they are they should say so on the package), and to cook with vegetable oils.

Carbohydrates, when broken down by digestion, become sugar. Sugar is necessary for the digestion of fats and proteins, which cannot be completely broken down without it. Carbohydrates are found in all vegetables, fruits and grains (and in small quantities in all foods). Important sources are: root vegetables, brown rice, flour, cereals and beans.

Refined Carbohydrates: Refined sugar, white flour, and white rice are all carbohydrates which have been artificially refined and which we tend to eat excessively. The refining process removes much of the nutritive value and most of the roughage. Refined sugar is the worst of them. It is so concentrated that we can easily eat a great deal without realizing it; the average daily intake of sugar in Britain is equivalent to eating $2\frac{1}{2}$ lb. of sugar beets per day, so it's easy to see why sugar is fattening. It is also acid-forming, and the acid rots our teeth and can damage our stomach lining; it lacks Vitamin B which it needs for digestion so it uses up any vitamin B in the body from other sources, often creating a deficiency. Each time sugar is eaten, insulin in the body is stimulated to release sugar already in the blood and deposit it elsewhere as fat. As it is metabolized very fast, the burst of energy which follows a dose of sugar will be followed by a drop in energy when it has gone, creating hunger or a craving for more sugar, and so the cycle continues, possibly upsetting the natural balance of insulin and resulting in diabetes (when the body can no longer produce insulin and it has to be artificially supplied). Because sugar satisfies hunger temporarily it stops us eating more nutritious foods. It is not necessary to eat refined sugar at all, as sufficient exists naturally in the other foods we eat. Most of us are pretty hooked on it by now and it is hard to give up but it is worthwhile trying to cut it down.*

White flour, and hence white bread still has some nutritive content other than carbohydrate; for many people it is regrettably a major source of protein and vitamin B. However, much of the real value of the grain is lost in refining, and like sugar it is a concentrated source of carbohydrate which satisfies hunger without fully satisfying food requirements. Much of the same can be said of white rice. Tooth decay and obesity are related to refined carbohydrate consumption. Without these foods we would be less likely to suffer from either.

Vitamins and Minerals: These nutrients help prevent diseases, strengthen bones, keep our hair and skin healthy, help our blood to clot and our wounds to heal and much more besides. They often work in combination, and we need only very small amounts of each. Our vitamin requirements should be met by eating a reasonable amount of fresh vegetables, whole grains, nuts, and milk products. Vitamin A is the only one that is found only in meat, but it can be manufactured by our bodies from carotene which is found in yellow and green plants. Vitamins C and B are both water-soluble so should be eaten every day as they cannot be stored in the body. Refined bread has a number of synthetic B vitamins added, but whole grain bread, or breads like Hovis or Vitbe, wheat germ, liver, leafy vegetables and dried beans are better sources.

Vitamin C is found in all fresh fruit and vegetables, but it is destroyed very easily through storage or heating so it is important to eat some produce which is grown locally to ensure that the vitamin C is preserved. Frozen foods, which are processed soon after harvesting when food has fully ripened, are often a better source of vitamin C than so-called fresh foods which have been in storage for months, but they must be used within an hour of thawing or most of the vitamin C will have disappeared. Vitamin E is found in corn, whole grains, peanuts and eggs. It is destroyed by iron supplements so they should be taken several hours afterwards. Though its function is unclear it is thought to play a part in protecting unsaturated fats. It is also thought to protect certain of the sex-hormones and is therefore important for menopausal women.

* Professor John Yudkin believes that sugar rather than fat is the cause of heart disease. See his book *Pure White and Deadly*.

Cooking methods are important if the vitamins are to be preserved. They will be lost if you wash vegetables for a long time in running water, or boil them in deep water which is then thrown away. The best methods are: steaming over boiling water, cooking in about one inch of water with the lid on the pan (allow them to simmer slowly or the pan will burn, and then keep any water to add to soups or stews), or cooking them in the liquid in which they will be eaten. The shorter the cooking time the less value will be destroyed by heat. It is a good rule to make raw vegetables a component of every meal.

Iron is a mineral that women often lack. It occurs naturally in a number of foods (liver, eggs, dried fruits, dried beans and peas, whole grains, dark green vegetables and brewers' yeast), but intake can be bolstered by using iron saucepans for cooking. Lack of iron, often lost through heavy bleeding, can cause anaemia. Calcium is another essential for pregnant and menstruating women: it comes in milk foods, green vegetables and eggs.

Cellulose and Water: Water forms an essential part of the tissues; it also contains trace minerals. Most people need 6–7 glasses of liquid a day, not including alcoholic drinks which dehydrate. Cellulose (roughage) is often lacking in our diets, which contain too much refined food. We need it to keep our intestinal muscles in trim and to prevent constipation. Roughage also keeps our teeth clean. Fruits, grains, whole grain bread and whole cereals all contain roughage. Anti-constipation medications are no substitute, as they take over from natural processes and allow the muscles to get flabby.

Beware of these foods*

1. Refined carbohydrates and all foods containing refined sugar (including brown sugar and molasses). (See under Refined Carbohydrates, p. 117.)
2. Animal fats (see under Fats), contained in most ice-cream, cakes, etc.
3. The following destroy vitamin B: sulphur dioxide (a preservative), alcohol and antibiotics (which kill vitamin B-producing bacteria in the intestine), coffee, tea and other diuretics (which cause excretion of water-soluble vitamins), and sleeping pills. Lack of vitamin B causes depression and irritability, so vitamin B supplements, especially yeast, may be useful if you are taking any of these substances. (See also Refined Carbohydrates.)
4. The following destroy vitamin C: alcohol, coffee, tea and diuretics, aspirin, smoking, long storage of foods, and heat.
5. The following destroy vitamin E: iron salts (they should be taken several hours before or after vitamin E supplements), rancid fats, chlorinated water and chlorine dioxide (a white bread preservative).

6. Mineral oil laxatives remove vitamins A, D, E and K which are fat-soluble.

7. Salt: we eat far too much of it and the excess has to be dealt with by the kidneys which can become overloaded. It also causes water retention, possibly hardened arteries, and can aggravate rheumatism and arthritis.

Eat more of these foods

1. Fresh vegetables and fruit eaten raw or cooked in very little water.

2. Brown rice, rather than white rice which is stripped of roughage and much of its vitamin and protein content. It takes longer to cook but it's worth it.

3. Dried beans (soaked overnight in lots of water and then cooked for about an hour) with your brown rice to give you complete protein.

4. Stoneground bread or, failing that, Hovis or Vitbe, as they all contain wheat germ and stoneground contains roughage unlike white bread. (Wheat germ and whole flour are 'unstable' — they cannot be stored for long unless they are refrigerated.)

5. Unsweetened natural yogurt and other milk foods; the flavoured ones are filled with sugar.

6. Wheat germ, bran, nuts and fresh fruit mixed with rolled oats provide a nutritious breakfast cereal, unlike the refined 'Sunshine' food sold commercially which is thought to contain little more nutritive value than the box it is in.

If you eat plenty of these foods the occasional binge probably won't do you much harm and you won't have to make a conscious effort to ensure that your meals are 'balanced'.

* Information in this box comes from *The Diet Revolution* by Jill Wordsworth, Gollancz, 1976.

A WORD ABOUT WEIGHT

Psychological eating problems are almost exclusive to women. They range from anorexia nervosa (compulsive self-starvation) to compulsive eating and compulsive dieting.

Eating patterns are learned in childhood. Many mothers overfeed their babies out of anxiety and without reference to their real needs. Childhood eating patterns have psychological as well as physiological repercussions. Eating is associated with good behaviour, love and comfort. Most children if set a good example and left to themselves with a reasonable range of food to choose from will eat well, but the system of coercion and reward which is built into meal times turns many children into food faddists at a very early age.

For girls particularly, the conflicts grow with age. We identify with sweet things (sugar, honey, etc.); much confectionery advertising is aimed at men for them to give to women, or at women to buy as a luxury, a treat. By adolescence many of us are well caught up in the conflict between our desire for sweet things and the fashionable need to be slim.

Obesity is a health problem; wearing a dress one size larger than a fashion model is not. Perennial dieting is as unhelpful as it is depressing. Food becomes entangled with morality; missing a meal becomes a matter for self-congratulation. Actual food consumption becomes wildly unbalanced and the attendant drop in necessary nutrients causes lethargy and depression. But more important, appetite becomes completely distorted and divorced from need. Ideally we should all be able to rely on our bodies to tell us what to eat. An appetite which is programmed on guilt and reward is incapable of making sound judgements about food.

What can be done? Support is an important factor in regaining self-respect and breaking out of the diet-binge cycle:

Since I've been in the women's liberation movement people have encouraged me to stop hating myself. It's amazing the sense of security it has given me. The women I know don't care if I'm fat. When I cared intensely about being thin, other people seemed to feel it too. Now that I'm less concerned about being fat the men I meet don't seem to care either.

I decided to learn to love my curves and stop trying to get thin. I got to know my body, to look at it and to like it, my feelings were transferred to others and I gained confidence. I haven't dieted for over three years and as if by magic I've dropped over a stone in weight and at least a size in clothes. Now I eat chocolate when I want to which is practically never and I don't like over-eating because it makes me feel sluggish and miserable. I like being thinner but not so that I look good to others, I really don't mind what they think, besides I'm now convinced that their opinion is only a reflection of my self-esteem.

We can help each other to start seeing food as necessary fuel, to re-educate our bodies and to separate our food needs from our emotional needs. For those of us who find it hard without help, the Women's Therapy Centre at 19a Hartham Road, London N7 (tel. 01 607 2864) runs group therapy sessions for compulsive eaters.

CONCLUSION

We don't have to be experts in nutrition to eat wisely. A diet which is based on mixed fresh and unrefined food will provide all the nutrients we need. For those who want to find out more about the different schools of thought on nutrition we recommend Jill Wordsworth's *The Diet Revolution* (see p. 142). It is a very straightforward account of the main theories, summing up their similarities and differences.

For those of us who have only ever eaten vegetables boiled or fried next to a hunk of meat, a good vegetarian cookery book could open up a whole new world of good eating at a fraction of the cost of eating meat. We've mentioned one or two good books in the bibliography, though once you know the basics, recipes give way to invention. Vegetable cookery is not complicated. It need not be more time-consuming either; soups, beans and rice, etc. can be made and stored in the fridge and then re-heated with the addition of a few fresh vegetables.

Our eating habits depend on what we can buy in the shops; dried lentils, mung beans, and wheat germ may not be available in your local supermarket (though in urban areas supermarkets do have a surprising range of such foods). Many people have started their own food co-ops, combining with a few neighbours or even a whole estate. Food co-ops are not difficult to start (see Bibliography). The responsibility for collecting foods from wholesalers and markets can be rotated, dried foods can be bought in bulk and stored, and though whole grain flour shouldn't be stored for long, unless it is refrigerated or in an airtight container, bulk buying and distribution among a number of people will bring the price down. It is not possible to buy 'whole' foods everywhere but we can choose the better (less processed) mass produced foods.

The co-op idea can be extended to baking batches of bread and growing vegetables in gardens or allotments. Most urban areas have some land allocated for allotments, and though there may be a waiting list it is worth contacting the council to find out. Alternatively, there is land all over Britain awaiting development and we should fight for the right to put it to use on a short term basis for growing food. For those who live in tiny flats and have no desire to dig, there is one kind of cultivation which is open to all – growing bean sprouts. You can do this on wet cotton wool in the kitchen; when the sprouts are about two inches high they make a delicious basis to salads and they are bulging with vitamins and minerals. Food can't get any fresher than that.

Exercise

How can I explain it? It gets to you, it is you! We have this notion that mind and body are separate – but how can you feel good in the head, really, if your body's like a limp rag? Before, my body would embarrass me – do clumsy things, because there wasn't a lot of muscular control, or it wouldn't do much at all. Now that I exercise I'm happier about my body, it acts and reacts in ways that please me — it's stronger, more real, more energetic. It's like being three-dimensional instead of two-dimensional; it makes me feel more complete, more whole.

In agricultural societies and rural areas the concept of exercise is fairly meaningless. The substance of people's lives is strenuous physical labour, with women doing as many (or more) of the heavy tasks as men. Today in the UK most people live in urban or suburban areas. Here a growing majority of jobs, and not just middle-class ones, require little physical effort although they may be extremely tiring. Even when time, money and opportunity exist, a strikingly small number of women incorporate vigorous exercise into their daily lives. There are many reasons. Many of us have to fight against the ideas that women can't do certain things and that we shouldn't do certain things.*

From early childhood on, many women are discouraged, subtly and sometimes not so subtly, from participating in strenuous physical activities.

Gillian Coutard, aged 12, of Thorne, near Doncaster, the only girl member of her school football team, was picked to play for the Thorne Democratic Club's Under-15 side. But the referee refused to let her play . . .

Baby girls are pampered and treated more delicately than boy babies. A woman we know sometimes introduced her baby girl as Danny. The adults who met 'Danny' encouraged her to play actively without worrying about a few bumps or even tears. But when she was introduced as Sara, people were more protective of her. No wonder many girls grow up scared to try out things with their bodies. Even local streets are usually the boys' turf. Growing up to believe that physical coordination is a male characteristic, boys will teach each other athletic skills but won't do the same with girls. Joanne told us: 'Sometimes the boys would let me join their games, but if several of us girls wanted to play, they would chase us away.' And organized sport is mostly a male world. Most men want to keep it that way, for sport is one area where they can assert their 'masculinity' by displaying their strength, skill and aggressiveness, or by identifying with and idolizing those who do.

---

* These prejudices affect most deeply middle- and upper-class women. Pre-capitalist and capitalist exploitation has never seen anything wrong with driving black and working-class women as hard as men. Sojourner Truth's famous outburst makes that abundantly clear: "The man over there says that women need to be helped into carriages and lifted over ditches, and to have the best place everywhere. Nobody ever helps me into carriages or over puddles or gives me the best place . . . and ain't I a woman? Look at my arm! I have ploughed and planted and gathered into barns, and no man could head me . . . and ain't I a woman? I could work as much and eat as much as a man when I could get it — and bear the lash as well . . . and ain't I a woman?" (From a speech to the Women's Rights Convention, Akron, Ohio, 1851.)

As we pass into and through adolescence, the pressures on us to be 'popular with the boys' reach epidemic proportions and often squash any remaining desire to exercise strenuously. We give up learning athletic skills in favour of learning to swing our hips. We're taught that popularity depends on 'femininity': muscles on a woman are considered un-attractive – to men, of course. In a recent pilot study in Scotland of children's attitudes to PE and sports, it was found that children have clearly defined ideas about 'suitable' activities for boys and girls. The girls who were relatively keen to take part in sports had encouragement from parents, but most of those in their teens had experienced some pressure from their peers to give up sports.

Alice told us: 'When I started studying karate my boyfriend got really upset: he was afraid I'd get muscular and not be his slim little lady any more. But that's his problem. I feel good now, and I'm not so afraid of a bruise or two.'

Many women have been taught that physical activity during menstruation is dangerous. Untrue! Women in fact can do all kinds of heavy work without injury to our reproductive organs or any other part of ourselves. Nell described arguments she had with her husband: 'Peter gets angry at me for moving furniture. "You'll hurt yourself," he says. He doesn't know now many heavy things I lift – like our thirty-pound son! I think he's scared that my being stronger will make me less dependent on him.'

A final deterrent to doing vigorous exercise is the clothing that we're expected to wear.

High heels damage our feet permanently. Our entire foot is meant to hit the ground – our arches are shock absorbers, and that function can't be carried out if half our foot is in the air. High heels also force our weight forward, making balance difficult, which is awkward as well as danger-ous. Tight shoes of any kind cramp our bones and prevent our feet from breathing.

Tight belts, corsets and girdles, over-tight panty hose and other restrictive garments impede our breathing, circulation and digestion. Bras of course fall into this category, but whereas many small-breasted women will enjoy the comfort and freedom that comes from not wearing a bra, larger-breasted women may always need to wear one for support or because it's painful without. Sometimes a bra is helpful while exercis-ing, especially at times of the month when the breasts can be particularly tender. If and when you wear a bra, be sure it allows you to breathe and move freely.

Very short skirts make it difficult to be active without worrying that this might lead to lecherous comments or even attack. Very long skirts bind one's legs and make it difficult to move or run.

THINGS ARE BEGINNING TO CHANGE

Many women have become as concerned with comfort and practicality as with style and appearance. Increasingly, women wear trousers. More and more, we are rejecting the ridiculous outfits (and postures) of the fashion world, outfits that have encouraged us to mistreat our bodies. A woman we know designed a pair of trousers for hiking and camping which had a zip going from the front to the back of the crotch. You just unzip the trousers and pee standing up – no need for the whole awkward and sometimes humiliating, production of taking your pants down!

There are similar trends in footwear – all of which keep the feet closer to the ground and allow them to live.

There has been a general increase in public athletic facilities – more public swimming pools, skating rinks and even tennis courts. It's no longer unusual to see women jogging along tracks where only men used to run. In almost every area of sports, women are seriously developing strength, confidence and ability. Daily papers are beginning to cover women's events for the first time on a more regular basis. We do not want to see women triumphing over women in ugly, masculine ways. Instead of turning talented people into superstars, we favour providing opportunity and encouragement for all. The Chinese (in the People's Republic), in their games, put friendship first, competition second. Like them we feel it essential that we develop ourselves to be the best we can, each and every woman.

CHOOSING AN EXERCISE

Select exercises that stretch and strengthen the entire body – arms, legs, torso, neck.

Pick activities that feel good, that give pleasure. All mammals need to play, and humans are no exception.

Select something that allows you to pace yourself, with which you can work at enlarging your own capacity, both in the frequency and intensity with which you do it.

For some of us it'll be important to find activities that can be done at home.

The total exercises, such as running or swimming, are the best because they use and therefore develop many different muscles; they keep bodily systems healthy as well as expanding their working ability. Bulging muscles alone won't create good health, but the more solid yet supple the muscle the better. Good back muscles reduce the likelihood of back problems; strong abdominal muscles are also necessary for a healthy back, as well as for holding internal organs in place, for good blood circulation and elimination, and they usually make childbirth and menstruation less painful. In general we'll sit or stand straighter and feel better; everyday tasks will be easier and less tiring.

A total exercise will help your breathing. The exertion of it should make you pant. One woman we knew was afraid that panting meant her body was breaking down. In fact the opposite is true. Working harder, you'll begin to breathe more slowly, deeply, and more regularly. Your lungs will develop a larger capacity for air. With vigorous exercise, blood that is ordinarily pooled in the organs of the body is drawn into circulation; the heart has to pump this increased amount of liquid around faster; over time this means that the heart, a muscle, will strengthen and be able to pump out a greater volume of blood with fewer beats. The contractions and relaxations of the muscles, especially in the legs, which have been called a second heart, will squeeze the veins, helping the blood return upward to the heart. Good circulation ensures that all the muscles and organs get a continually fresh supply of blood, which is essential to their survival and well-being.

Total exercise also helps our attitude towards food and improves our digestion. It regularizes eating habits: we eat more if we need to, but it helps curb the compulsive eating that is a problem for so many women. The movement of the body and its muscles speeds up the peristaltic (wavelike) action of the digestive organs. People who exercise regularly are less prone to constipation and kidney stones.

Exercise will help both body and mind relax and enjoy life. We are not suggesting exercise as a cure-all, as a substitute for changing this oppressive society into a human one we can live in, but we are saying that we need it to relieve the harmful effects of all the frustration, anxiety and anger we experience daily. Exercising regularly will help you sleep better (as long as you don't jog a mile just before bedtime). If your body has good tone and doesn't slouch, your mind will surely function better. Learning and practising many sports is not only a physical exercise but also mentally stimulating since it requires concentration, memorization and creative thinking.

Jogging, as we have said, is one of the best forms of exercise. A mile run in the morning will make you feel better all day long. Wear comfortable, loose-fitting clothes and sturdy, flexible shoes. Build up slowly: start at a slow pace and gradually increase speed and distance. At first walk, then jog, then walk again. As you get stronger, vary periods of slow running with periods of sprinting. This alternation is very good for circulation. Move naturally and let your arms swing. Try to relax, especially your neck and shoulders, and keep a good body posture. Stay off pavements (or run lightly) because the shock of your feet constantly hitting such hard surfaces may result in inflammation of the muscle tissue or cause the calf muscles to be torn away from the bone. Another benefit of running is that it helps varicose veins by pumping the blood up from the legs.

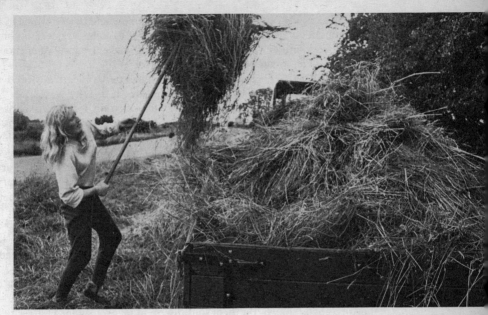

If you don't feel strong enough to try running, then begin to build up strength by walking daily. Get off the bus one stop sooner on the way to work or shopping and use stairs instead of lifts. Move briskly, with strong strides, using your entire leg (impossible to do in high heels!).

Bicycling is fine exercise, especially for the legs.

Swimming is another excellent general conditioner. Try to swim at least several times weekly. Start each session with one, four, or ten lengths, whatever feels comfortable, and build up by pushing yourself to do at least one more length than you think you can.

Group sports are also terrific exercise if done regularly. Netball, hockey, tennis and other ball games will build coordination and endurance and improve agility.

Self-defence arts such as judo, aikido, jujitsu and karate can be excellent forms of exercise. They improve balance, coordination, control and of course strength and endurance. (See also p. 227, 'Self-Defence'.)

Yoga exercises have been developed over many, many years to stimulate or, conversely, take the pressure off your internal organs as well as to improve muscle tone and control, limberness and flexibility. With focus on proper breathing, yoga helps you tremendously to relax and sends healing energy to all parts of your body. After a session of it you will feel revitalized and integrated – mind and body together. In our tense and aggressive society, yoga's total lack of competitiveness is a wonderful release.

Tai chi also stresses rhythmic, flowing body movements performed in a non-competitive way. It is a healthy system of exercise to develop your balance, coordination, flexibility and mental concentration. At a more advanced stage, it can be used for self-defence.

The *Alexander Technique* (see p. 134) can teach us to unlearn destructive physical habits and help us to use our bodies in a healthy way.

Dance can also be a strenuous and exhilarating form of exercise, especially when done regularly and in a disciplined way.

Working at home, there are many exercises you can do to develop strength and flexibility. Some suggestions:

Strengthening exercises include push-ups, leg lifts, sit-ups. There are many good exercise books available at your local bookshop or library that will provide variety and get to a lot of different muscles. When you're beginning to get in shape, try some elementary gymnastic stunts (headstand, cartwheel – there are hundreds) to keep the pure exercise routine from boring you to the point of abandoning it. Having goals to work towards is a great incentive, and there is no end to the challenges for your body.

Use dumbbells to build up arm, shoulder and torso muscles. There is a series of exercises to be done with three-pound weights (available in most sporting-goods shops). Do them faithfully and vigorously for best results. Weight-lifting with an adjustable barbell strengthens trunk and leg as well as arm muscles, and is more exciting. Find out how many presses you should begin with and work up.

Skipping is excellent exercise and doesn't take up much room. Try to jump steadily for a minute, pause to catch your breath, and jump another minute. Repeat three or four times.

Reassess the physical work you do during the day and make each motion using muscles so as to develop but not strain them. Try to build up both sides of your body equally; don't favour the strong side.

Don't bother with gimmicky home exercisers – save your money for healthy foods or real athletic facilities or camping trips or decent hiking shoes.

None of these physical activities is an either-or proposition. Running is a total exercise because it is so good for all your body systems and your leg muscles, but you may want to supplement it with a dumbbell routine to develop your arms. Stretching is very necessary, too. You want flexible muscles as well as strong ones – throughout your body. Joints freeze if you don't keep them moving in all the directions they are designed to move. Whatever you do, do it regularly. Short, frequent periods of practice are better than fewer longer ones.

It might be a good idea to work in a group: many of us lack the discipline to work by ourselves, at least at first. Others of us get lonely or bored. Exercising to music can help. Especially in the initial learning stages of many skills, some organized instruction is necessary (e.g. a keep fit group). In addition to providing technical information, a group can also provide support and encouragement. Women we know studying yoga agreed that they needed the discipline of a class when they began; as their skills and confidence grew, they found it easier to practise alone. In women's groups we can be more open, less self-conscious about our awkwardness or the shape of our bodies.

On the other hand, some women cite the advantages of mixed groups. Some female karate students found the experience of sparring with men valuable – it was realistic and prepared them better for an actual encounter.

SOME FINAL ADVICE

Start slowly and build up, in general and during each session. Muscle growth comes from pushing each muscle involved slightly beyond what you forced it to do the previous time. Stretching (for flexibility) is based on the same principle. But take care. When you're stiff and out of shape you can tear a ligament or even permanently damage a muscle by driving it too violently (this is *always* so). If you want to get into an activity that puts a lot of stress on joints, be sure that the muscles around them are strong (and coordinated) enough to support them; otherwise you may do real damage.

Taper off any period slowly. Never flop down from an energetic run, for example, without some transitional activity such as walking. Your body needs time to adjust its heartbeat, breathing and temperature; it needs to keep up good circulation in order to remove the wastes that have accumulated in the muscles during the run and to bring them fresh supplies of oxygen, glucose and protein. Sudden relaxation may cause dizziness and nausea.

Don't race out into the cold after exercising – that will cause undue stiffness. A hot bath or shower is ideal: it will relax your body, keep circulation up, and clean your body after all the sweating. A hot bath before exercising will increase flexibility.

Don't eat heavily before exercising. The stomach requires a large blood supply to digest food, and exercise diverts blood from the stomach to other muscles. The stomach's attempts to function actively with less blood than it needs may cause pain. Eat a variety of *healthy* foods (see 'Nutrition', p. 114) to meet the demands of greater physical activity and particularly to replace the calcium, sodium chloride and iodine lost through sweating. Except under extreme conditions, you don't need to take salt pills.

Never wear anything too tight or binding. In cold weather especially, wear an outfit (such as track-suit or long underwear) that keeps the heat in to prevent unnecessary stress or injury to joints and muscles.

Get plenty of rest. You'll probably need more once you start working your body harder, and you'll probably sleep better too. See if you can sleep or rest on a moderately hard, flat surface, using only a thin pillow.

Expect some stiffness. If you're really pushing your muscles they're bound to hurt the following day. But don't pamper yourself and stop. The best remedy is moderate exercise: this will increase circulation, which will help carry away the accumulated lactic acid causing the stiffness. Heat and massage applied to a particular muscle are also helpful. They are relaxants and they also dilate the blood vessels, bringing fresh nutrients and speeding waste removal. As you keep exercising, your body will gradually become accustomed to working harder and the discomfort will disappear. You'll be amazed at how much progress you'll make. Occasionally, though, you will overdo it and stretch the ligaments of a joint too far, maybe even tear them (a *sprain*) or pull a muscle or a tendon in much the same way (a *strain*). Unless the injury is severe, you can treat it yourself. Elevate the injured part and apply cold to it as soon as possible. This minimizes pain and swelling. After 24 hours or so, you can switch to moist heat. Rest it until it feels better; then when you are ready to begin exercising again, bind it evenly (not too tight) for support and take it easy. As you start getting in touch with your body you'll be able to sense what you can cure by yourself and what may need some professional help.

Just as you sort out natural soreness from real pain, you need to use judgement about sickness. Never be put off from exercising by psychosomatic symptoms. Many a headache, nervous stomach and fatigue that comes from tension or boredom or unhappiness has been driven off by some exhilarating physical activity. It won't hurt a cold either, but if you're really ill – with fever and other such symptoms – of course you shouldn't push yourself. After a long illness or surgery you need exercise. If you have any physical problem it would be wise to check with a doctor, although you might also get useful suggestions from other people (a physiotherapist, gym teacher, trainer, etc.) or want to experiment carefully on your own.

Exercise during a normal pregnancy is excellent. You'll feel better all the way through and the actual labour will be easier. If you haven't exercised much before getting pregnant, build up sensibly, as you would anyway, but don't worry about jiggling the foetus loose. Even a sport like netball is all right until the eighth month.

Women with special physical problems are often left out of sports or are made to feel so awkward they don't even want to try. We hope this will change. All of us are responsible for helping these women to develop the potential they do have. We know one woman with cerebral palsy who does a lot of swimming and has worked up a really strong punch with her good arm in a self-defence class.

A word about age. In our youth-oriented sexist society the line 'Life begins at forty' appears to be a cruel joke to many women. We may feel more that life ends at forty. In terms of physical activity, it is never too late. At any age you can build up strength, endurance, flexibility and coordination — it just will take a little longer, but it will come, provided the determination is there.

Be patient! It will be hard work and perhaps discouraging at first. You may come home exhausted and dripping wet from jogging one block. You may be frustrated by not being able to make your muscles work the way you want them to at the beginning. But exercise can help change our lives. It has already given many of us new energy, new confidence and greater independence. 'I have more respect for my body. It belongs to me now.' 'Dance has developed my muscles and stretch. It's beautiful to become aware of my capabilities, to grow.' 'Karate has made me feel stronger, more alive, more independent. I can run and dance and even climb a tree. Some days I feel I could fly.'

Alternative Medicine and Preventive Health Care

Most of us know so little about alternatives to orthodox Western medicine that we are quite incapable of assessing their usefulness. We are going to describe, briefly, a number of different systems. The one thing they all have in common is a view of health and ill-health which leads them to look at the whole body, not just its individual parts. They are for this reason particularly successful in curing the chronic conditions from which so many women suffer.

HOMEOPATHY

This system has been practised all over the world since the eighteenth century when it was invented by Samuel Hahnemann. The system was (and still is) scorned by traditional doctors although it was more successful at healing than their bleeding and drugging. Homeopathy is the treatment of 'like by like'. The pioneers of the system studied and documented in great detail the effects of various herbs and venoms on their own bodies. Treatment consists of matching the signs and symptoms of the patient with the substances which would most accurately reproduce those symptoms in a healthy person. This is thought to affect the body's immune processes which then fight off the disease (rather in the way that immunization produces antibodies in the blood ready to fight disease before it strikes). There is no one cure for one condition; the cure is matched to the person.

A good homeopathic doctor will study the patient in great depth, asking questions about life-style and eating habits, noting condition of hair, skin, etc. A really effective cure may make you feel worse before you get better. Few people are prepared to tolerate this and many homeopaths adapt their treatment to minimize bad effects. However a treatment which makes you feel bad for a while could cure a chronic condition for ever.

Every homeopathic doctor has to do a traditional medical course before he or she can register as a doctor. Few doctors train in homeopathy, either because they know nothing about it or because they are loath to spend the extra time studying. Since the practice of homeopathy requires detailed and careful history-taking and diagnosis, the NHS provides a further disincentive, as the payment per patient system discriminates against those who take more time with patients. (See Bibliography, p. 142, for more information on this subject.)

ACUPUNCTURE, ACUPRESSURE AND REFLEXOLOGY

Acupuncture was invented in China at least 5,000 years ago. It is still practised there alongside Western medicine. This system is based on a concept of duality which has its source in Taoism (Yin and Yang, the two poles which must be balanced to ensure harmony and therefore health.) When the balance is upset by unsound eating, bad posture, shallow breathing, etc., disease strikes.

Diagnosis is made by taking the 'pulses' (there are twelve of these relating to twelve different organs of the body), to find the weak points. There are also twelve 'meridians' in the body – nerves which run from one part of the body to the other – and along these 'life energy pathways' lie specific points which, when stimulated, help to balance the flow of energy.

Some of these points are quite familiar to Western medicine: for example, the painful area on top of the shoulder which indicates a spleen condition, or the pain in the left arm which in certain heart conditions follows the exact course of the heart meridian. If a needle is inserted in the right acupuncture point it will alleviate (sometimes cure) the condition, and it is widely used as a form of anaesthetic in which the patient is fully awake but has no sensation in a particular body part. (It is a much safer anaesthetic than that used in the West.)

Acupuncture is theoretically painless, but degrees of sensitivity vary enormously with each patient, and probably with each acupuncturist.

I always found it painful. A very distinct 'nerve pain' like a toothache which I experienced in different parts of my body. I was assured that statistically, women are usually more sensitive, younger women more so, but this is not always so.

For those of us who don't find ordinary acupuncture tolerable, Japanese needles are finer and less painful. If we are too sensitive even for these, another alternative is acupressure; no needles are used, the thumbs or fingertips are pressed quite hard on the relevant points.

Most ailments respond well to acupuncture treatment, but it seems to be most effective in those where the cause is rather obscure: asthma, persistent migraine, rheumatics, digestive disorders and general ill-health. In fact as a mere pick-up it restores energy, sometimes miraculously. It is also extremely valuable on a preventive basis. If the pulses show weakness, action can be taken before disease sets in.

Reflexology: This is similar to acupressure but the pressure points are all on the foot. Each area of the foot corresponds to a part of the body (see Bibliography, p. 143).

NATURE CURE OR NATUROPATHY

Naturopaths believe that ill-health is caused by germs but that they gain a hold only over those bodies which are weakened by bad eating and unhealthy living. They see most symptoms such as rashes, colds, fever, etc. as the body's natural defence mechanisms, a way of expelling the build-up of poisons in the body. If the defence system is run down, the germs will multiply. Treatment involves no use of drugs of any kind, relying on diet, sunshine, fresh air, water, exercise, manipulation and attitude of mind to maintain health. Naturopathy is not a recognized form of medical treatment and therefore naturopaths cannot register as doctors, nor can they practise within the NHS. However, training takes four years and there are plans to start an official state register to separate the trained practitioners from the untrained. See p. 143 for further reading and how to find a naturopath. There are some GPs who have made a special study of nutrition. They are not naturopaths but they are more likely to give sound information on preventive medicine than other traditional doctors. Many of them are members of the McCarrison Society, see p. 143.

HERBALISM

This is one of the oldest forms of healing. Much of it has proved its worth, if only because herbs form the basis of many modern medicines. It makes sense to take them in their natural (and gentler) form for some ailments. Although we can take herbal medicines on our own initiative we may make mistakes if we have no experience. We have listed helpful books in the Bibliography but it is also worthwhile consulting a herbalist, who should be a member of the National Institute of Medical Herbalists (see Resources, p. 144).

OSTEOPATHY

This is a 'first aid' treatment for symptoms caused by joints, slipped discs, etc. but it does not deal with the cause of these problems. Treatment is by manipulation of bones, muscles and tendons and it can relieve headaches caused by muscle tension as well.

THE ALEXANDER TECHNIQUE

The Alexander Technique was originated by F. Matthias Alexander in the late nineteenth and early twentieth centuries. The principle of this technique is basically that by 'un-learning' the habitual ways we have developed of using ourselves (e.g. the way we think, feel, worry, stand, sit, walk, talk, breathe, etc.), we can achieve a better way of functioning. This can have far-reaching implications for our general health, both physical and mental. The implications for women are particularly important, because women have been so pressurized over the years to misuse our bodies – to walk with mincing 'feminine' steps, to wear over-tight clothes and fashionable shoes, and to sit and stand in 'feminine', fashionable ways, all of which distort our whole bodies. No human being was designed to sit with her legs locked together, though many of us have been taught that only that way of sitting is 'permissible'. If we have been taught to misuse our bodies in such a way, it is not surprising that childbirth is for so many of us a painful experience. The Alexander Technique can help us in childbirth (see p. 419) as well as in any other situation – from bending over the sink, or playing a musical instrument, to performing at a job interview or any other potentially anxiety-producing situation. The technique can be *understood* from books (see Bibliography) but cannot be *learnt* from books, as the sensory appreciation (feelings system) is the part that needs re-education. At present we can only have lessons privately, except in rare instances when teachers are employed, for example, by music or drama colleges. However, many teachers operate a sliding scale of fees. The technique is gradually gaining recognition, so hopefully one day it will be more widely available to anyone, regardless of cost.

I started having lessons after I had almost permanent pain in my shoulder and back. The doctor couldn't or wouldn't help, and although a physiotherapist could get rid of the pain, as soon as I stood up and resumed my normal activities, it would return. Now I understand that physiotherapy could not deal with the cause of the problem. Soon after I started having lessons, the pain began to disappear. If it returned I was able to get rid of it by putting into practice what I had learnt. Then the pain disappeared altogether. If I ever get those pains now, I know that it is because I am causing them by my reactions and it is within my power to prevent them from occurring. But the A.T. also made me feel more healthy generally and more competent to act in the world. I can deal with situations which I never dreamed I could and in a way I could never have done. Gradually I am trying to apply what I have learnt to every aspect of my life. The A.T. really opened doors for me.

To find a teacher, see p. 144.

HYPNOTHERAPY

Hypnotherapy can be used in a variety of ways, for nervous conditions, habits such as smoking and personal problems. It can also be used as a way of reducing pain during minor surgery or childbirth. Some GPs practise hypnotherapy as part of general treatment. To find a hypno-therapist, see p. 144.

SELF-EXAMINATION TECHNIQUES*

This is a guide to examining our own vagina, cervix, etc. By examining ourselves regularly we build up a picture of what is normal for us at every stage in the monthly cycle. This helps us to know what is normal for us and spot changes very quickly. Self-examination is a form of preventive

* Adapted from *Second Wave*, Vol. 2, No. 3 (Summer, 1973).

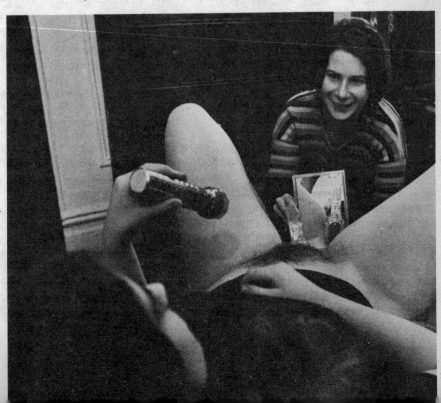

medicine which we can use to diagnose conditions and get treatment early. It is not a substitute for a medical pelvic examination which will be necessary if we need prescribed treatment. It is best to start self-examination in a group where you can discuss and compare what you see with other women, and break down taboos about touching yourself and looking at each other into the bargain. If you want to read more about self-examination read Nancy McKeith's *New Women's Health Handbook*, and for information on existing Health Groups contact WIRES (see p. 570).

You need for self-examination:

Directional light (a strong torch)
Speculum (plastic ones are inexpensive and easier to obtain)
KY Jelly (or similar lubricant, but not vaseline)
Mirror
Firm bed or table, or floor

It's a good idea to have your own plastic speculum to prevent the transfer of infection. Wash it in soap and warm water after each use. Go through the motions of opening and locking the speculum before you actually examine yourself.

1. When you are familiar with manipulation of the speculum, empty your bladder, position yourself comfortably, sitting or lying down with knees bent and feet placed far apart. You may want to prop yourself up on a pillow.
2. Lubricate the speculum with a small amount of KY Jelly. Holding the speculum closed, gently insert it sideways into your vagina, at the same angle you would hold a tampon.
3. When it is in all the way, slowly turn it so that the handle points up.
4. Then grasp the handle and firmly push the shorter, outside section of the handle towards you. This will open the blades of the speculum inside you. If you have not already heard a click, push down the outside section until you do. The speculum is then locked open.
5. If you have never done this before, or are in an awkward position, your vagina may tend to reject the speculum. Also, you may have to move the speculum around or reinsert it before the cervix pops into view. A friend can be very helpful here, particularly if your cervix is off to one side (a common occurrence).
6. It is often easier to have the light pointed at the mirror and the mirror held so that you can see into the tunnel that your speculum has opened up. This pink area, which looks much like the walls of your throat, is your vagina. At the end of the tunnel is a pinkish, bulbous dome-shaped protrusion. That is your cervix. If you don't see it, then gently draw out the speculum and push down with your stomach muscles. This usually causes the cervix to pop into view.

7. To remove the speculum, keep it open and slowly pull it straight out.

I had already been in a health group for some time when we decided to start doing self-examination. Even though it seemed very clear in our minds why we were going to do it, when the appointed time came, we were all pretty apprehensive. We had asked one woman to come and show us what to do, and after she had shown us slides and demonstrated to us, we all felt a lot more comfortable. However, it did seem a big step when the first woman volunteered to start. After that, we all quickly lost our inhibitions, and our first self-examination became an important experience. For many of us we were able to have a clear idea of anatomy for the first time. Our cervices were not at the end of a long dark tunnel, but were easily accessible to view. Doing this in a group was a very positive experience. We were sharing what we were learning, and breaking down taboos all at the same time.

We suggest that you use Chapter 2 on anatomy to help with your examination. Here are some ideas of what you can look for, from the San Francisco Women's Centre. Enter your different findings or comments on a chart, using drawings if necessary.

VULVA: colour of outer lips; colour of inner lips; clitoris; Bartholins glands — not normally seen or felt unless infected.

VAGINAL WALLS: hymen — sometimes seen about an inch in; colour of walls; texture — firm, puffy, ridged, smooth; surface — clean, tender, any discharge.

DISCHARGE: colour — clear, milky white, yellow, greenish; smell — yeasty, fishy, acidic, bland; consistency — thick, thin, stringy, foamy, chunky; amount — profuse, moderate, small. (Look in chapter on vaginal infections for possible reasons for these differences.)

CERVIX: colour — pink, red, bluish; discolourations — red patches, bumps; position of cervix.

OS: shape — dimple, slit; size — open/closed, usual shape; (IUD string length).

MUCOUS SECRETIONS FROM OS: colour; consistency — thick, thin, stringy; smell; amount.

MENSTRUAL BLOOD: Colour; amount.

GENERAL HEALTH INFORMATION: ease of speculum insertion; note if you went off Pill, had IUD removed, painful intercourse, day of cycle.

PELVIC-FLOOR (KEGEL)* EXERCISES

Another form of bodily self-help are Kegel exercises. These involve practising contracting your pelvic-floor muscles. This helps prevent or reduce sagging of the organs and urinary incontinence (losing urine when you cough, sneeze, or laugh), strengthens orgasms, and prepares

* After Arnold Kegel, a pioneering California physician.

for childbirth. Practised regularly, the exercises can help prevent prolapse of the uterus (falling of the uterus into a stretched vagina, which has lost its muscle tone), cystocele (a bulge of the bladder into the vagina) and rectocele (a bulge of the rectum into the vagina).

A good way to locate these muscles is to spread your legs apart while urinating and to start and stop the flow of urine — your ability to do this is one indication of how strong your muscles are. Another method is to try tightening against a man's erect penis during intercourse (this can help to enhance your pleasure, and he will enjoy it too).

Begin exercising these muscles by contracting hard for a second and then releasing completely. Repeat this ten times in a row to make up one group of exercises (this takes about twenty seconds). In a month's time, try to work up to twenty groups during one day (about seven minutes total). You can do this at any time — while sitting in a car or bus, while talking on the telephone, or even as a 'wake-up' exercise. Some of us have noticed improved muscle tone (and occasionally increased pleasure during intercourse) in only several weeks. For more detailed instruction on Kegel exercises, consult your local National Childbirth Trust group.

Physical Examination and Basic Tests

We have included these descriptions of an overall physical examination and pelvic examination as an example of what the Boston Women's Health Collective feels we should all have annually. This sort of care is rarely taken by British doctors even when we have symptoms, and it is practically unheard of as a preventive measure. Most of us expect a peremptory pelvic examination when we have something wrong in that region or when we are pregnant; we do not even get an examination as a matter of course when we are prescribed contraceptives.

- Thyroid palpation.
- Breast examination, including, if necessary, directions for doing a breast self-examination.
- Careful listening to the heart and lungs with stethoscope in several positions.
- Blood-pressure, weight and height measurements.
- Abdominal and pelvic examinations (including speculum, bi-manual and recto-vaginal examinations).
- Complete blood count (CBC), including blood test for cholesterol and triglyceride levels *or* haemoglobin test at a bare minimum.
- Urinalysis, and clean voided specimen if there are cystitis symptoms.
- VD tests.

- Pap test (cervical smear).
- Other tests as may be necessary for our individual health needs.

Ask to have a written copy of all test results.

THE INTERNAL (PELVIC) EXAMINATION

We should expect the following as part of the internal (pelvic) examination at a birth control, VD or antenatal clinic, or from a GP.

INSPECTION OF THE EXTERNAL GENITALS (THE VULVA): The doctor will check for irritations, discolouration, bumps and swellings, crabs, irregular hair distribution, size and/or adhesions of the clitoris, skin lesions and unusual vaginal discharge. You will be checked internally (usually with a gloved finger) and asked about cystoceles and rectoceles (see under 'Kegel Exercises' above), stress incontinence (you will be asked to cough to see if urine will involuntarily flow), presence of pus in Skene's glands (which are at the entrance of the urinary opening), presence of Bartholin's cysts, and strength of pelvic-floor and abdominal muscles.

SPECULUM EXAMINATIONS: With the speculum inserted in place (if metal, it should be pre-warmed), holding open the walls of the vagina, the examiner will look for unusual discharge and inflammation of the vaginal walls, unusual discharge from the cervix, signs of infection, damage or growths and abnormal mucous membrane colour.

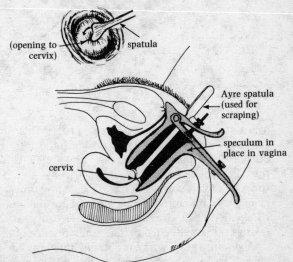

(opening to cervix)

spatula

Ayre spatula (used for scraping)

speculum in place in vagina

cervix

Placement of speculum for a pelvic examination. Spatula scrapes cervix for cervical smear (this is painless)

S/he will then obtain a scraping of tissue from around the cervix for a cervical cancer test. This does not hurt, though too much pressure applied against the cervix during the scraping (only a couple of seconds) may be uncomfortable. In addition, a smear of discharge for microscopic examination and for a culture to test for gonorrhoea should be taken at this time. (Speculum should have only water lubrication for this test.)

If you are curious and have not yet tried self-examination, ask for help to position a light and mirror so that you can see yourself (also see 'Self-Examination Techniques', p. 135).

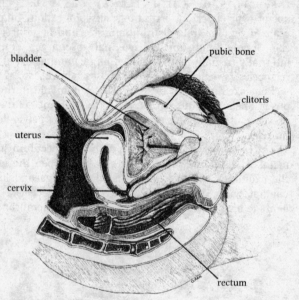

bladder

pubic bone

clitoris

uterus

cervix

rectum

Bimanual pelvic examination

BIMANUAL VAGINAL EXAMINATION: This involves the insertion of the index and middle fingers of one hand into the vagina and, on the outside, the palpation of the lower abdominal wall. The examiner will feel the size, shape, movability, consistency and position of the uterus, tubes and ovaries and will try to locate any unusual growths, pelvic pain, evidence of inflammation or other abnormalities.

Palpation of the uterus should cause no pain; often, palpation of the ovaries hurts a little (sometimes the presence of this pain is the only way the examiner knows s/he is actually touching the ovaries – they are *very difficult* to find). It helps both you and the examiner if you can relax; it may help to breathe through your mouth and to focus on relaxing your hands, neck and back, as well as your abdomen.

RECTO-VAGINAL EXAMINATION: The examiner inserts one finger into the vagina and one into the rectum to get more information about the tone and alignment of the pelvic organs and adnexal region (includes ovaries, tubes, and ligaments of the uterus); about rectal problems; and about the tone of the rectal sphincter muscle. This can be an unpleasant procedure for some women – talking about any discomfort you may have usually helps. Also, you may feel as though you are having a bowel movement as the examiner's finger withdraws from the rectum, but this will not happen.

There are wide variations in the skill and sensitivity of those who give internal exams; there are also differences in the ability of individual women to relax, which can make the same technique feel very different. You can do Kegel exercises (p. 137) and practise inserting a tampon or a speculum in advance of an internal, to help you learn relaxation.

Bibliography and Resources

NUTRITION

Bright, Spencer, 'Catering for the Community', *Time Out*, No. 347, 1976. A guide to starting a food co-op with information on wholesalers and existing co-ops in London.

Boyle, Godfrey, and Harper, Peter, *Radical Technology*, Wildwood House, 1976. Has a good section on nutrition.

Davis, Adelle, *Let's Eat Right to Keep Fit*, Allen & Unwin, 1971. She wrote many other books on the subject. Her theories are sometimes controversial, particularly in regard to her high-protein diet.

HMSO, *Manual of Nutrition*, 1970. Comprehensive, informative, with food charts and suggestions for how to plan diets.

Lappe, Francis Moore, *Diet for A Small Planet*, Ballantine, New York, 1971. Excellent book. Food combinations to produce high protein, good recipes. (Available from Compendium, see p. 573.)

McGuire, Thomas, *The Tooth Trip*, Wildwood House, 1973. A rather trendy look at dental care with particular reference to nutrition. It is clear, straightforward and would be good for children as well as adults.

Orbach, Susie, *Fat is a Feminist Issue*, Paddington Press, 1978.

Reekie, Jennie, *Everything Raw*, Penguin, 1978.

Samuels, Mike, and Bennett, Hal, *The Well Body Book*, Wildwood House, 1974. Oriented towards preventive medicine with a good chapter on food.

Shirley, Oliver, *The Future of Food*, Open University, Man Made Futures course, Design and Technology units 7 and 8, Future Access File 1975. A critique of food technology.

Thomas, Anna, *The Vegetarian Epicure*, Penguin, 1976.

Thompson & Morgan, Seed Catalogues, London Road, Ipswich IP2 0BA. Full information on sprouting peas and beans come with their seed packets, with some recipes.

Wordsworth, Jill, *The Diet Revolution*, Gollancz, 1976. A cool look at all the food theories, extremely informative and easy to read.

Yudkin, John, *This Slimming Business*, Penguin, 1965.

Yudkin, John, *Pure White and Deadly*, Davis Poynter, 1972. Main argument is against the consumption of carbohydrates.

Bruce, Liza, and Barber, Nicholas, *Alternative Cookery*, Tandem, 1975. Although many ingredients are American, the recipes are easy to follow and adapt.

The Bulk Buy Bureau, 18 Queen Anne's Gate, London SW1H 9AA (01 839 2846). Government-sponsored information on bulk buying, part of National Consumer Council.

EXERCISE

Morris, Margaret, *My Life in Movement*, Peter Owen, 1969. Dance therapy.

Rush, Anne Kent, *Getting Clear: Body Work for Women*, Wildwood House, 1974. A book for women on how to open ourselves up. Has a lot of good stuff on self-awareness through therapy and role playing, massage, relaxation, women's health, including the pelvic self-examination and so forth.

Times Science Report, 'Sport: Women catching up with Men', 23 March, 1976.

Women's Report, 'Women and Sport', Vol. 2, issue 6, 1974.

Women's Report, 'Further thoughts on Women and Sport', Vol. 3, issue 1, 1974.

HOMEOPATHY

Blackie, Marjorie G., *The Patient, Not the Cure: The Challenge of Homeopathy*, Macdonald and Jane's, 1976.

Chandra, Sharma, *Manual of Homeopathy and Natural Medicine*, Turnstone Press, 1975.

Ruthven Mitchell, G., *Homeopathy*, W. H. Allen, 1975. An interesting if wordy historical account — unfortunately rather sexist.

For a list of GPs who practise homeopathy in your area contact the Homeopathic Faculty at the **Royal Homeopathic Hospital** (see below), or, if you live near one of the following hospitals, make an appointment at their out-patient clinic.

Royal Homeopathic Hospital, Great Ormond Street, London WC1N 3HR (01 837 3091).

Glasgow Homeopathic Hospital for Children, 221 Hamilton Road, Glasgow E2 (041 778 1185). Also sees adult out-patients.

Glasgow Homeopathic Hospital, 1000 Great Western Road, Glasgow W2 (041 339 0381–2).

Glasgow Homeopathic Outpatient Department, 5 Lyndeoch Crescent, Glasgow C3 (041 332 4490).

Bristol Homeopathic Hospital, Cotham, Bristol 6 (0272 33068-9).

Tunbridge Wells Homeopathic Hospital, Church Road, Tunbridge Wells, Kent (0892 26111).

The **Mossley Hill Hospital**, Park Avenue, Mossley Hill, Liverpool L18 (051 724 2335).
The **Department of Homeopathy**, 1 Myrtle Street, Liverpool L7 7DE (051 709 5475).

ACUPUNCTURE

De Langre, J., *The First Book of Do-In, Guide Pratique*, Happiness Press, 1971. Excellent guide to self-help acupressure, available from Compendium (see p. 51) in English.
Ingham, Eunice, *Stories the Feet can Tell*, Ingham Publications, USA, 1951. On Reflexology, available from Compendium.
Irwin, Y., *Shiatzu*, Routledge & Kegan Paul, 1977. Explains how to do Japanese acupressure to yourself or to others; refreshingly uses feminine pronouns throughout.
Lawson-Wood, Joyce and Denis, *The Incredible Healing Needles*, Thorsons, 1974.
Mann, Felix, *Acupuncture Cure of Many Diseases*, Pan, 1973.
Thie, J. F., *et al.*, *Touch for Health*, De Vorss and Co., USA, 1973. Teaches you how to follow meridians yourself. Available from Compendium.

The **Acupuncture Association**, 2 Harrowby Court, Seymour Street, London W1. Can supply lists of acupuncturists.

NATUROPATHY

British Naturopathic and Osteopathic College and Clinic, 6 Netherhall Gardens, London NW3 (01 435 7830).
Tyringham Clinic, Newport Pagnell, Bucks (Newport Pagnell 610450). A charitable clinic which takes people who cannot afford fees.
Nature Cure Clinic, 15 Oldbury Place, London W1 (01 935 2787). Staffed on a part-time basis by registered doctors, this clinic offers treatment through diet, homeopathy and acupuncture.
Naturopathic Private Clinic for Women, 11 Alderton Crescent, London NW4 (01 202 6242).
The Kingston Clinic, 291 Gilmerton Road, Edinburgh EH16 5UQ (031 664 3435). Also provides information on trained naturopaths.
The McCarrison Society, c/o Dr Barbara Latto, 5 Derby Road, Caversham, Reading, Berks, for information on the research and education on diet in medicine organized by the Society.

HERBALISM

Beckett, Sarah, *Herbs for Feminine Ailments*, Thorson, 1973.
Culpeper, Dr Nicholas, *Culpeper's Complete Herbal*, Foulsham, 1952.
Kloss, Jethro, *Back to Eden*, Lancer Books, New York, 1976.
Loewenfeld, Claire, *Herb Gardening and Why and How to Grow Herbs*, Faber, 1964.

Loewenfeld, Claire, *Herbs for Health and Cookery*, Pan 1971.
Loewenfeld, Claire, *Herbal Teas for Health and Pleasure*, Health Sciences Press, 1968.
Potters New Encyclopaedia of Botanical Drugs and Preparations. Health Sciences Press, 1970. A comprehensive guide to treatment.
Rutherford and Warren-Davis, *A Pattern of Herbs*, Allen & Unwin, 1975.

The National Institute of Medical Herbalists, 68 London Road, Leicester. For lists of herbalists.
Society of Herbalists, 34 Boscobel Place, London SW1 (01 235 1530). A library. Members of the society get cheaper treatment.
Herbal suppliers: Culpeper House, Bruton Street, London W1; Crittens, 39 Park Road, London SE7; G. Baldwin & Co., 173 Walworth Road, London SE17.

OSTEOPATHY

The British School of Osteopathy, 16 Buckingham Gate, London SW1 (01 834 5085).
The Osteopathic Association Clinic, 25 Dorset Square, London NW1 (01 262 1128).

ALEXANDER TECHNIQUE

Barlow, Wilfred, *The Alexander Principle*, Gollancz, 1973; Arrow, 1975.
Maisel, Edward (ed.), *The Alexander Technique*, Thames & Hudson, 1974.

The Constructive Teaching Centre Ltd, 18 Lansdowne Road, Holland Park, London W11 (01 727 7222).
The Society for Teachers of the Alexander Technique, 3 Albert Court, Kensington Gore, London SW7 (01 589 3834).
Both these organizations can put you in touch with teachers.

HYPNOTHERAPY

British Hypnotherapy Association, 67 Upper Berkeley Street, London W1 (01 262 8852). Provides details of non-medical practitioners.
Society for Medical and Dental Hypnosis, 10 Chillerton Road, London SW17 (01 672 3025). Provides details of medical practitioners.

GENERAL

Benjamin, Harry, *Everybody's Guide to Nature Cure*, Thorson, 1973.
Brodsky, *From Eden to Aquarius*, Bantam, 1974. Several different alternative treatments.
Inglis, Brian, *Fringe Medicine*, Faber & Faber, 1964.
Kinnersley, Pat, *The Hazards of Work*, Pluto, 1973.

Leamington Spa Good Earth Society, 10a Beauchamp Avenue, Leamington Spa, Warwicks. The centre provides information and classes on various forms of alternative medicine.

The Whitecross Society, 82 Bell Street, London NW1 (01 262 0991). Seeks to provide 'alternatives to the use of unpredictable drugs and help the individual in an active personal pursuit of health'. Runs inquiry service and courses.

7 Common Medical and Health Problems. Traditional and Alternative Treatments

In this chapter we look at the most common conditions and infections which affect women specifically. The first section deals with non-infectious conditions, and the second section goes into all kinds of infection of the genitals and urinary tract. Most of us do not recognize the names of our afflictions so we have written a symptom guide at the end to help you find your way around the chapter (see p. 210). We couldn't include every condition which we can suffer from and proper diagnosis is usually essential.

For those of us who use self-examination of the vagina (see p. 135), or the breasts (see p. 152), many infections and abnormalities can be discovered at an early stage and treated before unpleasant symptoms arise.

Anaemia and Hypertension

Anaemia and hypertension are systemic (affecting all parts of the body) and may cause serious health problems if not cared for soon enough. Frequently we don't recognize the symptoms of these conditions and, as a result, don't do anything about them until we're very obviously sick. Many doctors don't recognize the symptoms either; they often attribute them to some psychological disorder.

ANAEMIA

Menstruating women need to anticipate iron-deficiency anaemia, which results from a shortage of red blood cells. The symptoms include pallor, extreme fatigue, dizziness, shortness of breath and occasionally bone pain. The best preventive is good nutrition, involving adequate intake of iron, calcium, vitamin C and the B vitamins, particularly B_{12} and folic acid. If you can't eat enough iron-rich food, there are many iron products for sale, so ask for the generic name – *ferrous sulphate* or *ferrous gluconate* or *fumarate* – that's the cheapest way of buying them.

A full blood count done in a lab on blood removed from a vein in your arm is the only accurate way to detect anaemia and to determine its cause. But there is one quick, simple test, called a haemoglobin test, which can be done in a doctor's surgery without going to a lab. It won't help much if you're borderline, but it will quickly pick up more serious anaemic conditions. It is a good way to decide whether a further, more elaborate test is needed.

HYPERTENSION

Hypertension means high blood pressure. It has been called 'the quiet killer' because even though just having high blood pressure doesn't kill you immediately, it can, if untreated, lead to heart disease and strokes, which *are* the leading killers of both men and women in Britain and the USA. Even younger women and babies are showing signs of hypertension. We do not yet know how early hypertension affects life expectancy. This unknown factor is becoming more important as larger numbers of women take the Pill, since about 25% of women who use the Pill develop hypertension (see Birth Control chapter, p. 248).

Hypertension may be accompanied by warning symptoms such as headache, dizziness, fainting spells, ringing in the ears, etc. The only way to get a sure diagnosis is to take periodic blood-pressure readings. (Sometimes specialized blood tests may be necessary.) Taking blood pressure is simple; many people could learn this basic skill, particularly those of us who have hypertension or have it in our families.

'Essential' hypertension is the name given to 95% of all cases of high blood pressure (those not caused by specific glandular or hormonal abnormalities). Causes are still being investigated. Apart from the Pill, they include the following:

1. Diet.
2. Obesity (excess weight).
3. Stress (from both emotional and life-style factors).
4. Hereditary links.
5. Water supply.

Diet can play a key role in controlling hypertension, by reducing salt intake in particular. The balance of protein and carbohydrates in our diets is another important factor. But the greatest tragedy about hypertension is the possibility that it is truly a disease of malnutrition and poverty. The fact that blacks, especially women, appear to be more susceptible than whites may simply mean that too many black people have tried to live too long on inadequate protein and protein substitutes. Foods that are high in fats and carbohydrates are often cheapest, so poorer people, of all races, have learned to survive on them; women usually feed themselves last. Also it can be difficult to give up high-salt and high-sugar foods that are giving so much (sometimes the only) pleasure in life to isolated and restricted people like the poor and the elderly. Unfortunately, most work on hypertension does not deal with these cultural and economic realities.

There is a remarkable correlation between high rates of hypertension and geographic areas where the water is soft. It is not yet fully understood whether this is because of something beneficial in hard water or something harmful in soft water. Evidence suggests that the acidity of soft water is the problem – that acid water attacks surrounding earth and rocks to extract trace elements, such as cadmium, which is strongly linked to hypertension. Although more research is needed, soft water is clearly more significantly related to hypertension than are such factors as socioeconomic background, education, stress, or smoking (all repeatedly investigated in the past, though with less significant results). Also, cadmium is one of the prominent trace minerals in refined white flour products. It may be that the combined amounts of cadmium in soft water and in white flour products have become harmful for many of us.

Hypertension is usually controlled by drugs; however, it can also be controlled by diet. 'Biofeedback' and meditation can help too. The former involves a special machine that signals bodily responses and can be used to teach control over them.

Breast Problems*

In this country breasts have an exaggerated sexual significance to both men and women. Breasts are displayed provocatively (but never fully exposed) as a way of titillating male consumers into buying everything from cars to whisky. Topless waitresses and dancers are the final step in this process. This exaggeration and objectification has a profound effect on many women, and fosters feelings of insecurity:

Going braless was for some of us an attempt to deal with the stereotyped image of women. It was a way of saying, 'This is my natural woman

Requests for breast augmentation surgery are increasing. A Manchester hospital doctor told the *Evening Standard* that women hope 'Improved femininity might rekindle sexual attraction where the husband is straying from the marital bed'.

* See also 'Breasts', Chapter 2, p. 24.

shape and I like it and I'm not going to push it into some distorted line or hide it just because it's "unfashionable".' But the braless look has since become fashionable, and for some men it has made breasts more titillating than ever. Meanwhile there are still strong taboos about breast-feeding in public.

If your breasts are young, they can probably go unsupported for a year or so without any long-term ill effects, but the sheer laws of physics are thought by some to cause a breast of any size to begin to sag eventually. Whether this matters is of course entirely up to you. There *are* times when many of us need to wear bras for comfort's sake, e.g. during sporting activities or while pregnant. There is a myth that breast-feeding causes breasts to sag, while it is just the failure to support the extra weight with a good bra.

Our breasts can be intensely pleasurable to us although this response varies tremendously from woman to woman. Some women experience orgasm from breast stimulation alone, or from nursing an infant. This sexual context makes it hard for us to think about breasts as functional parts of our bodies that need health care and attention from us. It also makes breast problems particularly disturbing.

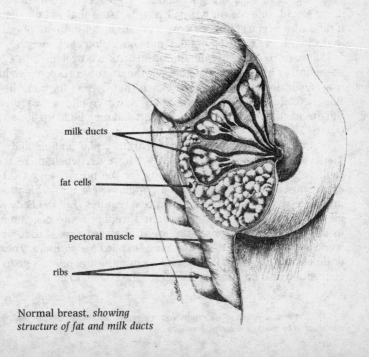

milk ducts

fat cells

pectoral muscle

ribs

Normal breast, *showing structure of fat and milk ducts*

COMMON BENIGN PROBLEMS

One of the most common problems is the monthly swelling and painful tenderness (*mastodynia*) that often precedes a period. Wearing a bra can be helpful, especially one of the stretchy types. Adopting measures to relieve pre-menstrual tension, of which breast tenderness is a part, can also help (see p. 172).

As we get older, many of us find that the swelling can become chronic and often includes a kind of lumpy texture. Sometimes after our period is over, some of the lumpiness remains. In fact, a certain amount of lumpiness is normal. If we have not been in the habit of examining our breasts each month after our period – and even if we have – we may suddenly discover what feels like a distinct lump that wasn't there before. While hundreds of women rush immediately to the nearest doctor, hundreds of others remain silent, afraid to go to a doctor because they are sure it *is* cancer and they can't face the thought of it. But the chances are (roughly nine out of ten) that the problem is caused by something far less worrying.

The problem of swelling and lumpiness affects many of us, particularly in our childbearing years. In its chronic, recurring state, this lumpy condition may be either *fibroadenosis* (multiple tiny nodules) or (chronic) *cystic mastitis*,* sometimes called 'fibrocystic disease'. A lump may be a *fibroadenoma* (a solid benign tumour). The label 'chronic disease' has a scary sound. One reason it is called a disease is that not all women have it, and also because it represents a failure or an inability of our systems to deal with the build-up of fluid and congestion each month.

Compare the breast with the uterus. As we explained in Chapter 2, the monthly build-up of the lining of the uterus in response to hormones is a preparation for pregnancy. When that doesn't happen, the lining is sloughed off and the cycle starts again. However, after a great many cycles the uterine lining may begin to thicken and may build up fibroid tumours (see p. 177).

A similar thing happens to the breast. It builds up fluid and glandular tissue in preparation for pregnancy. However, when there is no conception, there is no convenient way for the breasts to get rid of these extra substances. While there is a lymph system into which the breasts drain (see diagram, p. 151), the process requires that the body reabsorbs all this extra substance rather than shedding some of it immediately, as the uterus does. (Lymphatics are thin-walled vessels that form a network from the breast to certain glands called *lymph nodes*. These vessels drain tissue fluids from the breast.) As months and months go by without conception, it is harder and harder for the system to do this.

---

* *Mastitis* is an infection which results from a plugged milk duct in a breast-feeding mother, and is not to be confused with *cystic mastitis*.

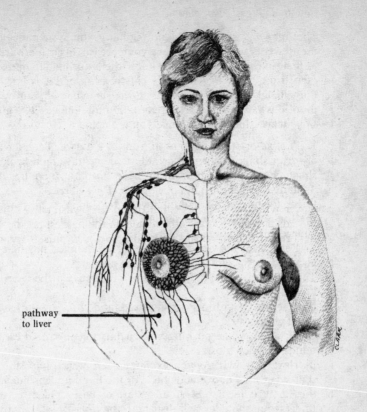

pathway
to liver

The lymphatic system of the breast, *showing drainages to nodes under the arms, under the breastbone, and pathways to the liver and neck*

Without pregnancy, some congestion may become more or less permanent (pregnancy usually clears this up). Fluids get trapped in the ducts to form sacs called cysts, which are rarely harmful, or solid lumps called fibroadenomas, which virtually never become cancers. Most of these benign lumps are approximately round, move around freely under the skin, and don't seem to be attached to the chest beneath. There is often an accompanying tenderness to the touch, though not always.

In over 80% of all cases one of these benign conditions causes the 'lumps'. Fibroadenomas are more common than cysts but don't usually disappear with pregnancy. Unlike cysts, they are less frequent with advancing age, becoming rare in our forties. Fibroadenosis is not serious and also tends to disappear with pregnancy.

How to do breast examination

The following should be done regularly and systematically every month. It is worth examining your breasts even more frequently at first, so that you can get to know them during all phases of your menstrual cycle. If you are of childbearing age it is best to do it immediately after your period, on the same day of your cycle each month, when your breasts are at minimum fullness. It is important to be warm and relaxed while you are doing it.

1. First sit or stand straight in front of a mirror. Look for changes of size or shape in each breast. Most people have breasts of unequal shape or size. It is important to make sure that there has not been a change in the normal appearance of *your* breasts.
Check for puckering or dimpling of the skin. You may have to lift the breasts to see underneath. Check nipples for changes or discharge but *don't* squeeze them.
2. Raise arms above head and check for changes, paying attention also to the area which goes up to the armpit.
Turn to each side slightly so that you can see the sides of your breast too.
Lean forward, with arms still raised, and check again for any unusual changes.
Check again while pushing your palms together or pressing your hands on your hips.
3. Next, lie down. As you examine each breast, have the arm on that side raised above your head or the hand under your head and the elbow lying flat. A small pillow or large folded towel placed under your shoulder will distribute the breast tissue more evenly. Also examine each breast with the arm lying along your side or hanging over the edge of the bed.

Feel your breast gently and systematically with the front part of the flat of your hand, keeping the fingers straight and together. If you use your fingertips, you can become confused, particularly if you have glandular breasts, since fingertips can pick up all sorts of irregularities. The flat of the hand should be able to pick up any abnormal lumps. It can be easier to feel your breasts in the bath, while your hands are soapy. Examine your breasts systematically. Some people recommend mentally dividing the breast into quarters or halves, others into three horizontal sections. Whatever you do, you must include all parts of the breast, including the nipple and under the arm. At first it is difficult to judge how much pressure to use, so it might help to ask someone experienced to show you. Do *not* squeeze or pinch the breast. Remember that it is *changes* that you are looking for.

BREAST EXAMINATION

Opposite is a summary of the best leaflets and booklets on self-examination. If you want a more detailed idea of what you are looking for and how to do it, with lots of pictures and diagrams, see 'Breast Cancer Self-Examination, an Aid to Early Detection', published by BUPA, or Rose Kushner (see Bibliography, p. 212).

Importance of Breast Examination

Although cancer is not the leading cause of death of women in Britain, breast cancer kills more women than any other cancer – over 11,000 annually in England and Wales – and it *is* the leading cause of death for women aged 37–55. Many of these deaths are preventable by early diagnosis and treatment. One woman in seventeen will develop breast cancer and this rate may be rising.

The importance of examining your own breasts both regularly and systematically cannot be over-emphasized. You are the best monitor of your breasts, better than any doctor, who cannot possibly detect changes in them better than you can. As one breast cancer specialist has said,

A large proportion of women who come to me diagnosed by a physician as having a breast lump do not have one, whereas 90% of those who come saying 'I have a lump I have found myself' do have one.

But even though many of us know that breast self-examination is important, we still cannot bring ourselves to do it. We can help each other break down lifelong attitudes and taboos by getting together and sharing our fears and difficulties. Women in consciousness-raising or self-help groups can meet with experienced people and learn together. Then they can help other women to learn.

What Are You Looking for in a Breast Examination?

Basically, you are looking for changes. That is why it is important to do this examination regularly, so that you get to know your breasts and can spot changes – like the following:
Unusual lump, thickening or local lumpy areas. (Many lumps give the feeling of rubbing the flat of your hand over a knuckle of the other one, but even soft lumps should be properly investigated.)
Unusual change in the size or shape of a breast.
One breast unusually higher or lower than the other.
Puckering or dimpling of the skin of the breast.
Unusual drawing back or turning in of the nipple.
Discharge from the nipple.
Skin trouble on or around the nipple, or change in skin texture.

Swelling of the upper arm.
Enlarged lymphatic nodes (see above, p. 150).
Pain or discomfort not felt before, and not confined to the time just before
or during a period.

If You Find a Lump

Most lumps you find will probably tend to get suddenly larger before
your period and then go down or even disappear altogether a week
afterwards. These are almost certainly benign, fluid-filled cysts. Once
you have got to know your breasts, you will immediately be able to spot
any changes, unrelated to your normal menstrual pattern. If, after a
month of noticing these changes, they don't disappear, you should then
take skilled medical advice without delay.

As in other areas of medicine, with breast lumps doctors can sometimes be dangerously unhelpful and incompetent. We must be prepared
for this. Some doctors do not know how to examine breasts:

*I went to the family planning clinic for my routine Pill prescription. I asked the
doctor to examine my breasts. I practically had to force him to do this and then
found out that he had no idea how to do it! He just got hold of them and
squeezed them.*

Others do not know what to do with a lump if they are shown one:

*I went to my doctor with a small, pea-sized lump. Without doing any tests, he
told me it was a milk lump and not to worry. Three months later I went
back because it had got bigger. He said the same thing. Three months after
that, the lump (now the size of a golf ball) became very painful. I went to a
different doctor who sent me to hospital straight away. It was cancer, and
my doctor had left it to spread. (Young woman in her mid-twenties)*

Sometimes doctors assume that because a lump is painful, or because
the woman is young, the problem is not cancer. A cancerous lump is
often painless but that does not mean that a painful lump should be
discounted. Similarly, although cancer in a young woman is relatively
rare, a lump should always be carefully investigated. A sore nipple can
be a skin disorder, but it could be cancer and again, should be investigated.

It is of course frightening to discover that doctors can be gratuitously
reassuring. But unless we are aware that this can happen, we cannot
begin to stand up for ourselves. We must learn from other women's
experiences. In the case of breast cancer, it can be very easy to be
reassured:

*It was my boyfriend who first noticed the lump in my left breast. He persuaded
me to visit a doctor which I did, albeit reluctantly. The local, male GP was*

reassuring. He examined my breasts, said that it was a swollen gland common among women taking the Pill (which I had been on for seven years) and told me not to worry. Over the next weeks I was relieved to find that the lump did seem to reduce in size. Looking back, I wonder how much of this was wishful thinking and imagination. A few months later I made a routine visit to the F P A. I mentioned to the doctor that I had a small lump in the breast. She did not seem keen to examine me but finally agreed. After examining both breasts she said that she had found nothing. Feeling over-anxious and fussy I began to question her further. She replied by reassuring me that if I had a 'cyst' she wouldn't be giving me the Pill. As she said this she signed me up for a six-month supply.

As I stood in the queue to collect supplies I decided to take out my treatment card and see what the doctor had written. To my bewilderment I read the words 'Nodule in left breast'. I still find this incident inexplicable. I couldn't face going back in to confront her so I collected the pills and went home feeling very shocked and puzzled. I picked up a leaflet as I went out which proclaimed 'Don't gamble with breast cancer!' The leaflet informed me that early treatment was essential and that anyone finding a lump should see a doctor immediately!

When I look back on these incidents I feel furious with myself for my spinelessness. Yet if the doctors would not take the lump in my breast seriously it was a great temptation for me to take their reassurances at face value. What woman does not dread that a lump will turn out to be cancer and that she will lose her breast and with it her sexual identity. These deeply repressed fears prevented me from fighting the apathy I encountered. I think this may be an important point in helping other women get treatment fast — to recognize the reluctance to fight an issue like this. (Lin Layram in Spare Rib, *37)*

In conclusion, if you find a change in your breasts and it is different from your usual cyclical changes after a month's observation you should expect your doctor to be suspicious and to refer you to a clinic or doctor specializing in breast problems. If your G P is unhelpful, you can try referring yourself to a clinic (see below). Some clinics allow self-referral. If yours doesn't, you can change your GP (see p. 557). Remember, very few G P s or family planning doctors are in a position to make a diagnosis: they haven't the facilities nor the expertise.

Diagnostic Tests

Usually, only a pathologist's microscopic examination of cells from the lump (a *biopsy*) will provide certain diagnosis. However, you do *not* necessarily have to undergo anaesthesia and surgical biopsy right away. This depends on which hospital you go to and who is in charge of your case. At present, all training in the U K involves seeing breast disease as a surgical problem. Only the most progressive clinics see it as a 'medical' problem, i.e. involving all sorts of experts. Thus, most GPs will refer you to a surgeon. However, you *can* ask to be referred to a centre specializing in breast problems, in which case you have more chance of seeing someone who is an expert in diagnosing – and treating – breast symptoms . . . not necessarily a surgeon. (You can find out about your nearest centre by consulting one of the organizations on p. 213.)

If you are referred to a surgeon at the local hospital, it is unlikely that he will perform any tests other than a surgical biopsy involving general anaesthetic (see below). But at a breast clinic a variety of tests are likely to be used. For example, Professor Forrest's breast clinic at Edinburgh Royal Infirmary sees about 1,000 women a year. Only about 300 of these need some form of biopsy (and only one quarter of this 300 will have cancer, incidentally). The other 700 are given one or other of the following diagnostic tests: *mammography*, similar to the type of X-ray used by dentists; *xerography*, or *xeroradiography*, similar to the above but producing a picture of the breast tissue which is easier to 'read' (it also involves larger doses of radiation at present); *thermography*, a totally harmless technique in which a heat-sensing device produces a 'picture' of any area where a high level of cellular activity is going on. None of the techniques is perfect; they are only as good as the people who use them.* Thus, there is no point in trusting anybody who says that you don't need a biopsy unless they are experienced in diagnosing breast diseases. It is of course difficult to ask doctors about their training and experience, but this is what it all boils down to, particularly in the case of breast disease.

X-ray tests should not be used on anyone under 40 unless there is a very pressing reason. Again, it is the judgement of an experienced person that counts. Most breast X-rays done once involve less radiation hazard than a chest X-ray. But the reason for caution is that once mammography or xerography has been used it is likely to be used again (at present, xerography should be used only when *absolutely* necessary). More government support is needed in order to develop low-dose X-ray techniques. As one specialist says, it is disgraceful that this support is not available. In some hospitals – particularly those that have specialist breast clinics – special equipment exists which enables minimum doses of radiation to be used. This is not necessarily the case elsewhere (see Rose Kushner, p. 212).

If your tests confirm that a lump is present, or if you don't want to trust your doctor's diagnosis, you will need a biopsy.

Needle Biopsy Often it is possible to have a 'needle biopsy' on a distinct lump right in the examination room. A needle is inserted directly into

*For more about these techniques see Jill Rakusen, *Spare Rib*, 42.

the lump, and a local anaesthetic is given. In a great many cases the lump then collapses, yielding fluid which can be drawn into the syringe (aspiration), showing the lump to be a cyst. (Other kinds of lumps require surgical biopsy – see below.) This fluid, which also contains some cells from the wall of the cyst at the point of entry, can be analysed in a laboratory for the presence of any abnormal cells (though these are rarely found). While it is of course possible for some cancerous cells to be present in another part of the cyst wall, this is extremely unlikely, particularly if there are no other signs or symptoms, or any history of pathology. When in doubt, your doctor can re-examine a drained cyst via air injection followed by a new mammogram. In any case, you *must* be examined again one month later: cysts can refill, or they can (rarely) become cancerous. Cysts may need to be aspirated for years!

If a needle biopsy is *not* offered before a surgical biopsy you could ask why. Mammograms should also be performed as well, in order to check the rest of the breast. The decision as to what procedure(s) to use should be made jointly between a woman and her doctor.

Surgical Biopsy   If the needle biopsy does not collapse the lump and reveal it as a cyst, it is probably a benign tumour, or fibroadenoma, but it should be surgically removed. In order to be positive it is not cancerous, a section of it must be examined under a microscope by a pathologist.

Unfortunately, most biopsies are performed as 'frozen sections': this means that the laboratory examination is done as quickly as possible while the woman remains under general anaesthetic, so that if cancer cells are found, the whole breast can be removed at the same time. Such haste is unnecessary. Apart from the dangers of anaesthesia and diagnostic error which although minimal, do exist with this dual procedure,* the psychological risks of this procedure are only now, after fifty years of use, being questioned. In any case, cancer treatment (see below) may not necessarily involve surgery.

If after a thorough explanation and discussion you agree with your doctor that a surgical biopsy must be performed, you will probably want to ask that the biopsy be done as an end procedure – that is, that no plans be made for further treatment until the results are known.† The argument that this procedure might 'knock' cancer cells into the system is no longer considered a valid excuse for the simultaneous procedure (see Rose Kushner, *Breast Cancer*).

* See Jill Rakusen, *Spare Rib*, 37.

† There has been discussion recently about the possible advantages of having a surgical biopsy under local anaesthetic, as some people think it is likely to be less traumatic than under a general. Others would disagree. If you prefer the idea of a local, for example, because it can be performed on an outpatient basis, you could discuss it with the specialist. It is, however, doubtful whether you should contemplate this procedure unless you are in the hands of an experienced specialist and, even then, few doctors – or women – would feel happy with a local unless the lump were easily accessible.

Whatever kind of biopsy you have, it is best that it is performed by a specialist in breast diseases rather than by a general surgeon. Again, you *can* insist on going to a clinic specializing in breast diseases, although you may need some support from your sisters if your doctor's feelings are hurt and he becomes difficult.

If your lump turns out to be cancer, there is no reason whatsoever why your breast should be removed at the same time as a biopsy is performed. Some doctors have even been known to remove the breast without properly warning the patient. In fact, there are very good reasons – apart from the psychological ones – against doing this. As Maureen Roberts of Edinburgh Royal Infirmary says, 'Before we do a mastectomy we first investigate to see whether the disease has spread beyond the breasts and we do this by performing X-rays, scans, blood tests and possibly urine tests. This is called "preoperative staging". If the cancer has already spread, there's really no reason to do a mastectomy.' These tests are standard at other specialist clinics (e.g. Guys Hospital and the Royal Marsden in London). In any case, delay rather than speed is now considered physically beneficial by some doctors.*

If you have to undergo a surgical biopsy, be careful to read the wording of the permission forms you sign.

BREAST CANCER

Causes

No one yet knows exactly what causes breast cancer. There are virus theories and immune-system-breakdown theories for cancer in general. In the case of breast cancer, many theories have been discarded along with old wives' tales; for example:
Cancer is not caused by sexual intercourse, childbirth, or nursing, nor by blows, bites, or bruises.
Cancer cannot be caught from another person like an infection.
Breast-feeding does not appear to protect against breast cancer.

The possible causes include the following:
Diet or environment – This is perhaps where the strongest evidence lies. For example, Japanese women have a low incidence of breast cancer, but if they migrate to areas where incidence is highest (e.g. in the USA or northern Europe) they begin to show a pattern like these countries in a generation or two. Thus, diet and/or environment are suspect. It is thought that by reducing the fat content of your diet you

---

* George Crile, 'What Women Should Know about the Breast Cancer Controversy', and Rose Kushner, *Breast Cancer* (see Bibliography).

may be less susceptible to breast cancer.†

Hormone levels – It appears, for example, that women who have had their ovaries removed have less susceptibility to breast cancer.

Synthetic hormones – the long-term effect of synthetic hormones, such as those contained in the Pill (see p. 249), in most hormone replacement therapy regimens and in Depo-Provera (see p. 260), is still not known, although of course the cancer-causing *potential* of oestrogens has been known for some years. However, with regard to diethylstilboestrol (see p. 284), there is an increased risk of vaginal cancer in daughters of women given the drug to prevent miscarriage. There is also now very suggestive evidence that the mothers themselves run a greatly increased risk of developing various cancers, particularly breast cancer.

Virus particles in breast milk – In animal studies virus transmission from mother to baby via breast milk has been demonstrated, but it has not yet been proven in humans.

Who Is at Risk?

The following factors are relevant:

1. A history of breast cancer on the mother's side. This does not mean that if a woman's mother has had breast cancer, she herself is bound to get it. Heredity is of far less importance than other known factors.

2. Age: the risk of breast cancer increases with each decade of life. The majority of cases are over 40; the commonest age range is from 45 to 60, although the number of cases, particularly in the 35 to 45 age group, is increasing.

3. Women who have had benign breast diseases apart from fibroadenoma seem to have a slightly higher chance of contracting breast cancer, but this theory is still open to question. (It is not yet known if fibroadenoma predisposes towards breast cancer since no one has yet researched into this). One textbook suggests that every woman with benign breast disease should be examined at intervals of three to six months. Mammography is also suggested at yearly intervals, although many experts would now disagree with routine annual mammograms.

4. The age at which a woman has children: If a woman is pregnant by the age of 20, the risk could be reduced by half. A woman who has her children after the age of 35 is in a higher risk group than the childless woman. If you are infertile, you have one and a half times the risk of a fertile woman.

5. If you already have cancer in one breast.

† For more about diet (and other factors) see 'Cancer: How to Cut the Risk', by Oliver Gillie, *Sunday Times*, 13 June 1976, and Rose Kushner, *Breast Cancer*.

6. Weight: this does not seem to be an important factor, although women with larger breasts could be slightly more at risk.

7. If you began menstruating very early and have been menstruating for a long time, the risks increase. (The average age for beginning menstruation is at present around $12\frac{1}{2}$.) The earlier the menopause, whether artificial (via surgery) or natural, the lower the risk.

8. Women who have taken DES. (See p. 284.)

There appears to be a slightly greater risk of developing breast cancer if you have the following (though nothing has been proven): earwax that is wet rather than dry; a hypothyroid (underfunctioning thyroid) condition; live in a cold climate; or have relatively high socioeconomic status.

Should All Women be Screened?

Some people have said that all women should be screened annually by palpation, thermography and mammography. With regard to *palpation* (manual examination), there is little controversy and, as we have said when discussing breast examination, each woman is herself the person most equipped to carry out this procedure on a monthly basis. Concerning *thermography*, there is again little controversy except in that many people are beginning to doubt the effectiveness of this harmless procedure. It is with *mammography* that there is now considerable concern, in respect of regular screening. In 1976 the National Cancer Institute in the USA halted its nationwide annual screening programme involving mammography, because of the radiation risk. Regular mammographic screening is now only recommended by the NCI for women who have symptoms or for women over 50 (who are particularly at risk). Other experts are less cautious and suggest regular screening for all high risk categories. However, there *is* a case for a *single* mammographic screening for women in slightly younger age groups, for such a test could provide some base-line information against which to compare any future developments. Even so, if you do not fall into a high risk category, you may want to avoid all radiation unless there is a clear justification for it, particularly if you suspect you have been exposed to too much in the past, and particularly if the only equipment available is old (which would mean that the doses of radiation might be higher than necessary and the tests less accurate). In any case, although mammography is especially useful for women past the menopause, or with large fatty breasts, it appears at present to be no more able to detect lumps in pre-menopausal women than a skilled manual examination; (manual examinations and mammograms *together* increase the accuracy rate). It is difficult to obtain screening on the NHS. If you want screening, keeping the above information in mind, you can contact the Women's National Cancer Control Campaign (see addresses, p. 213) to find out about facilities in your area. Contact the WNCCC and your Community (or Local) Health Council also, if you are interested in ensuring that government expenditure cuts do not interfere with the purchase of up-to-date screening equipment.

Different Breast Cancers and Their Alternative Treatments*

Breast cancer takes at least three or four different forms, each growing at different rates. A small lump may be very slow-growing, or the fastest-growing type may have spread (metastasized) throughout the body by the time the lump is discovered. In between there are slower-growing cancers which may have spread into surrounding tissues, but not to other body systems. Cancer of the breast usually spreads into the lymphatic system before it reaches the bloodstream. Lymph nodes can delay passage of cancer into the bloodstream. The nodes first affected are near the armpit, under the sternum (breast bone), or in the neck. (Enlarged nodes under the arm may or may not be cancerous and, as with breast lumps, only biopsy can tell for sure.) Adequate treatment of breast cancer must consider all these areas.

Since breast cancer takes many different forms and spreads through the body in different ways, there is no one treatment that would be best for all of them. Breast cancer tends to be divided into stages as follows:

Stage 0. The cancer is very small (microscopic) and is usually found accidentally, in biopsy of a lump which is predominantly not cancer but in which a few cancer cells are found. This type does not infiltrate (invade) breast tissue and is called *in situ* (in place) cancer. Women with this sort of cancer are at risk of having similar small (microscopic) deposits of cancer cells in other parts of the same breast and/or in the other breast. In time (2 to 25 years later) a percentage of these women will develop a lump all of which is cancerous. (The figures range from 10 to 30%.) Thus, it is difficult to decide whether just removing the lump (lumpectomy) is the best thing to do. Some surgeons feel this is all right, provided there is very careful medical follow-up, since most women (70 to 90%) will *not* develop such 'infiltrating' cancers.

Stage I. Here the lump is usually palpable (can be felt) but is still small (less than 2 cm.). These cancer cells do invade breast tissue. Sometimes (rarely) they also invade beyond to nodes. Occasionally the lymph nodes in the axilla (armpit) are felt to be enlarged, sometimes not. Only biopsy of such lymph nodes can tell for sure whether cancer has really spread there.

* With help from Dr Mary Costanza, Department of Oncology, Tufts New England Medical Center, Boston, and Dr Maureen Roberts, Edinburgh Royal Infirmary.

Again, treatment is very controversial. In some cases a small lump, particularly when located on the outer side of the breast, can be adequately treated by excision (lumpectomy – see below) with or without radiation therapy. More usually, removal of the whole breast (simple mastectomy) is considered necessary. Rarely, particularly in the UK, does a surgeon want to perform a radical mastectomy – see below. There is at present no difference in survival (or cure) rates between any of these methods of treatment.

Stage II. Here, the cancer is larger (2 to 5 cm.) when diagnosed. The axillary lymph nodes are affected as well. Treatment can involve any of the procedures outlined above, with or without radiotherapy. So far no 'best' way has been proven. The chance of cure depends in great part on how many lymph nodes are involved.

There is no firm evidence that, if lymph nodes are involved, removal (radical or modified radical mastectomy) will improve survival or chances of cure. Simple mastectomy plus radiotherapy may be better. Retaining the axillary nodes may maintain immunity against the spread of cancer, although since so little is known about this idea, it would probably be best at this point in time either to remove or to irradiate the nodes. Certainly from Stage II cancer onwards, systemic therapy, involving chemotherapy and/or hormone therapy (see below) can be very useful in dealing with metastases and forestalling recurrence (see p. 164).

Stage III. In this instance, when breast cancer is diagnosed it is large (greater than 5 cm.), and lymph nodes are almost always involved. The chances of cure are usually rather slim (though some women have large tumours and many positive nodes, and never develop a metastasis or even a recurrence). Nevertheless there are therapies which can help local control and prolong survival. Simple mastectomy or radiation therapy can control the local breast disease.

Stage IV. In this case, when first found, the lump is usually greater than 5 cm., the lymph nodes are usually enlarged, and most important, there is evidence that the cancer has already spread via the bloodstream beyond the breast and lymph nodes. Therapy can include removal of ovaries (for menstruating women), removal of adrenal glands (for post-menopausal women), hormone administration and/or chemotherapy. Advances are being made in extending useful, symptom-free survival time for women even when they have extensive disease: 'I have now met many women who – with proper follow-up after mastectomy – have lived for years even with recurrences and metastases' (Kushner, p. 166).

For information about follow-up, see below.

Treatment Procedures.
Simple Mastectomy removes only the breast, but all of it. This is the most common treatment procedure in the UK, with or without radiotherapy.

Radical Mastectomy involves taking all of the breast, all the axillary nodes, and the pectoral muscles under the breast (which also support arm function). This operation is relatively uncommon (unlike in the USA) and is on the whole considered unnecessary. Recent US National Cancer Institute reports indicate that this type of radical surgery is *never* necessary. Cure rates are not improved, and discomfort is worse. If performed well, with good rehabilitation afterwards, it should not interfere with arm function.

Super-Radical Mastectomy involves removal of the above, plus the underlying muscles of the chest wall, and the nodes under the sternum. This operation is now, thankfully, unheard of in the UK.

Modified Radical Mastectomy takes less or none of the chest muscles that connect the arm and removes the nodes. Radiation of remaining nodes may follow. Modified radicals are not uncommon, e.g. at Guys Hospital, where complication rates are low.

Partial Mastectomy removes the lump and some of the surrounding tissue and is often followed by radiotherapy. One breast will be smaller than the other afterwards, but breast reconstruction could be a possibility (see below).

Subcutaneous Mastectomy involves removal of the inner breast but leaves the outer skin and nipple. Again, implants are then possible.

Lumpectomy or *Tylectomy* involves removing just the lump and possibly doing a biopsy under the armpit to check the nodes. As in the case of partial and subcutaneous mastectomies, this procedure is not too common. It depends on what kind of cancer is involved, where it is and what stage it is at (the problem is being sure that all of the affected area has been removed), but above all, it depends upon the attitudes and expertise of the doctors involved. However, a few hospitals – such as the Royal Marsden in London – have been performing lumpectomies followed by radiotherapy for some years where women have refused to have mastectomies.

The amount and intensity of pain immediately after the operation and during the months that followed vary considerably. Some women whose surgeries were fairly recent told me they still felt nothing at all except numbness in most of the affected area. One young mother . . . was hitting tennis balls at a public court less than six weeks after her stitches were removed . . . I could never have done that. When I interviewed her (about a year after the mastectomy), she still had no pain. All she felt was tightness across the chest. (Kushner, p. 215)

The avoidance of unpleasant after-effects from the above procedures is yet one more reason for getting a specialist experienced in breast disease.

Oophorectomy or *Ovariectomy (Removal of the Ovaries)*: about one third of all breast cancers are strongly hormone dependent – thus, in pre-menopausal women, removal of the ovaries (which produce a lot of hormones) can have a dramatic effect if second cancers develop. Sometimes even the pituitary gland is removed as well – since this also produces hormones. Research is being conducted into *hormone assays* – a test for hormone dependency – which can then isolate those tumours which will benefit from removal of the ovaries and those tumours for which it would make no difference. The additional trauma of a premature menopause could thus be avoided in some women.

Radiotherapy as treatment for the disease is still being evaluated. But as long ago as 1946 it was recognized that radiotherapy did not help, and possibly even exacerbated the disease if given following a mastectomy when the nodes had been removed. (But radiotherapy was useful in the relief of pain.) With lumpectomies and simple mastectomies, it is still thought that radiotherapy is effective. The after-effects can be worse than from surgery, involving nausea, hair loss, swelling and pain, sensitive and 'weeping' skin, infection, and even paralysis of the irradiated area. But the newest equipment has been designed to avoid all these symptoms.

My eight weeks of radiotherapy were totally trauma-free . . . I happened to be treated at a London teaching hospital which favours non-traumatic radio-therapy. This means that they give smaller dosage over a longer period in the belief that this is just as effective as the more concentrated kind, which leaves you feeling and looking as though you've had a really bad sunburn. (Caroline Nicholson, Nova, March 1973)

But as Caroline Nicholson said, 'Expediency comes into it . . . The longer you take with a patient, the fewer you can treat. And many radiotherapy departments in Britain have long queues and a lot of out-dated equipment.' In France, radiotherapy is so advanced that in some cases the cancer can be cured by radiotherapy alone (see *Nova*, March 1973).

Chemotherapy (drugs that kill cells): as with X-ray treatment, this could cause cancer elsewhere, therefore it must be very carefully used, and only by an expert chemotherapist. Some doctors believe that biologically-active drugs are at their most effective when the disease is in its early stages, but as a rule, chemotherapy is only given when the disease is at Stage II or more. Chemotherapy in early breast cancer has not yet been evaluated over a long enough period of time, and it is one of the most controversial areas at present. As with all new treatments, the method of evaluation involves putting some women on it and using another set of women as 'controls' to monitor the results. It presupposes that women – the patients – should have no say in our treatment. Perhaps we as women, and society at large, have to begin to decide whether we are prepared to be guinea-pigs or whether we would rather be in charge of our own risk-taking. As Rose Kushner says, 'It might make sense to risk perhaps developing leukemia in 15 or 20 years instead of facing almost certain death from breast cancer in five or ten.' For a fuller discussion of the pros and cons of early chemotherapy, see her book.

Follow-up.   Breast cancer is a chronic disease. It *must* be monitored in order to catch early any recurrence or metastasis. If you are regularly monitored, the chances of missing a recurrence are very slim. Many doctors are alarmingly ignorant in this field:

I had my mastectomy performed at a local hospital in London. They did do regular check-ups but they only consisted of a cursory feeling around. Once or twice I mentioned lumps in the other breast, but they didn't take me very seriously. I didn't have much confidence in them. By accident, I found out about the Royal Marsden's breast clinic in London and asked my GP to refer me there. At my first appointment I had a very careful palpation plus mammography and thermography and a blood test. The atmosphere was such that for the first time I felt I could talk about my fears and feelings. I had a long chat with the specialist (a woman). She was fantastically helpful, very sympathetic and very honest.

Again, the importance of attending a specialist clinic with an experienced team is obvious.

Roughly speaking, you should be examined every three months for the first year, gradually lengthening to annually after five years (chances of recurrence decrease with time). In addition, you should regularly examine yourself, particularly around the incision itself – where recurrence can often occur. Signs of lung or liver problems should also be watched for, as should menstrual irregularities. Your check-ups should at least involve the following: skilled palpation (manual examination) of the operated area and of the other breast, liver palpation, close questioning as to general health, as well as comfort and psychological adjustment. A check on blood count once a year is advisable, and liver function tests can also be useful, possibly every six months. If there are symptoms such as a lingering cough or hoarseness, an X-ray would be called for and proper investigations made. Some people feel that an X-ray of the chest, pelvis and spine should be performed every six months; others feel that X-rays (including mammograms) should not be performed more than once a year, and even then, only if the person is not feeling well. If the cancer had not spread at the time of initial treatment and you are feeling well, it is probably best for your doctors to keep a careful watch and avoid X-ray screening.

If X-rays show up any suspicious spots, it is then advisable to perform bone scans. These, like X-rays, involve radiation but they should not be performed unless absolutely necessary as the dosage is much greater.

There should be women doctors available at a good mastectomy clinic, and you should be able to see the same doctor at each visit. The doctor should pay careful attention to psychological care, and to catering for each woman's needs.

How Can Women Decide?

If you suspect you have breast cancer, the earlier you act, the more options are open to you. If you are ever diagnosed as having the disease, you will be much better able to cope with it and decide what to do if you have done some reading and thinking beforehand (see Bibliography). Perhaps the most useful book to read is Rose Kushner's. She examines every aspect of the subject in some detail – impossible in a chapter of this length – and she writes extensively about what it feels like, coming to terms with the disease, and how to go about making decisions. She herself had to have a breast removed. However, even after you have read her book, a lot of questions will probably come to mind that need answering and detailed books about cancer tend to date fast.

When doctors disagree as much as they do in the case of breast cancer, they are poor sources of objective advice. In a case like this we women really make the final choice, because the kind of treatment we get depends on who we choose to treat us. Once you have read this chapter and the supporting material you can ask *why* a doctor wants to perform a particular procedure or whether another would be any better or worse (see 'Patients' Rights in Hospital', in Chapter 17, p. 552). It is most important that you be able to discuss openly with your doctors the various alternatives and their prejudices. Whatever happens, you should not have a mastectomy without preoperative staging (see 'Biopsy', p. 158).

As we have emphasized, the place to which you go is of prime importance. You should be able to insist upon going to a specialist breast clinic, and it should not matter where you live. For example, the Edinburgh clinic sees women from all over Scotland, and even in some cases from England. As yet there are only a few such breast clinics in the UK. Hopefully there will be more one day, but women will have to fight hard for them – together with those doctors who see them as important (for example, the British Breast Group). Information about clinics and hospitals can be obtained from your regional cancer service (see addresses, p. 213), or your local health authority. Be sure your doctor is up-to-date with current knowledge, has experience with many breast cancer patients, and is willing to discuss and learn about the different therapies.

You should be in a position to ask for the objective advice of at least two doctors, neither of whom has a particular axe to grind. For example, Rose Kushner quotes one doctor from the Royal Marsden breast clinic who, although he believes that women have the right to decide the kind of surgery they will have, will do 'everything' to persuade them to have some kind of radical mastectomy. Ideally, decisions about treatment should be made on the basis of joint discussion between all the relevant specialists (e.g. chemotherapist, radiotherapist, pathologist and surgeon).* But in some hospitals, particularly the smaller ones, the surgeon may reign supreme, with the power to decide whether or not even to *refer* to a specialist from another discipline.

I had my mastectomy at the local hospital. I was only seen by a general surgeon who told me 'There is no other treatment.' I never saw a radiologist or a chemotherapist.

Some doctors will be unhappy at the idea of a woman wishing to participate in a decision about her treatment. Some doctors don't believe in telling their patients that they have cancer — even if they indicate that they want to know (see *Spare Rib*, 37).

The radiologist told my client that the cancer was all cleared up. She was very relieved to hear this as she was a young single mother and needed to know if she would have to make arrangements for her children. I saw her GP who said, 'Well, you know, it's not true . . . They tell everybody that because you can't tell people the truth, can you? You tell them the truth, but not the whole truth.'

Even the strongest of us needs support at a time of crisis. Do not expect this type of support from your doctor (although it *may* be there and is much more likely in specialist clinics). Most doctors and nurses are too busy and may have different ideas from yours about what is important. If possible, get someone you trust to accompany you and act as an advocate for you. Get support from somewhere. It's your breast and your life.

If You Have Had a Mastectomy

Prostheses†. Some women prefer not to wear a prosthesis (false breast), particularly if their other breast is quite small. But often the lopsidedness resulting from not wearing a prosthesis and bra (the latter is necessary to hold the prosthesis in place) can result in backache.

In order to obtain these items on the NHS, a hospital doctor has to prescribe them for you. Unfortunately, there are still many areas in the UK where doctors will not prescribe the best prostheses (see *Spare Rib*, 37). *You have the right to insist on having a prosthesis and on choosing what feels*

---

* See *Women's Report*, Vol. 3, issue 3, p. 14.

† The Mastectomy Association can tell you where to get bras, prostheses and swimwear.

right for you. You should be given ample opportunity to try out the best prostheses and bras available. Only then can you come to the right decision as to what is best for you. No surgeon can possibly decide what is best, even if he does give you the opportunity to test the various kinds. Only you can make the decision.

Silicone gel prostheses are the most lifelike – and the most expensive. They are available on the NHS and any doctor who says the opposite is wrong. They are gel-filled with a smooth silicone skin which clings to the chest wall, is non-slip, and assumes the body's temperature. These prostheses can be washed as often as necessary, are not liable to leak, and last indefinitely (they are guaranteed for ten years). Women with a small breast might not find the right size to suit them, but the manufacturers are developing smaller prostheses in different shapes as well. The next best prostheses are fluid-filled, need to be replaced every so often and *can* leak. For a small breast they can be too heavy, but for many women they are fine.

The Mastectomy Association makes light 'temporary' ones for after the operation but many doctors have not heard of them. Small-breasted women often prefer these for permanent use.

Alternatively, you can make your own. Betty Underhill describes how to do this (see Bibliography). The advantage of a 'custom-made' prosthesis is that it can be made to fit the exact shape of the other breast. It can be sewn into bras, swimsuits or dresses and can be washed with each garment.

Many women use ordinary bras with ribbons sewn in to hold the prosthesis in place (see the Mastectomy Association's leaflets). But unless a bra is properly designed to hold the weight that non-existent muscles should be doing, backache can result. There are thus obvious grounds for the NHS to provide a bra. Again, the doctor at the hospital can – and should – prescribe one if necessary.

If a few women, with the support of women's groups, insist on good bras and prostheses, the NHS will start providing them for others as a matter of course.

Breast Reconstruction.   Breast reconstruction is being performed in some areas. At Birmingham General Hospital, half the women leave with a new breast implanted under the skin with nipple intact, although it is only possible if the growth is caught early and if there is little chance of recurrence. Implants can be done years after the original operation. Not all doctors approve of them – mainly because they have not yet been properly evaluated and it could be difficult to spot recurrences. The decision whether to have one or not would to some extent depend on the person doing it. Implants are available on the NHS, but you might have to wait even years. They are not always very lifelike, but many women are really happy with them:

I had to have treatment for depression. My spirits soared when I heard later about replacement surgery . . . I'm delighted to say the breast looks almost normal . . . I have so much to be thankful for . . .

Much more research needs to be done on breast reconstruction. For a fuller discussion of the pros and cons of this technique, see Rose Kushner.

Psychological Adjustment. Of the thousands of women who have had mastectomies, many have adjusted quickly and gone on to lead busy, active lives almost as if nothing had happened. Many have been helped by organizations such as the Mastectomy Association founded by Betty Westgate, a former mastectomy patient (address p. 213). Volunteers who have undergone mastectomy visit new mastectomy patients, help them with practical questions and offer psychological support and a living example of confident recovery. While some doctors gladly tell their patients about the Mastectomy Association, others have been known to withhold information about it or to be unaware of its existence. Very few women ever receive adequate preparation for the reality of mastectomy — from anyone. The Mastectomy Association would probably be three or four times as effective if the volunteers could visit mastectomy candidates *before* the surgery. Then prospective patients could learn in advance what to expect during the first hours, days and weeks afterwards.

They could also discuss in advance, both with the other women and with their partners, the doubts and fears about how the loss of a breast may affect their relationships.

My husband is now, if possible, more tender and loving than he ever was before. Our love life has a brand-new dimension that wasn't there until I had the mastectomy. It's as if he suddenly realized that I was something very precious that he almost — and could still — lose. This feeling of being 'cherished' like something very valuable, a treasure, is what has been added to our love.

We have never enjoyed each other so much.

I've had two lovers since and neither of them minded, but I've also had one sheer right off when I told him, and that hurts, it shakes your confidence.

They could be helped to anticipate the depression or grief that is a normal human response to the loss of any body part, but particularly such a uniquely female part as a breast. Deeper depression and rage may also be involved — rage at the disease itself, or at fate, or at the outside world for not caring more or doing more research. The depression may stir up normally hidden and controlled feelings of low self-esteem and convince us that we are forever unlovable.

I found myself looking at some particularly ugly, grotesque, or obnoxious woman and thinking bitterly, enviously, 'Why me and not her?' It was not a nice thought to have. I was so ashamed of myself for having it. Later, when I began interviewing post-mastectomy patients, I found this jealousy was not unique to me; everyone had felt it at one time or another. And everyone had been ashamed, too, and had never mentioned it, even to husbands, friends or close relatives. (Rose Kushner, p. 238)

Doctors do not choose to publicize 'unsuccessful' mastectomy patients nor encourage any serious research on how widespread such cases are. As one surgeon told Caroline Nicholson, 'British women will do pretty much what you tell them. They grit their teeth and go into depressions later.' In one of the few psychological studies of mastectomy patients* it was found that 'over one third of the women became very anxious and depressed, some becoming so low as to feel that life was pointless . . . Unfortunately, *as before biopsy, much of this distress remained undetected by the nursing and medical staff* (our italics). The study found that of the women who had been given time to adjust to the idea of having breast cancer, most viewed their operation constructively. But those women who had not accepted the idea, or had not been given a chance to, tended to be extremely upset. It is clear that many women need much more help than is ever offered.† Hopefully, then, the situation will change – when we as women change, demanding options and psychological care to meet our needs. We believe strongly that women can offer one another unique help by sharing experiences.

Menstrual Problems

(See Chapter 2 for description of the menstrual cycle.)

Most women experience some menstrual discomfort some time in their lives. Over 50% of women have painful periods.

The day before and sometimes the first day of my period my whole abdominal cavity feels unsettled. It feels like the membranes between my organs are disintegrating and everything is getting mixed up.

Medical textbooks pay far more attention to the rarer problem of amenorrhea (absence of periods – see infertility, p. 490) than to the more

* 'The Psychological and Social Consequences of Breast Cancer', by Peter Maguire – see *Nursing Mirror*, 3 April 1975.

† See also Rosamond Campion's *The Invisible Worm*, Macmillan, New York, 1972.

common problems which so many of us suffer from. In spite of their lack of knowledge we often find textbooks and doctors drawing conclusions based on nothing but supposition (see Jeffcoate's gynaecology textbook quoted on p. 548), and many doctors still think the problem is in our heads!

One doctor who has been researching the menstrual cycle is Katherina Dalton. In her book *The Menstrual Cycle* she says that menstrual problems are based on hormone imbalance, and her form of treatment involves hormone supplements. Recently this area of research has been taken up by at least two London hospitals (University College and St Thomas's).

Dr Dalton divides most problems into two categories; spasmodic dysmenorrhoea (characterized by *pain*) and congestive dysmenorrhoea (characterized by pre-menstrual tension).

SPASMODIC DYSMENORRHOEA

Symptoms: acute pains and cramps in the lower abdomen, occasionally accompanied by shakiness and nausea at the start of a period. It is most common between the ages of fifteen and twenty-five, and usually stops with pregnancy. Origin: Dr Dalton thinks that this problem is associated with excess progesterone compared with oestrogen and is tied to hormone levels of the ovulatory cycle.

CONGESTIVE DYSMENORRHOEA

Symptoms: heaviness and dull aching in the abdomen, nausea, water retention, painful breasts, constipation, headaches, backaches, irritability, tension, depression and lethargy. It can occur any time from puberty onwards and often increases with each pregnancy and continues until menopause (and according to Dalton, beyond). Origin: according to Dalton, an excess of oestrogen compared with progesterone. These categories make a useful base to work from; however, we are not all so easy to categorize. We know of many women who suffer from pre-menstrual tension *and* bad pains. This might be explained by the function of prostaglandin which we discuss under Medical Remedies, p. 173.

Alternative Remedies

For those of us who prefer to try alternative methods of treatment, here are some suggestions.

Rest: If we can arrange to take more rest before or during menstruation it helps. We can also try to avoid scheduling stressful activities at the times when we will feel worst. But this can be hard to arrange as our menstrual cycles are easily affected by stress.

Diet: We can reduce salt intake for about ten days prior to menstruation, as salt absorbs water and increases water retention, which causes breast pain and even headaches. Calcium either in food, such as milk products or almonds, or in calcium tablets, can supplement dropping calcium levels which are associated with hormone imbalance. (Adelle Davis says that low calcium *causes* the imbalance – see *Let's Get Well*, p. 219 – she recommends calcium tablets to relieve cramps.) Vitamin B$_6$ is also useful in reducing pre-menstrual tension and water retention (take at least 50 milligrams per day for 2 weeks before a period). It is likely that vitamin B and C levels will drop if we are taking diuretics to increase urination (see under 'Medical Remedies') because they are both water-soluble, so these supplements could be useful.

We should make a special effort to eat well at this time to keep up our energy.

Herbal remedies: For pain: bancha-leaf and tamari (soy sauce), Lady's Mantle, catnip and mint teas (all anti-spasmodic); for water retention and pain: raspberry leaf, marjoram and thyme teas. These are all available at Health food or herbal shops (see p. 144).

Body Work: This relieves pain for many people (for specific exercises see Hilary C. Maddux, *Menstruation* or Erna Wright, *Periods Without Pain*). The Alexander Technique (see p. 134) is also helpful, as is massage (see *Spare Rib*, 56).

Other Ideas: Heat (i.e. a hot water bottle) applied to the stomach and lower back, massage, drugs such as alcoholic drinks or marijuana, or acupuncture and homeopathic remedies (see p. 131); if your symptoms are relieved by heavy blood flow, an orgasm, sauna, or steam bath can speed it up. See also menstrual extraction, p. 28. If all else fails, painkillers such as aspirin, codeine or paracetamol can be used – sparingly.

Medical Remedies

Diuretics: Water retention (and, as a result, many of the other effects of pre-menstrual tension) can be helped by diuretics. These are drugs which act on the kidneys to increase urination. They often have quite a dramatic effect but can also make you excrete important minerals and vitamins. Potassium may be lost and most diuretics contain potassium because of this. (It is also found in ripe fruits such as bananas, oranges or figs). It may be wise to take supplements of other water-soluble vitamins as well. Diuretic pills are only available on prescription and should be taken once daily for about ten days before a period.

Hormone Treatment: If *pre-menstrual tension* is the problem, hormone treatment is complicated. Many doctors prescribe the Pill for this condition and it often makes things worse. According to Katherina Dalton, this is because most synthetic progesterones (progestogens) actually suppress the body's natural production of progesterone so even a progestogen-only pill won't work. (As natural progesterone cannot be taken orally it is not used in contraceptive pills.)

Those people who do get relief from the Pill may well realize later that it has merely evened out the rise and fall of their cycles so that though they no longer feel particularly bad just before a period the low feeling spreads throughout the month.

It was only when I came off the Pill for a totally different reason that I realized I had been feeling 10% under and not functioning acutely while I was on it. The PMT came back with a vengeance but at least I am now fully awake and alert for the rest of the month.

Hormone treatment can still be used and is effective in dealing with symptoms for many women, although as with other hormone treatments it is early days to assess the long-term risks. So far no problems have been discovered, but little research has been done. (However, there is some concern about the possible relationship between 'progestogen only' contraceptives, and ectopic pregnancies. Also, see Barbara & Gideon Seaman, *Women and the Crisis in Sex Hormones*.)

It appears that the most effective treatment is with natural progesterone administered in pessaries or by injection. Tests are also being done on an artificial progestogen called dydrogesterone which can be taken orally. As yet, few GPs are likely to prescribe either of these and it would probably be necessary to ask for a referral to a hospital.

Another hormone which seems to be involved in pre-menstrual tension is *prolactin*. An excess of this substance has been found to reduce progesterone levels. A relatively new drug called *bromocriptine* can reduce the level of prolactin and gives relief from PMT. Studies on this drug are also in their early stages.[*]

For *period pains* uncomplicated by PMT, combined contraceptive pills can be an answer because they suppress ovulation. However, the Pill carries its own risks (see p. 244). Research now seems to suggest that the production in the uterus of prostaglandins (hormone-like substances) causes uterine contractions and pain. Drugs which inhibit the production of prostaglandin (such as aspirin or flufenamic acid) can prevent pain caused by such contractions.

[*] According to *The Medical Letter*, 16 December 1977, this drug has serious adverse effects.

If you have trouble every cycle, or are having painful periods after having had relatively comfortable ones previously, you should check with your doctor to find out if you have endometriosis. You should also get a check-up if you have any abnormal (to you) bleeding.

Uterine and Ovarian Problems

CERVICAL EROSION

A cervical erosion is a rather scary name for a common phenomenon. It means that the soft dark pink cells from inside the cervix have grown outside. It looks like a small reddish area around the entrance to the cervical canal. An erosion grows in response to oestrogen so it is a normal occurrence in pregnancy and often occurs in women who take the Pill.

Erosions are rarely troublesome. Sometimes they cause a discharge and because of the fragility of the cells may be associated with slight bleeding after intercourse. The major problem is that an erosion can be susceptible to infection. If you suspect an infection or are worried about an erosion, a VD clinic will do a routine cervical smear. If there is infection, the treatment will be as for cervicitis, but it will not cure the erosion, only the infection.

It is probably better to leave well alone unless a discharge becomes troublesome or infections are recurrent. (Some doctors recommend action at an unnecessarily early stage.) A discharge can be helped by the vinegar or salt treatment mentioned on p. 188. If the infection is chronic it may be advisable to deal with the erosion itself, but this is only worthwhile if at the same time you cut down on the oestrogen which caused it in the first place. This means coming off the Pill or postponing treatment until after childbirth if you are pregnant. The most common treatments are cauterizing (burning the cells off) or cryosurgery (freezing them off). After either process, which should be painless unless you have a very sensitive cervix, you should not have sexual intercourse for 10–14 days to allow the new cells to grow over the area.

ENDOMETRIOSIS

The symptoms of endometriosis vary. Menstrual pain is the most common symptom, often getting increasingly painful after years of relative comfort. There may also be a dull, or even severe pain in the whole of the lower abdomen, often starting two or three weeks before a period and only slackening immediately after the period has come. Severe pain on intercourse is another distressing effect. Forty per cent of women with endometriosis are infertile in spite of apparently normal periods.

Endometriosis happens when fragments of the uterine lining (endometrium) leave the uterus and attach themselves to other parts of the pelvic anatomy. Wherever they find themselves these patches will continue to behave like the uterine lining, increasing every month and then bleeding during a period. However, when the bleeding occurs in the abdominal cavity there is nowhere for it to go, so it forms scabs where it lies, building up scar tissue which often causes adhesions (when organs stick together).

Present treatment methods do not guarantee cure. However, the best way to stop endometriosis (or to stop it increasing) is to stop periods occurring. This means either becoming pregnant, which often clears the condition completely, or taking artificial hormones to simulate pregnancy. Occasionally Depo Provera is used for this purpose; see p. 260 for the disadvantages of using this drug. (The Pill is not likely to be sufficient, although prolonged use of it may prevent the condition starting by decreasing the build up of the endometrium.) The disadvantage of hormone therapy is that some people react badly to it.

If this is not effective alone, or if the ovaries or fallopian tubes are already affected and you still wish to have children, minor surgery is probably necessary to remove the growth and free the trapped organs. Surgery of this kind should be accompanied by hormone treatment to prevent recurrence. However it is not always sufficient. If the pain still persists more radical surgery may be required; removal of the uterus and sometimes even the ovary may be the only effective treatment for some women.

I had been having painful menstrual cramps and went to the university health service. A doctor there, without giving any physical examination, told me my cramps were psychosomatic and implied they would go away when I got married and settled down and lived according to the conventional woman's role and conventional sexual morality.

Two years later the cramps had got very much worse, and my periods were lasting eleven days. I asked friends about private gynaecologists and one was recommended. He found I had endometriosis. I suggest that all women troubled by painful cramps and/or unusually long periods ask to be checked for this condition. Untreated endometriosis can lead to sterility, which can be prevented by early, proper treatment.

Diagnosis is hard in the early stages, and the condition is not usually suspected unless there is severe menstrual pain or an endometrial cyst (growth) big enough to feel.

If endometriosis is diagnosed and you want to have children, it would be best to have them as soon as is practically possible, as the ovaries and tubes could easily become blocked.

REPRODUCTIVE TUMOURS

The word 'tumour' is very scary to most of us. It is part of an older language of illness that was used by many of our grand-parents, both patients and doctors, to disguise the mention of cancer. Actually tumours are growths of cells which serve no purpose; however, over 90% of all tumours are benign and harmless (i.e. cysts, polyps, fibroids). No one knows exactly why the human body produces them (they have been known since ancient times), but fat consumption and metabolism have been linked to tumour production.

When we have tumours anywhere in our reproductive organs we are almost always afraid it is cancer. The chance of malignancy (cancer) increases with age, particularly after menopause. Reproductive cancers in women occur, in order of frequency, in the breasts, the cervix, the ovaries, the body of the uterus itself and the vagina.

As mentioned elsewhere, hormones, carcinogenic substances and the malfunctioning of the immune system have all been linked to cancer, which takes many different forms but remains mysterious despite extensive research. Our fear of this disease sometimes keeps us from learning even simple facts and habits which could help us to prolong our own lives or the lives of others. This same fear makes us vulnerable to suggestions of violent and dangerous treatments, many of which are not necessary, and keeps us from exploring our options and alternatives. Throughout this section we've tried to show ways our knowledge of both health and disease can free us from the trap of letting others make decisions for us.

OVARIAN CYSTS

Ovarian cysts are relatively common and often don't give any symptoms or discomfort. They are found by a bimanual pelvic examination and usually don't require any treatment at all (they disappear by themselves), though some types of cysts may have to be removed.

A cyst develops when a follicle has grown large — as one does every month during ovulation — but has failed to rupture and release an egg (see Chapter 2). Most of these cysts fill with fluid; others become solid tumours. Cysts may be accompanied by certain symptoms such as a disturbance in the normal menstrual cycle; an unfamiliar pain or discomfort at any point during the cycle; an unexplained abdominal swelling.

To determine whether a cyst requires treatment, simply wait a cycle or two for it to disappear. At one time abdominal surgery was the only way to tell whether a cyst that didn't disappear was benign, or a cancerous tumour which needed removal. Today laparoscopy or culdoscopy (see p. 287) may enable the doctor to make this examination with a minimum of interference and tissue damage, so that unnecessary abdominal surgery can be avoided. Be sure to ask which procedure will be used and why.

FIBROIDS, POLYPS AND OVARIAN CYSTS

Fibroids

One out of four or five women of childbearing age is likely to get fibroids, which are almost always benign and slow-growing. Only a very small percentage are cancerous, and these usually can be diagnosed early with a D & C (dilation and curettage) and cell analysis. Sometimes diagnosis can be made from a cervical smear. As cycle after cycle goes by without a conception, the uterus is less able to slough off the entire build-up of muscle-like tissues and lining each month. One possible result is that fibroids (myomas of the uterus) may develop.

Fibroids usually appear a few at a time. They can interfere with pregnancy in a young woman, either by blocking the tubes or by making a normal delivery difficult; however, most are too small to cause problems. Later, in older women, they can get large enough to cause menstrual irregularities – either bleeding between periods or an excessive flow, and may also push against the rectum or bladder or cause urinary tract infections. They rarely cause pain, though they may produce a feeling of heaviness in the abdomen.

When women who are past childbearing age get fibroids there is usually nothing to worry about, particularly since they usually shrink or even disappear at menopause.

If fibroids become large enough to cause problems, they can be removed by myomectomy, a surgical procedure which leaves the uterus intact. However, some women, and their doctors, feel that if childbearing is over, the uterus should be taken out. There is controversy on this point (see 'D & C and Hysterectomy', p. 183).

Polyps

Polyps are protrusions that grow from a mucous membrane. In women they may appear inside the uterus (endometrial polyps) or along the canal of the cervix, where they grow out of the glands lining the canal.

Endometrial polyps are more common. A polyp appears long and tubelike, but small, easily noticeable by the redness at the tip.

If you have had suspicious bleeding or menstrual flow that seems irregular, it may be caused by polyps. Aside from an abnormal menstrual cycle, bleeding at other times – between periods or right after intercourse – may indicate that there is a growth inside the uterus. This should be checked. A gynaecologist very often will discover a polyp during a pelvic examination (see p. 139). A D & C may be done to remove polyps, and further tests may be suggested to ensure that the specimen is not malignant, which they almost never are.

CERVICAL CELL ABNORMALITY (DYSPLASIA) AND CERVICAL CANCER

Cervical cancer can usually be diagnosed at an early stage (when it should be treatable), by a method of examining the cells of the cervix under a microscope to see if they are undergoing pre-cancerous changes. The examination is made from a scraping taken off the cervix with a wooden spatula. It is usually referred to as a *cervical smear*.

GPs are only paid to perform routine smears every 5 years, and only on women who are over 35 or who have had three or more pregnancies. The rationale is that these women are more at risk and that it usually takes 7–10 years for early signs of cell abnormality to develop into cancer. (Some cancers do spring up very fast, so fast in fact that even a yearly smear won't catch them, but they are rare.) However, experts now suggest that all women should have a first smear when they become heterosexually active, and a second one 6 months later in view of the possibility of a false negative. (Beware, positive results can be masked by substances like blood and spermicide.) Thereafter, they suggest smears every 3 years.

All women who have had herpes (see p. 203) should have more frequent smears (every 6 months to 1 year) because of the statistical link between herpes and cancer.

If you are registered at a 'cytology' clinic you should be recalled at the prescribed time for new smears, but if you want to have it done more regularly there are plenty of ways to get yearly check-ups within the NHS. Smears are (or should be) routine in all VD clinics because they are useful for diagnosing other conditions. Birth control clinics will usually ask when you last had a smear at your yearly check-up; they are unlikely to refuse you once you're being examined. Your GP can of course do them as well.

Basically the results will be either negative, meaning no abnormal cells are present, or positive, meaning that some abnormal cells have been identified and further investigation is required. There are five classifications on some NHS forms:

---

1. Negative – all clear.
2. Mild dysplasia (slight cell abnormality) – considered negative; treatment for infection would probably be prescribed.
2R. Borderline dysplasia – automatic recall and regular surveillance.
3. Suspicion of carcinoma in situ – automatic recall and surveillance.
4. Definite carcinoma in situ – recommendation for biopsy.

Forms differ from one place to another; some only have four categories, others are numbered differently, but basically the classifications correspond with those in the box.

If you get a positive smear you have not necessarily got cancer. This is only an early warning system, an indication that some cells are changing in nature, or have changed. Any results which cause the slightest suspicion will be referred back for a further check.

The first step will probably be a repeat smear. If you have very mild cell abnormality (dysplasia) most British doctors would only recommend continued surveillance, i.e. smear tests every few months until either the test reverts to negative or begins to show a development. In some cases a smear will remain 'borderline' (2R) for years and some doctors might then recommend a further investigation.

The second step would be a biopsy. This means removing a section of tissue from the cervix to allow further examination of 'cell architecture'. Biopsy may be recommended at the class 3 stage, but there is a tendency to wait until class 4 stage (i.e. malignant cells which are confined to a small area and are not affecting other cells), before taking any action which might damage the cervix unnecessarily. The decision to recommend a biopsy varies from one gynaecologist to another. You should find out exactly what your smear diagnosis is, and the gynaecologist's recommended plan of action. Make sure you are given all the information before agreeing to surgery.

There are several methods of doing a biopsy. A *punch biopsy* removes small pieces of tissue for examination; this is a fairly simple operation but it is not a treatment. A *cone biopsy*, which is nearly always done after a class 4 smear test, can be both diagnosis and treatment as it may totally remove the offending cells. Conization, as it is called, is done under anaesthetic in a hospital. It is a method of 'coring out' the tissue of the cervix, which is then tested. Conization does damage the cervix. It becomes very stiff and is no longer able to dilate naturally, therefore any future pregnancies might have to be delivered by caesarian. A cone biopsy is not usually carried out on a pregnant woman for this reason, and it can usually be safely left until after delivery.

If you have 'carcinoma in situ' the biopsy may remove all the abnormal cells and a D & C (see p. 183) will reveal any abnormality in the body of the uterus. Regular smears will be carried out afterwards to ensure that the malignancy has been eradicated. The question is whether the carcinoma will change and become *invasive* — i.e. start to invade other surrounding cells. In 20% of cases, carcinoma in situ becomes invasive carcinoma in 7 to 10 years.

The statistical relationship between carcinoma in situ and invasive carcinoma leads many doctors to recommend hysterectomy straight away. This is because once the cancer begins to move it is very hard to stop. If the entire organ is removed there is a high chance that the problem will be solved for ever. But hysterectomy is a frightening thing to face, particularly so for a woman who has not yet had children and would like to do so. It is of course possible to postpone hysterectomy in the early stages, but the condition would need very careful watching. While the cancer remains stable it would be quite possible to conceive and bear a child. If childbearing is over, or not in question, early surgery would probably relieve you of a great deal of worry in the future.

If cancer has already invaded other cells at the time of diagnosis, surgery may be advised straight away, and it will almost certainly be accompanied by radiotherapy. This is radiation applied directly to the malignant cells, usually done by inserting an implant of radium into the womb for 24 hours on three occasions over 3 weeks. It is extremely uncomfortable. This therapy has been able to stop cancer developing further in some cases, and delay its recurrence for several years in others. Radiation may be used alone if there is extensive spreading of the cancer cells. Radiotherapy is not effective in all cases and would not therefore be recommended instead of surgery at an earlier stage.

Chemotherapy, the treatment of cancer with certain drugs, is now being used quite extensively. The drugs have to be used under careful control because they are not selective and can damage good cells as well as cancerous ones. They also have a tendency to damage white blood cells and interfere with the body's immune system which makes you more vulnerable to infection. Chemotherapy is unlikely to be offered as an alternative to surgery in the early stages.

Once cancer is really advanced there is little that can be done except to administer pain-killing drugs and as much comfort as possible. The purpose of cervical smears and early diagnosis is to prevent any of us suffering the terminal stage. Remember, cancer can be stopped.

The cause of cervical cancer is not known. It may be a virus (genital herpes is one possibility). It is certainly related to class; working-class women are more likely to get it than middle-class women. This could relate to their access to preventive medical care, number of pregnancies, diet or living conditions — we do not know.

CANCER OF THE BODY OF THE UTERUS

Cancer in the uterine lining (endometrium) is quite rare. It is most likely to occur around or after menopause and there is some evidence that it could be inherited in some cases. Endometrial cancer often occurs after a history of menstrual irregularities. Hormone replacement therapy has also been strongly implicated as a cause (see chapter 16).

The most common symptoms are very irregular periods, heavy, prolonged bleeding, post-menopausal bleeding and spotting between periods. Irregularities in bleeding should be investigated. The only effective way to screen for malignant cells is to have a D & C (see p. 183), so that the lining of the uterus can be properly examined.

Treatment may include radiation therapy in the uterus and/or hormone treatment (progesterone), but the usual treatment is hysterectomy and removal of the ovaries.

CANCER OF THE OVARIES

Ovarian cancers are relatively rare (about 1% of all cancer cases), but they are dangerous. They occur most often in post-menopausal women, particularly in women who are infertile or have had ectopic pregnancies resulting in a build-up of endometrial tissue in the fallopian tubes.

Detection of ovarian cancer is difficult. Any lumps on the ovaries which are detected during pelvic examination should be investigated, particularly in post-menopausal women. The cancer cells will also release fluid into the pelvic cavity, so there may be a noticeable fullness in the abdomen.

As ovarian cancer spreads quickly, the best treatment is surgical removal of the affected organs (often both ovaries are involved). Radiation therapy may be used in more advanced cases.

Although removal of the unaffected ovaries (oophorectomy) is sometimes suggested as a preventive measure, particularly when other areas of the reproductive system have been treated for cancer, this treatment has very severe side effects because it brings on a very sharp artificial menopause (see Hysterectomy, p. 183).

VAGINAL CANCER

Until 1970 vaginal cancer was one of the rarest human cancers, virtually unknown in women under fifty. Since that time, it has been identified in several hundred young women (including some pre-adolescents), almost all of whose mothers were given diethylstilbestrol (DES) during pregnancy to prevent miscarriage. Almost all reported cases were in the USA. Tragically, it was already known as early as 1953 that DES, a synthetic oestrogen, did not prevent miscarriage; but many obstetricians continued to prescribe it for this purpose, and indeed some did so right up until the first link between DES and vaginal cancer was demonstrated in 1970. Vaginal clear-cell adenocarcinoma is fundamentally a new, iatrogenic (medically induced) disease.

The link between this oestrogen, when given even in small doses during the first 3 months and clear-cell vaginal cancer in female children is now clearly established. If you took DES, or suspect that you may have been given it and you have a daughter, insist that she be referred to a specialist for checks. If your mother was given DES (ask her!), you should be checked yourself. You cannot get access to your medical records in Britain, but your GP should have them; if he doesn't he can get them, and he can also ask for information from your mother's records. It may be difficult to find out, but if you have the slightest suspicion (e.g. your mother had treatment for recurrent miscarriages), you should push for this important information.

Abnormalities of the genitals have now been found in male children also. They are: small testes; infertility; subfertility; and, in some subfertile men, damaged sperm. No one knows how this would affect offspring. Though malignancy has not yet appeared in males, other effects may be discovered in their female offspring. All DES children should be watched. (See p. 284 for more on DES.)

Diagnosis

If you suspect you are at risk, diagnosis involves not only smears and routine vaginal examinations but also examination by colposcope (a device which brings light and magnification to the walls of the vagina). This examination should be repeated at six-month intervals to detect any cancer cells as soon as possible.

A second test involves painting the entire vaginal area with a stain (Schiller test) to reveal the presence of any abnormal cells.

These tests are vitally necessary, since most of the cases so far discovered have been fairly advanced at the time of diagnosis and *had not been picked up in previous routine gynaecological examinations.* Many women had been reassured that they were perfectly normal, only to have their cancers detected by these other techniques later.

Because this disease is so new, all treatments are by definition experimental. Some doctors believe it may be possible to stop or even reverse the progress of the disease with progesterone suppositories. Various types of surgical excision and cauterization as well as radiation have all produced some beneficial results.

Obviously treatment involves (or should involve) prevention of any additional exposure to oestrogen or DES specifically. This means avoiding the morning-after pill and may mean avoiding all oestrogens, in the contraceptive pill or in the form of oestrogen therapy, until more is known. If DES or oestrogen is taken as a morning-after pill for a suspected pregnancy and does *not* bring on menstruation, an early abortion could be sought to avoid the possibility of cancer in female children.

D&C AND HYSTERECTOMY

Dilatation and Curettage (D&C)

A D&C may be performed for many reasons. As a method of abortion, it has been largely replaced by the suction method. It may be performed for infertility (some doctors question its usefulness) and to prevent the spread of infection following an incomplete abortion or delivery. Some doctors perform one routinely before most major gynaecological operations. It is also used to diagnose cancer of the uterus and fallopian tubes, the cause of abnormal uterine bleeding or discharge, or a pregnancy outside the uterus.

In a D&C the cervical opening is first enlarged (dilated) by inserting several probes of increasing size. Care must be taken to keep from puncturing the uterus. The womb is then gently scraped with a curette, a metal loop on the end of a long, thin handle. A general anaesthetic is usually routine. Recuperation takes from six hours to two days. During this time there may be some bleeding.

Hysterectomy

Hysterectomy means surgical removal of the uterus. We use the term a lot, without being exactly sure whether it also means removal of the ovaries and tubes (that is *pan-hystero-salpingo-oophorectomy*, not a 'complete hysterectomy', as it is sometimes wrongly called). When the uterus is removed but the cervix remains the operation is called a 'partial hysterectomy'. The ovaries and tubes are left, and the woman continues to ovulate each month, but there are no more menstrual periods.

Another procedure also removes the cervix.* In a more extreme procedure, called 'radical total hysterectomy', the cervix and upper portion of the vagina are also removed. (This is usually only done in the case of cervical disease.) In Britain the removal of cervix and uterus is the most common procedure.

Hysterectomies can be done by abdominal incision, or through the vagina which eliminates an abdominal scar. This latter procedure has a higher rate of complication unless the surgeon is experienced in this procedure, because it is more difficult to perform, but the recovery time is quicker and there is less post-operative discomfort.

There is much medical controversy about hysterectomy. Most of it inevitably centres around how patients should be 'assessed' and treated rather than how women can be helped to decide for themselves. There are undoubtedly too many hysterectomies performed in this country: by the age of 75 one in five women is wombless* and many of these operations could have been avoided. One particularly worrying trend is that of routinely removing the ovaries of hysterectomy patients who are nearing menopause (sometimes as young as 40). The ovaries would normally continue to give out small amounts of oestrogen so that the change over from pre- to post-menopause is gradual. The sudden withdrawal of the hormone supply can greatly increase the discomfort of menopause, and the supply of artificial hormones does not entirely make up for the lack.

It is particularly important to ask before the operation if oophorectomy is intended, and to refuse it unless there is a good reason for it such as a verified malignancy.

According to many respected doctors these are the situations in which a hysterectomy is necessary:

1. A local malignancy of the cervix or in the lining of the uterus itself.
2. Symptomatic non-malignant conditions – e.g. excessive numbers of very large fibroids on the inside of the uterus (see 'Fibroids', p. 177), or possibly severe prolapse.
3. Excessive bleeding that does not respond to hormone treatments (see Menopause chapter) or D & Cs (see above), or in such cases when these treatments may not be appropriate for a particular woman.
4. Diseases of the tubes or ovaries which also require removal of the uterus.
5. Cancer of the uterus itself.
6. Catastrophe during childbirth (which requires removal of the uterus for the woman's survival).

---

* Whether or not the cervix is left, a regular smear test is still important.
* Oliver Gillie, *Sunday Times*, 8 December 1974.

Only a tiny percentage of hysterectomies are for cancer, and over 50% of the uteruses examined afterwards are found to be perfectly normal. Why then are there so many hysterectomies? This quote from an American doctor, Ralph C. Wright, could equally apply to some British doctors:

When the patient has completed her family, total hysterectomy should also be performed as prophylactic procedure. Under these circumstances, the uterus becomes a useless, bleeding, symptom-producing, potentially cancer-bearing organ and therefore should be removed . . . To sterilize a woman and allow her to keep a useless and potentially lethal organ is incompatible with modern gynaecological concepts. Hysterectomy is the only logical approach to surgical sterilization of women.

Hysterectomies are too often performed in the following instances:
1. To treat minor problems in middle-aged women such as small fibroids or even pre-menstrual tension.
2. As an abortion method; this is a dangerous practice which should have stopped when the Lane Committee on abortion condemned it.
3. As a sterilization method; this is no longer acceptable as it is far more dangerous than tubal ligation (see p. 287).

The reasons for this frivolous disposal of our wombs don't stand up to examination. It is illogical to carry out a major operation on hundreds of women to prevent the occurrence of cancer or further complications in a few. One cannot imagine similar logic being applied to the removal of any part of the male sexual anatomy.

If a doctor does not take the trouble to explore a woman's problems before referral to a gynaecologist, it is likely that she will be operated on simply because the consultant does not have the time (or inclination?) to discuss the matter fully.

Examination over, the Presence [the gynaecologist] explained that it was necessary for me to have my uterus removed soon, 'the thing anyway would be useless to you, quite useless' . . . at that time I had no idea what a uterus was. A womb was a womb, but a uterus? I thought perhaps some odd little organ like an appendix which one could take or leave. He inquired about my having a child and my lame 'no-but-' was interrupted by his observation that if I had really wanted 'em I would have had 'em by now . . . So that was that.*

After Effects. There are obviously situations in which hysterectomy is the right answer, and many women are considerably relieved to be rid of unpleasant physical symptoms. However, the loss of a body part is bound to cause some kind of reaction and the loss of those parts of our bodies which are uniquely female can have a devastating impact.

---

* Danks, Margaret, *British Journal of Sexual Medicine.*

Those women who have seen their roles primarily as mothers tend to react more strongly than those of us who have a variety of roles.

Physical Problems.   With all the practice they are getting, doctors are now very skilled at performing hysterectomy; the death rate is only about 1/10,000 (in America it is 1/1,600). However, it is major surgery and there is always an attendant risk from anaesthesia, haemorrhage, or shock. The complication rate is about ten to twenty times that of tubal sterilization. One of the more common complications is the accidental cutting of a ureter; this causes urination problems and possibly, if the accident is overlooked, urine could pass into the abdominal cavity.

Recovery time should be about one to three months; for many women it takes a year to recover completely. The physical pain after the operation is usually severe. If the ovaries have been removed some kind of hormone treatment is given, unless cancer is present when it would be prescribed with caution. Many doctors also prescribe tranquillizers to deal with the menopausal symptoms, and the combination can produce side effects.

Psychological After Effects.   In two separate studies, Dr Montagu Barker and Dr D. H. Richards found that women for whom hysterectomy solved a previously serious condition were far less depressed afterwards than those in whom no physical abnormality was found. Overall, these studies indicated that there is an increase in depression among women who have hysterectomies as opposed to other major operations.

Dr Richards speculates that this could be due to a formerly unsuspected interruption of normal hormone flow even when the ovaries are left intact. This theory is still speculation; however, if the depression is hormone-connected it could be treated in a similar fashion to menopausal depression (see Menopause, p. 519).

Sexual After Effects.   These vary enormously. Some women are more interested in sex once they are rid of the fear of pregnancy, for others there is no change, while others experience a loss of libido due to menopausal symptoms (see Menopause, p. 517). There are physical contributors too. Some women find that their vagina is too short, or that lubrication is insufficient. Doctors are not always sympathetic:

Occasionally a patient complains that the loss of the cervix has affected her libido during coitus but an assurance that a possible cancer bearing area has been removed should be enough to satisfy her . . .*

* Doctor quoted by Jean Robinson, *Spare Rib*, 30.

With all these things in mind it is clearly vital that we insist on a thorough investigation of all the possible causes of discomfort, and on the basis of that evidence decide for ourselves whether or not this operation is justified.

I'm in my thirties, married, have two adopted children, and although we don't have the birth control hassle, I have experienced the hysterectomy hassle — i.e. a doctor using a hysterectomy for what seemed insufficient reasons to me. I was lucky enough to find another doctor who spelled out my choices to me and let me make my own decision (the diseased ovary alone was removed). I feel very strongly about patients' participating actively in their own medical decisions and treatment.

It is important to talk about any major decision like this with other people, particularly those with whom you are close. If you are living with a man try to involve him in the decision. An amazing variety of negative feelings have been reported from men of all ages and backgrounds. For all of us it is helpful to talk with other women and have a good friend (our partner if we have one) to accompany us on visits to the doctors.

In my case I was glad to have the hysterectomy — no more worry about profuse bleeding, no more heavy feelings, no more mess and fuss. Since I cannot take hormones, I expected much more of a jolt. I was somewhat nervous and excited — but not much. Compared to other things that can happen in life, I think the 'problem' of menopause is much overrated.

If you have had a hysterectomy and feel good about it, we hope you will understand why we feel it is vital for women to think and discuss what we've written here before they make any decisions.

Vaginal and Urinary Infections and Venereal Disease

All women secrete moisture and mucus from the membranes that line the vagina. This discharge is transparent or slightly milky and may be somewhat slippery. When dry, it may be yellowish. When a woman is sexually aroused or ovulating this secretion increases. It normally causes no irritation or inflammation of the vagina or vulva.

Many bacteria grow in the vagina of a normal, healthy woman. Some of them help to keep the vagina somewhat acid and keep yeast, fungi and other harmful organisms from multiplying out of all proportion. In large amounts, the waste products secreted by these harmful organisms may irritate the vaginal walls and cause infections to develop. At such times we may experience an abnormal discharge, mild or severe itching and burning of the vulva and chafing of the thighs, and occasionally frequent urination.

Some of the reasons we get vaginal infections are: a general lowered resistance (from lack of sleep, bad diet, another infection in our body, and similar factors); too much douching; pregnancy; taking birth control pills, other hormones, or antibiotics; diabetes or a pre-diabetic condition; cuts, abrasions and other irritations in the vagina (from childbirth, from intercourse without enough lubrication, or from using an instrument in the vagina medically or for masturbation).

'Feminine hygiene sprays' (vaginal deodorants) may also damage the delicate skin of the vulva. They are at best unnecessary, often harmful, and should be avoided. Some infections, bacterial or viral, are very contagious and can be transferred through sexual contact.

Prevention

Here are ways to prevent recurring infections:

1. Wash your vulva and bottom regularly. Pat your vulva dry after bathing and try to keep it dry. Also, don't use other people's towels or washcloths. Avoid irritating sprays and soaps (use special non-soap cleansers for skin very sensitive to plain soap).
2. Wear clean, cotton underpants. Avoid nylon underwear and panty hose, since they retain moisture and heat, which help harmful bacteria to grow faster.
3. Avoid trousers that are tight in the crotch and thighs.
4. Always wipe your anus from front to back (so that bacteria from the anus won't get into the vagina or urethra).
5. Your sexual partners should also be clean. It is a good practice for a man to wash his penis daily, especially before making love. Using a condom can provide added protection.
6. Use a sterile, water-soluble jelly if lubrication is needed during intercourse (KY Jelly or birth control jelly – *NOT* vaseline). Even saliva can aggravate a chronic yeast infection.
7. Avoid sexual intercourse that is painful or abrasive to your vagina.
8. Don't put anything sharp in your vagina.
9. Don't put anything in your vagina that you wouldn't put in your mouth.

Here are some preventive measures which can also be used as cures, although their action is mild and they will inevitably take longer to work than drugs would once the infection takes hold. Their value is that they can be used much earlier, before the infection causes real discomfort.

1. Adding vinegar to bath water, a bowl of water big enough to sit in (ratio 1–2 tbspns per quart), or on a tampon, keeps the vagina acidic, a

less favourable climate for bacterial growth. (Use twice a day once infection has started.) You can also use salt or baking soda, diluted. You can also use a douche for squirting the mixture into your vagina although regular douching is inadvisable as it can upset the balance in the vagina and may spread infection. (A douche can be bought in a big chemist though they are not widely available in the UK.)

2. Applications of natural yogurt either with a contraceptive foam plunger, using a speculum and teaspoon, or on a tampon can restore the 'good' bacteria in the vagina if they have been destroyed by antibiotics. Some women find that yeast infections always go hand in hand with antibiotic treatment. Yogurt should restore the natural balance before the infection starts.

3. Some women have cured bacterial infections by putting a clove of garlic into their vagina every day for three days (garlic is known to be antibiotic) and then douching with vinegar.

4. Diet is also important. A blood-sugar malfunction can make you more susceptible to infection. The condition can be corrected by reducing carbohydrate intake and keeping up vitamin B levels (see Nutrition, p. 115).

All these cures are based on restoring the natural balance of the vagina. A healthy vagina in a fertile woman is always slightly acid. The balance changes during periods (blood is alkaline) and after menopause.

Clinics — Diagnosis and Treatment

Once any infection is established it is important to get it checked and cured. All infections of the genital or urinary tract (genito-urinary) are best treated at VD clinics. These clinics are well provided with diagnostic facilities, and specialist staff are more likely to take the right specimens from the right places than, for example, a gynaecologist. GPs and birth control clinic staff may spot an infection but they are not really adequately equipped to diagnose and may as a result prescribe wrongly.

Many people are reluctant to use VD clinics. Even those of us who have accepted our sexuality sufficiently to use birth control are embarrassed and ashamed if sex leads to disease. Our own individual discomfort is not helped by the attitudes of many clinic doctors and nurses who seem to have cast themselves in the role of guardians of public morality. These public and individual attitudes may prevent us from getting the best help. Happily, attitudes in some areas are changing. Some clinic workers have made a constructive connection with sexuality and provide a helpful supportive atmosphere which encourages people to make use of their facilities.

You can find out where your local clinic is by:

1. Checking behind the doors of a public lavatory (clinic times may be out of date).
2. Looking in the phone book under VD.
3. Asking in a health centre or Citizens' Advice Bureau.
4. Asking (or telephoning) the casualty department of any hospital and asking for the 'special clinic'.
5. Asking your GP.

You do not have to be referred by anyone so you can choose the clinic you prefer even if it is not in your immediate area. Some clinics operate rigid appointment systems, others are more flexible.

What Happens at the Clinic?   When you arrive at the clinic you will be given a card with your name and clinic number for future appointments; you then see a doctor who takes down a detailed 'case history'. This entails asking questions which may seem rather embarrassing but give some guidance to diagnosis. For example: do you have a regular sexual partner? Do you ever have anal or oral sex? Next you go into a consulting room with a couch. You will be asked to undress from the waist down and lie on the couch. The following tests should be done routinely.

1. A cervical smear.
2. Vaginal, cervical and if necessary anal and urethral swabs which will be examined on a slide and cultured (bacteria are encouraged to multiply so that they can be seen more easily) and examined microscopically.
3. A blood test.
4. A urine test.
5. A bi-manual pelvic examination (which they sometimes forget!), see p. 140.

This is the most rigorous check-up that you can get anywhere in the NHS system.

You will then be asked to wait for the initial test result. Even if this test is negative, cultures must be done for greater accuracy. This takes at least 48 hours and it is *imperative* that you return to the clinic within the next few days for your results, as it may take weeks to trace you if infection is found. Unfortunately you can rarely get test results over the phone.

When you are given your results you will not necessarily be told what you have by name. 'Don't worry, just a little bug' is the sort of information often supplied. This withholding of information should be strongly opposed. If you are not given a clear diagnosis just go through the possible list by name and get them to say yes or no. (One reason for withholding information may be that your partner has asked for it to be confidential!)

It is important to know exactly what you have and exactly what you are being treated with. Some clinics will prescribe medicine if you are a confirmed contact with infection even if test results are not positive. In the case of gonorrhoea you may welcome this, as it is hard to diagnose and highly infectious. However, the liberal prescription of antibiotics 'just in case' is a particularly bad habit of British doctors. You do not have to accept medication and it is often wise to wait for a definite diagnosis. This may mean coming back to the clinic several times if you are fairly certain that you have picked something up, because diagnosis is not always accurate the first time.

Any medication will be prescribed and given to you immediately, *without prescription charges.* Make sure you finish the whole course, or the infection may recur, and don't have sex until you are clear. If you have syphilis or gonorrhoea you will be asked to see a social worker or 'contact tracer'. There you will be given slips with the address of the clinic to pass on to possible contacts so that they can come in for tests. It is very important to cooperate; if you have passed the disease on it may have spread to others, all of whom will need treatment. Even if you haven't got either of these infections you may be asked to bring your partner in for tests. (This is particularly important if you have a recurring infection.) He or she should be checked because otherwise the infection may keep coming back. Although most infections are less likely to travel between women they can do, particularly syphilis and the less fragile organisms like thrush and trichomonas. Women partners should be informed if you have a confirmed case of V D.

Ways to Prevent V D

To most people V D means syphilis or gonorrhoea (although many other infections are sexually transmitted). Since the war there has been a sharp increase in the number of reported cases of these diseases, though recently the numbers have started to level off and syphilis is actually decreasing among all sections of the population, except homosexual males. This could be a result of greater efforts to trace contacts and halt the spread of the disease.

Both syphilis and gonorrhoea are very easily spread by close contact, but prevention is made difficult because social and sexual attitudes make it hard for us to take avoiding action. How do you ask someone you fancy if they have the 'clap'? The simplest form of protection is obviously to sleep only with people you know well enough to ask or who you trust enough to tell you if they have got V D. Failing that, the old-fashioned method of wearing a 'raincoat' can't be beaten. The raincoat in this case means a sheath and though *you* can't wear them you can make sure you have them at hand and provide them when necessary. This does put

women at a disadvantage because some of us would find it as hard to
offer a sheath to a new lover as to ask him if he's got the clap. Another
way is to use a contraceptive cream, preferably with a cap for added
protection, although the protection they offer is by no means foolproof.

Preparations which help prevent VD:

Delfen Foam   Ortho-Gynol Jelly
Emko Foam   Ortho Cream

Other products good for VD prevention but not for birth control:
Lorophyn Vaginal Suppositories
Progonasyl (by prescription only)
All these preparations can also be used in the anus and applied
over the urethra to help stop infections moving up to the bladder.
However, they have not been tested for anal use and may be less
effective because of the different rate of absorption.

Remember, preventive measures cut down your chances of catching
VD but they are not 100% effective. If you have been exposed to infection,
get a test and don't have sex until you know you are cured. One cure
does not give you future immunity. You will always be equally susceptible
to infection.

Research and the Future

It is clear that venereal diseases will spread more easily as monogamy
ceases to be the accepted standard. The more people you sleep with the
greater your chance of contracting disease and passing it on. Most other
contagious diseases are now controlled by vaccines, clearly the most
efficient form of prevention. Some work is being done in this field but
the study of VD is not popular and it is not given the attention or money
which, for example, is pumped into research and production of cures for
'the common cold'. The reason is partly that the big drug firms which
have a virtual monopoly of drug production find it rather more lucrative
to put their money into cures, such as modifications of antibiotics, rather
than prevention.

While there is no vaccine available we must use those facilities which
do exist and clinics must be pressured into responding sympathetically
to the needs of women. Many birth control clinics have adapted to deal
with changing social attitudes to sex (although they are by no means
perfect). It is ludicrous that a woman can be supplied with contraceptives
without fear of guilt or embarrassment and yet, when the result of her

sexual activity is infection, is forced to suffer humiliation as part of her treatment.

Venereal disease is dangerous and unpleasant. It is up to all of us to take preventive measures and try and control the spread of disease but, equally, it is up to the authorities to provide adequate information. It is no more shameful to have VD than it is to have sex and the sooner the subject comes out from the back of loo doors and onto public information notice boards, the nearer we will be to stopping the spread of disease.

GONORRHOEA

Gonorrhoea is caused by a bacterium shaped like a coffee bean which works its way through the genital and urinary organs. Gonorrhoea organisms live best in a warm moist place. They die in less than a minute outside the body and are spread by intimate contact, usually through vaginal, oral or anal intercourse. It is also possible to spread the infection from discharge in the vagina or penis via hands, particularly to the eyes. It is spread more easily from penile discharge than vaginal discharge.

Women have a 40–50% chance of catching gonorrhoea from an infected male partner after just one exposure to it. If you use the Pill the risk may be higher, unless of course you use some preventive method (see 'Ways to Prevent VD', above). The Pill also seems to hasten the spread of infection into the fallopian tubes as soon as 2–3 weeks after infection. Although lesbian women are far less likely to catch gonorrhoea, it is wise to get a test if your partner has an infection.

Symptoms

There are rarely any visible symptoms in women. The best indication is always being told about or noticing symptoms in a male partner. Note, however, that some men don't have symptoms.

Early Male Symptoms.   90% of men show symptoms within a week – a thick milky discharge from the penis and pain or burning while urinating. The symptoms are similar to non-specific urethritis (see p. 199) so diagnosis is vital. You may notice a slight crusting at the end of the penis if there is a discharge. There may also be enlarged and tender lymph glands in the groin, and in uncircumcised men the discharge may cause reddening and irritation of the penis.

Early Female Symptoms.   The minority (20%) who do develop symptoms do so anywhere from 2 days to 3 weeks after exposure. The cervix is the most common site of infection. The vagina is not affected after puberty. (The vaginal walls are made of cells different from the cervical cells.)

You develop a cervical discharge which is the result of an irritant released by the gonococci when they die. You may attribute first symptoms to other routine gynaecological problems or to the use of birth control methods, such as the Pill. The urethra may also become infected, possibly causing painful urination. As the infection spreads it can affect the Skene's (on each side of the urinary opening) and Bartholin's glands and the rectum. The rectum is infected by the vaginal discharge, which can easily get into it, or through anal intercourse. Symptoms include anal irritation, discharge and painful defecation.

Late Female Symptoms.   In women the disease is more likely to persist and spread than in men, because the cervix becomes inflamed. The endocervical glands (lining the cervical canal) drain poorly, not allowing the bacteria and pus to be passed out of the body readily. As the disease spreads up the uterus and fallopian tubes you can have pain on one or both sides of your lower abdomen. You may also have vomiting and fever. Your menstrual periods may become irregular.

The more severe the infection, the more severe the pain and other symptoms. These symptoms may indicate pelvic inflammatory disease (see p. 205). One type of PID is salpingitis. This is scarring and infection of the fallopian tubes, which can lead to sterility if the tubes become blocked. It is more likely to happen if your birth control method is an IUD. The discharge from the infection can irritate surrounding tissues. Another kind of PID is peritonitis, inflammation of certain abdominal tissues.

Seventeen per cent of the women known to have gonorrhoea develop PID. Of these women, 15 to 40% may become sterile after one episode with it. A less common complication is proctitis, inflammation of the rectum. Blindness can also occur if the eyes are infected. Rarer but very serious problems occur when the bacteria travel through the bloodstream and cause infection in the valves of the heart, acute arthritis, meningitis, or even death.

The disease can be treated at any stage to prevent further damage, but often damage already done cannot be repaired.

Remember that gonorrhoea can also be spread from a man's penis to a woman's *throat*. You may have no symptoms, or your throat may be sore or your glands swollen. The *mouth* does not provide the right environment for gonorrhoea bacteria to grow.

As early diagnosis is so difficult and advanced symptoms so serious it is particularly important that women take preventive measures (see p. 191) and try to keep some kind of contact with partners so that infection can be reported at an early stage.

Diagnosis of Gonorrhoea

If you have had sex with someone who has confirmed gonorrhoea or a suspicious discharge, go to a VD clinic immediately. Diagnosis is not easy and specialized staff will give you the best results. If diagnosis in a male partner is not already confirmed, ask him to go with you, or soon after, for tests. Diagnosis of his discharge will give a clearer basis for your diagnosis. Make sure the test is done *before* you take any medication as the treatment renders the test inaccurate. Don't douche before getting a test because you can wash all the *accessible* bacteria away, giving a false negative result.

You may be asked before the test is done whether you ever have anal intercourse. If you do, an anal swab will be taken automatically. However, although a swab from the cervix is the best single test (88–93% accurate), about 50% of infected women have infection in the anus also whether or not they've had anal intercourse, so it is worth asking for both tests to be done. If you have had a hysterectomy ask for a urethral culture; if you have had oral-genital sex, ask for a gonococcal throat culture.

Samples can be taken during menstrual bleeding, but the discharge can cover up monilia (thrush) and trichomoniasis, making the tests harder to interpret. We believe also, though this is not confirmed, that the presence of gonorrhoea can give a false diagnosis of abnormal cervical cells, so if you do have gonorrhoea have a cervical smear two months after the infection has cleared.

The accuracy of swabs is vital to correct diagnosis but even then gonorrhoea is hard to diagnose. If your test is negative but you are a confirmed contact you should be asked to return a week later for a re-test. Go back anyway if you feel uneasy about a negative test. Treatment is usually prescribed even after two negative tests if your partner has gonorrhoea.

Treatment

Some doctors prescribe antibiotics without a positive test from you or your partner – 'just in case'. It may be better in this case to wait for a positive diagnosis because the bacteria can build up immunity to antibiotics and they shouldn't be used unless it is clearly necessary. Also, if the infection turns out to be something different, the treatment should also be different. If you do decide to postpone treatment make sure you can easily get back for a re-test and do not have close physical contact with anyone until you are cleared of infection.

The normal treatment for gonorrhoea is high-dosage injections of penicillin. This has the fewest side effects for most people, and the dose for gonorrhoea can also cure a syphilis infection still in the incubation stage. Oral probenecid (1 gram) is recommended in addition, to reduce the urinary excretion of penicillin and allow the penicillin to remain in the bloodstream in a high enough concentration to effect a cure. Tetracycline and other 'mycin' drugs can be used by those allergic to penicillin. Some do not work against syphilis. Ask. See the *VD Handbook* for more information on drugs and their possible side effects. Particularly if you are pregnant.

Gonorrhoea has required increasing doses of penicillin or other drugs to cure. New strains seem to have developed since the introduction of penicillin, and the more virulent strains are the only ones that survive the dose given for treatment. This trend can be reversed by using sufficient doses to kill all possible strains. The total dosage required, however, is still far lower than those commonly used for several other kinds of infection.

Test for Cure of Gonorrhoea

It is important that every woman treated for gonorrhoea have three negative culture tests, including a rectal culture, a week apart before being considered cured. (The culture test, as mentioned before, is not totally reliable.) If cultures remain positive, retreatment is another drug or double the initial dosage of penicillin. Pockets of infection in the reproductive organs or rectum may be particularly difficult to cure.

If you have an IUD (coil) and the infection is resistant to treatment, it may be best to have it removed and replaced after the treatment is completed.

Reinfection can occur soon after treatment if your partner has gonorrhoea and is not treated simultaneously.

Be sure to have a syphilis test three months after treatment for gonorrhoea because sometimes the penicillin disguises early syphilis without curing it.

Pregnancy and Gonorrhoea

A pregnant woman with untreated gonorrhoea can infect her baby as it passes through the birth canal. In past years many babies became blind right after birth because of gonococcal conjunctivitis. The eyes of newborn babies are treated with silver nitrate or penicillin drops in order to cure this disease if it is present.

SYPHILIS

Syphilis is caused by a small spiral-shaped bacterium called a spirochete. Once these bacteria have entered the body the disease goes through four stages.

Symptoms of Syphilis

Primary.   The first sign is usually a sore called a *chancre* (pronounced 'shanker'). It may look like a pimple, a blister, or an open sore. It is usually painless. It will probably show up any time from 9 to 90 days after the bacteria enter the body. This sore usually appears on or near the place where the bacteria enter, usually the genitals. However, it may appear on the fingertips, lips, breast, anus, or mouth. At this primary stage it is very infectious, since the chancre is full of bacteria which can easily be spread to others. Sometimes the chancre never develops or is hidden inside the body, giving no evidence of the disease. This is particularly true for women, in whom the sore frequently develops inside the vagina or is hidden inside the folds of the labia. Only about 10% of the women who get these chancres notice them. If you examine yourself regularly with a speculum you are more likely to see one if it develops. (See Chapter 6, p. 135, 'Self-examination Techniques'.) In any case, the sore goes away in 1 to 5 weeks with or without treatment — but the bacteria are still in the body, increasing and spreading. The preventive methods explained before (p. 191) work only if the chemical or physical barrier covers the infectious sore. In some people glands in the groin enlarge painlessly.

Secondary.   The next stage occurs anywhere from a week to 6 months later. It usually lasts 3 to 6 months, but sometimes the symptoms of this stage can come and go for several years. By this time the bacteria have spread all through the body, and there are many possible symptoms. A rash may appear over the entire body or just on the palms of the hands and the soles of the feet. Sores may appear in the mouth. Joints may become swollen or painful, and bones may hurt. There may be a sore throat, mild fever, or headache (all flu symptoms). Patches of hair may fall out. An infectious, raised area may appear around the genitals and anus and lymph glands enlarge all over. Any sexually active person who is not monogamous or whose partner(s) is (are) not monogamous should watch for any of these symptoms. If any appear, s/he should get a routine test for syphilis. During the secondary stage the disease can be spread by simple physical contact, including kissing, because bacteria are present in the open syphilitic sores which may appear on any part of the body. The bacteria are smaller than the average pore size and can easily pass through pores. This is also the stage in which syphilis imitates other diseases. Sometimes the symptoms are so mild that they go unnoticed. Again, the symptoms disappear, but the bacteria remain active in the body.

Latent.   During this stage, which may last 10 or 20 years, there are no outward signs. However, the bacteria may be invading the inner organs, including the heart and brain. The disease is not infectious after the first few years of the latent stage.

Late. In this stage the serious effects of the latent stage appear. Depending on which organ the bacteria have attacked, a person may develop serious heart disease, crippling, blindness, or mental incapacity. With our present ability to diagnose and treat syphilis, no one should have to reach this stage.

What to Look for in a Man. The symptoms are similar to a woman's. The most common place for the chancre to appear is on the penis and scrotum. It may be hidden in the folds under the foreskin or under the scrotum or where the penis meets the rest of the body. In the primary stages men are more likely than women to develop swollen lymph glands in the groin.

Diagnosis of Syphilis

Syphilis can be diagnosed and treated at any time. Early in the primary stages a doctor can look for subtle symptoms, like swollen lymph glands around the groin, and examine some of the discharge from the chancre, if one has developed, under a microscope (darkfield test). Do not put any kind of medication, cream or ointment on the sore until a doctor examines it. Otherwise the syphilis bacteria on the surface are likely to be killed, making the test less accurate. Spirochetes will be in the bloodstream a week or two after the chancre has formed. They stimulate the production of antibodies which show up in a blood test, which from then on, through all the stages, will reveal the infection. If you have been treated for gonorrhoea with medication other than penicillin you should arrange for four tests one month apart to cover the possible incubation period of syphilis. Some drugs used to treat gonorrhoea do not cure syphilis. Remember, incubation can be as long as 90 days, so refrain from sex until you are clear. A good description of the different blood tests used is in the *VD Handbook*. If you or your partner are sexually active with more than one partner, you should have regular check-ups at a VD clinic where a blood test will be given routinely.

Treatment and Test for Cure of Syphilis

The treatment for syphilis is penicillin, or a substitute such as tetracycline for those allergic to penicillin. It may be one long-lasting dose or a series of smaller doses. Since people sometimes have relapses or mistakes are made, it is important to have at least two follow-up blood tests to be sure the treatment has been complete. The first three stages of syphilis can be completely cured with no permanent damage, and even in late syphilis the destructive effects can be stopped from going any further.

A few syphilis antibodies will remain in the blood permanently, even after total cure. In future blood tests the amount of antibodies will be important; if you contract syphilis again the number will increase.

Syphilis and Pregnancy

If a pregnant woman has syphilis she can pass the bacteria on to her foetus. The bacteria attack the foetus just as they do an adult, and the child may be born dead or with important tissues deformed or diseased. But if the mother's syphilis is treated before the sixteenth week of pregnancy, the foetus will probably not be infected at all. (Even after the foetus has got syphilis, penicillin will stop the disease, although it cannot repair damage that has already been done.) It is important that every pregnant woman get a blood test for syphilis as soon as she knows she is pregnant. Thus, if she has the disease, she can be treated for it before she gives it to her foetus. She should have the test repeated during pregnancy any time she thinks she may have been exposed to syphilis.

NON-SPECIFIC URETHRITIS

Non-specific urethritis (NSU) is usually relatively trivial in women, but it is troublesome for men and has a tendency to recur. Women should not ignore it because as carriers they can re-infect their partners. It is also associated with trichomoniasis which is similarly asymptomatic in men.

Symptoms

NSU organisms can cause cervicitis which produces a whitish discharge. In men the symptoms are similar to gonorrhoea and may well be confused without proper diagnosis – a thin greyish discharge from the penis and stinging or irritation when urinating.

Diagnosis

A swab taken from the cervix (or the urethra in men) is cultured and examined microscopically to differentiate from gonorrhoea.

Treatment

Tetracycline. During treatment avoid alcohol and abstain from sexual intercourse.

Complications

In some cases NSU is associated with a form of arthritis called Reiters syndrome. It is extremely difficult to cure and causes swelling and stiffening of the joints which can cripple. Once this syndrome has developed it can be re-activated with any further contact with NSU. This condition is rarer in women.

TRICHOMONIASIS

Trichomonas vaginalis, or trich, is a one-celled parasite found in men and very commonly in women, though often without symptoms. Usually women with trich have a thin, foamy vaginal discharge that is yellowish-green or grey in colour and has a foul odour. If another infection is present along with trichomoniasis, the discharge may be thicker and whiter. Trich can also cause a urinary infection. It is most often contracted through intercourse (thus trichomoniasis can be a venereal infection), but can be passed on by moist objects such as towels, bathing suits, underwear, flannels and toilet seats.

Though trich is nearly always asymptomatic in men it is associated with NSU which is similarly asymptomatic in women (see above). Sometimes treatment is offered for 'suspected' trich but it is important to have a proper diagnosis before accepting treatment. Between 30% and 40% of women who have trich are also found to have gonorrhoea.

Treatment

Trichomoniasis is usually treated with metronidazole (Flagyl) by mouth which is the most effective treatment. However, in various tests, metronidazole has caused gene mutations in animals, and cancer in rats and mice (in at least seven different studies). Its safety is clearly questionable, as is that of a similar drug, nimorazole (Naxogin).

Originally Flagyl was licensed by the American Food and Drug Administration, but following some independent research the FDA had to re-examine its findings. FDA officials later testified that the US manufacturers (G. D. Searle) had falsified their data to make it appear that the drug was not carcinogenic in humans.* Neither the FDA nor the UK Committee on Safety of Medicines have issued cautions about it.

The respected American medical magazine *Medical Letter* advises that Flagyl should not be used for trich infections that can be cured by other means. The medical profession, particularly in the UK, are ill-informed about this drug and tend to prescribe it liberally. The UK manufacturers

---

* See *Off Our Backs*, August/September and September/October 1974.

state that there are no contraindications for the use of Flagyl even in pregnancy, though the standard medical guide to medicines does warn against prescribing it to pregnant or lactating women.

If you are prescribed Flagyl keep the following in mind:

1. Flagyl should not be taken by mouth by anyone who has either peptic ulcers, another infection elsewhere in the body, a history of blood diseases or a disease of the central nervous system, and preferably not by pregnant or lactating women.

2. While taking Flagyl avoid alcohol as the combination can cause headaches, nausea, and other side effects.

3. Intervals of 4–6 weeks should elapse between courses.

4. The manufacturers suggest a blood test before and after treatment to ensure that the blood is normal.

5. Regular partners should be treated as well to avoid re-infection, and sex should be ruled out during treatment.

Other Treatment

Frequently vaginal pessaries (such as Floraquin) or vaginal gels can provide adequate treatment. To avoid recurrences one specialist recommends the following: regular baths throughout the menstrual cycle, nightly use of Floraquin pessaries (or a similar product), loose cotton clothing since exposure to air destroys the parasites causing the infection, and avoidance of tampons, ordinary douches and vaginal sprays.

YEAST INFECTIONS (ALSO CALLED CANDIDA, MONILIA, FUNGUS AND THRUSH)

Candida albicans, a yeast fungus, normally grows in harmless quantities in your rectum and vagina. When your system is out of balance, yeast-like organisms may grow profusely and cause a vaginal discharge that is thick and white, may look like cottage cheese, and may smell like baking bread. It can itch maddeningly and usually makes intercourse painful. If a woman has a yeast infection when she gives birth, the baby will get yeasts in its digestive tract. This is called thrush and is treated orally with nystatin drops or gentian violet.

Candida grows best in a very mildly acidic environment. The pH in the vagina is normally more acidic than this (4.0 to 50), except when we take birth control pills or some antibiotics, when we are pregnant, when we have diabetes, and when we menstruate (the pH rises to 5.8 or 6.8 because blood is alkaline). Obviously, we often find ourselves with a vaginal pH favourable to monilia.

The preventive measures for infection mentioned on p. 188 are particularly important in conquering recurrent thrush. Some people find that vinegar treatment can work as a cure if it is used early enough. However, once a yeast infection has really taken hold, particularly if it is very irritating, such procedures might be either too slow or simply ineffective. In this case you will have to see a doctor or go to a clinic (it is useful to have tests done to make sure it is thrush).

Treatment usually consists of some form of nystatin pessaries which are only available on prescription. Nystatin cream may be prescribed for your partner to stop him from reinfecting you. If the infection is really severe, oral nystatin may be prescribed, but it shouldn't be used in pregnancy and should only be used if it is really necessary because it kills off fungi of all kinds throughout the body. It also occasionally makes you feel nauseous.

Another method which is effective, but less popular these days because it is messy, is gentian violet. It should be painted over the cervix, vagina and vulva. Some people react against it but for the others it is a very effective treatment and a sanitary pad worn during treatment will stop your clothes turning purple. It is important to use an *aqueous* solution, not alcohol, which will burn.

One of the problems with using medications to cure thrush is that all the good bacteria are destroyed with the bad and unless the good ones grow back first we can become reinfected. A change in diet with a reduction in refined foods, combined with the preventive routine, makes more sense, and for those sisters on the contraceptive pill it might be worth coming off it until your thrush is cleared. (Do get an alternative form of contraception.)

For a long time I felt as though I were on a merry-go-round. I would get a yeast infection, take Mycostatin [a brand of nystatin] for three weeks, clear up the infection, and then two weeks later find that the itching and the thick white discharge were back. Finally, once while on medication I also douched with Lactinex* and carefully watched my sugar intake. This worked for me and the monilia has not recurred in many months.

Thrush can be transferred by hand; this is of particular importance in lesbian relationships. Men rarely get thrush symptoms but they can reinfect their partners, so it is worthwhile getting a tube of nystatin for a regular male partner to use while you are using pessaries.

* Lactic acid, available in some chemists.

GENITAL HERPES

Genital herpes is a common viral disease which has recently reached epidemic proportions, particularly among women.

Herpes appears as painful sores which look like blisters or small bumps. These sores may be inside the vagina, on the external genitals, thighs, in or near the anus, or on the buttocks. Sores also appear on the cervix, where they are not painful. The blisters can rupture to form open sores, or ulcers, which are often very painful. While the sores are open the herpes virus is thought to spread very easily to other people. The open sores are also subject to infection by other bacteria. Other possible symptoms are fever, enlarged lymph nodes and flu-like symptoms. The sores sometimes heal by themselves in anywhere from a week to a month. The virus then enters a latent stage during which it is not contagious. A new eruption can occur at any time, although it often appears to be related to stress, either physical or emotional. For some women the outbreaks recur after prolonged intercourse or are connected with their menstrual cycles. There does not seem to be a limit to the number of outbreaks, although for many people the first one is the worst. Men's symptoms look like women's. They usually appear somewhere on the penis or near the anus. Herpes is usually (but not necessarily) spread by sexual intercourse. It is caused by a virus known as *Herpes simplex*, type 2, which is closely related to *Herpes simplex*, type 1, the cause of cold sores or fever blisters. Type 2 seems to appear below the waist and type 1 above, although there is an estimated 10% cross-over, probably resulting from oral-genital sex. The way it is transferred and its incubation period are unknown.

Because there is a statistically higher risk of contracting cervical cancer if you have herpes it is wise to get regular smear tests (see p. 178). The infection may also lead to miscarriage or early delivery in pregnant women, and if a baby comes into contact with open sores during childbirth it could suffer brain damage or die.

Diagnosis is usually determined by the appearance of the sores. A more accurate diagnosis can be made by microscopic examination of a smear taken from the sore or from the cervix. Diagnosis is important, because herpes can be confused with cystitis as they can both give acute discomfort when you urinate. Some people try to avoid urinating because of the pain but this can lead to urine retention as well. The best way to alleviate the pain is to urinate in the bath. This doesn't sound very nice but the water will dilute the urine and prevent the burning sensation.

There is no known cure for herpes, only symptomatic treatment. You should wear loose clothing and cotton underpants, try to keep the area cool and bathe it with cold water. Sometimes a lubricated tampon used to separate the labia will help. You should see a doctor to have the sores examined for bacterial infection. Sometimes infection can cause a fever, in which case it is wise to get antibiotic treatment and go to bed. Sulpha creams may be prescribed for local application but these may cause skin irritation and make the discomfort worse. A doctor can also prescribe local anaesthetic gels or you can use painkillers.

There are two medical treatments which may be prescribed. Corticosteroids, usually in cream form, are effective in reducing inflammation and pain, but they should only be used in very small quantities because they suppress the production of the body's own corticosteroids which play a vital part in dealing with infection and stress. On no account should these drugs be prescribed over a long period of time for herpes, and they should at all times be used with caution; some people react badly in which case they can produce a worse condition.

Herpid (Idoxuridine) is a new drug which has not been carefully studied. It is an anti-viral agent which can affect the gene structure of a foetus. It should never be used in pregnancy and should not be prescribed to children. It is not even clear if it works at all and certainly it will have no effect once the sores have been established. It should only be used very early on in an outbreak.

We have heard about one woman who inserted vitamin E capsules into her vagina at the first warning prick of an outbreak. She says it stopped the development of the sores but we have had no corroboration from anyone else.

It is wise to keep in good physical shape to try and prevent recurrence, and men should wear condoms to prevent spreading the infection.

VENEREAL WARTS

Venereal warts, or *Condyloma acuminatum,* are very common. They are caused by a virus and may look like regular warts. Though they may be spread in other ways, sexual intercourse helps to transmit them. The warts, which don't hurt, appear 1 to 3 months after contact with an infected person, usually on the bottom part of the vaginal opening. They are also found on the vaginal lips, inside the vagina, on the cervix, and around the anus. When small, they look like little pieces of hard, raised skin. If they become large they can develop a cauliflower-like appearance. Warmth and moisture seem to help them grow.

On a man the warts usually occur towards the tip of the penis, sometimes under the foreskin, and less often, on the shaft of the penis or the scrotum.

Diagnosis is usually made by appearance. If the warts are small they can be dried up with an application of podophyllin, a dark ointment or liquid which is available on prescription. Wash this chemical off after 4 hours so that you don't get burns from it. Several treatments may be necessary. Apply *very* carefully. Podophyllin will burn normal skin. If you cannot see well enough to apply it yourself, go to a clinic or get a friend to help. Podophyllin should not be used during pregnancy. Small warts can also be frozen off (cryosurgery) with solid CO_2 (dry ice). This hurts very briefly. If the warts are large they must be removed surgically. If all the warts are not removed at the same time, the ones left will usually spread again. If you want to get rid of them completely, make sure all the warts, including those inside the vagina and on the cervix, are removed. Even after apparently thorough treatment the warts may reappear. You can also catch them again if your sexual partner is not treated at the same time. If the warts are only on the penis or inside the vagina, using a condom can help to keep them from spreading.

CRABS, OR PUBIC LICE

Phthirus pubis is a roundish, crablike body louse that lives in pubic hair and occasionally in the hair of the chest, armpits, eyelashes and eyebrows. You can 'catch' them by intimate physical contact with someone who has them, or from bedding or clothes that person has used. They are blood-suckers and can carry such diseases as typhus. The main symptom of crabs is an intolerable itching in the genital area. They shouldn't be confused with thrush (see p. 201), because crabs are visible without a microscope. The cure for crabs is a cream, shampoo, or powder called Lorexane or Quellada, available fairly cheaply over the counter in a chemist, on prescription from a doctor, or free at a VD clinic. It should be left on for 24 hours and then washed off. It is a quick effective treatment (Normal soap will not affect crabs.)

After treatment you should use clean clothing and bed linen. Crabs die within 24 hours after separation from the human body, but the eggs live about 6 days. Previously used bedclothes, towels, etc. are safe after a week without use. Anything dry-cleaned or washed in boiling water can be used immediately.

OTHER DISEASES

Other diseases generally considered sexually transmitted are chancroid, lymphogranuloma venereum (LGV) and granuloma inguinale. The last may not be venereal. None has been well studied. However, each is treatable with antibiotics. See *VD Handbook* (Bibliography, p. 214) for more information on these diseases.

PELVIC INFLAMMATORY DISEASE (PID)

PID refers to a group of several pelvic infections including parametritis (affects the uterus), salpingitis (affects the tubes), and salpingo-oophoritis (affects the tubes and ovaries). It can be caused by gonorrhoea, certain bacteria, or certain viruses. Symptoms of PID can include pelvic pain, increasing pain with intercourse and/or menstruation, irregular bleeding (spotting or flooding or passing clots) and occasional chills and fever. (These same symptoms also occur in an ectopic pregnancy and endometriosis, so a pregnancy test is a good idea whenever they are present (see p. 349).) Some women who have PID in its early stages (subacute) also report a sharp abdominal pain at the time of ovulation, a pain they don't usually have.

Treatment of PID can include either tetracycline or ampicillin (for about 10 days), lots of bed rest (complete rest for at least one full week is strongly advised), *no* sexual intercourse for at least 2 weeks (this allows the infected area to heal), and a well-balanced diet (it's a good idea to have friends cook for you, so you can stay in bed). Symptoms should clear up somewhat within a few days. If they don't, you will probably need a culture and sensitivity test, if this was not already done at your first examination. In this test, a smear of your cervical discharge is cultured on a plate to determine exactly what organism is causing the infection (though even this might not show what bacteria are present further up). That way you can know if you are taking an antibiotic that effectively destroys the organisms infecting you. Sometimes you will have to try a different drug to treat PID successfully.

In some women PID is recurrent and responds poorly to antibiotics. Sometimes a woman may have to be hospitalized, especially when she is unable to get adequate bed rest at home. When the tubes are involved and become sufficiently scarred, infertility may result. Also, scarred tubes may increase the chance of an ectopic pregnancy. The seriousness of PID is often underrated. Any infection in the pelvic area should be treated early. If you have a history of PID don't use an IUD.

My pelvic inflammatory disease (PID) was caused by my IUD, according to my doctor, though the IUD gave me no pain and I had no medical history which would predict trouble. The first episode of infection was cleared up by ampicillin. That was over ten months ago and I'm not well yet. When the infection came back I went through one antibiotic after another, living in terrible pain, fever and misery for over two months, while the doctor assured me that this medicine would surely cure me. Then they hospitalized me for intravenous antibiotics, looked in with a laparoscope, decided not to operate, and sent me home. Two months later the infection flared up again. This time they took out my tubes, leaving my ovaries, since they seemed all right. After I recovered from the surgery my abdomen was swollen. I had a lot of pain and enormous fatigue, and the fever prevented me from functioning very well mentally. Everything has been complicated by the fact that I took no extra time off from work and have two toddlers, and my husband is out of town four days a week. Today, four months after the surgery, I still have intermittent pain caused by inflammation in my ovaries and uterus and by adhesions, internal scar tissue binding my organs together. I have learned not to wear trousers or do much bending and to get extra rest; intercourse no longer hurts so much, but orgasm sometimes still does. I'm waiting for improvement now but don't know if this is wise, since there's no cure and some doctors say I may get better while others predict I'll end up with a total hysterectomy even if I wait six more months. It's a pretty dreadful disease.

CYSTITIS

Cystitis is an inflammation and/or infection of the bladder. Sometime in her life nearly every woman gets it, and it can be hard to eradicate permanently. It usually means that intestinal bacteria, such as *Escherichia coli* (*E. coli*), useful in the digestive tract, have got into the bladder. Trich can also cause cystitis. The symptoms can be really frightening, though it is not a serious condition. If you suddenly have to urinate every few minutes and it burns like crazy even though almost nothing comes out, you probably have cystitis. There may also be blood in the urine (haematuria) and pus in the urine (pyuria). You may have pain just above your pubic bone, and sometimes there is a peculiar, heavy urine odour when you first urinate in the morning.

If these symptoms develop, you should see a doctor – although the infection may disappear without treatment. You can help relieve the symptoms before you see the doctor by following the advice given below under 'Prevention'. Examination is important, as cystitis and herpes symptoms can be confused.

I had recurring bouts of cystitis for several months, always precipitated by intercourse but not attributable to any specific cause that could be found by a urologist. The first few times I had an attack my distress seemed drastically out of proportion to the actual physical pain. I did not really 'hurt', but the physical discomfort, especially at night, triggered a terrible restlessness and panic. Talking to other women in the hospital emergency room, I discovered that this kind of psychological reaction is commonly associated with the physical symptoms for many women. Other women described the feeling that they were 'climbing the walls' or 'climbing out of their skin' all night. Knowing what to expect, I began to relax more when I had an attack and stopped feeling ashamed of 'over-reacting' to the symptoms. I found that I was most uncomfortable lying down and preferred to lose sleep when I felt a need to be active or distracted at night.

The doctor will ask for a urine sample, so take a drink of water before your visit. Treatment may begin immediately with a sulpha drug, although it is often delayed a couple of days until the offending bacteria and the drugs they are sensitive to can be identified. Tetracycline, nitrofurantoin, Septrin (Bactrim), and ampicillin are also commonly used.

Full treatment may take 2 weeks, but the symptoms should disappear in a day or so. If they don't, return to the doctor. Some bacteria are resistant to, and even thrive on, some of the drugs. You may be asked to control the pH of your urine by drinking lemon barley water or taking vitamin C (both are acid) or Mist. Pot. Citrate which is alkaline. This is important, since some drugs do not work well when the urine pH is not in the right range. Vaginitis, thrush and some digestive upset are common side effects of the antibiotics and sulpha drugs. Nausea may be decreased by taking the medication with meals.

Like vaginitis, cystitis is more likely to occur when your resistance is low. Damage to the urethra from nearby surgery, childbirth, or intercourse may also make you more susceptible to infection. Women who urinate infrequently and people who are catheterized for a long period or frequently often develop cystitis. If your cystitis keeps recurring consult a urologist, as a serious abnormality may be present.

Cystitis is sometimes, though not always, sex-related. The first time you have intercourse with a particular man or have intercourse after a long period of abstinence, you may get a sudden attack of urethritis (inflammation of the urethra), often called 'honeymoon cystitis'. In some cases this can lead to true cystitis.

Prevention

If you are a chronic cystitis sufferer there are preventive measures which you can take:

1. Drink enough to urinate several times a day (every hour if symptoms have started).
2. Drink lemon barley water or marshmallow tea (from a herbalist) regularly.
3. Avoid tea, coffee, alcohol and spices, particularly when symptoms have started, as they irritate the bladder.
4. Ensure that the hands and/or penis of your sexual partner are clean and avoid intercourse positions which stretch or damage the urethra or put excessive pressure on the bladder (such as penetration from the rear), particularly while the bladder is still tender from recent infection.
5. Urinate before and after sex.
6. If you expect to be distant from medical help you can get a prescription for Pyridium, which relieves the symptoms though it doesn't affect the bacteria. It makes your urine bright orange and the stain can be permanent, so guard against drips.
7. If symptoms start, soak in a hot bath several times a day, or try a hot water bottle on your abdomen and back.

Regular urine tests should be routine for any woman who has had chronic cystitis or kidney trouble, because it is possible to have a symptomless infection which could lead to complications such as kidney infections, high blood pressure or premature births if it is untreated. All pregnant women should have routine urine analysis throughout their pregnancy.

After several months of nearly continuous cystitis attacks, my urologist slit a narrowed area in my urethra to help drainage (internal urethrotomy). I had only one infection in the next three years; then the same story began all over again. My second operation did not help at all.

I consulted another doctor, who, while recognizing the importance of checking for serious abnormalities, also stressed the benefits of drinking lots of water. I now drink enough to urinate every hour or two (ten glasses a day, sometimes more). Ten glasses! Impossible, I thought. But it is better than drugs and not too hard if you work up to it. Take a drink whenever you urinate. I also wash my vulva every day and keep my urine pH at about 5.9 to 5.5 to inhibit bacterial growth. [Use litmus paper, available in chemists, to check it.] In the year since I began this programme I have had only two infections — when I slipped up on my precautions — and nipped a minor one by using these tactics.

More information on prevention is given in Angela Kilmartin's book *Understanding Cystitis*, which is highly recommended. Ms Kilmartin has also started a club for cystitis sufferers called the U&I club. She will answer private inquiries for £1.00 a time (see Bibliography). Chronic urinary infections can be agonizing, and often sufferers are either ignored or given insufficient help and advice from doctors who see the problem as trivial and feel that women who suffer from it are 'over-reacting'. We should not have to put up with such inhumanity, and the best course may well be to switch doctors (see p. 557), although a VD clinic will do tests and give treatment.

NON-SPECIFIC VAGINITIS AND CERVICITIS

These are other infections which may also affect the vagina and cervix. Symptoms are: a discharge which may be white, yellow or even streaked with blood; sometimes also 'cystitis-like' symptoms (see above), and possibly lower back pain, cramps and swollen glands in the abdomen and thighs. Establish whether your discharge is viral or bacterial. One of the bacterial variety is called *haemophilus vaginalis*; its symptoms are similar to 'trich' (see p. 200), the discharge is creamy-white or greyish and particularly foul-smelling after intercourse.

Any clinic will make a culture from the walls of the vagina, which are probably cloudy, puffy with fluid and covered in pus. From the culture the laboratory technicians should be able to sort out the kind of bug you have. If it is bacterial you may be prescribed sulpha cream or Penotrane pessaries; and if no bacteria are found you may get tetracycline, as a non-bacterial infection will not respond to sulpha cream. If you are prescribed tetracycline it is important that your partner(s) should be prescribed a course as well.

ENDOMETRITIS

Not to be confused with endometriosis (see p. 174). Endometritis is an inflammation of the uterine lining. Its main symptoms are pelvic pain, heavy bleeding, and bleeding between periods. If you have a bi-manual pelvic examination (see p. 140) your uterus may feel tender. However, endometritis is sometimes without symptoms. A speculum examination often reveals a thick, foul cervical discharge.

The cause of endometritis is often an IUD which has irritated the uterine lining. In the beginning you may not feel this irritation. Treatment usually includes ampicillin or tetracycline (i.e. antibiotics) for about one week, lots of bed rest, and no sex for 2 weeks. As with PID (see p. 205), a culture and sensitivity test (if not originally taken) is required if the symptoms persist.

Symptom Guide

Pain and Discomfort

Pain on Intercourse. Pelvic inflammatory disease (p. 205); endometriosis (p. 174); ovarian cysts (p. 177).

Discomfort on Intercourse. Thrush (vaginal irritation) (p. 201); herpes (p. 203); cystitis (p. 207); trichomoniasis (p. 200) or any vaginal infection; insufficient lubrication.

Abdominal Pain. Ovarian cysts (p. 177); endometriosis (p. 174); cystitis (p. 207); pelvic inflammatory disease (p. 205); advanced gonorrhoea (p. 193); period pains (p. 170); IUD (p. 260); ectopic pregnancy (p. 506); endometritis (p. 210).

Back Pain. PID (p. 205); period pains (p. 170); IUD (p. 260).

Pain When Urinating. Cystitis (p. 207); herpes (p. 203); gonorrhoea (if in the urethra) (p. 193).

Painful Sores. Herpes (p. 203).

Itching in and around Vagina. Thrush (p. 201); crabs (p. 205); trichomoniasis (p. 200).

Discharge

Thick, white, yeasty – thrush (p. 201).
White, yellow, bloody or greyish with bad smell after intercourse – vaginitis or cervicitis (p. 209).
Yellowish-green, thin, foamy, foul-smelling (fishy) – trichomoniasis (p. 200).
Thin, transparent – ovulation, cervical erosion (p. 174) or early gonorrhoea (p. 193).

Lumps, Bumps and Blisters

Hard raised skin on genitals – warts (p. 204).
Painless open blister or sore – primary syphilis (p. 196).

Abdominal lumps. Ovarian Cysts (p. 177); endometriosis (p. 174); ovarian cancer (p. 181).

Uterine lumps. Fibroids (p. 177).

Breast lumps. Fibroadenomas (p. 150); fibroadenosis (p. 150); cysts (p. 150); breast cancer (p. 158).

Bleeding Problems

Unusually heavy periods, bleeding between periods or spotting is most likely to be caused by pregnancy or menopause; however, all irregular bleeding should be checked. It could be:

Bleeding without Other Symptoms. Anaemia (p. 146); polyps or fibroids (benign uterine growths, p. 177); uterine cancer (mainly in older women) (p. 181); and other conditions which we haven't been able to go into. Sometimes there is no apparent reason for bleeding problems although hormone abnormalities and stress could be the cause.

Bleeding and Pain. Pelvic inflammatory disease (p. 205); endometritis (p. 210); ovarian cysts (p. 177); ectopic pregnancy (p. 506); endometriosis (p. 174).

Pain

Associated with Periods. Endometriosis (progressively increasing pain over a number of years) (p. 174); pelvic inflammatory disease (p. 205).

Bibliography and Resources

BREAST CANCER

Anglem, Thomas J., 'Management of Breast Cancer: Radical Mastectomy', *Journal of the American Medical Association*, Vol. 230, No. 1, 7 October 1974, pp. 99–105.

Anglem, Thomas J., 'Management of Breast Cancer: Radical Mastectomy – In Rebuttal to Dr Crile', ibid., pp. 108–9.

Bonnadonna *et al.*, 'Chemotherapy in Early Breast Cancer Patients', *New England Journal of Medicine*, 19 February 1976.

Breast Cancer Self Examination: An Aid to Early Detection, available from BUPA Medical Centre Ltd, Pentonville Road, London N1. Provides a clear guide to the breasts, on the basis that if you understand their anatomy and how disease develops, you'll have a good idea how to examine them.

Crile, George, Jr, MD, *What Women Should Know About The Breast Cancer Controversy*, Pocket Books, 1974.

Crile, George, Jr, MD, 'Breast Cancer: A Patient's Bill of Rights', *Ms* Magazine, Summer 1974, pp. 95–8.

Crile, George, Jr, MD, 'Management of Breast Cancer: Limited Mastectomy', *Journal of the American Medical Association*, Vol. 230, No. 1, 7 October 1974, pp. 95–8.

Crile, George, Jr, MD, 'Management of Breast Cancer: Limited Mastectomy – In Rebuttal to Dr Anglem', ibid., pp. 106–7.

Drama of a Medical Rip-Off, Publish Yourself Press. The sexism of the medical profession as seen through the eyes of a potential mastectomy patient. Available from 20 Hanover Terrace Mews, London NW1.

Evans, Joy, 'Mastectomy – the Patient's Point of View', *Nursing Mirror*, 3 April 1975.

Forrest, A. P. M., and Kunkler, P. B. (Eds.), *Prognostic Factors in Breast Cancer*, Livingstone, 1968.

Gillie, Oliver, 'Cancer: How to Cut the Risk', *Sunday Times*, 13 June 1976.

Harris, R. J. C. (ed.), *What We Know about Cancer*, Allen & Unwin, 1970.

Kushner, Rose, *Breast Cancer: A Personal History and Investigative Report*, Harcourt Brace Jovanovich, New York, 1975. 'Exhaustively researched, readable and full of empathy . . . while the book appears to be about breast cancer, it is also about the politics of health care. Information is power: make sure your library has a copy.'

Layram, Lin, 'To Lose a Breast Seemed More Terrible than Dying', *Spare Rib*, No. 37, 1975. Personal experience of breast cancer.

Maguire, Peter, 'The Psychological and Social Consequences of Breast Cancer', *Nursing Mirror*, 3 April 1975.

Mortimer, Penelope, *My Friend Says It's Bullet-Proof*, Penguin, 1969. A novel.

Mustakallio, S., 'Conservative Treatment of Breast Carcinoma – Review of 25 Years Follow-up', *Clinical Radiology*, 1972, *23*, pp. 110–16.

Nicholson, Caroline, 'Cancer Need Not be a Death Sentence...', *Nova*, March 1973.

Rakusen, Jill, 'The Diagnosis, Treatment and Aftercare of Breast Cancer', *Spare Rib*, No. 37, 1975.

Rakusen, Jill, 'Breast Cancer Screening – A Critical Guide', *Spare Rib*, No. 42, 1975.

Scott, Anne, 'Joan Scott – Living Her Dying', *Spare Rib*, No. 57, March 1977. A moving but positive account of mother and daughter living through the last months of terminal cancer. Highly recommended.

Seaman, Barbara, 'Liberating Yourself from Your Gynaecologist', *Free and Female*, Coward, McCann & Geoghegan, 1972.

Underhill, Betty, 'A Do-it-yourself Prosthesis for Mastectomy Patients', *World Medicine*, 8 September 1976.

Women's Report, 'Breast Reconstruction', Vol. 3, issue 5.

Women's Report, 'Cancer Detection, New Finds', Vol. 2, issue 4.

Women's Report, 'Delays in Diagnosis and Treatment', Vol. 4, issue 5.

Women's Report, 'Joint Decisions Concerning Treatment', Vol. 3, issue 3.

Women's Report, 'Screening', Vol. 3, issue 2.

Women's Report, 'Screening', Vol. 4, issue 2.

ADDRESSES

British Breast Group: a small group of doctors involved in investigating and treating breast cancer. They would be happy to receive inquiries. Contact Maureen Roberts, Secretary, British Breast Group, Royal Infirmary, Edinburgh.

British Cancer Council, 2 Harley Street, London W 1 (01 274 4002). Also gives information.

Cancer Information Association, Gloucester Green, Oxford OE1 2EQ (0865 46654).

CARE (Cancer After-Care and Rehabilitation Society), Lodge Cottage, Church Lane, Timsbury, Bath, Somerset BA3 1LF (Timsbury 70731). Self-help group which visits, gives advice and practical help, and publishes a newsletter.

Marie Curie Foundation, 124 Sloane Street, London SW1 (01 730 9157). Send s.a.e. Provides various leaflets on cancer, including breast cancer. It encourages women who would like further assistance to write to the Rehabilitation Officer. Stresses that all inquiries are answered by 'professionals' – which may or may not be a good thing.

Mastectomy Association, 1 Colworth Road, Croydon CRO 7AD (01 654 8643). Send s.a.e. 'Strictly non-medical, and concerned to complement medical and nursing care by giving information about bras, prostheses and swimwear, and by psychological understanding and support'. The support is only short-term, however. There is as yet no longer-term support network.

National Society for Cancer Relief, 30 Dorset Square, London NW1 (01 402 8125).

Regional Cancer Services: there are four of these, in Manchester, Leeds, South West Thames and Wessex (addresses can be obtained from your Area Health Authority or the British Cancer Council). One of their main aims is to bring together the various disciplines (e.g. radiotherapy, chemotherapy, surgery) to get the right decision for treatment. They provide an advisory and information service for anyone, including patients.

Women's National Cancer Control Campaign, 9 King Street, London W C 2 E 8 H N (01 836 9901). Provides free leaflets, for example on breast screening. A pressure group.

HYPERTENSION

Pickering, Sir G., *Hypertension: Causes, Consequence and Management*, Churchill Livingstone, 1972.

Sharper, Andrew G., 'Soft Water, Heart Attacks and Stroke', *Journal of American Medical Association*, 7 October 1974.

Williams, H., *You and Your Blood Pressure* (B M A Family Doctor Booklet).

Women's Report, 'Increase of Incidence of Heart Disease in Young Women', Vol 3, issue 2.

MENSTRUAL PROBLEMS

Beckett, Sarah, *Herbs for Feminine Ailments*, Thorson, 1973.

Boston Women's Health Book Collective, *Easing the Cramps* (on massage), *Spare Rib* 56, 1977.

Dalton, Katharina, *The Menstrual Cycle*, Pelican, 1969. Out of print, but may be in libraries. Comprehensive book. Her preferred treatment (hormones) may not be for everyone, but her analysis makes sense.

Dalton, Katharina, *The Pre-Menstrual Syndrome and Progesterone Therapy*, Heinemann, 1978.

Davis, Adelle, *Let's Get Well*, Allen & Unwin, 1974. You might not agree with her view of women, but she provides interesting information on menstrual and other female problems.

Lacey, Gillian, 'Periods', *Spare Rib*, No. 47.

Lanson, Lucienne, *From Woman to Woman*, Penguin, 1977. Very much 'from doctor to woman', but does cover menstrual problems in some depth.

Maddux, Hilary C., *Menstruation,* Tobey Publishing Co., 1975. Available from Compendium. Section on exercise good, rest of book fair, underlying attitude about menstruation negative.

Palaiseul, Jean, *Grandmother's Secrets*, Penguin, 1976. Useful on herbal remedies.

Seaman, B. & G., *Women and the Crisis in Sex Hormones*, Rawson Co. (U S A), 1977.

Weideger, Paula, *Menstruation and Menopause: The Physiology and Psychology, The Myth and the Reality*, Alfred Knopf, New York, 1975.

Wright, Erna, *Periods Without Pain*, Tandem Books, 1966. Very cheap. Written by an ex-sufferer in a maternal, decidedly non-feminist, though well-meaning way. Gives practical advice on exercises and how to help ourselves by treating our bodies with care and respect.

VD

Catterall, R. D., *The Venereal Diseases*, Impact, 1967.

Cherniak, D., and Feingold, A., *VD Handbook*. Montreal Health Press, 1975. Available from Rising Free and Compendium (see p. 573).

'Flagyl', *Off Our Backs*, Aug./Sept. and Sept./Oct. issues, 1974.

'Homosexual Love may be Less Dangerous to the Health than Heterosexual Love', *Monthly Extract*, May/June and Sept./Oct. issues, 1973.

Kilmartin, Angela, *Understanding Cystitis*, Heinemann, 1973.

Kilmartin, Angela, *Self Help in Cystitis and Thrush*, from U & I Club, 9e Compton Road, London N1.

Rakusen, Jill, 'Use of Flagyl in the UK', *Spare Rib*, No. 28, p. 21.

Stauber, Ann, 'Trichomonas', *Monthly Extract*, Vol. 2, issue 3.

HYSTERECTOMY

Barker, Montague, *British Medical Journal*, 2, 1968, p. 91.

Gillie, Oliver, *The Sunday Times*, 8 December 1974.

HMSO, The Lane Report on Abortion, 1974.

Richards, Dr D. H., *The Lancet*, ii, 1973, p. 430.

Robinson, Jean, *Spare Rib*, No. 30, p. 10.

8 Violence

Battering

WHAT IS IT?

The battering of women is widespread, both nationally and internationally. It is not the prerogative of men of any class background, age group, or any other social classification. It is spread across the whole social spectrum. There is a great need for much more research into the problem, and for a clarification of underlying assumptions about it. (National Women's Aid Federation, *Battered Women Need Refuges*)

Women are battered by husbands, boyfriends and even sons. It has been estimated that in one in 100 marriages, the women suffer *severe* violence – in other words, 140,000 in the UK.* The Royal Scottish Society for Prevention of Cruelty to Children has found that 20% of its cases throughout Scotland involved the battering of women, sometimes severe. Out of 10,000 readers of *Women's Own* questioned in 1975, 17% had been battered by their husbands. From 1971 to 1974, one large refuge dealt with about 25,000 women. Here are just three examples of what we are talking about.

A woman awakens and tugs at a blanket on the bed; the next thing she knows, her husband is attempting to suffocate her with a pillow. A husband finds a photograph in his wife's wallet; five minutes later he places a hot iron on her arm in an attempt to make her confess to having an affair. A man complains of his wife's untidiness and they have an argument; he goes and works all day, but when he returns the argument continues, he beats his wife and throws her and the children out into the cold. (Marsden and Owens)

Battering often has links with sexual violence, although the law does not recognize rape within marriage. Other forms of brutality include attempted strangulation, repeated punching, kicking, the use of weapons, boiling water, etc. Battering can involve mental torture and humiliation:

Being told how useless you are (and if you are told often enough you start to believe it). (Battered Women Need Refuges)

* Marsden and Owens, *New Society*, 8 May 1975.

Battering is not a new phenomenon – a pamphlet on 'Wife Torture' (by Frances Power Cobbe) appeared in the 1870s. But battering did not become a recognized 'problem' until the first refuge was set up in Chiswick in 1971, when women kept on arriving in order to escape. The recent publicity about battering has enabled women to talk about it, often for the first time, to start questioning men's behaviour, and the setting up of refuges has at last given many women the means to escape. But we still don't know the true extent of battering.

WHY DOES IT HAPPEN?

It is not uncommon for people – even women – to say of a battered woman, 'she must have asked for it', 'she must be violent too', 'she's a nag', or 'she must like it – otherwise she'd leave'. We do not believe that such violence is in any way excusable. This kind of simplistic and ignorant attitude not only fails to explain why battering happens, it also reinforces in women's minds the idea that, as with rape, we actually cause it!

To understand – and prevent – battering, we need to understand the complexities involved in our relationships to each other and to society at large. We cannot examine these complexities in any depth in this book, but we can try to put battering into some kind of perspective and point out at least some of the links between battering and women's oppression in general. For further reading, see Bibliography, p. 233.

The way our society is structured affects all human relationships. Outside the home we have a system of power relationships: worker/ employer, individual/state, etc., and most people feel powerless outside the home to a greater or lesser extent. People can feel particularly powerless if their specific situation is beyond their control: for example, if they are unemployed, scraping a living, working at unpleasant jobs at unpleasant hours, or if they have to 'be' people they don't want to be (such as a man 'having' to be a breadwinner or a woman 'having' to be a housewife). The resultant stresses and strains need outlets.

There are many different kinds of outlets. We can use our anger or frustration by directing it constructively – into changing society. But many people drown their feelings in drink, for example, or go into a depression, or perhaps lash out. Many of us are inclined at least sometimes to take out our frustration on people nearest us. The limitations of private family life can act like a hot-house, increasing frustration so that we lash out in our various ways.

The kind of destructive outlet that a woman uses may be physical – either against her husband or children – but more often it is psychological (against her family or herself). If the violence is against the man, he still has the ultimate sanction: he can walk out. The kind of oppressive violence a woman can persistently use is more often directed towards her children – because they cannot walk out. It is interesting that while the law has protected children for some years, it is still equivocal in the protection it gives battered women. Commonly, women turn violent feelings inwards: twice as many women as men suffer from depression. Women who live in deprived areas, who don't go out to work, are, not surprisingly, the most vulnerable to depression.

As far as men are concerned, they have been brought up to use their fists – and even encouraged to do so. It is not surprising, therefore, that a man's outlet can, in its extreme form, involve physical violence against his wife and family. Many women do not have the ultimate sanction: we cannot easily leave home. Men – even the most oppressed men – have a semblance of legal and economic power in areas such as housing, employment, education, child care, fertility control. Women are in comparison relatively powerless. We would like to examine some of these areas more closely.

In many marriages, the home is in the husband's name. If a woman wants to leave home, she may find it very difficult to find another one, because of prejudice against women in general or against women with children in particular, or of course, because she is on social security or very low pay. Furthermore, if a woman leaves home with children, they are likely to be taken into care – while she, on the other hand, is not considered 'homeless'. After all, as the reasoning goes, she still has a home with her husband! If she leaves home alone, she is even less likely to be housed. Even if a woman is in the fortunate position of being able to kick the man out of the home (and, even harder, keep him out), she can still be held liable for her husband's rent arrears. So, many battered women don't leave home because they can't.

Women are also expected to look after children – even though we have no real choice about whether, when or in what circumstances we want them. Many women are consequently totally reliant on their husbands' incomes, or earn a pittance at part-time, low-paid jobs. Fathers, on the other hand, are not ultimately seen by society as responsible for the care of their children. A man can still drink all his earnings if he wishes. One of the reasons some women put up with battering for so long is because they are concerned about how they could bring up the children with little money on their own if they left. Often, women finally leave only when they fear that their children are themselves in physical or mental danger from their fathers.

I have left my husband in desperation five times but have had to return for my children's sake, as he didn't take care of them in my absence. (From Pizzey, *Scream Quietly or the Neighbours Will Hear*)

If a woman does have a job, or if she manages to find one if and when she leaves the home, the pay is unlikely to be much. The average female wage is only 60% of that of the average man; the lowest-paid jobs are done by women; many women have to work part-time and consequently for little money because they are expected to have full responsibility for children; there are very few facilities for children – crèches, nurseries or after-school facilities – provided by the state or by employers; maternity pay and maternity leave are rarely adequate.

All these factors conspire to confine a woman in a battering situation. They shed considerable light on the reasons why women 'put up with' battering and other forms of unsatisfactory marriage.

There are also enormous pressures on women to remain married, to 'try harder', as women can be told by psychiatrists. As one Women's Aid worker points out, 'Local councillors don't think women should leave their husbands.' Women somehow feel responsible, ashamed and guilty for being beaten or raped.

REFUGES

While many women are working to eliminate the causes of battering, it is still essential that enough refuges are provided to enable women to escape and to start making a new life. The National Women's Aid Federation believes that there should be at least one refuge in each town. Such refuges must operate not only as a sanctuary but also as a means by which women can discover their strength and recognize that battering is not a personal but a political problem. The N W A F coordinates refuges in Britain. Contact them to find out about refuges in your area and for help in setting up new ones. (See Bibliography and Resources, p. 233.)

While we can eliminate battering – by women simply not being there to be battered – this will still not solve the problem of frustration and aggression. This is a problem we all face in an oppressive, patriarchal, capitalist society. We need to create a more equitable society where all people – women and men – can fulfil themselves according to their own needs. The 'problem' of battering is everyone's problem!

Rape

Rape is a crime against women and children (far more children are victims of rape than most of us realize). It is the ultimate expression of contempt for women of all ages.

Although most of us think of rape as a clear-cut, unjustifiable sexual act forced on a woman against her will, many people, especially men (but not only men), have misconceptions about what rape is and what it isn't. In their minds 'rape is rape' when it happens in an alley, when it's committed by a stranger, or when there are bruises and signs of physical violence; but for them rape is not really rape when it happens in a bed, when it's committed by a friend or acquaintance, or when a woman appears not to be physically harmed. Many of us women know that these latter rapes are just as much 'real rape' as the former. More men need to understand this too.

Rape is an exaggerated acting out of some of our society's conventional ideas towards women. Women are supposed to 'belong to' a man, so we are often considered 'fair game', or to be 'asking for it', if we are not visibly protected by a man. Women are often viewed as passive sex objects, 'there to be violated'. We hope that as attitudes like these change we will begin to eliminate rape and to have better treatment for rape victims — better law enforcement approaches, better medical and psychiatric care and more humane courts.

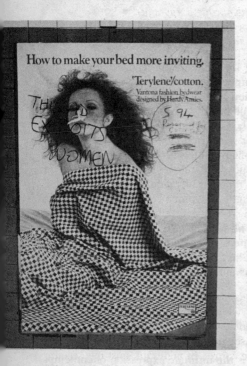 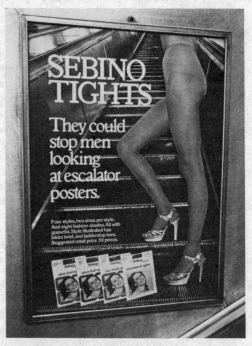

WHO GETS RAPED: WHEN, WHERE, BY WHOM AND WHY

Children as young as six months and women as old as ninety-three years have been raped. Rape can happen to any woman — rich, poor, young, old, of any racial or ethnic background. Even the 'good girl' (long a destructive stereotype in our society) can be raped.

The woman is a nineteen-year-old student at university. It is about two o'clock in the afternoon and she is in an isolated part of one of the buildings. Her attacker is a young married man who is a lecturer at the university.

The woman is seventeen, a school student. It is about four o'clock in the afternoon. Her boyfriend's father has picked her up in his car after school to take her to meet his son. He stops by his house and says she should wait for him in the car. When he has pulled the car into the garage, this thirty-seven-year-old father of six rapes her.

The woman is thirty-nine, separated from her husband, the mother of five children. Her attacker breaks into the house in the middle of the night. He turns out to be a friend's husband, the father of several children.

The woman is twenty and has recently got a new job. The boss asks her to come in on a holiday to help with the inventory. When she arrives, there is no one else there. Her boss, a man of about thirty, rapes her.

*The woman is sixteen, still at school. She has a date with a college student she knows fairly well. He drives her to an isolated area and rapes her.**

Although rape in Britain is not (yet?) a problem of the dimensions that it is in the USA, it is growing. *Reported* rapes have increased from 869 in 1969 to 998 in 1973. In America the official rate for 1973 was 51,000 and it has been estimated that only 10–25% of rapes are reported there. It is probable that a similar number of rapes go unreported here.

Experience suggests that the most common form of rape in this country occurs between people who know each other. This is clearly the most difficult rape to prove unless violence has been used. Many women have to face the humiliation of court procedures and see the man who attacked them acquitted. If the man is known to a woman and her friends life can be made intolerable and women have been known to leave the area rather than face the rapist again. In one province of Australia the idea that women accuse men of rape out of revenge has been enshrined in law. If a rapist is acquitted, the victim can be charged with making a false complaint.

Rape can happen with people around, sometimes even watching the crime. This is just one indication of how the rape problem extends far beyond rapists: there are many who themselves would never commit a rape, but who continue to condone or accept others' rape crimes. They often blame the victims, and they see no need for significant changes in law enforcement procedures, or the courts. In addition, most men realize at some level that the existence of rape tends to keep women dependent on them for 'protection'. Unfortunately, many of these men wish to perpetuate such dependence.

Who are the rapists? Many are married and have apparently 'normal' sex lives. The rapist often knows his victim and usually plans the rape

* Thompson and Medea, *Against Rape*, (see Bibliography).

(he is not, as one of the current myths would have it, 'in the grip of an uncontrollable sex drive'). Several studies have indicated that 60 to 70% of rapes are premeditated. Some psychological testing of rapists has indicated that they tend to express more violence and rage than the 'average' male, but their sexual personalities do *not appear to differ from the average male.*

Many rapists and non-rapists have similar fantasies about rape, but there is an important difference between having a fantasy and acting on it. We are angry that so many men feel free to act on their rape fantasies. This is another example of how rape reflects a much bigger problem than the act itself — it reflects a prevalent social attitude towards women that continues to undermine more humane relationships between men and women.

Rapists seem to have many different motives. Here, one rapist speaks of his own motives:

Other people think they know why I do the things I do.

One witch doctor [psychiatrist] I talked with told me that I rape women because I fear them and cannot adequately cope with the games they play. Another said that I am incapable of having normal sexual relationships because I view sex as nothing more than an energy release and not as a means of expressing/sharing my love for a particular woman. Another put forth the theory that I used rape to strike back at my mother.

There's truth in what they say. I often quote them when the need arises to justify/rationalize my behaviour. But there's a thing which most people, including the witch doctors, overlook. The main reason why I do the things I do is that I find rape enormously stimulating and very exciting.

*It's fun.**

There is also evidence of a significant (not surprising) relationship between alcoholism and rape. In one study at an American treatment centre for convicted rapists, 35% of the rapists were alcoholic and 50% had been drinking before the rape offence.

Some rapists need to feel powerful; some need to prove their 'manhood' to themselves or to their peers; some need to 'violate' another man's 'property'; some need to be physically violent in order to achieve sexual satisfaction; some feel that they are simply taking their 'due' from girlfriends, dates, or acquaintances. None of these reasons can justify the act of rape. We look forward to a time when there are fewer men with such distorted needs.

* J. B. & J. Csida, *Rape. How to Avoid it and What to do about it if You Can't*, Chatworth, Calif. 1974.

WHAT TO DO IF YOU HAVE BEEN RAPED

Your first instinct may well be to go home, have a bath and pretend it didn't happen. It is understandable that we should react in this way to such an experience, but unfortunately the law doesn't see it that way. Your instinctive reaction may be seen as an attempt to falsify evidence. Your best action would be to call a friend straight away for comfort or support, or to call the Rape Crisis Centre in London (see p. 234). It really helps to confide in someone rather than brood on it alone.

Should You Report the Rape to the Police?

You are under no obligation to do so, but remember, he might rape someone else and the next time he could be more violent. Your evidence could protect others, and, if he can be caught immediately, he is more likely to confess and spare you the misery of cross-questioning in the dock, although recent changes in the law to some extent protect us from unfair questioning and publicity. In addition, every rape that goes unreported reinforces the idea that rapists can get away with it.

Reporting the Rape

Go to the police as soon as you can. If necessary go there first and ring from the police station to get a friend to come down and help you. Speed is important because your behaviour and appearance immediately after the rape could be used by the police as 'corroborating evidence'. As rapes are rarely witnessed, evidence of distress, disarrayed clothing, etc. can be important, and the police are more likely to be considered impartial observers of your condition than your mother or husband.

You will be questioned by the police, often for hours and rarely with tact and sympathy. Many policemen still believe that women ask for rape.

They treated me like a criminal; they kept asking me, 'What where you wearing, were your trousers tight?' They were oblivious to how upset and scared I was. I had to cry before they took me seriously.

Everyone seemed to believe that I was lying or exaggerating. I was beginning to realize that when you open your front door to a man, it is the same as inviting him to rape you in the eyes of the police and society. *

The police still expect you to fight for your 'virtue', even though they themselves admit that resistance could be more dangerous. It is quite wrong that the police should feel it their duty to test your story to this degree. The test is supposed to take place in court, not in the police station,

* From 'Freedom from Rape', Women's Crisis Center, Ann Arbor, Michigan, USA (but our police are no different).

and it is not the victim's innocence which should be questioned, but the rapist's.

The police will arrange for you to be examined by a doctor. This is to establish whether intercourse has actually taken place and to gather medical evidence for a possible prosecution. This examination may also be a humiliating experience. The doctor has often to be called out late at night, he may be asked to examine you in a place which is not suitable, and he may not be kind or sympathetic. He will ask questions about your gynaecological history, if you have had an abortion, if you are on the Pill, etc. Some of the questions relate to physical conditions which may affect the evidence, others are irrelevant and have in the past been used by the defence to cast doubt on your morality.

The purpose of these humiliating experiences is for the police to get a set of statements which will be used at the trial. You will be asked to dictate your statement which you should then read over and sign.

Medical Attention

Whether or not you report the rape, you must see a doctor as soon as possible to be checked for V D and pregnancy. Obviously it is impossible to find out if you are pregnant immediately. You might be offered a 'morning-after pill'. This is a high dose of oestrogen which would stop the implantation of a fertilized ovum if it is taken within 48 hours of the rape. It has unpleasant side effects and should be used cautiously (see p. 283), so you might prefer to wait until you can get a pregnancy test and decide whether or not to have an abortion.

A suitable dose of penicillin given immediately after the attack should take care of possible V D. An additional check-up six weeks later is also advisable. The doctor should examine you for any tearing, bruising or general damage both internally and externally.

Again, if you have no obvious signs that force has been used, you might find the doctor somewhat sceptical about rape.

When one woman we know reported a rape to her G P he angrily told her not to try and cover up an illicit affair with a story like that. If you have a friend with you it is less likely that a doctor can behave in this way.

Emotional After Effects

A rape is usually traumatic. It is important to have supportive friends and/or counsellors to talk to about your feelings. Sometimes women feel too embarrassed or humiliated to speak about their rape experience — this can be a difficult burden to carry alone. Women who have been raped and have talked about it afterwards are apt to feel less guilty and ashamed, because they were able to express their anger and discuss the crime as something that happens to many women. We must remember that rape is *not our fault*. Because rape violates our self-respect, anger is a most appropriate response. We need to help one another to feel and express our anger about rape, since we can suffer a lot from turning these feelings inward. One woman who was raped was severely depressed for six months, until she could finally express her rage at what had been done to her. Many women have joined anti-rape groups to use their angry energy in positive ways.

A rape victim, and often her family, will need follow-up counselling to cope with difficult feelings. Humiliation, embarrassment, guilt, disgust, horror and anxiety – these are all possible reactions to rape. Sometimes a close friend has the skills and ability to help a rape victim express and work through her feelings, but in some cases a woman should see a counsellor, ideally someone who is experienced with the needs of rape victims. Hospital psychiatric departments are sometimes helpful. Groups organized by local rape crisis centres (let's start more of them!) can be a good way for rape victims to share their experiences and support one another. Women who have been raped and have had the opportunity to work through their feelings can be especially helpful to a recent rape victim. We cannot overemphasize the importance of talking to an understanding person.

A rape victim needs support and understanding for what may be the first traumatic experience in her life, especially if she is a younger woman. Many fathers, boyfriends, husbands and lovers feel violent anger towards the rapist, often because they see the rape as a personal violation of themselves (this is especially true of men who view women as their 'property'). When this reaction to rape is not accompanied by sympathy and support, it can be demoralizing for the rape victim. Other men are more casual and insensitive to the seriousness of the act ('Why are you so upset? After all, he didn't hurt you'). Fortunately, more and more men (and women) are beginning to understand the serious consequences of rape and are learning to be supportive and sensitive to the rape victim regardless of their own reactions.

Very young rape victims have special needs. A little girl may not understand what has happened to her or that the rape was somehow a 'bad thing'. Her reactions depend largely on the reactions of those around her: if everyone gets very upset, then she will be very upset; if others express strong anger towards the rapist, she may feel that this anger is directed towards her or is somehow her fault – this response to anger is common in children. Whatever our own feelings about the rape of a child, we must try not to express them in ways that will only add to a child's fear and trauma.

Teenage rape victims often feel tremendously embarrassed and/or guilty. Sometimes they keep the rape a secret for many years, until they finally feel okay about sharing the experience or can no longer bear the burden alone. They often feel that they will be blamed for what happened or that 'no boy will ever come near them again'. Parents must try to be sympathetic and supportive to teenage rape victims, even though other feelings, of anger, dismay and self-pity, may make this difficult to do (especially for fathers).

The experience of courts and the functioning of the law are a further agony for most rape victims, though recent changes in the law should protect women to some degree from having their past sexual histories dragged through the court. But however the law is changed it is unlikely to *prevent* rape. If women are to be protected from violence of all kinds we must set about changing society's view of us and we must learn to defend ourselves.

Preventing Attacks

Protection against rape is usually seen in terms of limiting our freedom, withdrawing into dependency or trying not to attract attention. If we accept such protection we are encouraging the myth that women cause rape and that we must be locked away if rape is to be prevented. If we want to hitch-hike, to live alone, to walk home alone at night, to enjoy the solitary freedom of city parks, to do things that most men take for granted, we must learn to protect ourselves against unwelcome attention from men, violent or otherwise. We can use a number of devices to increase our safety from attacks:

1. Make contact with friendly neighbours and keep a list of their phone numbers at hand. If possible arrange a special signal (whistle, hooter, etc.) to bring help. We can also keep the phone number of the local police station by the phone.
2. If we list only our initial in the phone book and put names of fake flatmates by the door bell we will not be automatically picked out as female and alone.
3. Good, safe locks on doors and windows with bars on ground floor windows are a worthwhile investment.
4. We should keep doorways and landings well lit; pressure the landlord to do so if it is his responsibility, and badger the local council to do the same for dark alleyways and secluded streets. We should avoid fumbling for keys at the door – have them in your hand as you arrive.
5. If you are alone don't let strangers in.
6. When hitching (particularly alone) we should avoid taking lifts if there is more than one man in the car. Never sit in the back of a two-door car. Check that you can open the door from the inside. Try to make a note of the registration number and make of the car and whenever

possible take lifts from lorries or vans rather than private cars. A professional driver has a schedule to follow, a reputation to keep and is easier to identify. We should try to avoid hitching at night.

7. A purposeful and confident air is our best protection when walking alone. If you are followed, walk up to a house and if necessary break a window.

But the best defence of all is the knowledge that you are fit and know how to fight. Learning self-defence (see below) will give you confidence (and confident women are less likely to be attacked than frightened ones) as well as keeping you fit and teaching you to use your strength to advantage.

Self-Defence

Many of us are reared in protective environments where fighting among girls is discouraged. As a result, we feel helpless and vulnerable and even go so far as to question our right to defend ourselves. We believe it's essential that women begin to take self-defence seriously. We need to build up and maintain strength and endurance to accomplish this (see p. 122). That strength alone, however, will not equip us to fight. Most women are afraid of pain and violence, and we have little sense of the potential power of our bodies. The physical and mental togetherness that comes from exercise and self-defence training not only teaches us this but also gives us added confidence in all areas of our lives.

'I used to feel as though I became public property whenever I walked in the city. Now I feel a private space around myself.' 'My fantasies are changing since I joined the class. When I think about situations that make me angry, I visualize the kinds of things we've learned to do, not just a vague blur of wanting to struggle.' 'It's especially mind-blowing for a short person like me. I've always felt totally helpless and walked around as if waiting to be victimized. Not any more.' (Taken from *Self Confidence/Defence* by Sarita Cordell)

CLASSES

For obvious reasons, it is best to learn techniques that include fighting. Judo, aikido and karate can all train us in fighting techniques. Jujitsu and some other martial-art styles train you to do combinations of the above in confrontation situations. This approach seems ideal. But rather than recommending any one particular style, we suggest that you pick the school or class with the best attitude towards its students.

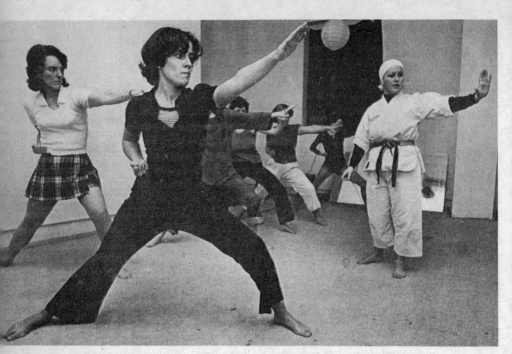

In some areas, special schools exist, for example in judo or karate. You can look them up in the phone book under the relevant technique. If no classes exist in your area, or you do not like the ones that do, you can ask your local authority to provide you with classes provided there are at least ten people interested. It's also worth approaching your local branch of the Workers' Educational Association, Colleges of Further Education, University Extra-Mural Departments or even your union. Try to find an instructor who takes women seriously. If at all possible classes should be taught for women by women who understand where we are coming from physically and emotionally, as well as where we have to go. A useful way to begin physical training is in a supportive atmosphere – to begin building your confidence. Ideally, a women's group can join a class or start a class together. The Women's Free Arts Alliance in London has been running courses; perhaps there will be many more by the time this book comes out. Some older women may need classes especially designed to go at the pace best suited to them; others will feel fine in any class. One woman we read about started at the age of sixty-two and at seventy-two had two black belts – in judo and aikido! Girls, of course, should be taught from the earliest years how to take care of themselves and then should join a class that's right for them when they are ready. The school system must begin taking responsibility for this.

Many male instructors give women a watered-down version of karate that allows no body contact. It could be helpful to arrange extra women's classes to work on techniques that are particularly hard or useful to the women there and to discuss ways of coping with the day-to-day sexism you face in the school. There are, of course, advantages in a mixed-class: you learn how to fight men and see that they have weaknesses, too. A lot of male instructors know useful stuff about how women can effectively fight men, and if it's a good school they should teach it to you in a decent way as fast as you want to absorb it.

If there are no opportunities for you to go to a class, get a couple of books on self-defence (see Bibliography) and learn some techniques from them.

SOME THINGS YOU CAN DO

Self-defence is a skill that can be learned. It is also a matter of common sense and learning to think strategically. Practise with friends. Think through possible situations. What would you do if someone came up and grabbed you from behind? How would you respond if someone approached you while you were in a telephone booth? Suppose a man's hand started creeping up your knee in a tube train? Take turns in playing the attacked and the attacker. Work at breaking out of holds or wrestling on the floor, and punching and kicking (not too hard) to help break down some of the fears and inhibitions women have about striking out and getting hit. Cheap boxing gloves are wonderful for punching – you can hit without fear of injury. But don't neglect your legs – kicks to the shins, knees, groin are essential; they are a surprise and they hurt. Practise on a hard pillow or stuffed laundry bag. If you're not used to expressing your anger verbally when you would like to, do some of that – it relieves a lot of tension. Get your partner to make some obscene comment so that you can retort.

If you work with a friend you'll be much less likely to panic in a real situation, since you will have prepared yourself and built up some confidence in your ability to fight back. Fear is a deadly emotion that may keep you from remembering what you can do.

On the street, especially at night and in unfamiliar surroundings, be alert at all times. If a threatening situation develops, don't try to ignore it as we've often been taught to do. Start assessing it as you move along quickly with an air of determination and direction. If things get worse, the safest response is to run, unless you're *really* confident that you can defend yourself. Head for a shop, building, or lighted area where people are likely to be.

If you're caught by surprise or have nowhere to run, you can fight off an attacker in a number of different ways. He comes at you from the front: you kick his knees (or shins), *hard.* If he grabs you before you can kick, ram your knee up into his groin. If your arms are free, use them: chop or punch at his head – temple, eyes, right under the ears, mouth, nose. If not, you can spit or bite. If he grabs you from behind, move your hips so that you can drive your elbow back into his solar plexus (the sensitive region of the stomach, under the breast bone and between the first ribs), then finish him off with a blow to the groin with the back or side of your fist. Some people advocate grabbing his balls instead, and pulling them down sharply. If this is impossible kick back hard into his knee with your heel, then slide down the shin and stamp on his instep. Be prepared with more than just one technique – it may take a series of accurate hits to be successful. Be calm but quick, make your hand or foot *tight,* and put your whole body into the blows while keeping your balance. Remember, in dangerous situations we often respond with a power we didn't know we had.

Although it is illegal to carry any kind of weapon in Britain, some women like to carry for ready use (not tucked away in the depths of a handbag) a pepper shaker, an artificial plastic lemon filled with lemon juice, vinegar or some other burning substance, or a deodorant spray. The problem with all these is that you have to be really speedy to use them. If you hesitate, the attacker has time to disarm you and may use the object against you. Nevertheless, we know women who have warded off attacks with a spray. It is also possible to use (depending on what's available) an umbrella, handbag, bottle, hammer, or the like as a weapon; but this is tricky, so you should know exactly what you intend to do with it. At home, don't be embarrassed to sleep with a weapon nearby if it makes you feel better. Whatever kind of counter-attack seems best, do it with a yell – not a scream for help, but a loud, blood-curdling battle cry. This will give you a psychological boost and will scare your attacker. Once you're free of his grasp, don't hang around to see how he is. Run, fast. If you're at home call friends to help, or the police. If necessary call from next door.

Unfortunately there may be more than one attacker, and then you really have to keep your cool. Break away through the weakest link in their approach and run. Yell 'fire' rather than 'help', knock on some-one's door, or throw a stone through a window to attract attention. Verbal tactics sometimes work: one friend of ours talked off a bunch of men by telling them very matter-of-factly about how shitty her day had been and now here they were bothering her to cap it all. Another friend went into a 'crazy' act and got rid of two men following her. Of course it's safer to travel in twos or groups, but nothing is foolproof, so discuss with your companions what you might do together in a crisis. Fighting in pairs or more has to be planned and practised, too.

Your use of these techniques depends upon your being able to move quickly and effectively. Clothes often inhibit movement. It's easier to defend yourself if you're wearing trousers (not too tight) and shoes that stay on your feet. Clothes like these will give you more confidence in your ability to take care of yourself.

In all bad situations you have to decide how aggressive or defensive you want to be. You have the right to stop a physical attack (after trying to escape) – not, though, to injure the attacker beyond what is necessary to stop him from injuring you. But since the law does not concern itself with the anger of oppressed people, it rules against the force we may feel compelled to use against the brutal, degrading and low-level harassment that endlessly comes our way. In some situations you can pick your time and place. Be aware of resources the man might have to find you later and retaliate, of who else is around, and so forth. It's one thing to let loose at a single stranger in a park miles from home, if you're feeling confident of your ability to handle him, and quite another to take on a gang of neighbourhood boys or your drunken husband. Other times there will be no choice: you do what you have to do – as best you can – no matter how it turns out. Women who fight back, as some always have and more and more are starting to do, are forcing the white, male court system to deal seriously with our right to meet violence with violence in our own defence. One woman, Juanita Greening, was in a phone box phoning the police after her husband had beaten her up, when he came in and attacked her again. In the ensuing struggle she strangled him with the telephone wire. She was then charged with murder. A request for a lesser charge of manslaughter (in self-defence) was refused. She was even refused bail, although she had good sureties and a petition signed by over 100 people who were personally aware of the treatment she had received from her husband. When her case came up for trial the judge began by saying that clearly no one could have any sympathy for her. Much emphasis was placed on the relative heights and weights of Ms Greening and her husband. The judge referred to her as a Big Woman, saying she looked as if she could look after herself. As *Spare Rib* commented on the trial, to be a legitimate battered wife you are evidently expected to be a passive victim.

But the outcome of the Greening trial is, we hope, a precedent. Although the authorities treated Ms Greening as a dangerous woman – by refusing her bail – the jury only convicted her of manslaughter. The judge, evidently swayed by the support she received, gave her a suspended sentence. As women become more confident, more of us will begin to fight back. We must continue to help and support women in these situations in all ways possible.

Not all violence comes from men. Women do, of course, fight one another, and we will as long as we are angry, frustrated, afraid, confused and separated from each other. People lash out most often at someone they can hurt without fear of reprisal – in the case of women, that usually means other women and children. All responsible self-defence training should include political education to help us work out where our anger should *really* be aimed, so that power and fighting skills won't be used in destructive ways.

The police and courts can be pressured to become more understanding of our problems – but we must *never* rely on them for our ultimate protection. At every opportunity we should point out the ways our society encourages men, from boyhood on, to make sex and violence an inseparable pair, and to see women as sex objects up for grabs, as helpless victims, or as creatures who have to be punished and kept down. If men must be taught a whole new sense about human relationships, we women must grow up to be strong and self-reliant people aware of our needs and resources, ready to stand up for ourselves and each other, any time, anywhere.

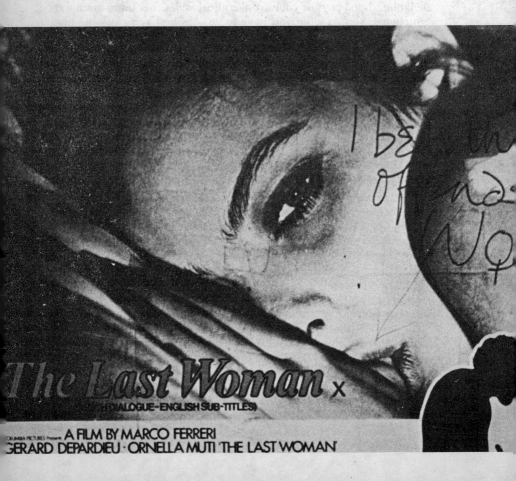

Bibliography and Resources

BATTERING

Brown, George, *et al.*, 'Social Class and Psychiatric Disturbance among Women in an Urban Population', *Sociology*, May 1975.

Catholic Aid Society, *What Chance a Home?* Report on housing situation faced by one-parent families, available from the Society, 189a Old Brompton Road, London S W 5.

Dobash, R. and R., 'Battered Women: The Importance of Existing Perspectives', presented to the British Sociological Association Study Group on Women, 1975.

Gayford, J. J., 'Wife Battering: a Preliminary Survey of 100 cases'. *British Medical Journal*, 25 January 1975 (N B: see Wilson, below).

Glasgow Women's Independence Group, *Women and Housing* (women in Scotland, and Glasgow in particular). Obtainable from Rising Free.

H M S O, *Report from the Select Committee on Violence in Marriage*, House of Commons paper no. 553, 1975.

Holt, Ruth, *Do-it-yourself Injunction Kit for Battered Wives*, Paddington Neighbourhood Law Centre. Obtainable from Rising Free.

Interaction, *Battered Women and the Law*. Available from Rising Free (see p. 573).

Marsden, Dennis, and Owens, David, 'The Jekyll and Hyde Marriages', *New Society*, 8 May 1975.

National Council for Civil Liberties, *Battered Women: How to Use the New Law*, 1977.

National Women's Aid Federation, *And Still You Have Done Nothing* (address below).

National Women's Aid Federation, *Battered Women, Refuges and Women's Aid* (address below).

Nichols, David Ian, *Marriage, Divorce and the Family*. An introduction to *Scots* family law available from Rutovitz, 31 Royal Terrace, Edinburgh.

Pizzey, Erin, *Scream Quietly or the Neighbours Will Hear*, Penguin, 1974.

Scott, P. D., 'Battered Wives', *British Journal of Psychology*, 125, 433–41, 1974.

Scottish Women's Aid, *Battered Women in Scotland: Your Rights and Where to Turn for Help* (address below).

Snell, J. E., *et al.*, 'The Wifebeater's Wife: a Study of Family Interaction', *Archives of General Psychiatry*, August 1964: typical of those studies which attempt to 'prove' that battering is psychogenic.

Swansea Women's Liberation Group, *Getting Unmarried*. 'All you need to know about divorce, separation, maintenance, S S, getting a place to live, going to work, day nurseries, etc.'; very cheap. Obtainable from Rising Free.

Wilson, Elizabeth, *The Existing Research into Battered Women* (National Women's Aid Federation): critique of current research and, in particular, that of John Gayford.

Women's Report, 'Violence in Marriage'. Analysis and critique of H M S O. *Report from the Select Committee on Violence in Marriage*, Vol. 4, issue 1.

Women's Report, 'Women's Aid: Social Work or Societal Revolution?', Vol. 3, issue 3.

FILMS

Battered Wives (produced with notes) – Camera Talks Ltd, 31 North Row, Park Lane, London W 1.

Scream Quietly or the Neighbours Will Hear, Concord Films Council, Nacton, Ipswich, Suffolk.
That's No Lady . . . (produced with teacher's notes by Sheffield Women's Film Co-operative in conjunction with NWAF): available from NWAF.

National Women's Aid Federation, 374 Grays Inn Road, London WC1 (01 837 9316). Refuges can be contacted via this address or via local Social Services Departments, Citizens' Advice Bureaux, the Samaritans and similar agencies.
Scottish Women's Aid, Ainslie House, 11 St Colme Street, Edinburgh EH3 6AA (031 225 4606).

RAPE

Brownmiller, Susan, *Against Our Will*, Penguin, 1977. Very good American book, but heavy going.
Coote, A., and Gill, T., *The Rape Controversy*, National Council for Civil Liberties pamphlet on suggested legal changes. (See NCCL address, p. 570.)
Medea, Andra, and Thompson, Kathleen, *Against Rape*, Noonday Press, USA, 1975. Excellent, readable, with sound feminist analysis and practical advice.
Toner, Barbara, *The Facts of Rape*, Hutchinson and Arrow, 1977. An attempt to provide information about rape in Britain, which falls down because of the author's general view that 'most rape is an opportunist crime arising from sexual confusion'. Read Brownmiller or Medea & Thompson first.

Rape Crisis Centre, 01 340 6145. PO Box 42, London N6 5BU.
'Reclaiming the Night Groups' have been started in many areas. Involved in action to raise consciousness on violence against women. Contact WIRES, p. 570, for addresses.
Women Against Rape, 38 Mount Pleasant, London WC1 (01 837 7509). Shares premises, and many members, with Wages for Housework Campaign.

SELF-DEFENCE

Belden, Jack, 'Gold Flower's Story', *China Shakes the World*, 1949, now available in new (paperback) edition from Monthly Review Press, New York. The story of a group of peasant women who banded together against their oppressive families.
Butler, Pat and Karen, *Judo and Self Defence for Women and Girls*, Faber, 1971.
Cordell, Sarita, 'Self Confidence/Defence', *Second Wave*, Vol. 2, No. 4, 1973.
Hudson, Kathleen, *A Woman's Guide to Self Defence*, Collins, 1977.
Lomax, Maggie, 'Self Defence', *Spare Rib*, No. 16.
Nakayama, M., and Draeger, Donn F., *Practical Karate: For Women*, Tokyo, Japan, and Rutland, Vt: Charles E Tuttle, 1965.
Offstein, Jerrold N., *Self Defense for Women*, Mayfield, USA, 1972.

Parker, Rosie, 'Self Defence', *Spare Rib*, No. 55, 1977.

Short, Pauline and Paula, *Fight Back! A Self Defence Training Program for Women*, Portland, Oregon, Andersons PMS, 1974.

Tegner, Bruce, and McGrath, Alice, *Self Defense for Women, A Simple Method*, Thor, USA, 1977.

British Karate Control Commission, 4/16 Deptford Bridge, London SE8 4JS (01 691 3433). Provides information on clubs.

9   Birth Control

Introduction

In 1882 the diaphragm was invented; an important year both for the history of contraception and for the liberation of women. It was the first time that a reliable and safe method of separating sex from procreation had been put into our hands. Some contraception today is easier to use and more effective, but, unlike the diaphragm, more recent methods have sprung from a desire to control populations rather than to free women. It is in this atmosphere that a doctor can say:

The dangers of overpopulation are so great that we may have to use certain techniques of contraception that may entail considerable risk to the individual woman.*

We in the women's movement totally reject such a rationale. We also oppose the attempts by rich Western countries to impose policies of population control on poorer nations rather than changing exploitative economic policies. Unlike the population lobby we want to see fertility control placed firmly in the hands of women.

We often hear it said that 'no responsible woman today should get pregnant accidentally'. Figures from the Pregnancy Advisory Service† show that the majority of women requesting abortions had been using some kind of contraception, and over 30% were regular users – contraception methods are not foolproof.

Many women are restricted from choosing methods with a low pregnancy rate, for medical reasons, or because they feel unhappy using drugs on a daily basis or otherwise interfering with their natural processes. Those of us who would use a more effective method are often prevented from doing so because we don't have information about it or

* Doctor Frederick Robbins, quoted in 'The Doctors' Case Against the Pill', by Barbara Seaman.
† A Study of 1000 patients: Socio-Medical Reasons for requesting Abortion, 1973.

because prevailing attitudes of morality make us feel embarrassed about asking for advice.

For young people, information is particularly hard to find. Some schools have good straightforward sex-education programmes, others deal with the subject only in terms of conception and say nothing about preventing it. Where there is good sex education it is usually the responsibility of individual teachers who understand its importance. Teachers in the women's movement are organizing to change attitudes to sex education, and some local groups organize discussions on contraception and abortion in schools and youth clubs.

We are not helped in our efforts to gain control over our fertility by the attitudes of many doctors and drug companies. When contraceptives started to be supplied free through the NHS (April 1974), GPs were encouraged to participate in prescribing them. Due to the fuss kicked up by the British Medical Association, they were also awarded extra payment for the 'non-medical' prescription of contraceptives. Immediately many previously unsympathetic doctors took up birth control work. There was no onus on them to have birth control training as well, indeed relatively few of them have had any. They rely instead on advertising and information from drug companies. Contraceptives are of course sold for profit, so sales material is not an unbiased source of information.

This has very serious implications for women, who may be on the Pill for years without so much as a blood pressure test or may be fitted with an IUD by an untrained person. Even those who are trained may not take the trouble to keep up with the latest information or bother to take the time and trouble to pass it on clearly to us.

Doctors see contraception as something they prescribe and we take. Taking the Pill or using other kinds of contraception should in fact be a decision which we make together with our doctor, based on experience of our own needs. Without this cooperation many of us stop using contraception altogether. We are then categorized as *irresponsible* if we become pregnant. Those of us who experience side effects from the Pill or IUD are not even free to use abortion as a back-up to the safer (to us) mechanical forms of contraception (see Abortion chapter).

MEN AND BIRTH CONTROL

The attitudes of the men we are sexually involved with have much to do with how we use and feel about birth control. Both men and women these days seem to see contraception as a woman's responsibility because it is our lives which will be most affected by an unwanted pregnancy.

For those of us who can talk about birth control to our partners many of these problems are reduced; a caring man will be prepared to take his share of the burden and of the responsibility, he will recognize that unprotected intercourse holds a greater danger for women. His attitude counts; two people prevent pregnancy better than one.

WOMEN AND BIRTH CONTROL

For many of us the most stubborn resistance to birth control comes from within us. If we have grown up amid repressive attitudes to sex it is often difficult for us to accept our sexuality and take responsibility for our sexual behaviour.

Here are some of the personal reasons why we sometimes have trouble using birth control or don't even use it at all:

- We are embarrassed by, ashamed of, confused about our own sexuality.
- We cannot admit we might have or are having intercourse because we feel (or someone told us) it is wrong.
- We are romantic about sex — sex has to be a passionate, spontaneous sharing, and birth control seems too premeditated, too clinical, and often too messy.
- We hesitate to inconvenience our sex partner. This fear of displeasing him is a measure of the inequality in our relationship.
- If we are using natural birth control we sometimes have a hard time abstaining during our fertile days because we fear our partner will get angry and find sex elsewhere.
- We feel, 'It can't happen to me. I won't get pregnant.'
- We have questions about birth control and sex and don't know whom to talk with.
- We hesitate to go to a doctor or clinic and face the hurried, impersonal care or, if we are young or unmarried, the moralizing and disapproval that we feel likely to receive.
- We are afraid of having a pelvic examination (see p. 139).
- We don't recognize our deep dissatisfactions with the method we are using and begin to use it haphazardly.
- We want a baby and can't admit it to ourselves. Or we feel tempted to get pregnant just to prove to ourselves that we are fertile, or to try to improve a shaky relationship.

BIRTH CONTROL AND SEXUAL FREEDOM

Wide availability of contraception has brought with it some new problems for women. Where before we could retreat from unwanted sex by pleading fear of pregnancy, we now have to learn to be honest and simply say 'no' without feeling guilty and embarrassed. It isn't always easy to do, and we may feel tempted to give in rather than be thought puritanical and old-fashioned. By pressurizing us to have sex against our will, many men are turning our new-found freedom into a new oppression.

HELPING OURSELVES

If we talk to each other openly about our difficulties with sex and contraception we will help each other to gain the necessary confidence for genuinely taking responsibility for our sexuality. With confidence we will feel more able to bring up these things with our male partners and put our relationships on to a more open and equal basis. Together we can also organize to change things not only for ourselves but for and with other women in our area. We can pressurize birth control clinics to provide better information on contraception, we can organize group discussions in clinics, schools, colleges and youth clubs. (For more on this see p. 563.)

CONCEPTION — THE PROCESS TO BE INTERRUPTED

During sexual intercourse, sperm are ejaculated through the man's penis into the woman's vagina. If uninterrupted, some of the sperm swim through the cervical opening, through the woman's uterus and into the fallopian tubes. It is also possible for sperm deposited in or near the lips around the vagina during sex play to swim into the vagina and follow the route to fertilize the egg. (This is possible even if the woman has an intact hymen or has never been penetrated!) If the sperm encounter an egg in the outer third of the fallopian tube, a sperm may penetrate the egg (fertilization). The process of an egg and a sperm uniting is called *conception* (see Chapter 2, 'Anatomy', for more about this). Although it is unusual, *a woman can get pregnant from having intercourse during her period.*

The Sperm. Sperm are made in the man's testicles ('balls'). Sexual stimulation makes blood flow into erectile tissue inside the penis, causing the penis to get stiff, hard, erect. A few sperm can come out in the drops of liquid that may come from the penis soon after the erection occurs. Continued sexual stimulation can cause the man to have an orgasm. As his orgasm begins, the sperm travel up the sperm ducts, over the bladder, and through the prostate gland into the urethra. Here the sperm are picked up by about a teaspoonful of seminal fluid (from the prostate and seminal vesicles) and are propelled out of the urethra by rhythmic contractions which are very pleasurable to the man. This is called ejaculation. (See diagram on p. 24 in Chapter 2.)

About 300–500 million sperm come out in one ejaculation. So many will die on the way to the egg that this great number is needed to ensure that reproduction can occur.

Sperm come out fast, usually headed straight for the entrance to the cervical canal. They swim an inch in eight minutes – so a sperm may reach an egg in as little as thirty minutes. Sperm can move more quickly in the few days around ovulation because of the nature of the cervical mucus at that time. See 'Natural Birth Control', p. 277, for details.

The acid environment of the vagina is hostile to sperm, so sperm in the vagina die in about eight hours. Once sperm get to the uterus, however, they can live for four to five days.

Monthly Fertility Cycle

Uterine lining, fully developed by about day 25, starts to disintegrate from day 26 to day 28

Bleeding (shedding of uterine lining) from day 1 to day 5

AN AVERAGE MENSTRUAL CYCLE (28 DAYS) (NO PREGNANCY)

Egg development and preliminary build-up of uterine lining from day 6 to day 13

Ovulation of ripe egg usually occurs between day 12 and day 16

Since sperm live 4 to 5 days, most fertile time is from day 7 to day 16 (although cycle varies, so no time is really safe for unprotected intercourse)

CHOOSING YOUR BIRTH CONTROL METHOD

Each of the currently available contraceptive methods has disadvantages as well as advantages. Some methods we find to be a nuisance, others may make us sick. Many may have long-term dangers still unknown. The choice usually involves deciding where we are willing to make a compromise. We can weigh whether effectiveness, safety, or convenience matters more to us, and most important, what method we feel the most comfortable with and which one we will use the most consistently. We will choose differently according to where we are in our lives — no one method is likely to be satisfactory enough to carry us all the way through our fertile years.

Approximate Number of Pregnancies during the First Year of Use Per 100 Non-Sterile Women Initiating Method*

Method	Used Correctly and Consistently	Average US Experience Among 100 Women Who Wanted No More Children
Abortion	0	0+
Abstinence	0	?
Hysterectomy	·0001	·0001
Tubal Ligation	·04	·04
Vasectomy	·15	·15+
Oral Contraceptive (combined)	·34	4[a]–10[b]
IM Long-Acting Progestogen (injection)	·25	5–10
Condom + Spermicidal Agent	Less than 1·0	5
Low Dose Oral Progestogen	1–1·5	5–10
IUD	1–3	5[a]
Condom	3	10[a]
Diaphragm (with spermicide)	3	17[a]
Spermicidal Foam	3	22[a]
Coitus Interruptus	9	20–25
Rhythm (Calendar)	13	21[a]
Lactation for 12 months	25	40[c]
Chance (sexually active)	90[d]	90[d]
Douche	?	40[a]

* From Contraceptive Technology 1976–77 by Hatcher & Stewart. Halstead Press (USA). 1977.

[a]Ryder, Norman B., 'Contraceptive Failure in the United States', *Family Planning Perspectives* 5: 133–142, 1973.

[b]Oral contraceptive failure rates may be far higher than this, if one considers women who become pregnant after discontinuing oral contraceptives, but prior to initiating another method. Oral contraceptive discontinuation rates as high as 50–60% in the first year of use are not uncommon in family planning programmes.

[c]Most women supplement breast feedings, significantly decreasing the contraceptive effectiveness of lactation. In Rwanda 50% of non-lactating women were found to conceive by just over 4 months postpartum. It might be noted that in this community sexual intercourse is culturally permitted from about 6 days postpartum on. (Bonte, M. and van Balen, H., *Journal of Biosocial Science*, 1 : 97, 1969).

[d]This figure is higher in young couples having intercourse frequently, lower in women over 35 having intercourse infrequently. For example, MacLeod found that within 6 months 94·6% of wives of men under 25 having intercourse four or more times per week conceived. Only 16·0% of wives of men 35 and over having intercourse less than twice a week conceived (MacLeod: *Fertility and Sterility* 4: 10–33, 1953).

When choosing a method we should bear in mind that failure rates vary according to consistent or average use (see chart above) and that the theoretical rate, usually shown on the package, gives the contraceptive effectiveness in laboratory conditions. When choosing a contraceptive remember that the failure rate on the package will be the *theoretical* rate, and that when your chosen method is controlled by you (e.g. diaphragm, pill, foam) the rate will depend very much on how effectively you use it. The chart shows how much effectiveness varies with personal motivation. The more difficult the method is to use *correctly* the more likely it is to fail; foam sprayed directly on to sperm in a laboratory may work perfectly but in practice the two might never meet! In methods which are not so much affected by human error (IUD, sterilization), consistent use rates and average rates are much closer. Methods that are controlled by your partner will also be as effective as he is able – or inclined – to make them.

In the table above, a 3% pregnancy rate, or failure rate, which is the same as a 97% effectiveness rate, means that studies in the past have shown that 3 women out of 100 using that particular method have become pregnant in one year. Note that, in comparison, sexually active women using no method at all have a 90% pregnancy rate.

There are other things apart from effectiveness which you must take into account. How do you rate your memory? Will you remember to take pills every day, to take diaphragm or pills with you when you go away? How do you feel about using abortion as a back-up, and how possible will that be in your area or on your income? Your relationship with your partner(s): will you feel able to stop and put your diaphragm in, will you feel able to discuss and share contraceptive methods? Where you live: is there a place where you can easily store supplies, and will it matter if others find them? Different birth control methods are discussed later in this chapter.

WHERE TO GO FOR CONTRACEPTIVES

For most of us there are three options:

1. A birth control clinic.
2. Our own GP.
3. Another GP who is prepared to see and prescribe birth control for patients who are not on his list.

If your GP is trained in contraceptive work, it might be sensible to get contraceptive advice from him or her rather than to divide off another area of your body and take it to another place (see p. 556 for questions to ask your doctor). If your GP is not trained in this work or if you feel reluctant to discuss this with your own doctor, a contraceptive clinic is the best solution. The doctors there should be trained in contraception and they will have had a certain amount of experience in dealing with various complications and side effects. If you cannot go to a clinic, consult p. 556 for how to find a doctor who will prescribe for you.

The Clinic

You can find the telephone number and address of your nearest clinic through the Community (Local) Health Council, Citizens' Advice Bureau, Local Library, or under Family Planning in the Yellow Pages. It is best to ring first for an appointment. In some areas you may be asked to wait for several weeks for the first one, though they may offer you sheaths and spermicides to tide you over in an emergency (see p. 273).

Your first visit to a clinic may seem a little intimidating; most of us feel embarrassed the first time. A nurse or counsellor will ask you questions: name, address, job, etc., and also one or two questions about your relationship: are you married, do you have a 'steady relationship', etc. These questions are asked partly for irrelevant statistical purposes but also as a guide to what kind of method would suit you. They would of course be unnecessary if they explained all the methods detailing different problems and asked *you* to decide. You will then be weighed, and have your blood pressure checked. This provides a basis for measuring any increase in blood pressure or weight if you go on the Pill. The next visit is to the doctor, who asks questions about your medical history and examines you internally (see p. 139). Many women are very apprehensive about internal (pelvic) examinations. It seems like a terrible invasion of our privacy, and more so if we have never touched that part of our bodies ourselves. If you read Chapter 2 (Anatomy) and do a little exploring yourself before going to the clinic you may feel less worried about being examined. And remember, the vaginal muscles are very strong; if you're tense you will squeeze them together involuntarily and examination will be difficult and possibly even painful. If you can relax and breathe naturally, it will be much easier.

After the examination you discuss various methods of contraception with the doctor. It is at this point that communication often breaks down. Make sure that you are given time to think about each alternative and that you make the final decision about the kind of contraception you want, and are told clearly how to use it. If you feel at all doubtful, ask. If you don't remember what to ask until you get home, ring up later. Clinics are there for our convenience. You may prefer to go with someone else for your first visit — many women do. Don't be afraid to ask the doctor if your companion can stay with you during the examination.

Birth Control Pills

COMBINATION PILLS

These are the most widely used pills. They interrupt the menstrual cycle (see Chapter 2) by introducing synthetic versions of the female hormones.

Combination pills prevent pregnancy primarily by inhibiting the development of the egg in the ovary. During your period, the low oestrogen level normally indirectly triggers your pituitary gland to send out F S H, a hormone that starts an egg developing to maturity in one of your ovaries. The Pill, if taken according to the instructions on the packet, gives you just enough synthetic oestrogen to raise your oestrogen level high enough to keep F S H from being released. So, during a month on the Pill your ovaries remain relatively inactive, and there is no egg to be fertilized by sperm. This is the same principle by which a woman's body checks ovulation when she is pregnant: so in a way, using much lower levels of hormones, the Pill simulates pregnancy, and some of the Pill's side effects are like those of early pregnancy. If ovulation occurs, it is because your body needed a higher dose of oestrogen than your Pill gave you to inhibit F S H (if you are overweight, for example, you may need larger doses of hormones), or because you have missed one or more pills. Progestogen, synthetic progesterone, is the other hormone in the Pill. Progestogen provides two extra contraceptive effects: increased thickness of cervical mucus, and altered development of the uterine lining.

Effectiveness

Combination pills have the very low theoretical pregnancy rate of 0.34%. In actual use they show a failure rate of 4–10%. Pregnancy can occur if you forget to take your pill for one or more days; if you try to juggle your pill schedule; if you don't use a back-up method of birth control for your first two weeks of pills in the first packet, and occasionally when you change from one brand of pill to another (but see pp. 255–6 for details). Until recently, women were invariably blamed for any Pill pregnancies. But now it is becoming clear that failure to take a pill is relatively rare. Instead it has been discovered that if we have an upset stomach, causing vomiting or diarrhoea, this can prevent the pill from being absorbed. This possibility appears to be more real the earlier in the cycle you are ill and the longer you are ill, although pregnancies have been known when the stomach upset occurred for one day only and after more than 12 tablets had been taken. The *Handbook of Contraceptive Practice*, published for the use of doctors by the D H S S, does not mention these possibilities. If you do have diarrhoea or vomiting, it is best to take extra precautions for the rest of the month.

It is also possible for other drugs to cancel out the effectiveness of the Pill, and this becomes theoretically more possible as the doses of the Pill become lower. So far, Rifampicin (an antibiotic used for the treatment of TB) has been shown to do this; certain other antibiotics (ampicillin, phenoxymethylpenicillin, neomycin, nitrofurantoin), analgesics including aspirin, phenacetin and caffeine, and the anti-epileptic drugs are suspected too. If you experience breakthrough bleeding while taking these drugs, it is advisable to use extra contraception until the end of your cycle.

Reversibility

If you want to become pregnant, stop taking pills at the end of a packet. It may be several months before your ovaries are functioning regularly, and your first non-Pill periods may be late, or missed completely. While most women do have successful pregnancies after going off the Pill, it is now clear that there is some temporary infertility in a few women (permanent infertility has yet to be studied). In their recent 'Long-term Follow-up Study of Women Using Different Methods of Contraception', Vessey and Doll *et al.* show that after 30 months of trying, 16% of women who had been on the Pill had still not given birth, compared with 11% who had never used the Pill (a 50% difference). Length of time on the Pill appeared to be irrelevant. But in women who had already had a child there was no difference at all.*

Some women, especially those who menstruated irregularly before taking the Pill, have difficulty conceiving after they go off the Pill, but they may have been sterile or subfertile already. It may be best for such women to use a different method of contraception. Women with low body-weight, either because they are under-weight or simply small, may be slightly more at risk from infertility after taking the Pill. This could possibly be because their bodies do not need the standard doses found in most contraceptive pills. If you fit into this category, it might be best to use a particularly low-dose Pill such as Loestrin 20 (see 'Differences Among the Several Brands of Pills', p. 258). But as one study concludes, such women should possibly not take the combination pill at all. For women who do have difficulty conceiving after coming off the Pill fertility drugs can be given to induce ovulation, although they do not always work and can occasionally result in multiple births.

Safety

A lot of the information we receive about the Pill appears to be contradictory. On the one hand there are 'scares' which cause some of us to panic and come off the Pill immediately, possibly getting pregnant as a result. On the other hand we are told that the Pill is perfectly safe and

* Their more recent study, published in the British Medical Journal (4 February 1978) has found no evidence of *permanent* sterility in women taking the Pill.

there is nothing to worry about. Whatever we hear about the Pill we have to bear in mind who is saying it, and what their vested interest might be. Those people who play down or ignore the possible risks may well represent, or be funded by, drug companies. Or they may be concerned to prevent unwanted pregnancies at all costs, such as some family planning doctors and, it can be argued, the FPA itself. Those people who emphasize the risks may be primarily concerned about 'promiscuity' and sex education in schools (see *Safety and the Pill* by Dr Margaret White, published by the Responsible Society.)

The conclusions of an influential study – *Oral Contraceptives and Health*, performed by the Royal College of General Practitioners – have been widely used to encourage women to use the Pill *and to stay on it.** It was welcomed almost universally in the medical and lay press, being referred to, for example, as the 'recent all-clear on safety given to the Pill' (*British Medical Journal* leader, July 1974). The report appears to be a long-term study of 46,000 women, half of whom were on the Pill and half who weren't. But the longest any women in the study had been on the Pill was 5 years, and about half of those came off it before the study was completed. Moreover, most of the Pill takers had already been established on the Pill before the study began – so they had already been proved as 'tolerant' of it to some extent. It is very difficult to deduce these important facts from the report itself, which is disturbingly unscientific in many other respects, such as in its use of statistics and in the biased way that 'facts' are presented.† So we need to take with several pinches of salt the conclusions of this 'impartial and scientific study' (to quote the Family Planning Association – *F.P. News*, June 1974). *There is no easy answer to the question 'Is the Pill safe?'* It is often argued that the Pill is safer than pregnancy. Indeed, the risk of death from thrombosis due to pregnancy is about 20 times greater than that from the Pill. But this argument is too misleading to be entirely reassuring. Firstly, pregnancy is not the only alternative to the Pill. Secondly, a generalization is of little relevance to the individual. The relative risks depend, for example, on your general state of health, family and medical histories, your age, where you live, whether and how much you smoke, and the competence of your doctor. If, for instance, you smoke and you have a history of blood clots in your family, you are considerably more at risk than another woman of the same age. Thirdly, death rates are no indication of the significant number of women who have suffered from crippling strokes or other non-fatal blood clots,

---

* The conclusions in this study have since been somewhat overruled by the latest report by Beral and Kay (see Bibliography), which indicated that there was a much higher risk of death from circulatory disease than had previously been estimated by the RCGP (see 'Complications and Side Effects', below).

† See Jill Rakusen, 'Information or Propaganda', *Spare Rib*, 32

who develop diabetes on the Pill or who become debilitatingly depressed.

Birth control pills are dangerous for some women, and in quite a number of other women can cause side effects ranging from nuisances to major complications. Although most women have taken the Pill with no major immediate side effects, many of us are uneasy about taking a synthetic drug every day for months and years when its effects have not been conclusively tested and it has been in wide use for only 15 years. Yet the dangers of the Pill can be considered alongside the dangers of other drugs taken all the time, or air pollution, poisonous food additives or crossing the road. And effective protection against pregnancy is a very important tool for us as we start to take control of our lives. Many women will continue to decide to use the Pill, if only because we don't want to get pregnant and, because of restrictive laws, we cannot rely on getting an abortion if we use a less effective method. In our collective we prefer to use other methods whenever possible, if we feel we can use them effectively. The fact remains that we cannot make a real choice about the Pill unless we have access to reliable information and competent doctors, and until we have come together and won the fight for free, safe contraception and abortion for all who want it.

Complications and Side Effects

It is not surprising that the Pill can have many effects: it enters your bloodstream and travels around your body, affecting many tissues and organs just as natural hormones do. Undoubtedly some of the side effects can be psychosomatic. There is a tendency to blame mental and physical problems on something concrete, such as the Pill, especially if there has been a lot of publicity about it, or if we aren't sure we want to take it. We have a right to know all the possible side effects of the Pill, but we should keep in mind that many women notice no side effects other than some nausea at the beginning, and that, having weighed up the risks, some may still decide this is the best method for them. However, some women might begin to experience side effects after several years on the Pill. If you get an unpleasant side effect from one brand of pill, you might find that it disappears if you try another one.

Blood Clots. Blood clots can lead to pain, hospitalization and sometimes death. While the great majority of women on the Pill do not encounter problems with blood clotting, all women on the Pill run a considerably greater risk of incurring them. At worst, the risk is between 9 and 11 times greater for women on the Pill than for those who aren't. While the risk for each individual is difficult to assess, it does seem to be higher if you smoke, have a family history of any form of thrombosis in a young relative, if you are over 35, have been on the Pill for 5 years or more, have varicose veins or have had clotting problems in the past. It is even higher if all of these risk factors are involved. While the risk of death from blood clots is probably less than 3 per 100,000 per year in women on the Pill, clotting is very serious and could lead to a stroke, for example, with some kind of permanent impairment or paralysis of one side of the body. Clotting of the artery leading to the eye can lead to blindness. Each year one out of every 2,000 Pill users is hospitalized for thrombosis.

After operations, the risk of deep-vein thrombosis is higher if you have recently been on the Pill. It is advisable to come off it for at least one month before undergoing surgery, although coming off it for as little as 3 days would probably reduce the risk to some extent. It has been suggested that Heparin – a drug which stops clotting – can be given instead of a woman having to come off the Pill for an operation. This drug is itself dangerous unless its use is absolutely necessary, as it can lead to un-controllable bleeding. It is disturbing that doctors may be prepared to expose women to Heparin rather than to suggest that we come off the Pill and use another method of contraception.

The risk of blood clots with Pills containing 50 mcg. of oestrogen or less *may* be lower than with higher-dose Pills.

Heart Attacks. Two recent studies strongly suggest that women on the Pill run a 3–5 times higher risk of heart attack (coronary thrombosis) than non-users. The risk seems to be higher for women with certain predisposing risk factors: heavy smoking, obesity, diabetes, hypertension and age (over 35) – although the risk even in young women appears to be higher in Pill takers. In women over 30 the risk of heart attack is greater than that of clots. Deaths from heart attacks due to the Pill are estimated at 3–4 per 100,000 women per year in the 30–39 age range and 20 per 100,000 per year in the 40–44 age range. The length of time a woman is on the Pill, i.e. 5 years or more, also appears to increase the risk.

Hypertension (rise in blood pressure). The Pill causes an increase in blood pressure in a certain percentage of users. The incidence of high blood pressure tends to increase with age, weight and increased duration of Pill use. If left, hypertension could eventually lead to death as a result of heart or kidney failure or stroke. It is therefore very important to have your blood pressure checked regularly if you are on the Pill. Going off the Pill brings blood pressure down; so do anti-hypertensive drugs, but staying on the Pill and taking these drugs is not recommended, since they carry their own dangers and side effects and should only be taken if absolutely necessary. Switching to a progestogen-only Pill (see p. 257) is said to eliminate hypertension, but this has never been evaluated and women with severe hypertension should consider going off the Pill entirely.

Other Circulatory Diseases. The Pill is now thought to increase the risk of other circulatory diseases (as well as those above) to women over 35 and/or women who have taken the Pill for over 5 years. (See V. Beral and C. R. Kay in the Bibliography.)

Cancer. As yet there is no proof that the Pill either causes or protects against cancer of the breast, uterus or ovaries. The studies that exist so far are for 2, 3, or 4 years only, while the possible cancer-inducing effects of a drug may not show up for 20 years. A recent study (Stern, 1977) indicates that the Pill increases the risk of cervical cancer in women who already have abnormal cells (see p. 178) before starting on the Pill and whose cells do not return to normal within 6 months. After 7 years, 6 times as many of these women had cancer, which in some cases appeared as soon as 2 years after starting the Pill.

All Pill users should have regular smears. If even minimal abnormality exists tests should be done every 3–6 months. You would be wise to stop taking the Pill if there is any worsening in this condition.

The Pill does seem to reduce the incidence of benign breast tumours. If you already have *cystic mastitis* – a benign breast condition – it may not be a good idea to go on the Pill since there is a slight chance that the condition could become malignant; with fibroadenoma, another benign breast condition, it is probably all right to take the Pill. Oestrogen can aggravate an existing cancer, so make sure you are regularly checked (see 'How to Get Pills', p. 255); it is also important to examine your own breasts regularly every month (see 'Breast Self-Examination, p. 152). A family history of breast cancer is not usually considered a contraindication to use the Pill.

Your Children. There may be an association between ingestion of sex hormones in the first trimester of pregnancy (or just before) and congenital abnormalities. However, the incidence of such abnormalities is extremely low and there have not been enough studies to verify this yet. It is advisable to come off the Pill for about 3 months before trying to conceive. There also may be a higher rate of neonatal jaundice among infants whose mothers had taken the Pill before pregnancy. Children who find Pills and eat them probably won't be hurt, but tell your doctor.

Headaches. Some women on the Pill develop migraines or other frequent headaches. Blood vessel changes in one part of the body, causing relatively 'minor' problems such as headaches, may parallel changes in other parts of the body which could be more serious, such as strokes (see Grant in Bibliography). Migraines can be a warning signal for impending stroke and should cause a woman to switch to a lower-dose oestrogen Pill or to stop taking the Pill altogether.

Diabetes. In some women, the Pill, like pregnancy, can precipitate diabetes.

Depression. Some women experience increased irritability or a tendency to feel depressed while on the Pill. These symptoms often continue instead of improving with succeeding cycles, and can grow on you without your being aware of them. A Pill with a less potent progestogen may help (see below). Vitamin B_6 may help depression in some women who become deficient in it.

Change in Intensity of Sexual Desire and Response. Many women experience an increase in sexual desire as soon as their fear of pregnancy is removed. But increasing numbers of women on progestogen-dominant, low-dosage oestrogen pills are complaining of lack of sex drive, lack of vaginal lubrication, decreased sensitivity in their vulval tissues, and decreased ability to have orgasms. A higher-dosage oestrogen pill, such as Ovulen, can help but it does mean a higher risk of thromboembolism.

Nausea. A common early side effect of the Pill, nausea usually goes away after 2 months; taking the Pill with a meal or just before bed will usually give relief.

Fatigue. If tiredness or lethargy occur, they usually last only 2 or 3 months while your body gets used to the different hormone levels.

Vaginitis and Vaginal Discharge (see p. 187). This does not always occur, but any of the Pills could make the vagina more susceptible, particularly to monilia (thrush). Vaginitis is treatable, but if it persists you may have to go off the Pill. Increased vaginal discharge is fairly common, can be due to oestrogen, and does not necessarily indicate infection – though if it is bothering you, you should have it checked.

Venereal Disease. Some people think that women on the combination pill are more likely to catch gonorrhoea when exposed, and women on the Pill who do get gonorrhoea seem to develop dangerous pelvic inflammatory disease more quickly – in other words, the disease spreads up into the uterus and fallopian tubes more quickly.

Urinary Tract Infection. Women on the Pill also tend to have more infections of the bladder and urethra, the tube which leads urine out of your body. The infection rate is higher with higher oestrogen doses.

Changes in Menstrual Flow. Your periods will be lighter with most Pills (oestrogenic pills cause more normal flow). Occasionally your flow may be very slight or you may miss a period. Missing a period when you haven't missed a pill rarely means you are pregnant; if you miss two periods in a row, consult a doctor.

Breakthrough Bleeding. That is, vaginal bleeding or staining between periods. If there isn't enough oestrogen or progestogen in the Pill to support the lining of your uterus at a given point in your cycle, a little of the lining will slough off. (This may also occur if you miss a pill.) It usually happens in your first or second Pill cycle and often clears up as your uterus gets used to the new levels of hormones. If breakthrough bleeding doesn't stop after a few months, or if you begin to experience it after some time on the Pill, see a doctor to find out whether you need to try a different brand of Pill or whether you may have another problem. Breakthrough bleeding does not mean that the Pill isn't working as a contraceptive.

Breast Changes. Increased breast tenderness might occur, but it usually lasts for only one or two cycles. Breasts may also increase in size.

Weight Gain. Progestogen-dominant pills, such as Norlestrin or Gynovlar, can cause appetite increase and permanent weight gain because of the build-up of protein in muscular tissue. Oestrogenic pills (e.g. Ovulen) can cause fluid retention because of increased sodium. This effect is temporary and usually cyclic. It can often be reversed by changing your brand of Pill. Some people who retain fluid take a diuretic drug to stimulate their urine production, but diuretics have their own side effects (they rob the body of potassium, for instance), so use them sparingly if at all.

Skin Changes. Can be caused by the Pill. They usually clear up after stopping it or possibly switching to a progestogen-only brand. Disorders that can be caused by the pill include: *chloasma* ('giant freckles'); *itching of the skin*; extreme sensitivity to *sunlight* (even through glass); oily skin and *acne* (a progestogen-dominant Pill can cause or increase these problems in some women while an oestrogenic Pill can decrease acne); *erythema nodosum* (nodules under the skin). Most of them are quite rare although they should always be investigated since apart from the latter problem they could be indicative of *hepatic porphyria*, a serious though rare liver disorder.

Gum Inflammation. The Pills, like pregnancy, foster the development of gum inflammation. Women on the Pill should brush their teeth extra carefully, use dental floss regularly, and see a dentist every 6 months to a year.

Gall Bladder Disease. An increased incidence of gall bladder disease has been found among Pill users and may increase with higher progestogen dosages.

Epilepsy. A higher incidence of new cases of epilepsy has been reported in one study among women taking the Pill. In addition, the Pill could aggravate existing epilepsy. The woman should stay under close medical supervision.

Allergies. Allergies such as eczema or asthma can be either aggravated or improved by the Pill.

Liver Tumours. These tumours are extremely rare, particularly in young women, but even though a small number of cases have been reported recently in young women taking the Pill, this is a big increase in percentage terms. The recent increased incidence is leading people strongly to associate liver tumours with the Pill and particularly with its long-term use. One writer computes that the risk increases 25 times after the Pill has been used for 5 years. She comments that 'fortunately', most women only take it for about 2 years. Virtually all the tumours that have been discovered have been benign, but they are still extremely dangerous and can easily lead to haemorrhage and death. They also appear to be related to blood vessel changes and, as we have already pointed out, it is possible that 'minor' vascular changes may be precursors of more serious problems. Some doctors are suggesting that examination of the area round the liver should be routine, particularly for women who have been on the Pill for 5 years or more.

Virus Infections. An increased incidence of chicken-pox and other viral infections among Pill users suggests that the Pill may affect your body's immunity.

A number of other connections have been suggested between the Pill and conditions such as changes in liver function, sometimes leading to jaundice; pleurisy; suppression of bone growth in young women; visual disturbances; ulcers in the mouth; bruising; vitamin deficiencies, e.g. B_{12}, B_6, folic acid, ascorbic acid; lupus erythematosus, a disease of unknown origin which may be caused by an allergic reaction; and abnormalities in the cervix. There is no conclusive proof that the Pill causes these effects. But if you encounter one of these problems, it might be connected with the Pill.

(For more detailed descriptions of the side effects see the *Birth Control Handbook* from the Montreal Health Press – listed in Bibliography.)

Beneficial Side Effects

Menstrual cramps and occasionally pre-menstrual tension can be decreased, but in the case of pre-menstrual tension, the problem can even be aggravated by the Pill. Iron deficiency anaemia is less likely, probably because of the decreased menstrual flow. Benign breast growths are seen less frequently among women on the Pill, although this could be because women with benign breast disease tend to be recommended another method of contraception.

Warning Signals

Any side effect that lasts more than two or three cycles should be reported to the doctor. More serious symptoms of adverse reactions are: severe leg or chest pains, swelling of the legs, shortness of breath, sensation of flashing lights, severe headache, sudden blurred vision. They are signs of incipient thromboembolism and mean that you should stop taking the Pill. If you experience any of these symptoms, contact your doctor *immediately* and remind him that you are on the Pill. (Note on leg pain: the kind of pain we are talking about is not like cramp although it is usually in the calf; it is extremely painful and if you touch your leg, you'll know about it!)

Who Should Not Use the Pill?

Women who have certain pre-existing conditions which are exacerbated by the Pill are more at risk of developing serious complications if they take it. They should only take the Pill if there are very good personal reasons for doing so. Women with any of the following conditions or risk factors should think very seriously about whether or not to take the Pill. They are arranged more or less in order of importance:

Age. Women *over 35* run a statistically higher risk of circulatory diseases and other complications when taking the Pill, and an even higher risk if other predisposing risk factors are present (see above, pp. 247–8).

No woman over 40 should use the Pill. Women over 30 should reconsider, especially if they smoke or have been on the Pill for 5 years or more.*

Smoking. Anyone who smokes has an increased risk of suffering serious diseases of the heart and blood vessels. For Pill-takers, the risk is further increased. It is because of this that the US government has decided that all women should be warned against using the Pill if they smoke.

Any Disease or Condition Associated with Poor Blood Circulation or Excess Blood Clotting: bad varicose veins, thrombophlebitis (clots in veins, frequently in the leg), pulmonary embolism (clot which has travelled to the lung), stroke, heart disease or defect.

Cancer of the breast or of the reproductive organs. (See also *Cancer* above concerning abnormal cervical cells.)

Undiagnosed Abnormal Genital Bleeding.

Hepatitis or Other Liver Diseases. As the liver metabolizes the steroids in the Pill, no one with liver disease should take it until the disease is cleared up. Use a good alternative method of contraception, since pregnancy can be a great strain on the liver. A woman who tends to get jaundice during pregnancy should not use the Pill.

Diabetes or Pre-Diabetes. Sugar metabolism is extensively altered in women on the Pill. Progestogen tends to bind the body's insulin and keep it out of circulation, which increases a diabetic woman's insulin requirement. If you are a diabetic, or if close relatives are diabetic, you should have regular blood tests if you go on the Pill. Many doctors put diabetic women on the Pill because pregnancy is especially hazardous for them, but another method of contraception would be safer.

Kidney Disease.

Circulatory Conditions such as high blood pressure or mild varicose veins (see 'Hypertension', p. 248).

---

* The Tietze report, comparing death rates, found that in women over 35 the safest contraceptive was a mechanical method such as the cap plus abortion as a back-up (see Bibliography).

Sickle-Cell Anaemia or Trait. There is an increased risk of blood clotting with both sickle-cell anaemia and the Pill. Black women planning to go on the Pill should have a sickle-cell test. If it is positive for sickle-cell trait (not in itself as serious as the anaemia), discuss with your doctor the possible hazards of your taking the Pill.

Epilepsy and Asthma (see p. 251).

Migraine Headaches (see p. 249).

Certain Benign Breast Problems such as cystic mastitis (see p. 249).

Uterine Fibroids.

Tendency to Severe Depression or any Serious Psychiatric Problem.

Cystic Fibrosis.

Lactation. The Pill may dry up the mother's supply of milk, especially if taken soon after she gives birth. Even if it does not dry it up, the Pill decreases the amounts of protein, fat and calcium in the milk. Some oestrogen will also come through into the milk. At present this is a controversial subject; most nursing mothers are advised not to take the Pill, even low-dose Pills (see Breast-feeding, pp. 463–4).

In conclusion, the Pill is dangerous for certain women and you should be checked for each of the above contraindications. If you do have one of the problems we have mentioned, particularly one of the first nine, you would be unwise to take the Pill at all. Whether you have any pre-existing problems or not, you should take the Pill only under responsible medical supervision.

How Long To Take the Pill

You may feel you want to enjoy the freedom of the Pill indefinitely. Yet if you take the Pill for many years at a time, you are in a sense part of a huge experiment on the long-term effects of daily hormone ingestion in healthy women. Your decision depends on a lot of factors. If a pregnancy would be physically dangerous to you, you may choose to stay on the Pill. If you want to have a baby at some point later on, you may choose not to stay on the Pill for more than 2 to 4 years at a time. Keep in mind that the older you get, the greater the risk. The cumulative effect of the Pill has not been adequately studied, yet the incidence of at least some side effects is now known to increase over time.

We are 'spoiled' by the simplicity of the Pill. Yet we must face the fact that it is *not* a method we can use for ever. We need discussion, information and support in making a switch to another method.

How to Get Pills

Since certain physical conditions would make taking birth control pills very dangerous, it is in our interest to go to a competent doctor or family planning clinic for a prescription. The current 'Pill off prescription' lobby appears to be more concerned with preventing pregnancy at all costs than with looking after our well-being. Make sure that you are examined carefully. The ideal consultation should include an internal pelvic examination, breast examination, cervical smear and blood pressure test. Blood and urine tests and an eye examination would also be useful in long-term users and older women. The interview should include questions about you and your family's medical history of breast cancer, blood clots, diabetes, migraines and so on. *Too many doctors prescribe birth control pills hurriedly; it's up to you to make sure you are carefully checked for each one of the contraindications.* When you are on the Pill you should see a doctor every 6 months to a year for the same tests and examinations, except perhaps the smear which does not always have to be done so regularly.

How to Use Pills

Combination Pills come in packets of 21 or 28 pills and, less commonly, 20 to 22 pills. There is no real difference between any of these regimens, but you must follow the required regimen for your particular brand of Pill. With 21-day Pills you take one pill a day for 21 days and then stop for 7 days, during which time your period will come. With 28-day Pills, which give you 21 hormone pills followed by 7 different-coloured placebos (without drugs), you take one pill a day with no pause between packets. Your period comes during the time that you are taking the 7 different-coloured pills. The 28-day Pill is good if you feel you would have trouble remembering the on-and-off schedule of the other Pills.

Start the first pill on the fifth day after your period starts, counting the day you start your period as day one. Or, as the FPA has recently suggested, start your pills on the first day of your period, counting that as day one. Take one pill at approximately the same time each day, and carry a spare packet of pills with you in case you get caught away from home or lose pills.

It is possible to take the 21-day Pill continuously. By doing this, we don't bleed. (When we bleed on the Pill it is not 'real' menstruation.) Women should treat this idea with caution, particularly following recent studies concerning hormone replacement therapy and possible association with endometrial cancer (see chapter on the Menopause, p. 522).

If You Forget a Pill

These may not be the instructions you would get from your doctor; they are a combination of the best advice we could find.

Low-dose Pills (50 mcg. of oestrogen or less): If you forget one of these for less than 12 hours, take it, and take the next pill at the appointed time. If you forget it for more than 12 hours, don't take it because by taking a pill close to the next time you should be taking one, you could actually trigger ovulation! Instead, simply skip the one missed pill, take the next pill at the appointed time and carry on with the rest of the pills as usual. It is unlikely that you'll get pregnant.

High-dose Progestogen Pills (such as Gynovlar and Anovlar): If you forget one of these for more than 12 hours, you would be unlikely to ovulate because of the high dose of progestogen, so you can still take your missed pill right up to the time you are supposed to take your next one.

All Combination Pills: If you forget two pills, ovulation may occur. Read the instructions on the packet: with some pills, you can take a double dose for the next two days and carry on as before; with others, you will need another method of contraception up to the first 2 weeks of the next cycle. You may have some spotting. If you forget three pills or more, stop taking your pills; start on a new packet after you have been off for 7 days, during which time you should have a period. Use another method of birth control from the day you realize you forgot the pills through two weeks of the next cycle. If you miss a pill or two and skip a period, get a pregnancy test. If you've been taking your pills correctly and you skip a period, it is unlikely, though not impossible, that you are pregnant.

Protection. Your first packet of pills may not protect you perfectly if you start on the 5th day of your period, so use another method of birth control for at least the first 2 weeks. However, if you start the Pill the same day your period begins, additional precautions should be unnecessary. After your first month on pills you will be protected against pregnancy all month long, even during the days between packets.

Advantages and Disadvantages of the Combination Pill

Advantages. Almost complete protection against unwanted pregnancy.

Regularity of bleeding – every 28 days.

Lighter flow during periods. This effect pleases some women, bothers some.

Relief of pre-menstrual syndrome in some women.

Fewer menstrual cramps or none at all.

An oestrogenic Pill will clear up acne for some women.

The Pill often brings a sense of well-being and a new enjoyment of sex because the fear of pregnancy is gone.

Taking the Pill has no immediate physical relationship to lovemaking. This is especially relaxing if you are just starting to have intercourse and have a lot to learn about your body and his. Later on when you are more comfortable with sex and more able to communicate openly with your partner, a diaphragm or foam and condoms will not seem like such interruptions.

Disadvantages. Most of the disadvantages have been described under the section on side effects. If you do become pregnant on the Pill, it could be a long time before you find out. The only disadvantage to add is that you do have to remember to take a pill every day. Younger women who live at home and feel a need to hide their pills from their parents sometimes leave them behind or are unable to take them on time.

SEQUENTIAL PILLS

Sequential Pills use oestrogen alone for the first part of the cycle and then combine oestrogen and progestogen for the last 5 or 6 days. They are *less effective* and because of their high oestrogen levels they carry a higher risk of blood clots. They should not be used except in rare cases of overreaction to progestogen in combination Pills.

PROGESTOGEN-ONLY PILLS

These are sometimes called 'mini-pills'. They contain small doses of progestogen. They contain no oestrogen. You take one a day continuously, starting on day one of your period, at the same time each day (particularly important), without stopping during your period.

It is unknown exactly how they work, but progestogens cause changes in cervical mucus that make it hard for sperm to get through; inhibition of the travel of the egg through the tubes; partial inhibition of the ability of the sperm to penetrate the egg; partial inhibition of implantation; and sometimes inhibition of ovulation.

Effectiveness. The theoretical pregnancy rate is 1 to 4%, higher than the combination Pill. The actual failure rate is of course higher than this. The pregnancy rate may be lower for women who switch from the combination Pill to the progestogen-only Pill than it is for women who have never taken the combination Pill. Efficiency tends to decrease with duration of use. These Pills do *not* prevent ectopic pregnancy (see p. 506). Any pelvic pain should be investigated with this possibility in mind.

Unfortunately, the symptoms of an ectopic pregnancy can be very similar to the effects of this Pill.

Possible Side Effects.   Side effects are being reported for the progestogen-only Pill, such as change in weight, cervical erosion and change in cervical secretion, jaundice, allergic skin rash, chloasma, depression, gastrointestinal disturbances, breast changes. A common complaint is that menstrual bleeding is very irregular in amount and duration of flow and length of cycle. (If you don't have a period within 45 days of your last one, get a pregnancy test.) Furthermore, not enough research has been done to establish, for example, whether or not these Pills have the same effect on blood-clotting as combined Pills. However, good side effects include less frequency of painful periods. These Pills have not been used long enough for any conclusions to be drawn about their desirability. You may feel safer taking them knowing they have no oestrogen and a very small dose of progestogen, and that they may have about the same rate of effectiveness as an IUD or a properly-used sheath or diaphragm. On the other hand, the irregular cycles may get you down, or you may not wish to be one of the testers of a very new Pill.

Differences Among the Several Brands of Pills

Different Pills have different kinds, strengths and quantities of synthetic oestrogen and progestogen in them. The Committee on Safety of Medicines warns that high-oestrogen Pills are more likely to give us blood clots. It advises that only products containing 50 mcg. or less of oestrogen should be used. (The FPA recommends only 30 mcg.) 50-mcg. Pills include Ortho-Novin 1/50, Norinyl 1, Demulen, Norlestrin and Gynovlar 21. Pills with more than 50 mcg. include Ortho-Novin 1/80, Ortho-Novin 2, Ovulen, Conovid-E, Conovid 5 and all sequential Pills.

Pills with doses of oestrogen lower than 50 mcg. ('low-dose' Pills) include Eugynon 30, Ovranette (both 30 mcg.) and Loestrin 20 (20 mcg.). These Pills may produce more spotting between periods, and the pregnancy rate with Loestrin 20 may be a bit higher.

High-dosage oestrogen Pills can be useful if a woman has had bad side effects from a higher-dose progestogen Pill or if there is an indication that she will have them (see below). In these cases the doctor should inform the woman of the higher risk of blood clots. The kind of side effects that a particular Pill is likely to have is related to the amount and potency of the progestogen relative to the oestrogen in that Pill. Strongly progestogenic Pills such as Gynovlar and Anovlar have a larger safety margin to allow for missed tablets. Unfortunately, all strongly progestogenic, low-oestrogen Pills are more likely to cause depression. On the other hand, weakly progestogenic Pills are more likely to cause irregular cycles or amenorrhoea. Certain progestogens such as norethisterone and norethisterone acetate (used in Ortho-Novin, Norlestrin, Norinyl, Gynovlar and Loestrin), tend to produce *androgenic* ('male') effects, such as hairiness, scanty periods, acne, permanent weight gain. With Pills in which the oestrogen dominates (Conovid, Demulen, Ovulen), either because of a lower progestogen-to-oestrogen ratio or because of the use of a less potent progestogen, the effects tend to be *oestrogenic* (or 'female'), such as heavier periods, fluid retention, breast swelling and tenderness.

It is not always possible to predict the oestrogen or progestogen potency by the dose because the synthetic compounds vary. There are two kinds of synthetic oestrogens, ethinyl-oestradiol and mestranol, which are offered in equivalent doses but may not be equal in strength. Some studies have suggested that ethinyl-oestradiol is more potent than mestranol and that it is also implicated more often in side effects such as strokes and urinary infections. All the 'low-dose' oestrogen pills (below 50 mcg.) use ethinyl-oestradiol. Progestogens in some Pills have an oestrogenic effect; others appear to have an anti-oestrogenic effect.

The exact effects that a given Pill will have on your body, if you experience side effects at all, depend on your normal oestrogen and progesterone levels. These levels are hard to test accurately, but you and the doctor can judge them in a general way. For instance, if you have a lot of body hair and scanty menstrual periods, you can guess that in your normal non-pill body chemistry there is a predominance of progesterone over oestrogen. A low-dosage oestrogen pill is likely to accentuate your progesterone-related characteristics, and you might experience one or more of the progestogen-excess symptoms — scant menstrual flow, changed sex drive, poor vaginal lubrication, susceptibility to monilia vaginitis, appetite increase and permanent weight gain, acne, depression, or fatigue. A more oestrogenic pill would be likely to balance your natural excess of progesterone.

On the other hand, if you have heavy periods or large breasts that get tender before your period, or if you tend to retain fluid and often feel bloated, you are probably oestrogen-sensitive or have a natural over-balance of oestrogen in your system. A low-dosage oestrogen or high-potency progestogen pill would be good for you, whereas a high-oestrogen pill would be likely to give you nausea, bloating, breast tenderness, leg cramps, chloasma (see p. 251), irritability and heavy periods.

Since it is not yet possible to predict side effects in any given case, use these guidelines when you can. Bear in mind, however, that some women are sensitive to all Pills and, while others might tolerate the Pill for several years, it is still possible to develop side effects at a later date.

Injections

DEPO-PROVERA

Depo-Provera (Depot Medroxyprogesterone acetate) is the most commonly used, though others are being experimented with.

Depo-Provera is an injection given every 3 or 6 months which suppresses ovulation. As with most hormonal methods of contraception, there are many questions concerning Depo-provera (DP) that remain to be answered. The oral form of DP was banned for use in the USA when it was found that DP could cause cancer in beagle dogs. The injectible form was left on the market, not because it was safer, but because it was argued that there was no alternative to the injectible form whereas there was to the oral form (i.e. the Pill). An association has also been found between DP and cervical cancer. That is all that is known about DP and cancer to date . . . except that two oral contraceptives were taken off the UK market in 1976 because they were implicated in studies similar to those carried out on DP. They both contain progestogens derived from the same source as DP.

DP has similar side effects to the Pill. Apart from increased incidence of blood-clotting, there appears to be a possibility of infertility, especially if DP is taken for some time. Disruption of bleeding can also be very disturbing. Some countries are concerned enough about the question of infertility to give DP only to women who have completed their families. But although the Committee on Safety of Medicines at the time of writing has not given DP a blanket licence for contraceptive use, it is still on the market and is being used as a contraceptive on hundreds of women. Some young women with no children have been given this drug. In some cases, the women were not even aware what the injections were for. One woman had terrible worry from bleeding problems that went on for ages after her baby was born. No one bothered to tell her it might have been the injection she'd been given after the birth.

Given what is known to date, we do not recommend this method of contraception, particularly over long periods of time, and particularly if you might consider having children in the future.*

IUD, or Intra-uterine Device: Coil, Loop

DESCRIPTION

Most IUDs are small white plastic devices of different shapes and sizes. They should be placed inside the uterus by a trained person. One or two strings extend from the uterus into the upper vagina so that you can

---

* For more details about DP, and the way that Third World women are being used as guinea-pigs, see Jill Rakusen. *Spare Rib*. Nos. 42 and 47 (see Bibliography).

check that the device is still in place by feeling for the threads. Once the IUD is inserted, nothing needs to be done other than checking, unless there are problems or you want to get pregnant. It should also be removed by a trained person.

HOW THE IUD WORKS

No one is absolutely sure how the IUD works to prevent pregnancy. Currently the IUD is believed to cause a local inflammatory reaction inside the uterus. The inflammation which occurs is a reaction to a foreign body (the IUD) and to irritation and does not necessarily mean there is an infection, even when there is an increase in vaginal discharge.

Some people find it a little unsettling that no one knows exactly how the IUD works. Others, uneasy with the Pill's more generalized effects and the pregnancy rates of other methods, choose the IUD. At least the effects of the IUD are local – if something goes wrong, your uterus usually hurts and you seek medical help.

THE DIFFERENT TYPES OF IUD

The most commonly used IUDs today are the Lippes Loop, Copper 7 (Cu-7) and the Saf-T-Coil.

A never-pregnant woman can have a hard time tolerating the IUD: a uterus that has not been stretched by pregnancy tends to react to one of these devices with cramping, backache and expulsion.

Some of the so-called 'second-generation' IUDs which have been developed are slightly smaller plastic devices with an active substance, usually copper, added to increase their effectiveness. The Cu-7 now in use has copper wire coiled around a small plastic device. These devices seem to be effective, to have a low expulsion rate even in never-pregnant women, and, because of their smaller size, to cause less pain during insertion as well as less blood loss during menstrual periods. They have the drawback of needing replacement every two years. Also the long-term effects of even these small amounts of copper are unknown. In mid 1976 a device was introduced containing a progestogen which is released into the uterus in tiny quantities. It has been withdrawn by the distributors pending further tests because trials indicate that of those women who do become pregnant with this IUD in place, 20% will have ectopic (tubal) pregnancies. A big increase in the rate noted with other IUDs (see below).

Effectiveness

Second only to the Pill (and, some people feel, matched by the diaphragm when the diaphragm is used perfectly). Pregnancy rates for the currently used types of IUD vary from 1 to 7%. The published rates are not

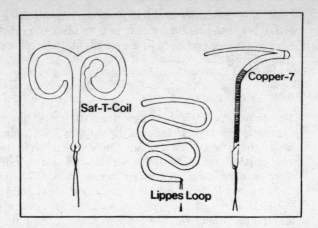

entirely comparable because they are based on studies of different quality. (Drug company representatives tend to give a lower failure rate for their devices.) Approximate pregnancy rates for the large (Size D) Lippes Loop and the Saf-T-Coil are 3%. So far, the copper devices, especially the Cu-7, have lower pregnancy rates, but they have not been tested very extensively. Pregnancy rates are lower among women over 30 and those who have given birth. For greater protection, contraceptive foam, cream or jelly can be used with the IUD, either all the time or for 7 to 10 days at mid-cycle (see 'Natural Birth Control', p. 277). Use a supplemental birth control method for the first 3 months with an IUD, as that is the time when conception seems to take place most often and when the IUD is most likely to be expelled. If you do become pregnant with the IUD in place, a miscarriage can be caused from 25 to 50% of the time simply by having the doctor remove the IUD.

Drugs and IUD Effectiveness.   Observations of IUD failures over the past few years have given rise to a suspicion that both *aspirin* and *antibiotics* (e.g. penicillin, tetracycline) may *lower* IUD effectiveness. Aspirin may hamper the action of contraction-causing prostaglandins (see p. 171) stimulated by the IUD's presence in the uterus. Antibiotics may interfere with the contraceptive effect of the IUD's irritation of the uterine lining. If you have an IUD, you may want to avoid taking pain killers containing aspirin and to use extra birth control (foam, condoms) while taking antibiotics.

Reversibility

Chances of becoming pregnant afterwards are generally the same as before using the IUD.

Safety and Side Effects

IUDs cause more complications than the Pill, although the Pill causes more deaths (see *Women's Report*, 4/2, p. 10).

Perforation. Perforation of the uterus, occurring in 1 out of about 1,000 women, is primarily the result of faulty insertion. Occasionally the IUD will slip out through a perforation in the abdominal cavity, where it can cause dangerous inflammation or adhesions, so it is important to check the strings and report their absence to the doctor.

*Infection.** There is an increased risk of uterine infection for the 2 weeks following insertion, and the infection rate remains somewhat higher than for women without the IUD. For your safety, have yourself checked for gonorrhoea, vaginal infection and pelvic inflammatory disease before getting an IUD.

If you feel abdominal tenderness or pain when the penis goes in deep, report it to the doctor. If you catch gonorrhoea while the IUD is in place, there is a chance that you won't be able to be cured until the IUD is removed, and the effects of the infection may be aggravated.

If you get a vaginal infection it may be caused by some tampon wool caught on the IUD string; it should be checked.

Long-term Effects. Like the Pill, the IUD has not been in wide use for long enough for us to know its long-term effects. There is some concern that an IUD left in for more than 4 or 5 years may cause changes in the lining of the uterus.

IUD and Pregnancy. If you get pregnant with an IUD in place, chances are very high (about 50%) that it will cause a miscarriage which may be accompanied by infection. Recent publicity about the Dalkon Shield focused attention on the hazards of getting pregnant with an IUD in the uterus: the rates of pregnancy complications, infections, uterine perforations, intestinal obstructions and haemorrhage are greatly increased and have led to some deaths. These problems also occur with other IUDs but seem to be more prevalent in women using the Dalkon Shield. Although the Dalkon Shield is no longer being distributed in this country, the DHSS is not recommending the recall of women who already have them inserted. However, they will advise immediate removal of the IUD if you become pregnant. If you do have a Dalkon Shield we urge you to take great care not to get pregnant, or to have it removed.

---

* See Daniel R. Mishell, Jr, 'Assessing the Intrauterine Device', *Family Planning Perspectives*, Vol. 7, No. 3 (May/June, 1975), for a clear, moderately pro-IUD discussion. And leader, *Lancet*, 25 September 1976: 'Pelvic infection seems to be about four or five times more likely among IUD users than other women.' The risk seems to be even higher among young women who have never had babies. (See also Westrom *et al.*, *Lancet*, 31 July 1976 and subsequent correspondence.)

There is such a high risk associated with all IUDs if pregnancy occurs that we feel that all women should have the IUD removed as soon as possible and be automatically offered an abortion if they want one in these circumstances.* If you only have the IUD removed, associated miscarriage would probably take place within the next fortnight, and if you do not miscarry the pregnancy should proceed normally and the foetus is unlikely to be affected.

It now seems that the IUD can occasionally cause tubal pregnancies (fertilized ovum implants in fallopian tube — see 'Some Exceptions in Pregnancy and Childbirth', p. 506). Recent reports suggest that IUD-associated infections may cause tubal blockage resulting in tubal pregnancy. This has not been proved. If you have an abortion because of an IUD-failure, have the uterine contents checked for foetal material.

Expulsion. A major drawback of the IUD is the expulsion rate, which is about 4 to 8 or 13 to 19%, depending on the study. The IUD is usually expelled, if at all, in the first 3 months of use, and usually during the menstrual flow. It often comes out without your knowing it or feeling it, so check your tampon or sanitary pad every time, and be sure to feel for the strings at the entrance to your cervix a few times a month, especially after your period.

Bleeding and Cramping. Some women experience little discomfort with the IUD, particularly if they have already had a child; others experience considerable pain and bleeding. Check with your doctor if it goes on for more than a couple of days after insertion. Different doctors and clinics report that from 5 to 20% of IUDs are removed because of pain and bleeding. The bleeding may be heavier during menstruation, or occur between periods; periods may be irregular. Prolonged menstrual cramps are possible, or cramping and back pain may occur between periods. These symptoms are usually more intense during the first 3 to 6 months of using the IUD and then tend to decline. The following is a subjective account of a probably rare occurrence; but you never know because such reports rarely get into the literature.

For about four months after I had my IUD inserted I felt that a white-hot wire was cutting through my uterus whenever I got aroused or had orgasms. I told the doctor who inserted it about this occurrence of pain, and he replied 'impossible'. I knew three other women who had gone to him for a Dalkon Shield, and they all said that they had felt foolish and hadn't mentioned that symptom to anyone, but they certainly felt it, too.

The attitude of the medical profession towards women can cause real problems for those of us who suffer from IUD side effects. Too often complaints of pain are ignored, we are told to 'be patient' and give it a

* In Boston the death rate from spontaneous abortion in women who have IUDs in place is found to be 50 times higher than among other women (*New England Journal of Medicine*).

chance to settle down. While it is true that for many of us the pain diminishes over time, and for most of us it only occurs at the start of menstruation, nevertheless we have different levels of pain tolerance and for some people it is simply unbearable. IUDs should always be removed on request. If your doctor refuses to remove yours, change your doctor and/or contact your local women's group.

I changed to the IUD because I was fed-up with messing around with a cap. Although I have bad cramps for a few hours at the start of every period, I prefer this kind of birth control to the Pill because the pain is local, I understand it and I don't feel slightly blurred and bovine as I used to on the Pill.

Other Possible Effects. The possible side effects of the copper in the Copper-T and the Copper-7 are unknown. Reports suggest it may produce an allergic skin reaction. One investigator has suggested that the copper may have an inhibitory effect on gonorrhoea, but don't count on it.

Who Should Not Use the IUD

IUDs should not be used by anyone with the following conditions: pregnancy, endometriosis, venereal disease, any vaginal or uterine infection, pelvic inflammatory disease, prohibitively small uterus, excessively heavy menstrual flow and/or cramping, bleeding between periods, large fibroids, uterine deformities, use of anticoagulants, anaemia and sickle-cell disease.

How to Get an IUD

The IUD must be inserted by a well-trained person. All contraceptive clinics can arrange this and in almost all cases insertion is performed by a doctor. If your GP offers to fit it, check that s/he is both trained to insert IUDs *and* has clinic experience which would ensure adequate practice in insertion. (If a mistake is made you could suffer great discomfort.) If s/he is not sufficiently experienced you would be better off at a clinic.

You should have a medical history taken in addition to a pelvic examination, cervical smear and VD tests before the device is inserted. If insertion is not done during a period a pregnancy test should be done as well. In many clinics these precautions are not taken in advance; evidence of infection may only come to light at your next examination.

IUDs are usually fitted during a period. Some clinics insist on this because if you are already pregnant (i.e. the fertilized egg is *implanted*), the IUD insertion could cause a septic miscarriage. In addition, your cervix is slightly dilated at this time so the insertion is a little easier. However, there has been concern recently that blood reintroduced into the uterus during a period might cause infection. The doctor does a

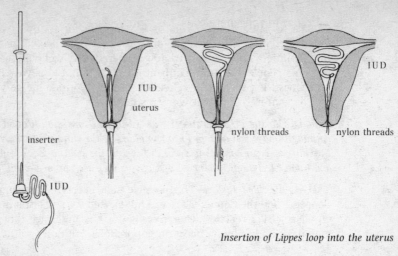

Insertion of Lippes loop into the uterus

sounding of the uterus which measures its depth, shape and position. The IUD can be put into a tipped uterus. Just before insertion, the Saf-T-Coil, Lippes Loop and Copper-7 are straightened out in a plastic tube like a straw; remember, the diameter of the cervical opening is the size of a thin straw. The doctor gently puts the tube into the vagina and up into the uterus through the cervix. Then the IUD is pushed through the tube and being made of 'memory plastic' springs into shape within the uterus.

The process can hurt, sometimes a lot, because the uterus is stretched and irritated by the device. You may have cramps during the insertion and for the rest of the day. Bring a friend with you if you can, and take aspirin beforehand, or a tranquillizer if they work for you, or try shallow panting to take your mind off it. The plastic IUD can stay in place for several years but you should have it checked every 6 months to a year. The copper IUDs must be replaced every 2 years because they appear to be less effective after this time.

Checking Your IUD

At first, check your IUD before intercourse (you may want to ask your partner to do it) and after each period. After 3 months or so, once after each period is enough.

Squat, to shorten the length of your vagina, bringing your bottom down near your heels, and reach into your vagina with your longest (clean) finger. Bearing down while you are sitting on the toilet will also bring your cervix within reach. You might be confused by the folds of your vagina, but when you reach your cervix you will know it; it feels rather like the tip of your nose. Find the dimple in your cervix; this is the entrance to your uterus, and the strings of the IUD should be sticking out a little way. Some days your uterus will be tipped in such a way that you can't reach the cervix or find the hole; try again the next day. If the string feels a lot longer, particularly if your cervix also feels more rigid than usual, it may be coming out. If you feel plastic protruding it is definitely coming out. Go to a clinic or doctor as soon as possible and use some other contraception in the meantime.

If the string has disappeared, and you cannot feel it over a few days, the IUD may have slipped out, or up, or possibly even worked its way through the wall of the uterus. You should definitely see a doctor.

Advantages and Disadvantages of the IUD

Advantages. You don't have to fuss with birth control at the time of intercourse (unless you are using foam or condoms at mid-cycle for closer to 100% protection).

You don't even have to remember to take a pill. If you are forgetful, or if your life is too hectic for you to keep track of pills, the IUD may be a better method for you than the Pill.

Disadvantages. Heavier periods, spotting and more frequent cramps make some women give up the IUD.

Some people don't like the idea of wearing something inside them all the time.

Side effects and possible complications as discussed above.

If you have a retroverted uterus the strings may irritate your partner's penis.

Diaphragm (Cap) and Spermicidal Jelly or Cream

A lot of people make a face when a diaphragm is mentioned. 'It's messy . . . It's a hassle . . . It fails all the time.' Yet many of our mothers used it for 30 years without a slip. Whether our mothers *enjoyed* using it is a different question. Today our more positive feelings about our sexuality, and our increasing ability to communicate openly with the men we sleep with, make us more able to use the diaphragm happily. If you are just starting to have intercourse you may not want to add a diaphragm to your sex life immediately, but in a few months, when you are more easy about sex, you may be glad to get off the pill or the IUD for a method that is effective if you use it well and that has no side effects at all.

The diaphragm is not used as much as it might be for a variety of reasons; because doctors rarely fit them they don't bother to mention them, we tend to be pushed towards more 'effective' methods and therefore many women don't even know of their existence. However, all contraceptive clinics can fit caps.

Description

A diaphragm, *which must always be used with spermicidal cream or jelly*, is made of soft rubber in the shape of a shallow cup. It has a flexible metal spring rim. When properly fitted and inserted, it fits snugly over your cervix, locked in place behind the pubic bone and reaching back behind your cervix. It comes in a variety of sizes measured in millimetres (mm.), ranging from 50 to 105 mm., or 2 to 4 inches, depending on the size of your upper vagina.

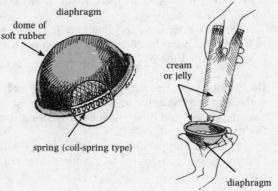

How It Works

When the diaphragm is in place, holding spermicidal jelly or cream up to your cervix, the sperm cannot make it into your cervical canal. The sperm that swim up around the rim of the diaphragm run into the cream or jelly, which kills them. The sperm that remain in the vagina die in 8 hours, as the vagina is a hostile environment to sperm. Never use the diaphragm without cream or jelly: they are the important contraceptive, and the diaphragm exists only to hold them in the proper place.

Effectiveness

If the diaphragm is used properly it is about as effective as an IUD. However, if you are not very careful its effectiveness drops to about 85–90% (see chart, p. 241).

The main points in using a diaphragm are to use it every time, and always to use a cream or jelly with it. Failures do occur about 3% of the time even when the diaphragm is properly used.

Reversibility

The diaphragm doesn't affect your fertility at all. Simply don't use it if you want to become pregnant.

Who Shouldn't Use the Diaphragm

A woman with a severely displaced uterus (severe prolapse, for instance) cannot use a diaphragm. If your uterus is tipped forward or backward slightly, the doctor can choose one of the three kinds of metal spring rim (arcing, coiled, or flat) to fit your particular anatomy. A woman with protrusion of the bladder through the vaginal wall (cystocele) or other openings in the vagina (fistulas) cannot use this method.

A virgin, since her diaphragm size will change with intercourse, should use a different method (foam and condom) the first few times and then go to be fitted.

If you don't feel comfortable touching your genitals and do not think you can get used to it *at this time*, you would most likely have trouble using a diaphragm effectively and should choose a different method. You can buy a diaphragm inserter if your diaphragm has a flat spring; but you will still need to check whether the diaphragm is covering your cervix, and you have to remove it without the inserter. (You may feel very squeamish and embarrassed the first time you put your finger into your vagina, but as you get used to it and realize that your body is yours to touch, you should get over any uneasiness about inserting the diaphragm.)

How to Get a Diaphragm

The size of diaphragm you need depends on the size and contour of your vagina. In this country it is usually a nurse who 'fits' you for a diaphragm. When you have been measured and fitted, you should practise putting in the diaphragm right there so the nurse can tell you if you have put it in right. (Or go home, practise, and come back in a few days with the diaphragm in place.) You can reach in and feel what it feels like when it is in right, and get help right then if you have problems, so that when you actually use it you won't be 'experimenting'. Sometimes this important step is neglected but it is routine in most clinics. You will normally be given the right size diaphragm at the clinic with an appropriate brand of spermicide (and pessaries if you want them). However you can buy both cap and spermicide at a chemist (you need a prescription for a cap).

Supplies from clinics are free, but some clinics try to limit the amount of spermicide you can have according to *their* idea of your needs. They have no right to do this, and your Community (or Local) Health Council should be informed if they do.

How to Use a Diaphragm

Putting it in the first time may seem awkward but once you've got used to it you'll probably find it quite simple. Some women feel they should go off and put it in privately so that they appear ready for spontaneous sex. If you are comfortable about using it you may prefer to put it in together with your partner so that it becomes a shared responsibility. However, if you feel likely to get carried away and forget it, you might be better off inserting it in advance.

Whichever method you choose, it must be put in no more than 2 hours before intercourse, or if you use pessaries or an applicator, you can put the cap in earlier and then insert a couple of pessaries behind and in front of the diaphragm a few minutes before intercourse. Since spermicides lose their potency over time inside you, the closer to intercourse you do it, the better.

Preparation and Insertion: Put about 2 inches of cream or jelly into the shallow cup, or on the dome side, whichever side you put against the cervix. Then put more cream around the *inside* of the rim. Now squeeze the cup together by pressing the rim firmly between your thumb and third finger. You can squat, or stand with one foot raised. With your free hand spread apart the lips of your vagina and insert the diaphragm, jelly uppermost into your vagina. Remember that your vagina angles towards your back, so push it backwards until it is right in and the lower rim is resting above your pubic bone.

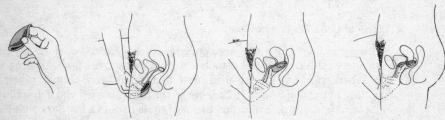

Insertion of diaphragm   *Checking of diaphragm*

You should then check with your finger to make sure you can feel the outline of your cervix through the rubber. Add some more cream or a pessary in front of it when it is in place (or you can put some on the outside of the cap as well as the inside before you start if you don't have an applicator). When it's in right and fits properly you will hardly feel it. (Some men notice that the tip of their penis is touching soft rubber instead of cervical and vaginal tissue, but this is not painful or bothersome.) Never use vaseline with a diaphragm, as it corrodes the rubber.

Leave the diaphragm in for at least 6 to 8 hours after intercourse, because it takes the spermicide that long to kill all the sperm. You can leave it in up to 24 hours. Douching is unnecessary, but if you want to douche you must wait 6 or 8 hours.

Subsequent intercourse. If you have intercourse again within the 6 hours, you *must* add spermicide. Put it into your vagina, leaving the diaphragm in place.

Care. Wash the diaphragm with mild soap and warm water, rinse and dry carefully, dust it with cornflour if you wish (but never talcum powder), and put it in a container (away from the light). Don't boil it. *Check it for holes* every so often by holding it up to the light or filling it with water and looking for leaks, especially around the rim.

Life of Product

Get your diaphragm rechecked every year. You will need a new size if you gain or lose 10 pounds, and after a pregnancy, abortion, or miscarriage. The diaphragm will last a couple of years with proper care. Spermicides lose their potency over time so don't bulk buy.

Brands of Jelly and Cream

In choosing one brand over another, you should consider factors of effectiveness, smell and taste (for oral-genital play), and any allergic reaction of yours or the man's. If you don't like the brand you're using, feel free to change. Unless they specifically mention on the pack or in the instructions that the product can be used with a cap don't use it; some forms of spermicide corrode rubber (e.g. Rendells pessaries; *Which* report, 1971).

Here is a list of F P A-approved products for use with a cap;

Foams (supplied in aerosol containers)

Delfen Foam (*Ortho Pharmaceutical Ltd*)
Emko Foam (*Syntex Pharmaceuticals Ltd*)

Creams (supplied in metal tubes)

Antemin (*Napp Laboratories Ltd*)
Duracreme (*L R Industries Ltd*)
Orthocreme (*Ortho Pharmaceutical Ltd*)

Jellies (supplied in metal tubes)

Duragel (*L R Industries Ltd*)
Ortho-Gynol Gel (*Ortho Pharmaceutical Ltd*)
Preceptin Gel (*Ortho Pharmaceutical Ltd*)
Prentif Compound (*Lamberts (Dalston) Ltd*)
Staycept Jelly (*Syntex Pharmaceuticals Ltd*)

Pessaries (for use with condoms, diaphragms and caps)

Orthoforms (*Ortho Pharmaceutical Ltd*)
Staycept Pessaries (*Syntex Pharmaceuticals Ltd*)

Advantages and Disadvantages of the Diaphragm

Advantages.   A good method if you have intercourse with a regular sex partner who is cooperative and helpful about using it.

No side effects or dangers.

Very effective if well used.

The diaphragm is helpful if you want to have intercourse during your period and don't want a heavy menstrual flow to interfere. It will hold around 12 hours' menstrual discharge, depending on your flow.

Using the diaphragm can be a good kind of body education. If you are unfamiliar with what your vagina feels like, using a diaphragm will teach you! And in the long run, the more familiar you are with your body, the more you will enjoy sex.

It is a good method for those who have sex infrequently, as long as you always carry it with you, and are perfectly at ease using this method with a man you do not know well. If you have infrequent sex within a relationship a cap may be a good bet, but again it might seem difficult to stop the flow and spontaneity of the moment, if the moments are rare.

Disadvantages.   Closely precedes sex act. If either you or your partner feels that sex must be absolutely spontaneous, with no interruptions, putting in the diaphragm may seem like a hassle. You must remember to use it every time, be sure not to run out of cream, jelly or pessaries, be sure to have it with you when you need it.

The discharge of spermicide can be a nuisance, although it does not stain. Try different brands and, if necessary, use a tampon, pad, or Kleenex for leaking after intercourse.

Some women have mentioned that they experience less cervical stimulation during intercourse when they use a diaphragm. Some like this, other don't. Since most people are not aware of cervical stimulation anyway, this will not be a factor for everyone.

Condom (Sheath, 'Durex')

Condoms were popularized for protection against conception and VD in the eighteenth century. A condom is a sheath, usually made of thin, strong latex rubber, designed to fit over an erect penis to keep the semen from getting into the woman's vagina. A condom usually comes rolled up, unrolls to about $7\frac{1}{2}$ inches; the open end has a $1\frac{3}{8}$-inch-diameter rubber ring around it to help keep the condom on the penis, and the closed end is either plain or teat-ended with a little nipple that catches the semen and helps to keep the condom from bursting. 'Skin' condoms (made of lamb membrane) are more expensive but tend to cut down less on sensation. (Some rubber ones are better than others.) Lubricated rubber condoms minimize the risk of tearing, but tend to slip off the penis more easily and must be used extra carefully.

If you buy them from a shop or machine make sure that they have BSI stamped on them (tested to British standards), and don't buy 'seconds' sold cheaply in bulk. If you are asked what size you want, this refers to the number in the box, *not* the size of the condom which is standard. If you or your partner are allergic to rubber, the FPA sells an allergenic brand. (They do mail order, see p. 292.)

Here is a list of FPA recommended products. They also market their own brands.

Non-lubricated Condoms

Durex (*L R Industries Ltd*)
Durex Allergy (*L R Industries Ltd*)
Prentif (*Lamberts (Dalston) Ltd*)
Transyl (*L R Industries Ltd*)

Lubricated Condoms

Atlas (*L R Industries Ltd*)
Durex Black Shadow (*L R Industries Ltd*)
Durex Fetherlite (*L R Industries Ltd*)
Durex Gossamer (*L R Industries Ltd*)
Durex Nu Form (*L R Industries Ltd*)
Lamberts (*Lamberts (Dalston) Ltd*)
Conceptrol Shields (*Ortho Pharmaceutical Ltd*)

Effectiveness
Used every time as directed a good-quality condom is 97% effective; but in actual use the effectiveness is around 80 to 90%, depending on how carefully it is used. We suggest combining condoms with a spermicidal foam, cream, or jelly for close to 100% protection. Good with IUD or diaphragm for extra protection at mid-cycle.

How to Use.   The man or woman unrolls the condom onto the erect penis before intercourse − *not* just before ejaculation, since long before ejaculation the male may discharge a few drops with enough sperm for pregnancy to occur.

Cautions.   Leave space at the end of the plain-ended condom for the semen: a half-inch of air-free space between the end of the penis and the condom will keep the ejaculate, which comes out fast, from bursting the condom. Catching air in the end may also cause bursting.

If you do not use a lubricated condom, use a lubricant to prevent it tearing − spermicide, or KY Jelly, but *never* vaseline. Saliva is always available but may increase your chances of developing a monilia infection. Apply the lubricant after the condom is on the penis.

The man or woman must hold the rim when he withdraws his no-longer-erect penis after ejaculation; otherwise the condom might slip off, and sperm could get into the vagina.

In case of accident, use spermicide as quickly as possible. Do not douche. Also see 'The Morning-After Pill', or IUD, p. 283 and 284.

Responsibility

This is the only effective temporary means of birth control that the man can use. As with the methods that are primarily the responsibility of the woman, use of the condom is much more enjoyable if both partners join in putting it on as part of the sexual foreplay. For a couple who sleep together more than a few times, condoms are a good way for the man to share the burden of birth control. In a shorter-term relationship, in which you may not know whether you'll be having intercourse or not, condoms can be very convenient. But if you expect that the man will have a condom in his pocket, you may be disappointed. If you don't know the man well enough to trust that he'll have a condom with him, it makes sense for you to carry something to protect yourself. Ideally, you could carry condoms with you, although for many of us, at least today, it would be hard to pull out a sheath and suggest that the man use it.

Advantages and Disadvantages of the Condom

Advantages.   As well as being available free, though in limited numbers, at family planning clinics, it is available fairly cheaply in slot machines and chemists.

It is a method of birth control that gives some protection against VD and other infections. It also prevents partners from infecting and re-infecting each other.

If the man tends to ejaculate too quickly, a condom can decrease the stimulation of his penis enough to help him delay ejaculation and prolong intercourse.

A condom catches the semen, so if the woman wants to go somewhere right after intercourse, she won't feel drippy.

Disadvantages. The condom has to be used right at the time of intercourse. For some couples this ruins the spontaneity of sex, unless the woman puts it on the man and makes it part of sex play.

It often cuts down on the man's sensation, as his penis is not directly touching the vaginal walls. Many men resist using condoms for this reason, forgetting the effects that women's birth control methods can have on a woman's enjoyment of sex.

The condom can irritate the vagina. Use of the lubricants mentioned above can help eliminate this problem.

Foam — Aerosol Vaginal Spermicide

Description

Foam is a white aerated cream (rather like shaving cream in consistency) which contains an effective spermicide. It comes in a can with a plunger-type applicator.

How it works

When deposited outside the entrance to your cervix the foam forms a barrier to the sperm and kills them.

Effectiveness

It is not considered as effective as the diaphragm or condom though it is useful in combination with the condom, IUD, in the first weeks of a course of pills or in an emergency. Used alone it is more effective than all other kinds of spermicide (see Birth Control Methods That Don't Work Very Well, p. 281), and recent studies in the USA seem to indicate that when used with extreme care it is reasonably effective (see chart on p. 241). However if you do have to use it alone, use at least 2 full applicators as close to the time of intercourse as possible. If it is very important to avoid pregnancy it is not wise to rely on foam alone.

How to Use Foam

Insert no longer than fifteen minutes before intercourse. Shake the can very well (at least 20 times): it is the bubbles which block the sperm, and the spermicide settles at the bottom of the container so it needs to be mixed. Put the applicator on top of the can, then when it is full, lie down, use your free hand to spread the lips of your vagina and insert the applicator three to four inches before pushing the plunger. If you have never used tampons before you may want to practise inserting the plunger before you use the foam (see Anatomy, p. 20). Your aim is to deposit the foam on the entrance to the cervix, not beyond. Use 2 full applicators. Wash the applicator in warm water with soap before putting it away (you don't have to do it immediately).

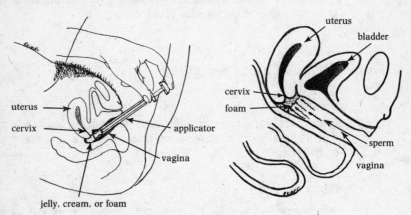

jelly, cream, or foam

How to insert sperm-killing foam, cream or jelly

Cautions

Put more foam in every time you have intercourse, no matter how soon.
Leave the foam for 6–8 hours before washing or douching.
Keep an extra can on hand as you can't tell when it is running out.
Use foam with a condom for maximum effectiveness.

Side Effects

Foam irritates some vaginas.

Advantages. Easily obtainable without prescription from a chemist, it's quick to use, less drippy than cream or jelly and helps prevent VD (see Chapter 7).

Disadvantages.   It is not very reliable alone.
It can cause a brief interruption of sex unless it is seen as part of it. Many people think it tastes terrible.

Brands.   The most widely used brands are Delfen and Emko.

Natural Birth Control

A number of groups are researching and testing methods of 'natural birth control'. Most of these are Catholic groups, interested in natural birth control because the Catholic Church opposes mechanical or chemical contraception.

Natural birth control methods are a possibility *for certain women* – for those of us who are able to pay careful attention to the phases of our menstrual cycle; for those of us who are willing not to be perfectly spontaneous in sex for part of our menstrual cycle; and those whose partners want to work with us in preventing pregnancy. They are methods that require above all a sense of personal responsibility. But a reasonably dependable birth control method without side effects is appealing.

Description

The methods of natural birth control depend on a woman's *recognition of bodily signs* which indicate to her whether she is in a fertile or unfertile phase of her menstrual cycle. During the fertile time (unsafe time) she can, with the cooperation of her partner, either abstain from all penis-vagina contact (according to the Catholic view) or use effective mechanical birth control.

When is the fertile or unsafe time? The method assumes that a woman releases only one egg each menstrual cycle; that the egg has 12 to 24 hours in which it can be fertilized; and that under favourable cervical-mucus conditions sperm can survive for 4 to 5 days inside the uterus and fallopian tubes. The actual fertile time is therefore approximately 6 days long, although for pregnancy prevention 2 'unsafe' days are added on at either end as an extra safeguard, extending the number of fertile days to 10.

It is difficult to determine ahead of time when ovulation will occur, since everyone – especially teenagers, pre-menopausal women, nursing mothers – has irregular cycles at one time or another. In natural birth control a woman uses one or both of two primary indicators of fertility: cyclic variations in her cervical mucus, and cyclic variations in her basal body temperature.

Awareness of Cervical Mucus Cycle (Ovulation Method).   You are perhaps already aware that your vaginal discharge changes consistency — tacky, stringy, etc. — at different points in your menstrual cycle. These reflect changes in your cervical mucus. As developed by two Australian doctors, Evelyn and John Billings, the ovulation method teaches a woman to become more familiar with the pattern of variations in her cervical mucus.

   a. Menstruation. Since menstrual discharge could mask mucus symptoms, these are not necessarily safe days.

   b. In some cycles, menstruation is followed by one or more days of no noticeable mucus discharge. (This does not happen in a short menstrual cycle, in which mucus has begun during the menstrual flow.) Symptom is a sensation of dryness in the vaginal area. The Billingses say that intercourse is *relatively* safe during these 'dry days'.

   c. At mid-cycle, sensation of dryness ends, followed by appearance of mucus. Mucus starts whitish or cloudy, and tacky. It usually increases and becomes clearer, until one or two *peak days* when the mucus is clear, slippery, stringy, resembling raw egg white. On the peak days there is often a definite sensation of vaginal lubrication or wetness. Within 24 hours after the last peak day ends, ovulation will occur. From the first sign of mucus until the *fourth* day after the peak symptom, the woman is fertile and must avoid unprotected intercourse.

   d. From the fourth day after peak until menstruation (about 10 days in a 28-day cycle) are unfertile, or safe, days. Mucus, if present, will be cloudy or white.

   From their experience with hundreds of women in Australia, the Billingses believe that every woman can be taught to recognize these symptoms if she checks her mucus regularly (inserting a finger into her vagina, observing underpants and toilet paper, or using a plastic speculum) and if she knows what to look for. They encourage woman-to-woman teaching of the method and daily recording of the mucus changes on a calendar. For details of how to practise this method, see the Billingses' book, listed in the Bibliography.

Awareness of Basal Body Temperature (Temperature Method).   There are slight temperature changes in a woman's body around the time of ovulation. Just before ovulation the temperature dips slightly. After ovulation, because of the ovary's secretion of progesterone, it rises several tenths of a degree and remains up until a day or so before menstruation. By taking your temperature on a special basal body temperature thermometer (calibrated in tenths of a degree) just as you wake up each morning, and recording it on a chart, you can tell when you have ovulated. You can get a thermometer and charts from your local family planning clinic.

From 3 days *after* the rise in temperature until your menstrual period starts (about 10 days) you are unfertile. This method by itself is of no use in determining safe days *before* ovulation in a given menstrual cycle.

The Sympto-thermic Method. This method combines the ovulation and temperature methods with the chart-keeping of the traditional calendar rhythm method (see below) and can thus be more effective. The sympto-thermic method is often taught on a couple-to-couple basis, as the man's role in the method is considered as important as the woman's.

The traditional *rhythm method* combined temperature-taking with keeping a chart of the menstrual cycle for 12 consecutive cycles. Not effective when used alone, the calendar method can be used with the sympto-thermic method as a means of establishing a clearer picture of a woman's menstrual patterns. Here's how to do it: count the first day of menstruation as day one of the cycle. At the end of 12 cycles, work out the number of days in the shortest and longest cycles. Subtract 18 from the number of days in the shortest cycle: this determines the first fertile or unsafe day in your average cycle. Subtract 11 from the longest cycle: this determines the last fertile day in your average cycle, the day on which your safe days begin. In a 28-day cycle, ovulation normally occurs about day 14, and absolutely unsafe days are from day 9 to day 17.

Effectiveness of Natural Birth Control

Effectiveness depends greatly on motivation of the couple and quality of the teaching they receive. The Canadian sample of a 2-year prospective study on the sympto-thermic method showed a rate of 1·1 conceptions per 100 woman-years in couples desiring to *prevent* pregnancy as compared to a rate of 14·9 conceptions per 100 woman-years for those intending to *space* their next conception.*

Fertility awareness can be used to *increase* the effectiveness of another birth control method, such as the IUD, diaphragm with cream or jelly, or the condom/foam combination.

Advantages and Disadvantages of Natural Birth Control

Advantages
1. No side effects.
2. Many of us enjoy being more aware of our body's cycles.

---

* Presented by Claude A. Lanctot, M.D. (Associate Professor of Community Medicine, Faculty of Medicine, University of Sherbrooke, Sherbrooke, Quebec, Canada) in a paper at the 25th Congress of the Federation of French-Speaking OBS-GYN Societies, Montreal, 26 September 1974.

3. In certain relationships the cooperation that is necessary in this method brings understanding and closeness between the partners.
4. Can lead, during unsafe days, to exploration of other ways of giving and receiving sexual pleasure – such as mutual masturbation and oral sex (be sure to avoid *all* penis to vagina contact).

Disadvantages
1. Major disadvantage: risk of pregnancy if you do not practise it diligently.
2. For some, it takes time to learn the method and feel confident with it.
3. Impractical for anyone not in a committed, cooperative relationship with her sex partner.
4. If abstention is practised, it can be sexually frustrating for those who want to have intercourse when they feel like it and who do not feel comfortable with alternate forms of sexual activity.

(The Bibliography lists resources for more information on natural birth control.)

Astrological Birth Control

Astrological birth control involves another level of fertility awareness which might be added to the tools of natural birth control. This method has not been widely tested or proved, but it is a subject of controversy and interest to many. It was first developed in Czechoslovakia by Eugen Jonas.

In addition to the fertility period whose signs are the temperature and mucus changes described above, the Jonas system assumes a second fertility period: the astrological, sometimes called 'cosmic', fertility period. This 24-hour period occurs each time the sun and moon are in the same angular relation to each other as they were when the woman was born. The angle recurs once each 29½-day lunar cycle. It may or may not coincide in any given month with the menstrual cycle's fertility period.

With a safety margin included, the astrological fertility period is 4 days long. To prevent pregnancy a woman must abstain or use dependable mechanical birth control during *both* fertility periods.

Effectiveness

This method is still essentially in the theoretical stage. It has not been proven that observation of this second fertility cycle is necessary *in addition to* the ovulation and sympto-thermic methods described above.

Advantages and Disadvantages

Same as for natural birth control methods discussed above. Fewer days are safe for unprotected intercourse.

For more details on astrological birth control and for information on how to calculate your own astrological fertility period, see the books listed in the Bibliography.

Birth Control Methods That Don't Work Very Well

SPERMICIDES FOR USE ALONE. JELLY, CREAM, PESSARIES, FILM

There are a number of different kinds of spermicide which are at present sold for use alone (without a cap or condom). It is likely that in the next year or so the Department of Health will insist that these products carry clear warnings on the package that they should not be used without additional protection (e.g. cap or condom). Until then, many more women will be taken in by the promises of effectiveness on the packaging.

None of these products is sufficiently reliable to be used alone as a long-term contraceptive method.* On their own they should only be used as a stop-gap before getting a more reliable form of contraception.

Foaming pessaries are more effective than the rest (they cannot be used with diaphragms). The other products are only effective if you manage to get the stuff on the cervix and it actually stays there during intercourse. The only effective way to keep the spermicide where it is meant to be is with a cap.

How to Use Them

All these products must be deposited at the entrance to the cervix. They must be used as soon as possible before intercourse (up to 20 minutes, and not less than 5 minutes before in the case of pessaries which must have time to melt). The spermicide must be reapplied before every act of intercourse and if intercourse is prolonged.

Jellies and creams (*less effective than foam*).   Use with an applicator as above; again, apply two applicators full.

Pessaries (*non-foaming pessaries are extremely ineffective alone*).   Insert by hand not less than 5 minutes before intercourse to allow them time to melt. Push them up as far as you can, ideally onto the entrance to the

---

* See *Women's Report*, Vol. 2, issue 4.

cervix. If they are the foaming kind, make sure that they *are* foaming and discard any that are not.

Film (C-Film). A 2-inch square piece of waxy film which must be applied by hand – ignore instructions which suggest that it can be applied on the penis, it's too risky. The film must be inserted shortly before intercourse on a dry finger as it will melt instantly on contact with moisture. The object is to get it on to the cervix *before* it melts. The enormity of this task for anyone with a damp hand or vagina is obvious. C-Film did so badly in the FPA tests that they do not supply or recommend it at all; however it does kill sperm if it actually comes in contact with it and could be used with the cap, it has the added advantage of not being drippy, but it isn't cheap and cannot be obtained free.

After Intercourse

All these products must be left untouched for 6 to 8 hours after intercourse. *Do not bath or douche during this time.*

Warnings

These products are not date-stamped but they do deteriorate over time, particularly in hot or damp places. It is difficult to say just what storage time is reasonable but it is probably better to get a new can/tube/box than to finish up the remains of some you found in the back of a drawer left over from the summer before last! Be wary about instructions. Remember that even advice is a form of advertising and the problems are usually put last in small type, if at all.

WITHDRAWAL (COITUS INTERRUPTUS, OR 'TAKING CARE', OR 'PULLING OUT')

Description

Withdrawal of the penis far away from the vagina just before ejaculation ('coming'), so that the semen is deposited outside the vagina and away from the lips of the vagina as well.

Effectiveness

Withdrawal is not highly effective because the drops of fluid that come out of the penis after it becomes erect can contain some sperm, enough to cause a pregnancy. Also, withdrawing at the last minute can be difficult, and the man cannot always get out in time to avoid contact, not only with the vagina, but also with the vaginal lips (sperm can swim all the way from the vaginal lips up into the fallopian tubes). Multiple acts of intercourse in a short period of time increase the likelihood of failure, since more sperm are mixed in with the lubricating fluid. Withdrawal has a pregnancy rate of 20 to 30%.

Responsibility

The man is responsible for withdrawal. The woman is dependent on his control over his ejaculation and must trust him greatly in order to be free of anxiety.

Disadvantages of Withdrawal

Withdrawal is the only last-minute method other than abstinence, but it has a number of drawbacks in addition to its high failure rate. The man must keep in control and therefore cannot relax and lose his self-consciousness. When used over a long period, it may lead to premature ejaculation by the male. Withdrawal can also be hard on the woman: the man might have to withdraw before she reaches orgasm, interrupting the flow of her sexual response; also, a part of her consciousness is wondering whether he's going to take it out on time, so that she, too, cannot entirely relax into her sexual feelings. Some couples who have used withdrawal for a long time have been able to work out these problems.

Avoiding Intercourse

Sex play such as mutual masturbation, in which you and your partner stimulate each other manually or orally until you both reach orgasm, can be pleasurable and satisfying. Take care that sperm do not get near your vagina, as they can move inside and go on to fertilize.

There is nothing wrong with abstinence. In fact sometimes it is just what we want. It is the most effective form of birth control, has been used for centuries, and is still very common.

After Unprotected Intercourse — 'The Morning-After Pill'

The morning-after pill is a series of very high dose synthetic oestrogens which must be started *within 3 days* of unprotected intercourse. The most common treatment is 205 mg. of diethylstilboestrol (DES) [or ethinyl-oestradiol] taken over a period of 5 days (two 25 mg. pills a day). The effectiveness in preventing pregnancy has not been determined, perhaps in part because of the relatively low rate of pregnancy involved: about 4 out of 100 women who have a *single* act of unprotected intercourse during the month get pregnant.

There is now evidence of a sharp increase in the rate of cancer, in particular breast cancer, among women who were treated with DES to prevent miscarriage in the 1950s. It has already been noted that many of the female children of those pregnancies have developed rare cancers, sometimes as early as 8 years old* (see p. 182). Because of this link with cancer and because there has been no study of the one-time use of DES on the user, DES is best avoided even in an emergency.

So far ethinyloestradiol has not been implicated in the same way as DES, but we feel it should also be treated with caution as a high dose, morning-after treatment.

The immediate side effects are the same as those of the oestrogen in birth control pills but magnified because of the high dosage (see 'Combination Pills' on p. 245). They are: severe nausea and vomiting, headache, menstrual irregularities and breast tenderness. In addition, women taking DES should be on the lookout for the symptoms of blood-clotting disorders: severe headaches, blurring or loss of vision, severe leg pains, chest pain, or shortness of breath. If any of these occur, the pills should be stopped immediately and a doctor notified. The doctor *should* take a full medical history before prescribing the morning-after pill, to check for contra-indications to the use of synthetic oestrogen (see 'Combination Pills, p. 255).

The morning-after pill is prescribed in many clinics across the country if there has been a single act of unprotected intercourse at the fertile time of the month. However, although abortion is a more difficult thing emotionally, and it is not always available, it may be safer in the long run. Those people who choose to restrict abortions, also choose to forget facts like this.

The 'Morning-After IUD'

In some places doctors are tending to use this method instead of the massive doses of oestrogen in the morning-after pill. It involves insertion of a small (second generation) IUD which should *prevent* implantation of

---

* Senate Health Subcommittee Hearings on DES (27 February 1975); testimonies available from Senate Health Subcommittee, Room 4228, New Senate Office Blg, Washington, D.C. See also Arthur Herbst, M.D., 'Clear Cell Adenocarcinoma of the Genital Tract in Young Females', *New England Journal of Medicine*, Vol. 287, No. 25, 21 December 1972.

a fertilized ovum and provide long-term contraception. The value of this method is that the IUD is functioning exactly as it would normally and in addition provides more than 'one-off' protection. However it is not suitable for all women, and is used mainly for those who have not had children. (See p. 260 for discussion of IUD.)

Non-Methods — Myths

Some women douche with water or other special solutions immediately after intercourse — trying to remove semen from the vagina before sperm enter the uterus.

Douching does not work. Sperm swim fast, and some will reach your uterus before you've reached the bathroom; and the douche, which is liquid squirted into your vagina under pressure, will push some sperm up into your uterus even as it is washing others away.

Douching is the least effective of all methods.

Some people think that in order to conceive, a woman must have an orgasm. This is false. One of the major differences between men and women in reproduction is that a man must have an erection to cause a pregnancy, whereas a woman can conceive without any sexual arousal. Avoiding orgasm won't prevent pregnancy!

Some people still think that the following are birth control methods: standing up during intercourse, only fucking during a period, holding your breath, not allowing the penis to go right in, jumping up and down afterwards, and the old one, it can't happen to me. They are not!

Sterilization

Sterilization is a virtually 100% effective, usually irreversible form of birth control, available for men and women. Most doctors are conservative about it and require the person to be a certain age, have a certain number of children, and get the spouse's signed consent, etc. To get an NHS sterilization you must be referred by your GP to a local hospital. Men have the additional choice of referral through a family planning clinic.

Waiting lists are very long, particularly for women because it is considered an inessential operation. It is quite wrong that people should be kept waiting for so long with the constant fear of an unexpected pregnancy to add tension to their lives. As a result, many people who can barely afford it get private treatment. Advice on low-cost private care is available through family planning clinics or the British Pregnancy Advisory Service (see p. 332); prices range from about £65 upwards for women and £28 upwards for men.

Choosing to get sterilized is a big decision. You have to deal with other people's possible adverse reactions as well as your own deeply internalized feelings.

The week before my sterilization I was very nervous, irritable and jumpy. I'd yell at my husband. I tried to pull out of myself all my fears about having an operation: I would die, there'd be a mistake, I'd be out of control, I'd get the wrong anaesthetic; and fears about this particular operation: my husband would think that I wasn't a real woman any more, he'd leave me for a fertile woman, I'd get all dried up and wrinkled. I felt angry at my husband for not wanting to deal with his feelings of loss of manhood by having a vasectomy (though that was a little irrational on my part, for his vasectomy couldn't give me my sexual freedom if I wanted to make love with another man).

Now, almost two years later, I am glad I made the choice I did. I feel much freer when I make love, and I am healthier in general. I am interested to discover that most of the sexual problems I had, had little to do with my use of birth control.

I did feel very alone during the whole experience, and even my husband's support did not reach to the deepest places in me, where I knew I had to live through this alone. That loneliness was emphasized because I couldn't make clear enough to my women friends that I felt I had passed an important milestone in my life and wanted to communicate the experience to all of them. I was no longer even sharing with them the hassles of birth control.

A life change like being sterilized must be carefully thought about, and it must be voluntary. There have been many instances of working-class women being forced to accept sterilization as a condition to having an abortion. In fact, abortion should never be accompanied by sterilization at the same time because of the increased risk of complications. In America, involuntary sterilization of black women is so common that it is referred to as the 'Mississippi Appendectomy'. Our right to *choose* sterilization must be protected.

There are a number of different sterilization procedures for women. Hysterectomy (see p. 183) is not often used for this purpose in this country (except in the private sector) and should never be, unless there are strong indications that the womb should be removed for other reasons.

One procedure is *tubal ligation*. There are two ways to perform a tubal ligation. In one, a fairly large abdominal incision (*laparotomy*) is made, a piece of each fallopian tube is cut out, and the two ends are tied off and folded back into the surrounding tissue. This method is now used most commonly immediately after childbirth. Tubal ligation can also be done entering the body through the vagina, although this method is somewhat less effective and has a slightly higher complication rate.

Another method is the *endoscopic technique*, in which a tube with mirrors and lights is inserted and the fallopian tubes are visually

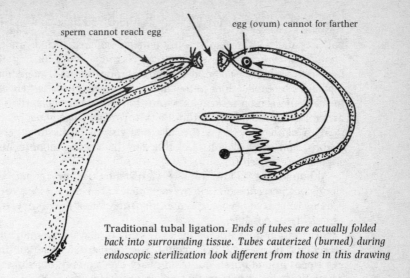

sperm cannot reach egg

egg (ovum) cannot for farther

Traditional tubal ligation. *Ends of tubes are actually folded back into surrounding tissue. Tubes cauterized (burned) during endoscopic sterilization look different from those in this drawing*

located and then cauterized (burned) with a small instrument. These methods have three names, depending on which route the instrument enters the body: *laparoscopy*, which enters through an abdominal incision; *culdoscopy*, which enters through the vagina; and *hysteroscopy*, in which the instrument enters the uterus through the vagina. The burning instrument is sometimes entered through a different incision or may be attached to the endoscope. The endoscopic techniques have a somewhat variable effectiveness rate. More recently, experiments have been done in which a clip or ring is put on the fallopian tube to hold it closed. Some methods cause the tube to close permanently and others are reversible.

A *laparoscopy* (the most common endoscopic technique) requires a hospital stay of only 1–2½ days. It is done on an outpatient basis in some clinics. Gas is pumped into the abdomen before insertion of the endoscope so that the surgeon can see what he is doing. This can cause bloating and pain afterwards. With *laparotomy* (tubal ligation) the hospital stay is about 4 days, and you will have some post-operative pain. A modified version of the laparotomy has recently been introduced, called the *Minilap*. It is a more minor operation than the laparotomy (it can be done on an outpatient basis), involving a smaller incision just above the pubic hair line. It also obviates the need for blowing gas into the abdomen which occasionally causes complications, the surgeon can see better, and cauterization with its attendant risks (see below) need not be used.

Side Effects and Complications. With both laparoscopy and laparotomy, excessive menstrual bleeding and pain are reported, particularly with laparoscopy using cauterization. In studies at the Royal Hampshire Hospital (see Neil *et al.*, 1975, and Noble, 1975) 7.4% of laparoscopy patients and 5.4% of laparotomy patients suffered complications severe enough to warrant subsequent hysterectomy, while during the same time only one woman in the control group had a hysterectomy. The increase in complications in the laparoscopy group was largely attributed to the cauterization technique, which has now been replaced in this unit and many other places by the use of reversible *Hulka-Clemens* clips.

With cauterization there is also the risk of burns to other internal organs, and some doctors feel that for this reason alone cauterization should not be used.

Although the failure rate of sterilization is low (about 1–2%), a significant percentage of such pregnancies are ectopic (see p. 506). This is dangerous, so it is wise to report any subsequent pregnancy to a doctor as quickly as possible.

Sterilization does not, as far as is known, affect a woman's hormone secretions, ovaries, or her vagina. Her menstrual cycle continues. An egg ripens in and bursts out of an ovary every month but stops part way down the tube, disintegrates, and is absorbed by the body. Her sexual response, which depends on her hormones, clitoris and vagina, is not lessened at all, and in fact may improve when she no longer fears pregnancy.

Sterilization for the man, called a *vasectomy*, is usually done in a clinic. The whole procedure requires about three visits – a preliminary visit (which often includes the wife), the operation, and a follow-up visit weeks later for a test of the sperm count, which may have to be repeated at intervals until no sperm are left in the seminal fluid – this can take as long as 6 months. The operation takes about half an hour. The doctor applies a local anaesthetic, makes one or two small incisions in the scrotum, locates the two vas deferens (tubes that carry sperm from testes to penis), removes a piece of each, and ties off the ends.

Vasectomy leaves the man's genital system basically unchanged. His sexual hormones remain operative, and there is no noticeable difference in his ejaculate, because sperm make up only a small part of the semen. Some men, even knowing these facts, are still anxious about what a vasectomy will do to their sexual performance. Talking with someone who has had a vasectomy can help allay such anxieties. For fuller discussion of the choice to have a vasectomy, see the books on vasectomy in the Bibliography at the end of this chapter.

In some men, antibodies to their own sperm can be found after vasectomy. This finding has led to the suggestion that vasectomy may lead to certain diseases of the immune system. Yet many fully fertile men also have such antibodies, and so far this suggestion is without support.

Future Methods of Birth Control

MALE CONTRACEPTIVE RESEARCH

A few years ago a birth control pill was developed for men, but in addition to its contraceptive effect of decreasing sperm production, it interfered with a man's ability to have an erection. Now researchers in Sweden and California are working on a sperm-incapacitation pill which would stop the sperm's ability to penetrate the egg. There is also a new small-scale study on a pill with synthetic androgen which causes reduced sperm counts. Other methods of male hormonal contraception have been suggested — such as a silastic implant injected under the skin which would release hormones slowly — but none of these methods has reached serious clinical trial.

One method which might be used by either a man or a woman but which is far from development is somehow causing the person to produce antibodies to sperm, rendering them dysfunctional. There is fear that antibodies would be difficult to control.

Compared with efforts directed at women, very little research is being done on contraceptive methods for men. Many women have been talking about lobbying for more research on male methods. We suspect that male scientists and doctors would be unwilling to offer men a contraceptive that exposed them to as many side effects and potential risks as the Pill or IUD does to women.

But what if there were a pill or injection for men? Not all of us are in situations in which we can absolutely trust our partners to keep us from getting pregnant. As part of the active-passive, pursuer-pursued, predator-prey, male-female stereotypes that we act out in sex, men say many persuasive things to women to get us into bed. If the man lied about taking birth control pills, the woman would still be the one to get pregnant. Even in a marriage a man might not have the incentive to remember his pill that the woman has: the threat of unwanted pregnancy and responsibility for child care. Getting men to share the burdens of birth control involves a lot more than finding methods for them to use. For now, many of us prefer to keep the control in our hands.

FEMALE CONTRACEPTIVE RESEARCH

With current means of birth control as unsatisfactory to us as they are today, it is clear that extensive research must be done to develop methods that are both safer and more effective. Drug companies do a lot of research, but we question whether they have our interests as a top priority. Because we are women and the people who fund and do research are often men, and because no preventive health care is valued very highly in this country, adequate research will not be done unless we join together in effective ways to insist on it. None of the methods listed below is free of side effects, although recent experiments on more convenient forms of barrier methods do sound hopeful.

Prevention of Ovulation, Implantation, or Sperm Entrance into Uterus by Use of Hormones.   These experimental methods are just variations on birth control pills in that they introduce synthetic hormones into the woman's body:

Subdermal (under the skin) implants of capsules containing progestogen that would leak into the blood a little every day, achieving the same effects as the progestogen-only pill.

Once-a-month-pill with oestrogen and progestogen in particular compounds that store in fatty tissue and are slowly released.

Morning-after progestogen pill, taken over 5 days, twice a day.

Progestogen-coated vaginal ring that would fit like the rim of a diaphragm. The ring releases enough progestogen every day to suppress ovulation. The ring is removed for 7 days once a month to allow cyclic bleeding to take place.

New IUD design.   An IUD filled with saline (salt water) is being developed. It is non-rigid, and the saline is injected after the device is placed, supposedly to 'custom-fit' the uterus.

Prostaglandins.   These substances cause uterine contractions and are now used to induce labour and to cause second-trimester abortion. Another use is to put them in a vaginal tampon or gel so that they can act locally to make the uterus contract, bringing on a period, or early abortion if the woman is pregnant. It is not always successful, and the side effects are still considerable, including nausea, cramping and diarrhoea.

Bibliography and Resources

Most of the books are available from the FPA (see address below).

GENERAL

Billings, Evelyn L. and John J., and Catarinich, Maurice, *Atlas of the Ovulation Method*, Advocate Press, Australia, 1974. Probably at Compendium.
Birth Control Handbook, Montreal Health Press, 1975. Available from Compendium or Rising Free (see p. 573).

Consumers' Association, 'Sex With Health', *Which?*, November, 1974. Guide to contraception, abortion and sex-related diseases.

Demarest, Robert, and Sciarra, John, *Conception, Birth and Contraception*, McGraw Hill, 1969.

Draper, Elizabeth, *Birth Control in the Modern World*, Penguin, 1972.

FPA, *Clinic Handbook*. Reference book intended for medical professionals.

FPA, *Current Literature in Family Planning*. A bi-monthly classified review of recent literature.

FPA, *Family Planning*. A quarterly journal.

Hatcher & Stewart, *Contraceptive Technology 1976—77*, Halstead Press (USA), 1977.

Neil *et al.*, (report on laparoscopic sterilization), *Lancet*, 11 October 1975.

Noble *et al.*, (ditto), *Lancet*, 25 October 1975.

Peel, J., and Potts, M., *Text Book of Contraceptive Practice*, Cambridge University Press, 1973. Very informative though rather population-conscious.

Rosenblum, Art, and Jackson, Leah, *The Natural Birth Control Book*, Aquarius, 1973.

Snowdon, Robert, *The IUD, a Practical Guide*, Croom Helm, 1977.

PILL

Beral, V., and Kay, C. R., 'Mortality among Oral Contraceptive Users', *Lancet*, II, 727, 1977.

Grant, E. C. G., 'Changing Oral Contraceptives', *British Medical Journal*, 27 December 1969.

Grant, E. C. G., 'Hormones and Headaches in Women', *Migraine News*, March 1974.

Grant, E. C. G., 'Venous Effects of Oral Contraceptives', *British Medical Journal*, 11 October 1969.

Kistner, Robert W., M.D., *The Pill*, Dell, New York, 1969. Dr Kistner is a great believer in the Pill, and tends somewhat to de-emphasize risks and side effects. So take what he says with a grain of salt, but read his book if you want to know in detail how the Pill works and what it does.

Prescribers' Journal, DHSS, Vol. 13/4 and Vol. 15/5. Gives lists of different Pills and their contents.

'Questions and Answers about the Pill', compiled by a women's group: send s.a.e. to 150 Moselle Avenue, London N22.

Rakusen, Jill, 'Information or Propaganda?', *Spare Rib*, 32. Critique of the following.

Royal College of General Practitioners, *Oral Contraceptives and Health*, Pitman Medical, 1974. Biased.

Seaman, Barbara, *The Doctors' Case Against the Pill*, Peter H. Wyden, New York, 1969. Ms Seaman is alarmed by the dangers of the Pill and cites numerous case histories to show that the Pill can 'cripple and kill'. A good antidote to the pro-Pill, 'almost-anyone-can-take-the-Pill' attitude in such books as Robert Kistner's *The Pill*. You should read both sides.

Stern, Elizabeth, *et al.*, (study concerning cervical cancer), *Science*, 24 June 1977.

Tietze, Christopher, *et al.*, 'Mortality Associated with the Control of Fertility', *Family Planning Perspectives*, 1976, Vol. 8, no. 1.

Vaughan, Paul, *The Pill on Trial*, Penguin, 1972. Examines the way the Pill was developed, lack of research, and what is still unknown about the Pill.

Vessey and Doll, *et al.*, 'A long-term Follow-up Study of Women Using Different Methods of Contraception' — an interim report, *Journal of Biosocial Science*, October 1976.

White, Margaret, *Safety and the Pill*, Responsible Society, 1974. Biased against the Pill.

INJECTIONS

Rakusen, Jill, 'Third World Women Not Told This Contraceptive is on Trial', *Spare Rib*, 42, p. 22.

Rakusen, Jill, 'DP: Still for Sale', *Spare Rib*, 47, p. 26.

ADDRESSES

Brook Advisory Clinic for Young People. A sympathetic service on everything to do with sex for young people. Main address: 233 Tottenham Court Road, London W1 (01 323 1522/01 580 2991). They have clinics in S E London and in Birmingham, Bristol, Cambridge, Coventry, Edinburgh, Liverpool. (The service is free.)

Family Planning Association, 27–35 Mortimer Street, London W1 (01 636 7866). Mail order service, research, sex education, etc.

Family Planning Association of Northern Ireland, Bryson House, 28 Bedford Street, Belfast 2 (Belfast 662618).

Irish Family Planning Association, 59 Synge Street, Dublin 8 (68 24 20).

Well Women Clinic, 108 Whitfield Street, London W1 (388 0662). This used to be the Marie Stopes Clinic; it is now run to provide a wider range of medical care for women at a small fee. (It is non-profit-making.)

Women and Education Newsletter, 4 Cliffdale Drive, Manchester 8 (for list of local W & E groups).

Women's Abortion and Contraception Campaign (see p. 297, 'Abortion').

For local clinics look under *Birth Control* or *Family Planning* in the phone book.

10 Abortion and Unwanted Pregnancies

Introduction

One of our most fundamental rights as women is the right to choose whether and when to have children. Only when we are in control of that choice are we free to take a full part in society. Birth control is the single best tool for implementing this choice, but as Chapter 9 makes painfully clear, birth control methods are still not effective enough for us to be able always to avoid unwanted pregnancy. And our society's attitudes towards sexuality, sex education and health care make it hard for many of us, especially the very young, to choose, obtain and use methods of birth control that will work for us. So right now, for many of us, a second indispensable tool for taking control of our fertility is *abortion*, the termination of a pregnancy by medical means.

The decision to have an abortion is rarely free of conflict. Even though a pre-twelve-week abortion performed by a trained person takes only 10 to 15 minutes and is medically very safe, most of us would much rather *prevent* a pregnancy than end one. We believe that women must be free to *choose* between abortion and childbirth. We want all abortions to be legal, free, voluntary and safe, done in a supportive atmosphere with sufficient information-sharing and counselling.

We know that a number of women and men believe sincerely that abortion is wrong. We cannot agree with them that an unborn foetus has more rights than the pregnant woman who is carrying it. Further, many of us who choose abortion believe that the quality of life we offer our children — which includes our emotional and situational readiness for a child or another child — is as important as the life itself.

We defend any woman's right *not* to end a pregnancy if she feels abortion is wrong for her. But some who are against abortion for themselves want to restrict others' freedom. We believe they are wrong to try to impose their beliefs on us. The 'Abortion Today' section of this chapter (p. 295) will describe some of the tactics of the anti-abortion movement and ways we can defend our newly established legal right to abortion.

HISTORY OF ABORTION LAWS AND PRACTICE

The anti-abortionists sometimes argue that abortion violates an age-old natural law. But for centuries abortion in the early stages of pregnancy was widely tolerated. In many societies in Europe and later in America it was used as one of the only dependable methods of fertility control. Even the Catholic Church took the conveniently loose view that the foetus became animated by the rational soul, and abortion therefore became a serious crime at forty days after conception for a boy and eighty days for a girl. (Methods of sex determination were not specified.) English and American common law, dating back to the thirteenth century, shows a fairly tolerant acceptance of abortion up until quickening, the moment sometime in the fifth month when the woman first feels the foetus move.

Most of the laws making abortion a crime were not passed until the nineteenth century. In 1869 Pope Pius IX declared that all abortion was murder. In the 1860s, in this country, new legislation outlawed all abortions except those 'necessary to save the life of the woman'.

These mid-nineteenth-century abortion laws did not succeed in curbing our strong natural sexuality. But history has shown that women will seek abortion whether it is legal or not, and the new laws obliged increasing numbers of women to get abortions illegally. The trauma of illegal abortion is a part of our collective history as women that deeply agonizes and angers us. There was a high rate of complication, infertility and even death among women who desperately tried to abort themselves, or who were forced underground for dangerous illegal operations. There were illegal profits to back-street abortionists, who charged high prices for non-medical procedures done in unsanitary conditions. There was blatant discrimination against poor women, who had to risk back-street abortions while their wealthier sisters could often find and pay a cooperative doctor. And those unable to end their unwanted pregnancies too often found their lives, and those of the children born, twisted by the hardships involved.[*]

Agitation against these laws started in earnest in 1936 with the formation of the Abortion Law Reform Association. It took ALRA 30 years to get a law through Parliament. Finally, David Steel's Abortion Act was passed in 1967. It does not apply to N. Ireland where women are still forced to use illegal methods or travel to England for private treatment. This law does not repeal previous legislation, it only outlines

---

[*] A Swedish study of children of women denied abortion 20 years earlier revealed them to be (as compared to a control group) in poorer health, with histories of more psychiatric care, and with a higher rate of alcohol use. Hans Forssman and Inga Thuwe, 'One Hundred and Twenty Children Born After Application for Therapeutic Abortion Refused', *Acta Psychiatra Scandinavica*, 42 (1966), pp. 71–88. See Garrett Hardin's *Mandatory Motherhood*, pp. 105–33, for sections of this study.

specific cases where to give or procure an abortion would no longer be a crime. They are:

1. When the continuance of the pregnancy would involve risk to the life of the pregnant woman, or injury to the mental or physical health of the pregnant woman or any existing children of her family, *greater than if the pregnancy were terminated.*
2. When there is a substantial risk that if the child were born, it would suffer from such physical or mental abnormalities as to be seriously handicapped.

Under these conditions termination is legal up until 28 weeks (this could be reduced to 24 or 20). In order to comply with the law, *two* medical practitioners have to certify 'in good faith' that the conditions above have been satisfied. They may take into account present and future environment in making their decision.

This law can be interpreted in many different ways. Some doctors still refuse to perform an abortion unless there is a real risk of death for the mother. Others will only do it if the patient accepts sterilization at the same time. At the other end of the scale there are concerned doctors who believe in the woman's right to decide. These doctors tend to interpret the law very liberally, on the basis that early abortion is always statistically safer than a pregnancy taken to term and will therefore always fall within the terms of the act.

ABORTION TODAY

These extremes in interpreting the Abortion Act have led to an inefficient, inadequate service throughout the National Health Service. At present only about half of all abortions are carried out through the Health Service. In a few areas, e.g. Aberdeen, Newcastle, and Camberwell in London, abortion is easily obtained free because hospitals in those areas have organized facilities to cope with the increased demand since the act came into force. In Birmingham, the West of Scotland, and Croydon in London the opposite is true and the majority of women seeking abortion are forced to use the private sector.

There is no doubt that there are still doctors in the private sector who are making fortunes out of abortion, because in spite of extended debate on the working of the abortion law, talk of 'tightening up the loop holes', 'curbing the abuses', no legislators have made any attempt to attack the real root of the problem – the appallingly inadequate NHS facilities. It is clear that if women were able to get abortions free, simply, without trauma, and early in their pregnancies, late terminations would be rare and they wouldn't use the private sector, so financial exploitation would disappear.

The partial legalization of abortion has provided a service for thousands of women over the past ten years. But women were not themselves given the right to choose – the decision was left to doctors and hedged about with rules and regulations. The growing liberalization of medical attitudes which followed has paradoxically endangered even this partial reform. Anti-abortion groups are attacking the law on the grounds that it is being abused by doctors who interpret it liberally and that it should therefore be restricted.

Our right to abortion will never be ensured until we have won the repeal of all legislation which can be used against women or the people who help us to get abortions.

THE ANTI-ABORTION MOVEMENT

The two major organizations are 'Life' and the Society for the Protection of Unborn Children (SPUC). These organizations are strongly supported by the Catholic Church, although they both claim to be non-denominational. The basis of their argument is that the foetus is a person from the moment of conception and that abortion is therefore murder. On this assumption they would like to deny the right to abortion to all women.

As soon as the abortion law was passed the anti-abortion forces began work. Initially they tried to get amending laws through Parliament. When that failed, they called for a committee to be established to look into the working of the law. When that committee came down firmly in favour of the law as it stands they declared that it was biased. They then started to organize a vast 'grass-roots' campaign with highly emotive literature, huge demonstrations and organized letter-writing to members of parliament. Their demonstrations include large contingents of nuns, Catholic schoolchildren and church-organized bus loads from all over the country.

On the crest of this wave of support James White, the MP for a largely Catholic marginal constituency in Glasgow, introduced his amendment Bill in February 1975. This time, instead of the previous outright rejections, the bill passed its second reading (each bill is read in parliament three times, with two debates and voted on at each stage), and was referred to a special 'select committee' for further examination.

THE PRO-ABORTION MOVEMENT

It was only at this point that a coherent national organization in support of the Abortion Law was started. The National Abortion Campaign consists mainly of young female activists working at local level throughout the country, and coordinated in London (see box). Other, smaller organizations already existed and they have either joined in with NAC

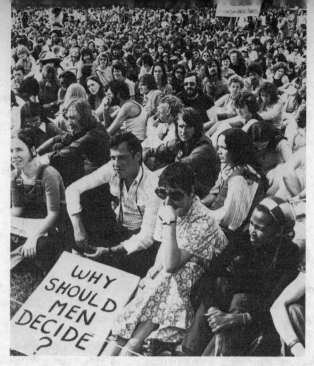

(for example the Women's Abortion and Contraception Campaign) or are working alongside in slightly different fields. The old Abortion Law Reform Association changed its policies and its name in 1975 to become 'A Woman's Right To Choose Campaign'. It is, together with NAC, pledged to fight for a change in the law to give women instead of doctors the right to choose. (For other organizations see box.)

The National Abortion Campaign is at 374 Grays Inn Road, London WC1 (01 278 0153). It organizes local and national events; participation is welcome both locally and nationally.

A Woman's Right to Choose is at 88a Islington High St, London N1 (tel. 01 359 5200/5209).

Committee in Defence of the 1967 Abortion Act, c/o The Birth Control Campaign, 27–35 Mortimer St, London W1A 4QW (01 580 9360). An umbrella organization for all organizations fighting restrictions to the Abortion Law (mainly establishment-oriented).

Women's Abortion and Contraception Campaign, c/o Merseyside Women's Centre, 49 Seel St, Liverpool 1. Publishes a newsletter which services local groups. Ongoing campaign within the women's movement.

Doctors for a Woman's Choice on Abortion, 8 Magdala Crescent, Edinburgh EH12 5BE.

At the time of writing a new amendment bill has been introduced in place of the 'White Bill' and several small and restrictive changes have been made in the law. It is more difficult to get late abortions and doctors are now more vulnerable to prosecution than before. Many other restrictions have been suggested and may go through, if not now then by later attempts at private members' bills.

If you do not know what the current state of legislation is, contact one of the organizations listed in the box. They will be glad to help, and glad of any help from you.

IMPROVING ABORTION SERVICES

In many areas National Abortion Campaign groups are campaigning for out-patient facilities in their local hospitals. Out-patient clinics, properly run, would allow the maximum number of women to get the help they need at an early stage in pregnancy. These clinics would also be cheaper to run than the current facilities, which often necessitate a two-night stay in hospital.

Some hospitals already run clinics of this kind. They tend to be set up by doctors who care about women and this care is reflected in the service provided. It is crucial that any abortion services should be organized not on the basis of saving money but of giving service. All patients should have the option of talking to a counsellor, and wherever possible that counsellor should be available to stay with a patient throughout the operation if local anaesthetic is used (see p. 314).

How to Organize

It isn't easy to tackle the monolith of the NHS, but within a NAC or women's group there are a number of things you can do.
1. Write leaflets and hand them out to staff and patients at the local hospital.
2. Try to contact members of hospital staff, particularly those who are active in unions, i.e. Confederation of Health Service Employees (COHSE), National Union of Public Employees (NUPE), Medical Practitioners' Union (MPU). If it is a teaching hospital, medical students will be in the National Union of Students. Trade-union members can work through their own unions to establish policy on out-patient clinics.
3. Organize meetings inside the hospitals with the help of staff, to discuss the issue of abortion with those people who are involved.
4. Contact your Local or Community Health Council (see p. 540), and Area Health Authority (see p. 538, 'Women & Health Care') and push them to support your campaign.

In some areas (e.g. Cardiff) out-patient facilities already exist but are not being used because of the attitudes of the local consultant gynae-cologist. If this is the case the waste of public money should be exposed and the hospital should be pressured into employing staff who are willing to carry out abortion.

There is no point in forcing medical staff to participate in abortion services against their will — the result would be disastrous for those women who were treated by them — rather they should be encouraged to allow others to take over these responsibilities.

For further information see 'Campaigning for Better Abortion Facilities in Your Area', from AWRTC (see Box, p. 297).

Statistics confirm that voluntary legal abortion is improving women's physical and psychological health. The Joint Program for the Study of Abortion* and New York City Department of Health statistics† show that during the first four years of New York's new law:

● the infant mortality rate dropped

● abortion-associated deaths dropped

● hospital admissions for incomplete (illegal) abortions dropped

● mortality and complication rates of legal abortion dropped steadily

● the mortality rate for early abortion was well below that for full-term pregnancy and delivery.

Studies on the psychological effects of legal abortion consistently show that women feel more happy than sad, more relieved than depressed, after having a voluntary legal abortion.‡

The mortality rate from abortion in the US was lower at the time of these studies than in Britain because it was then more freely available. A survey on abortion patients in Britain was started by the Royal College of General Practitioners in September 1976. So we should soon have more reliable follow-up statistics of our own.

---

* Joint Program for Study of Abortion reports can be found in *Studies in Family Planning*, a periodical of The Population Council, 245 Park Avenue, New York, NY 10017.

† J. Pacter, MD, Director, Bureau of Maternity Services, New York City Department of Health, cited in *Effects of New York State's Liberalized Abortion Law*, pamphlet prepared and issued by Abortion Rights Association, Inc. (National Abortion Rights Action League), 250 W. 57th St., New York, NY 10019.

‡ Joy D. Osofsky, PhD, and Howard H. Osofsky, MD, 'The Psychological Reaction of Patients to Legalized Abortion', *American Journal of Orthopsychiatry*, Vol. 42, No. 1 (January, 1972); Kenneth R. Niswander, MD, Judith Singer, PhD, and Michael Singer, PhD, 'Psychological Reaction of Therapeutic Abortion', *American Journal of Obstetrics and Gynecology*, Vol. 114, No. 1 (1 September, 1972).

If You Think You Are Pregnant

As soon as I missed my period I knew that I was pregnant. I felt differently than I ever had before. There was the going to the toilet, of course. I have always had a very weak bladder, but it was now weaker and more sensitive than ever. My energy seemed to be dwindling.

I sometimes miss my period anyway, or it comes really late. So when it didn't come this time I didn't even notice for a while. Then when I did notice, I thought 'That couldn't happen to me.' So I ignored it a while longer. [These words, from a sixteen-year-old, could also come from a woman nearing menopause.]

The most common sign of pregnancy is a missed menstrual period. Nausea and vomiting, breast tenderness, frequent urination, tiredness, may also be early signs. For some women, the vital sign of a missed period doesn't occur immediately. Some of us have as many as three 'periods' after conception and some women bleed regularly throughout pregnancy. 'Periods' during pregnancy are usually different from normal periods, often much lighter and lasting a shorter time, but any bleeding irregularity can be a sign of pregnancy.

If you have just come off the Pill, periods may take a while to return to a normal cycle, and for women who have irregular periods or very long cycles, the reassuring start of bleeding may not be a sufficiently dependable sign to rely on. If pregnancy is a possibility and/or you have any of the signs shown above, the best thing to do is to get a pregnancy test – see p. 349.

If your pregnancy test is 'positive' it means that you are almost certainly pregnant and should see a trained medical person to verify the existence and stage of pregnancy with a pelvic examination (see Pregnancy, p. 351, for how your uterus and cervix will change). If you have a negative test and your period doesn't come, you should have another test in a week – *and keep using birth control*, for if you aren't pregnant you can get pregnant! After two or three negative tests, you'd better have a pelvic examination, as some pregnancies never give positive results.

Deciding What to Do

If you are pregnant, it is first important to determine how far along you are in pregnancy. Medical people calculate the weeks of pregnancy from the first day of your last menstrual period and not from the day(s) you think you conceived. For example, if your period is 2 weeks overdue and your menstrual cycle is about 28 days long, you are considered 6 weeks pregnant even though it has probably been only 4 weeks since you conceived. Thus when we say a 'pre-12-week abortion', we mean an abortion done within 12 weeks from the first day of the woman's last menstrual period (12 weeks LMP), or possibly 10 weeks since she became pregnant.

If you are even considering terminating your pregnancy, remember that there is a time limit for your decision. *The earlier an abortion is done, the safer it is!* Complication rates for early procedures, while all low, do become higher with each week of pregnancy. The induction procedure (16 to 28 weeks) carries three to four times the risk of earlier abortions. Also, as the foetus becomes more developed, abortion becomes more emotionally upsetting both for you and for the medical and counselling staff (see 'Having an Abortion by the Induction Method', p. 320).

So, 8 to 10 weeks LMP should be your outside limit for a decision and immediate action.

If you are pregnant and it is still early in your pregnancy, you have some time – not a lot, but some – to make your choice about what to do. You can:

1. go ahead with the pregnancy and keep the baby;
2. go ahead with the pregnancy and give the baby to another family either temporarily (foster home) or permanently (adoption);
3. terminate the pregnancy by having a legal medical abortion.

For many women this is a painfully difficult choice to make.

FEELINGS ABOUT BEING PREGNANT

Most of us experience a powerful mixture of feelings when an unwanted pregnancy is confirmed. We may fear that our families will find out and punish us; fear that we won't be able to decide what to do; fear that we'll be all alone in trying to decide; fear the prospect of motherhood. We may also fear abortion even though we know it's legal and safe: Will it hurt? Will it cost more than I can pay? Will I be punished by having some dreadful complication and maybe even be made sterile? Will I feel guilty? Will I later wish I had the baby?

We feel a lot of anger too. We may feel angry with ourselves or our partners for not being careful enough about birth control. Often, however, we have been using birth control and it has failed:

When I found I was pregnant, I was frightened and angry that my body was out of my control. I was furious that my IUD had failed me, and I felt my sexual parts were alien and my enemy. I felt I was being punished for my femaleness.

We may be angry and sad that we don't have the money, relationship, or living situation that would allow us to go ahead and have a baby. We are angry that all the consequences of sexual intercourse fall on us. If we do not have the support and understanding of our lover or husband, we feel betrayed. We feel anger and confusion if we are pressured by our parents or friends or sexual partner to do something that we don't want to do, whether it be to have an abortion or to continue the pregnancy. And we feel angry if there are laws and procedures that restrict our right to choose freely what we will do.

We also almost always feel ambivalent. No matter what we choose to do, we will have some conflicting feelings. It helps to realize that our ambivalent feelings about the pregnancy are natural. If we decide we most want to go ahead with the pregnancy, we will still have moments of resentment and fear and uncertainty. On the other hand, if we choose abortion there are also opposing feelings within us. Even if our strongest and clearest feeling is 'I cannot have a child now', if it is a first pregnancy, it may feel exciting to know that our body 'works'; even when we absolutely don't want a child, there is a feeling of pride in our body processes that may confuse us if we don't know how natural it is, and make us question our decision for abortion. If we already have children, there's the feeling that we know what a child of ours would be like, and it feels cruel to say no to that possibility. We may feel selfish, especially in the face of our society's emphasis on motherhood or our children's or husband's desire for a larger family. We may feel guilty, especially if our religion disapproves of abortion or if we feel morally opposed to ending life. And there are wishes, too, that make us feel ambivalent. Maybe, married or unmarried, we or our partner or both are filled with romantic feelings that having a baby would 'make everything all right' in our relationship.

With all these mixed feelings and not much time, deciding what to do with an unplanned pregnancy can feel like an impossible task. It may help somewhat to know that after you make a decision, the ambivalence and mixed feelings tend to subside. Whatever we decide, it is important for us as women to make an *active* decision, one which is ours, rather than passively slipping into one choice or another. There are a few things we can do to help ourselves make decisions that we will be able to live with.

Find Someone to Talk With

Many of us have found that it really helps to talk out our feelings about being pregnant, about having to make a choice, about the decision itself, with someone who cares about us. We have often been surprised, once we speak, at the supportiveness of the very friend or relative we had been scared to tell. But sometimes there is no one close to us whom we feel we can trust to be *calm* about the pregnancy, and not to try to talk us into what they think we should do. Even then it is both possible and important to find someone to talk with. You can call a local women's centre, or go to a family planning clinic or Brook clinic. If you have a pregnancy test done at the FPA, Brook, or BPAS you should be given a chance to talk to someone as well. They can give you information about abortion if that is what you want but they should not try to push you into doing anything you are unsure about. Beware of rip-off referral agencies who demand money before giving you a chance to think about anything. If you are at school or college talk to a friendly teacher or welfare officer. If you have a good sympathetic doctor go to him/her straight away.

Many of us want to involve the man we got pregnant with. If we do not share with him the hassle and pain of the unplanned pregnancy, we allow him to avoid his responsibility or even prevent him from assuming it. We also deprive him of the opportunity to share his feelings and to give support. Of course some men will not face their involvement, and either leave us or withdraw emotionally. This is when we have to turn to a friend or counsellor for all of our support. It is perhaps hardest when our partner disagrees with what we feel we need to do. His feelings are important, but it's our body, and in this society the parenting will be primarily up to us – so the decision must finally be ours.

Check the Alternatives

ADOPTION

For some of us, continuing the pregnancy and then giving up the baby for adoption seems preferable to abortion, and sometimes the decision is left too long and then adoption may appear to be the only alternative. It is best to look into it as early as possible so that you are not submerged in red tape at the time when you have least energy.

1. Register with a doctor in your area who can organize antenatal care and a hospital bed (see 'Pregnancy' chapter). Antenatal care is essential both for your health and that of the baby.
2. Contact the National Council for One Parent Families, 255 Kentish Town Road, London NW1 (tel. 01 267 1361). If you are not certain whether to keep the baby or give it up for adoption they will help you decide and pass you on either to an adoption agency or to your Local Welcare unit. They can also find a place for you to stay for the remainder of your pregnancy if you cannot stay at home.
3. You can go directly to a voluntary agency or local Welcare unit (part of the Social Services Department) to arrange adoption. It is no longer legal to arrange it through a third party, and you may only arrange

adoption directly if the adoptive parents are relatives (you can of course adopt your child yourself.) The Association of British Adoption Agencies, 4 Southampton Row, London WC1 (tel. 01 242 8951) can provide a list of agencies in your area.

4. You must arrange before the birth to have the baby fostered if you do not want to care for him or her yourself for the first 6 weeks before adoption. At the end of the 6 weeks you will be asked to sign a consent form and, provided that the interviewing social worker feels that your decision is definite and you are not being pressured, you will not have to do anything else. The adoptive parents will be given the original birth certificate and when the child is 18 years old, he or she will have the right to see it with your name on it. It may be worrying to know that your child may try to find you in years to come, but to your child the information may seem very important.

Offering a baby for adoption can be a very difficult experience emotionally, with a sense of loss which can last for years. But for some of us it may be the least upsetting and most positive of the three alternatives.

Susan became pregnant in her second year at university. It was pre-1967 and she didn't think of trying to get an abortion. She took a term off and stayed with a friend. Now, eleven years later, she doesn't think about it much, just remembers a sense of pride at actually managing to produce a child.

Anna was only sixteen when she had her baby. She didn't really want it to be adopted but was too young to put up much of a fight. Now, she knows where he lives and goes around every day to watch him playing, just stands there and watches him.

BRINGING UP A BABY ALONE

For more and more women this is becoming a realistic option, socially, if not financially. Since 1967 the illegitimacy rate has risen and the number of babies for adoption is falling all the time. Increasingly the choice is between single parenthood and abortion. However, even if it is more 'socially' acceptable it isn't any easier. Money will be a constant source of anxiety, isolation will be hard to avoid and as the baby grows up single mothers often feel totally dislocated from society.

It is important to talk to other mothers about their experiences. If you are living in a communal situation your problems should be very much lessened but make sure that other members of your household really understand what it means to have a child around.

Read 'Parenting Alone' in Chapter 11, 'Considering Parenthood', and for a complete guide to the trials and tribulations of single motherhood and what to do about them read *A Single Woman's Guide to Pregnancy and Parenthood* by Patricia Ashdown-Sharp. Before you decide on an alternative it might be helpful to read the chapters on Pregnancy and Childbirth.

FIND OUT ABOUT ABORTION

Sometimes not knowing what happens in an abortion – what are the risks, procedures, prices – can keep us from making a clear decision for or against. The rest of the chapter should help you to find out, and it always helps to talk to someone who has had an abortion recently.

Non-Medical Techniques for Abortion

Abortion is a relatively safe procedure provided it is carried out by someone who is trained to do it. Historically there have been many so-called abortion methods which are dangerous and inefficient:

1. There is no known substance which will safely cause an abortion if swallowed. Most pills and potions that are sold for this purpose are poisonous.

2. Gin, hot baths, jumping from a height are only likely to dislodge a foetus if you were going to miscarry anyway.

3. Sticking sharp instruments into your uterus may well dislodge the foetus, but it is quite likely to kill you or damage the foetus as well. The same is true of introducing fluids into the uterus.

Medical Techniques for Abortion

In pregnancy, the woman's fertilized egg attaches itself to the lining of her uterus about one week after conception (see Chapters 2 and 9 for discussion) and continues to grow. When the embryo is one month old (about 6 weeks LMP) it is a pea-sized mass of tissue. A mass of tissue called the placenta is developing to nourish the embryo. By the end of the second month (10 weeks LMP) the growing embryo, by this time called a foetus, is about one inch long and is beginning to assume human shape. A 3-month foetus (14 weeks LMP) is about three inches long. A fluid-filled sac, the *amniotic sac*, surrounds and helps to protect it. By about the 20th week, the foetal heartbeat can be discerned with proper instruments, and the mother can start to feel the foetus move. Sometime between the 24th and 28th weeks the foetus reaches a point at which it might live for at least a short while under intensive hospital care if the mother had a miscarriage.

In an abortion, the contents of the uterus (foetus, placenta and built-up tissue on the lining of the uterus) are removed, leaving the uterus in an unpregnant state. Different methods are used, depending on how large the foetus has grown. These are outlined below. Since improvements are being made in abortion procedures, keep in mind that some of the information presented here may be out of date by the time you read it.

ENDOMETRIAL ASPIRATION

Also called *menstrual regulation*, and *pre-emptive abortion* (means: done before verification of pregnancy just in case you are pregnant). Improperly called 'menstrual extraction' (see p. 28).

This method is (as far as we know) rarely officially used in Britain. The reason is bound up with our restrictive abortion laws. Lawyers are at present uncertain about the legal implications of using this technique. Under certain circumstances it is legal in Scotland but the position is unclear for the rest of the UK.

This method is the safest and least disturbing form of abortion. It should be widely available at Family Planning clinics and doctor's surgeries, but until the abortion law is liberalized this is unlikely to happen.

When. Done any time after menstrual period is due until positive pregnancy is determined (about 4–6 weeks LMP up to 72 days LMP).

Method. A small flexible tube is inserted through the cervix into the uterus without any dilation (stretching) of the cervix. The outside end of the tube it attached to a source of suction – an electric or mechanical pump, or in very early pregnancy, a syringe – which gently sucks out the tissue from the wall of the uterus. (This is a similar technique to that used for menstrual extraction – see p. 28 – but in ME, a more gentle suction is used which is not at all disturbing.)

What comes out is the 'endometrium', or lining, that has built up over the four weeks of the menstrual cycle, plus the tiny bit of foetal tissue if the woman is pregnant. It takes only a few minutes. Cramping can be mildly painful but is brief. Anaesthesia (local) rarely necessary.

Risks and complications. Not much data available yet, but seems to have a very low rate of complications, risks, side effects. The flexibility of the tube means less risk of scarring or perforating the uterus. Since it is done without dilating the cervix there is probably less risk than there is in later abortions of adversely affecting the cervix's ability to perform properly in subsequent pregnancies.

Advantages. Can be done by a trained paraprofessional; expense and waiting of pregnancy testing eliminated; minimal complications; takes little time; relatively cheap; early emotional relief for the woman. Some women, however, would prefer to wait to know for sure whether they are pregnant, so as to deal with their feelings about it.

Disadvantages. In many cases it may be done unnecessarily: many women with a period a week overdue are not in fact pregnant. Secondly, perhaps because the foetal tissue at this stage is so tiny, it is hard for the abortionist to be totally certain that it was removed: it is occasionally missed and the woman remains pregnant. Because of this slight risk of continued pregnancy it is advisable to get a pregnancy test a week or so afterwards.

Contraindications. A pre-emptive abortion probably should not be done if you have Rh negative blood, because of the remote possibility of Rh sensitization (see p. 315 and Chapter 15).

DILATION AND EVACUATION (D&E)

Also called *vacuum suction,* or *vacuum curettage.*

When. From 7 to 12 weeks LMP.

Method. The cervical opening is dilated (stretched) until the tip (*vacurette*) of a non-flexible tube can be passed through into the uterus. Size of tip goes up to 12 mm., depending on duration of pregnancy and size of foetal tissue. The free end of the vacurette (in the vagina) is attached to a flexible tube leading to the vacuum aspirator, an electric or sometimes mechanical pump. The suction of the aspirator frees the foetal tissue from the uterine wall and pulls it through the tube and out of the body into a small container within the aspirator. The procedure takes about 10 minutes. For fuller description, see 'Having a Vacuum Suction Abortion', p. 315.

Risks and complications. Minor risk of perforation, infection, haemorrhage, incomplete abortion. Full discussion on p. 318.

Advantages. Quick and easy to perform, can be done by trained paraprofessionals (not legal at this point); low complication rate; little discomfort for most women; relatively cheap.

Disadvantages. Slightly more complications than for very early abortion.

Availability. This is the most widely used method although some doctors who do not perform abortions very often might still use D&C.

DILATION AND CURETTAGE (D&C)

When. From 8 to 12 and occasionally 15 weeks LMP.

Method. The cervix is dilated as with the suction method. As a rule, for the D&C slightly more dilation is necessary. After dilation the doctor uses a curette, a metal loop on the end of a long thin handle, to loosen the uterine lining, removing the foetal tissue with forceps.

Risks and complications. Perforation, infection, haemorrhage. Somewhat more bleeding than with D&E.

Advantages. No advantages over suction method for 7–12 weeks LMP. From 12–15 weeks it's the only method currently used.

Disadvantages. More dilation, more bleeding, more discomfort, necessity for general anaesthesia, all put D&C at a disadvantage to the D&E before 12 weeks.

Availability. The D&C is a standard gynaecological procedure used for such conditions as infertility, persistent menstrual irregularity and excessively heavy periods. The D&C used to be the best method for abortions up to 12 weeks. Now it has been virtually replaced by the quicker, easier and slightly safer D&E which can be done with local anaesthesia.

A doctor who does not do abortions frequently may want to do a D&C rather than a D&E because s/he feels more comfortable doing a familiar procedure. A few places do a 'late D&C' up to 15 weeks LMP. If you are 13 weeks pregnant, it would probably be much easier on you emotionally if you could terminate the pregnancy with a late D&C rather than wait until 16 weeks for an induction abortion. But medical opinion is very divided on the advisability of late D&C so many NHS hospitals do not even offer it. However, both the major charity services provide it. The method does require a great deal of skill and experience so there are not many doctors who are competent.

INDUCED LABOUR WITH INTRA-AMNIOTIC INFUSION:
SALINE ABORTION, PROSTAGLANDIN ABORTION. ALSO
CALLED LATE ABORTION

When. From 16 to 28 weeks LMP.

Method. As a pregnancy progresses beyond 12–15 weeks, the uterus expands and tilts and the walls become thinner, softer and more spongy, making perforation and excessive bleeding more likely with the vacuum suction and D&C procedures. The foetus becomes too large to be safely removed by suction or curettage. The preferred technique after 16 weeks is to cause the woman to go into labour so that the abortion occurs through the natural process of uterine contractions and cervical dilation as in full term labour and delivery. An abortion-causing solution is injected ('instilled') into the amniotic sac, or 'bag of waters', which surrounds the foetus. (Before 16 weeks LMP this sac is not large enough to be located accurately, so the induction procedure cannot be used safely until this time. In a newer method the solution (prostaglandin) is introduced into the uterus, outside the amniotic sac, with fewer side effects. Several hours later, contractions cause the cervix to dilate and the foetus and placenta to be expelled. (For details, see 'Having an Induction Abortion'.)

Until recently the most commonly used abortion-causing solution was hypertonic saline (salt) solution. Recently, prostaglandin has been approved for this method. Prostaglandins, contraction-causing hormone-like substances found in most body tissue, appear naturally in a woman's body at the time of full-term labour and delivery. Comparison of these two abortion-inducers appears in 'Having an Induction Abortion'.

Risks and complications. Higher than for earlier abortions. Very slight risk with saline of emergency shock or bleeding disorder (see p. 322). For both, possible haemorrhage (10 out of every 1,000 salines in New

York City*); retained placenta (40 per 1,000 salines in New York City, higher for prostaglandins); infection. With intra-amniotic prostaglandin, risk of damage to the cervix and uterine walls.

Contraindications. Saline: liver or kidney problems, cardiac failure, hypertension, sickle-cell anaemia. Prostaglandin: history of convulsions, epilepsy, asthma.

Advantages. Safer than the other late abortion method, hysterotomy (see below).

Disadvantages. Medically, higher risk and complication rate than for early abortion. Emotionally, can be a harrowing experience: for fuller discussion see 'Having an Induction Abortion'. Delivery of dead foetus is upsetting to woman and to staff. Delivery of live foetus, possible with prostaglandins and increasingly likely as pregnancy gets later, is even more upsetting. Costly, outside the NHS.

Availability. In a few private clinics usually only up to 20 weeks of pregnancy and by private gynaecologists in NHS hospitals. Most hospitals where abortions are performed can do inductions but many doctors are reluctant to do late abortions unless there are very strong medical reasons. However, in some areas, waiting lists are so long that many women are forced to go through this harrowing experience.

HYSTEROTOMY (*Not to be confused with hysterectomy*)

When. Can be done any time from 10 weeks or so. Usually done from 16 to 28 weeks. Rarely used at all.

Why. Done if induction method is contraindicated or has been tried unsuccessfully several times.

Method. Like a caesarean section (see p. 437). The foetus is removed through a small abdominal incision, usually below the pubic hairline.

Risks and Complications. Highest complication and mortality rate of all abortion methods. General anaesthesia, which is used, carries its own risk. Does not affect reproductive system.

Disadvantages. High risk; several days' hospital stay required; very expensive; can limit woman to caesarean births thereafter.

Availability. Privately at high cost or occasionally through the NHS.

Regulations Governing Clinics

All private clinics or nursing homes are licensed. At the time of writing, the only two private sector agencies which are allowed to do out-patient abortion are the two large charitable organizations BPAS and PAS.

* New York City Department of Health, July 1972–June 1973.

No clinic or nursing home may perform terminations after 20 weeks unless they have resuscitation equipment available for the aborted foetus. (This new regulation was aimed at stopping late abortion and many doctors will not now take on patients after 18 weeks to give themselves a margin of error. As a foetus is unlikely to live before 28 weeks this regulation is an unnecessary restriction on the Abortion Law.)

All clinics should be inspected regularly and may have their licences removed if they are not up to standard.

How to Find the Best Abortion Clinic for Your Needs

It is scandalous that in a country which prides itself on having a fully socialized National Health Service it should be necessary to discuss the facilities of the private sector. However, 50% of women seeking abortions are forced to go outside the NHS. If you are seeking an abortion the first avenue to explore is the local hospital, via your GP.

General Practitioners

If you have a good, well-informed, caring doctor you are much more likely to get an abortion. Some of us are afraid of discussing abortion with our doctor because we feel that s/he might tell our parents, look down on us, or because we feel too guilty and ashamed to talk to anyone who might have any contact with us in the future. For a number of reasons which we discuss further, it is worth approaching your doctor if it is at all feasible. Remember 75% of GPs are in favour of the 1967 Abortion Act so there is a reasonable chance that yours is one of them.*

Go to your GP as soon as you suspect you might be pregnant. S/he may laugh it off as 'hysterical' or appear noncommittal and tell you to come back for a test when you are two weeks late. S/he may also prescribe pills to bring on your period, particularly if s/he thinks you are unduly anxious. It is better to avoid them (see p. 350); they do not work if you are pregnant anyway.

Find out at this point how long a pregnancy test would take. Some GPs have testing equipment in their surgeries and can do a urine test while you wait. As this is a cheap and easy process they should all have the equipment, but many don't. There is no reason why you should have to wait more than 24 hours for results but some hospital services take up to two weeks. If it is going to take that long you would be better to save

* Gallup Poll – *Doctor* newspaper, 28 November 1974.

time and go elsewhere (see p. 350). If you are already convinced that you wouldn't want to go ahead with the pregnancy, say so. His/her reaction will be a good indication of how s/he will treat a request for termination. If you feel quite certain that s/he will not help you, you might as well start another channel of investigation straight away. If s/he seems noncommittal or sympathetic go back for a test when you are 2 weeks overdue or when pregnancy is confirmed elsewhere.

This is what your GP *should* do:

1. Act as a counsellor, helping you to make up your mind what to do, give you all the information you need and advise on the *medical* aspects of the different possibilities. S/he is not your moral adviser and should not act that way.

2. Sign a 'green form' (H.S.A.1) if s/he considers 'in good faith' that you fall within the terms of the Abortion Act (see p. 295). Many GPs will fob you off by saying that you are 'not eligible' for an NHS abortion and will make no effort to get you one. There is no difference in eligibility between the NHS and the private sector, merely a difference in practice. GPs should make it their business to know which hospitals in the area are sympathetic and which consultants are more likely to do terminations 'on social grounds'. They should be able to send patients directly to the right person on the right day. No woman should be sent to a consultant who is known to ill-treat women requesting abortion. However, with the best will in the world no GP is likely to be able to get you an NHS termination if you live in an area where abortions are not done on 'social grounds' at all and many of them are ill-informed about NHS procedure.

3. Your GP should make the appointment for you at the hospital, s/he should not ask you to do it. S/he is after all supposed to know the ropes.

4. The hospital will write to you with the date and time of your appointment. That shouldn't be more than a week later. However, waiting lists may be much longer, and some hospitals use their waiting lists as a convenient way of refusing an abortion *before* seeing you. If you will be more than 10 weeks pregnant by the time you go to a hospital you should consider 'going private'. You can always make an appointment at a pregnancy advisory service for the day after your NHS appointment in case you are refused an abortion. The earlier an abortion is done the better it will be for your health.

If your doctor refuses to help you, or you are unable to get an NHS appointment, or are turned down for an abortion you will have to try outside the health service.

Pregnancy Advisory Services

There are two major non-profitmaking organizations who can arrange an abortion for you where you will not be harassed or forced to do anything you don't want to do.

THE BRITISH PREGNANCY ADVISORY SERVICE
Main office: Guildhall Buildings, Navigation Street, Birmingham B2 4BT (tel. 021 643 1461).
Branches: Wistons, 138 Dyke Road, *Brighton,* Sussex BN1 5PA (tel. Brighton 509726).
Coundon Clinic, Barker Butts Lane, *Coventry* CV6 1DU (tel. Coventry 51663).
Fifth floor, Harley Buildings, 11 Old Hall Street, *Liverpool* L2 1BB (tel. 051 227 3721).
Second floor, 8 The Headrow, *Leeds* LS1 6PT (tel. Leeds 443861).

THE PREGNANCY ADVISORY SERVICE
40 Margaret Street, *London* W1 (tel. 01 409 0281).

THE ULSTER PREGNANCY ADVISORY ASSOCIATION
338a Lisburn Road, *Belfast* (tel. 667345).

These organizations employ counsellors to discuss feelings about pregnancy, help you to make a clear decision and to describe the process to you. (See 'Counselling', below.) BPA S and PAS also employ doctors on a sessional basis who will do the necessary examination and can sign your 'green form' if your GP has not done so. You can go to them direct if you would rather not contact your own doctor, though they do prefer you to have some contact with a GP in your area. You will then be referred to a second doctor (or gynaecologist) who will examine you again and add the second signature to your form. You will then be booked in at a clinic. It usually takes a week to ten days from first contacting the service to leaving the clinic.

Cost (at time of writing)
Consultation fee £12.50; Operation: PAS: £65 up to about 16 weeks pregnancy (occasionally a little longer), no facilities for induction. BPAS: £64 up to 14 weeks (occasionally later), induction, £118, hysterotomy, £150.

There are other smaller organizations which can help. Because of their size they can take longer with each patient. Occasionally they can arrange abortions on the NHS, although they might have to refer you to one of the above services.
RELEASE: 1 Elgin Avenue, London W9 (tel. 01 289 1123). A free service helping with a wide range of problems.

HELP: 79 Buckingham Palace Road, London SW1 (tel. 01 828 7495). Free service including free pregnancy tests.

Local Women's Centres: addresses from 'WIRES' (see p. 570 for address). Many local women's centres give referral advice and free pregnancy tests.

The prices quoted above are the most you should have to pay for an abortion (at the time of writing). Private gynaecologists outside the charities may well charge much higher fees and they are no better qualified. Try not to leave it too late — late abortions are much more difficult to get. Many doctors who are otherwise very liberal about abortion referral will refuse to sign the form after a certain time and it is increasingly difficult to get abortions anywhere after 20 weeks.

Counselling Before and If Necessary After the Abortion

All the good pregnancy advisory services offer counselling to every patient. Some NHS hospitals also employ counsellors (they are usually hospital social workers), but far too many of them offer no discussion other than an initial, and often brief, interview with a doctor. There should be pressure on all hospitals to provide unbiased counselling, particularly those which provide local anaesthetic out-patient abortions.

A counsellor should not force you to discuss things you would rather not mention or push you into taking any kind of action which is not determined by you. She should give any information you require and brief you about the abortion itself.

Questions to ask are:

1. Can contraception be prescribed by the operating doctors? If so will they provide supplies and can you have an IUD fitted at the time of the operation? (Some doctors prefer not to do this as they feel it may disguise early signs of infection.)

2. Ask about emergency back-up procedure. Serious complications are rare but you should be prepared in case. Both PAS and BPAS will give you an emergency number to ring if you are worried but they will encourage you to inform your own doctor so that you can be treated locally if necessary. If you are going to a hospital find out whether you can contact the ward direct in an emergency or whether you have to go through your GP.

3. If you are 10 weeks pregnant or less, the charitable clinics will give you the choice of in or out-patient procedure provided that you live relatively close to the clinic and have informed your GP. If your local hospital has an out-patient clinic you would automatically be admitted on an out-patient basis at this stage, provided there were no medical problems.

4. If there is a choice between local and general anaesthetic you will be able to choose which you prefer. (See below.)

In addition to formal counselling we have found that a lot of support and encouragement can come from the other women who are having abortions with us.

The two rooms where the abortions were done opened onto the porch where the six of us were waiting. One girl from our group, who had said she had never had even a pelvic examination in her life, was just coming out of the abortion room. She had just had her abortion, and she looked okay. That was comforting. A seventeen-year-old girl came in. She was very very scared. I held her hand and comforted her. I hadn't had my abortion yet and was scared too (though I'd had one operation, two children, and a D&C). Something amazing happened when I held her hand. Any fear I'd had disappeared as if it were drawn out of me from all sides. We were all such different women who for varying reasons were having the identical physical thing done to us.

Local anaesthetic can be used up to 12 weeks with D&E abortion. It does not put you to sleep. You can walk into the operating theatre and lie down on the couch. You will then have an injection in the cervix which numbs it, so that it can be stretched without causing pain. You do feel some pain, similar to period cramps, while the suction is in progress but it doesn't last long (5 minutes or so). One advantage is that the doctor is forced to be slower and more careful if you are awake and reacting to what he does. However, if you are very tense and frightened it may be difficult for the doctor to complete the operation properly. The success of local anaesthetic depends on a careful, gentle doctor and the presence of a counsellor or nurse to keep you company and reassure you during the operation. This emotional support is unfortunately not always provided.

General anaesthetic is widely used in this country, too often for the convenience of medical staff who do not want conscious patients so that they can work faster and are not therefore prepared to explain the relative merits of local or general anaesthesia.

The general anaesthetic will probably be light and last only about half an hour, so you wake up with little awareness of what has happened. The disadvantage is that you may feel nauseous and groggy afterwards; it can affect you for a few days. General anaesthetic also carries a slight risk of serious complications for those with blood or heart conditions.

Preparation for the Abortion

Take some sanitary towels with you to the clinic as you will probably bleed after the abortion. (You should not use tampons.) You will be asked not to eat for several hours beforehand if the operation is to take place on the day of admission (some NHS hospitals admit women a day early to do preliminary tests) – this is in case you should feel nauseous. It is particularly important if you are having a general anaesthetic, and most hospitals prefer you to be prepared for a general in case it should be necessary.

Medical Preliminaries

A detailed medical history and pelvic examination (see p. 139) should be taken at the time of referral to the clinic, then some tests (these may be done in the hospital).

The questions will cover: the number of full-term pregnancies you have had and previous abortions or miscarriages or caesarean births; a history of TB, heart disease, asthma, acute kidney disease, bleeding or clotting problems, epilepsy or a recent major operation.

The tests will be: a urine test to check again whether you are pregnant and for your general state of health; a blood test to check for anaemia (if you are anaemic the doctor will have to be very careful about blood loss. If this test is done in advance you may be prescribed a course of iron pills before the operation) and to check for sickle-cell anaemia; another blood test determines your Rh factor.

Rh Factor. Everybody's blood is either Rh positive or Rh negative. When an Rh negative woman carries an Rh positive foetus (which will usually be the case if the father is Rh positive), either birth or abortion can cause antibodies to build up in the woman's blood. These antibodies may react against a foetus in a future Rh positive pregnancy. If you have Rh negative blood and plan to have children in the future, unless the father of the foetus is Rh negative you should be given a shot of a blood derivative called Rhogam within 72 hours after the abortion. Rhogam will prevent the antibodies from forming in your blood.

Your blood pressure should be taken before, after and during the procedure. A change in blood pressure during the abortion can indicate internal bleeding.

Having a Vacuum Suction Abortion

The majority of abortions are carried out between 7 and 12 weeks of pregnancy. We want to describe that process step by step. We hope that our outline will give an idea both of what to expect and what to ask for by way of good medical care and emotional support.

In most NHS hospitals abortion, even at this stage, is an 'in-patient' procedure, often requiring a 2-night stay. In most of the private sector a

24-hour stay is required by law, although the two big non-profit organizations (BPAS and PAS) are allowed to run out-patient clinics.

For in-patient treatment you will automatically be offered a general anaesthetic unless there are medical problems, or you specifically request a local anaesthetic. Most NHS out-patient clinics and the PAS clinic give a choice of local or general anaesthetic; BPAS does not provide local anaesthetic.

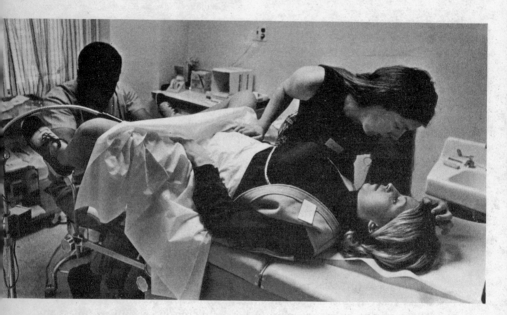

THE ABORTION

If you are having an anaesthetic you may be given 'pre-medication' which will make you feel drowsy, or you may be wheeled straight into the operating theatre before getting any medication. In either case, once on the operating couch you will be given an injection which sends you to sleep immediately. The operation is the same for local or general anaesthetic, except that those who have a general will be unaware of what has happened, so we will describe the rest as for a local anaesthetic abortion.

You will lie down on the couch with your feet in stirrups or your legs supported by knee pads. The doctor performs a bi-manual examination, inserting two fingers into the vaginal canal, holding the cervix with the fingers and placing the other hand on the abdomen above to feel the size and position of the uterus. At this point you may be given a tranquillizing injection to help you relax. The vaginal area is thoroughly cleaned with

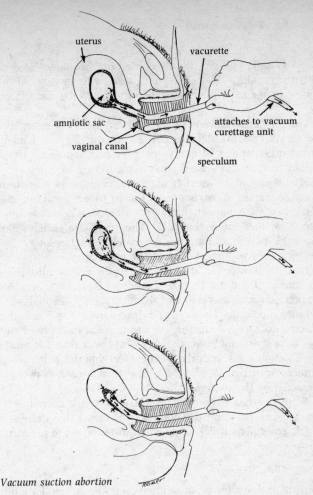

Vacuum suction abortion

antiseptic solution. It is unnecessary to shave off the pubic hair.

The doctor then inserts an instrument called a *speculum*, which keeps the walls of the vagina apart and allows a good view of the cervix (the mouth or opening of the uterus). This does not hurt, but it can feel like pressure.

The cervix is then grasped with a *tenaculum*, which feels like a slight pinch. The tenaculum will be held throughout the rest of the procedure to keep the cervix steady.

A local anaesthetic is injected into the cervix. This numbs the cervix. The injection is usually relatively painless, as the cervix is a muscle and has few nerve endings in it.

The cervix is then dilated (opened) slowly with sterile, generally stainless steel, instruments called dilators. They are from 6 to 12 inches long and vary in diameter from the size of a matchstick to the width of a piece of chalk, and are slightly curved on the ends. The cervix is dilated with the smallest dilator first and then with larger and larger dilators until it is opened wide enough for the tip of the vacurette to enter the uterus.

You may experience what feel like very heavy menstrual cramps while the cervix is being dilated. If the cervix has been dilated before (e.g. during miscarriage, delivery, or previous abortion), the cramping is usually less. Dilation usually takes less than 2 minutes.

The aspirator, or suction machine, consists of a vacuum-producing motor connected to two bottles. A hollow tube several feet long is attached to the bottles. A variety of different-sized sterile hollow tips (vacurettes) can fit on the end of this tube. These tips are either stainless steel or disposable plastic and are approximately 6 inches long. The diameter of this tip varies with the length of the pregnancy.

This tip is inserted through the open cervix into the uterus. The machine is turned on. The foetal material is removed by gentle pulling on the uterine walls, and is drawn through the tip, through the plastic tube, and into the bottle. The aspiration takes from 2 to 5 minutes.

Some doctors will then insert a thin metal instrument called a curette and move it around inside the uterus to check that it is completely empty (see 'Dilation and Curettage'). Others feel that this extra procedure causes unnecessary extra bleeding, and use tiny forceps to pull out any tissue not taken by the suction.

As the uterus is emptied of foetal material it contracts back to its original size. These muscle contractions may cause quite strong cramps, which generally subside 10 to 30 minutes after the procedure is over.

RECOVERY

You will lie down (or sit, depending on how you feel) for a half hour to an hour afterwards, in a recovery room where clinic staff can check your vital signs, such as blood pressure, temperature, etc. Then in many clinics you will be asked to sit in a lounge or waiting room for a while longer to make sure you are fully recovered, with no excessive bleeding, before you leave.

COMPLICATIONS

Physical complications do sometimes occur after a medically performed legal abortion. Here are the possible complications and their symptoms so that you will know what to look for. Seek medical help immediately if any of these signs should occur after you leave the clinic.

Perforation. Occasionally one of the instruments may poke through the uterine wall, making a small hole or perforation. These generally heal themselves with time. If a large perforation occurs the doctor usually knows right away by the amount of bleeding and pain during the procedure and recovery time.

Haemorrhage. A haemorrhage could be caused by laceration of the uterine wall or perforation of the uterus with the dilator, vacurette or curette. A heavy flow of blood accompanied by heavy clotting (not to be confused with the slight spotting that follows most normal abortions) could also indicate that not all the foetal material has been removed or that the uterus has not contracted to normal size.

Infection can occur if your resistance is low after the abortion so that an infection present before the abortion can spread. It can occur if the instruments used were not properly sterilized. It is most likely to occur if you douche, use tampons, or have sexual intercourse too soon after the abortion, thereby allowing germs to enter the uterus through the vaginal canal before the uterus has had a chance to heal completely. Nausea, vomiting, heavy cramping, abdominal tenderness, an unusual or bad smelling discharge, or a temperature of 100·5 degrees Fahrenheit or more are all signs of possible infection.

Incomplete abortion. This results when a doctor fails to remove all foetal material from the uterus. The abortion may then have to be completed in a hospital with a D&C (see p. 183). The danger signs to watch for are a foul-smelling vaginal discharge, cramping, nausea, vomiting, persistent heavy bleeding or haemorrhage as described above.

Unsuccessful Abortion. A very small number of abortions fail to remove the foetus from the uterus. Continued pregnancy symptoms – nausea, breast tenderness, etc. – would be the warning signals. There are also rare cases of ectopic pregnancy (see Chapter 15), in which the pregnancy is not in the uterus at all and continues to develop after the abortion, requiring an emergency operation at a later time.

To minimize the risk of both *incomplete* and *unsuccessful* abortion, abortion clinics should always examine the tissue removed from the uterus. If it isn't clear that all the foetal material has been removed, they should send the tissue to a pathology lab for analysis. Many clinics and doctors are not careful enough about this. One reader reported to us that her clinic, which had otherwise treated her very well, did not inform her that no foetal tissue had been removed. She had an emergency operation for ectopic pregnancy when severe abdominal pains took her to a hospital a few weeks later.

AFTERCARE

1. Because of the chance of infection, many doctors prescribe an antibiotic such as tetracycline (some prescribe Flagyl for this purpose; women should avoid this drug, see p. 200). Some advise you to take it

straight away, others to use it later if symptoms of infection develop. This is a rather dubious procedure as the doctor cannot know what type of infection may develop and the prescribed medication may not work for the infection you get. The result may be that the infection is masked by an insufficient dosage of antibiotic.

If *tetracyline* is prescribed don't eat for an hour before or after taking it and avoid dairy products – the calcium prevents full absorption of the drug. Sometimes *ergometrine* is given. It helps to contract the uterus to its normal size, cutting down the chances of haemorrhage and infection.

2. People's recoveries vary, but it is a good idea to rest for the remainder of that day and not to push yourself or do strenuous physical exercise for a day or two afterwards.

3. Keep an eye on yourself for danger signs: excessive bleeding or vomiting, fever, bad cramps or a foul smell from your vagina should be reported to the clinic or doctor.

4. To avoid infection: no douching, tampons, or sexual intercourse for 2 to 3 weeks after the abortion, so as to avoid getting any infectious germs into your vagina and up into your uterus before you are healed.

5. You will probably have a bloody discharge like a menstrual period for several days and you may have mild 'period' pains a few days after the abortion as the uterus contracts to its normal size. On about the third day a heavier blood flow is often reported; it should not persist. Your period will start about 4 to 6 weeks after the abortion.

6. See a doctor within a week if possible for a post-abortion check-up and for birth control if you did not get any at the time of your abortion. Many clinics and hospitals suggest a check-up 6 weeks later. This is better than nothing but later than it should be after the abortion.

Having an Abortion by the Induction Method

Having an induced-miscarriage abortion from 16 to 28 weeks of pregnancy is a more difficult experience both physically and emotionally than a pre-12-weeks abortion. Physically, as described below, you can go through several hours of discomfort as the uterus contracts to open the cervix and expel the foetus. The complication and mortality rates, though no higher than for full-term pregnancy and delivery, are higher than for earlier abortions.

Emotionally, too, it tends to be a hard experience, even when you are very sure you do not want to have a baby and are feeling great relief at the prospect of being free of pregnancy after long weeks of worry. The pain, the length of time it takes, the similarity of what you go through to what delivery of a baby would have been like; the fact that you have carried the pregnancy for many weeks and probably even felt the foetus move inside you; the fact that a very vocal part of society says what you are doing is 'bad' — all these factors can make late abortion much more upsetting than early abortion.

The very fact that you were not able to have an early abortion probably means that you have had a struggle already. Maybe you had hassles with, or fears about, doctors and hospitals which kept you from getting help until this late; perhaps you ran into opposition or lack of support from someone close to you; perhaps you had felt too confused to make up your mind whether to have an abortion or not; maybe for many weeks you had pretended to yourself that you were not pregnant because you felt you could not face it. So you come into the experience somewhat emotionally exhausted already.

As we mentioned earlier, it is very difficult to find a hospital which will accept you for a late abortion without strong medical grounds. NHS hospitals tend to be slightly more generous to women who are under age (below 16 years) or who have a history of severe psychiatric disorder. But many hospitals regularly perform inductions on women who, having been accepted for termination early in pregnancy, have been kept waiting so long that the simpler methods cannot be used.

The quality of care and degree of personal attention vary greatly. Some hospitals insensitively place abortion patients in with women who are having babies. In some hospitals you will be left alone a lot, not told clearly enough what is being done to you, not offered enough pain relief medication (if you want it). Talk to the doctor and find out exactly what the process will be before you go into the hospital.

If you have to go privately you will have the choice of Wistons clinic in Brighton (through BPAS) or a private gynaecologist operating in hospital. In both cases you can be sure of being only in the company of other abortion patients, or alone.

A COMPARISON OF SALINE AND PROSTAGLANDIN ABORTIONS

We suggest that you review the brief introduction to the induction abortion procedure on p. 308. In an induction abortion a miscarriage-causing solution is usually injected into the amniotic sac. The solutions used are a saline (salt) solution, which usually causes foetal death, uterine swelling and contractions, or the prostaglandin $f_2\alpha$, which causes contractions. What follows is a discussion of the advantages and drawbacks of each method. For medical reasons against each, see p. 309.

Saline solution, in longest use, currently has the advantage that doctors are more familiar with it. It also has fewer side effects, a lower rate of re-instillation (done if labour fails to begin in 48 hours), and a slightly lower rate of incomplete abortion and consequent D&C. Disadvantages of saline: labour takes longer to begin and goes on longer before delivery (see below); slight risk of serious emergency — *shock and possibly death* if careless instillation allows salt to enter blood vessel; *a bleeding disorder* probably caused by the release of material from the injured placenta (this can also occur in cases of foetal death not induced by abortion).

The prostaglandin $f_2\alpha$ has come into use more recently. Advantages: works more quickly; does not have the risk of serious emergency carried by saline. Disadvantages: more side effects like nausea, vomiting and diarrhoea (although experiments suggest that these side effects are reduced by extra-amniotic administration); higher rate of unsuccessful instillation; slightly higher rate of excessive bleeding and retained placenta (requiring immediate D&C). There is a likelihood that the foetus will be expelled with signs of life and not expire until shortly afterwards — this is why the prostaglandin method is not often used beyond 20 weeks LMP. There is also a risk of the cervix tearing in too-rapid dilation caused by the quick and sharp contractions.

PREPARATION

Similar to preparation for vacuum suction abortion (see p. 314). Plan to be at the hospital for at least 36 hours. Ask what to bring with you. If you are travelling far for the abortion, make sure before you go that you have the name and phone number of a doctor or clinic to call in case of complications.

MEDICAL PRELIMINARIES

Same tests and examinations necessary as for vacuum suction. In taking your medical history, the doctor should check for conditions which would contraindicate use of saline or prostaglandin methods (see p. 309).

THE PROCEDURE

What follows is a step-by-step version of the experience. It should be read along with the introductory description on p. 308.

There are five phases in an induced abortion: instillation, waiting, contractions, the expulsion of the foetus and placenta, and the recovery period.

Instillation. The process is started when the doctor cleans your abdomen, numbs a small area with a local anaesthetic, then inserts a needle or narrow plastic tube, usually through the abdominal wall a little below the navel (sometimes through the cervix), and injects the miscarriage-inducing liquid into the uterus. (Often in a saline abortion some amniotic fluid is removed before saline solution is introduced.) This does not hurt, although there may be a bloated feeling. In a saline abortion this instillation procedure must be done very slowly and carefully, because salt injected into a blood vessel by mistake could cause shock and death. You must let the doctor know immediately if you feel waves of heat, dizziness, backache, extreme dryness.

Waiting. It will take several hours for contractions to begin: with saline, at least 8 or 12 and sometimes over 24 hours; with prostaglandins, less. With saline you will feel very thirsty. With prostaglandins you may feel nausea and diarrhoea. If the waiting period is too long with saline (or occasionally with prostaglandin method), you may be given an injection of pitocin or oxytocin to bring on contractions or to speed them up.

Contractions. As contractions begin they will feel at first like mild cramps. At a certain point you may feel a gushing of liquid – this is the bursting of the amniotic sac. After this, and especially for the last few hours before the foetus is expelled, contractions will be stronger and more painful. With a prostaglandin abortion or when a drug like pitocin is used, the contractions are quicker and sharper.

As a rule the contractions are not as strong as those of full term labour and delivery, but they can cause you considerable pain. The breathing techniques mentioned in Chapter 12, 'Pregnancy', should help make the later contractions more tolerable. No general anaesthesia is given, but tranquillizers and pain medication should be offered.

Expulsion. At the end of about 8 to 15 hours of contractions (less for prostaglandins), the foetus, and then in a few minutes the placenta, will be expelled. With saline, the foetus is almost always dead. With prostaglandins, the foetus often will show some signs of life for a few minutes. It is likely that afterwards the doctor will recommend a D&C (see p. 183) to ensure that the abortion is complete.

RECOVERY

You will generally stay in the hospital for 24 hours or so after the procedure.

AFTERCARE

Most of the possible complications have been discussed earlier. In addition there is the possibility of haemorrhage at the time of expulsion, and infection can occur later. For discussion of these complications and description of aftercare see p. 315, 'Vacuum Suction Abortion'.

Birth Control After an Abortion

There is a temptation for us to say after an abortion, 'I'm never going to have sex again, so I don't need birth control.' Or, if we were in fact *on* some method of birth control when we got pregnant, we may feel angered and confused by the whole business of choosing a method again.

I lost my faith in birth control methods and finally began to take the Pill, which I hadn't wanted to take but which was by now the only thing I felt any sureness with.

Most of us feel that, yes, we will be wanting to have sexual intercourse again, and that despite the drawbacks of the current methods of birth control, we do not want to go through another abortion. So we have to make the choice.

If you are in doubt about a method, you can read Chapter 9, 'Birth Control'. For some of us, the counsellor and staff at the abortion clinic may be the first people who have given us a clear idea of what the methods are and how to use them.

Some clinics will insert a plastic IUD at the time of early abortion. (Some doctors do not insert any IUD at this time as IUD side effects of cramping and bleeding might mask the symptoms of an abortion-related infection.) If you plan to take birth control pills, it is a good idea to start taking them right after the abortion so that you will be fully protected by the time you have intercourse 2 to 3 weeks later. If you plan to use a diaphragm, wait until your post-abortion check-up to be fitted or re-fitted. You can use a combination of foam and condoms if your check-up is delayed.

Feelings After the Abortion

For most of us the end of an unplanned pregnancy is a tremendous relief. We feel glad to be able to go on with life in the way we need to, and proud that we have made and carried out an important decision. Sometimes the experience of working out the best solution with our lovers, friends or family is a very positive one. We discover strengths and weaknesses which we had not anticipated, both in ourselves and others. It can precipitate discussions which we might otherwise feel unable to start. It is a time for concentrating on our own needs, and for many of us, that may seem a unique experience. At the same time some of us experience a return of some of the same mixed feelings we had in deciding whether to have the abortion. Even the most positive feelings afterwards tend to be mixed with negative ones.

I left the clinic with my friend, feeling two ways about the whole experience: one, that I'd had as good and supportive an abortion experience as a woman could have; and two, I would never put myself in the position of having to go through it again.

Immediately after the abortion there can be a reaction which, like the depressed feelings a woman often has shortly after a full-term delivery, may be related to the lowering in our body of the hormone levels of pregnancy. We may have feelings of inconsolable sadness and periods of crying.

I was so relieved not to be pregnant any more that I didn't think I had any sad feelings at all. Then a few days later, on my way to a friend's house, I saw a young couple walking a new baby and I burst out crying right there on the street.

While society does not allow us a real right to choose by providing material support for those of us who want children, there are bound to be some of us who feel real grief after an abortion. Others of us feel sadness because the experience has brought home for the first time how hard life can be.

There are sometimes also hangover feelings of guilt about what we have done. They are not surprising in a society which has for so long told us that abortion is wrong. Those of us from religious backgrounds may feel particularly guilty. It may be a comfort to realize that thousands of other women whose lives have also been dominated by religion have had to make this same decision in the past. Women have always had to face the contradictions between man-made religious laws and the pragmatic decisions that they have to make for themselves and their families.

Even after the punishment of the operation itself I expected that in some way the odds would be evened in my life for the presumptuous thing I had done. When my favourite aunt got very sick I took it as a sign that I had done something wrong. I felt a nagging fear that I wouldn't ever be able to conceive again.

If we have been able to work through our mixed feelings before we have an abortion by talking to others we are unlikely to feel seriously depressed. In fact severe depression after an abortion is rare (studies in both America and at Kings College Hospital in London have conclusively proved this); even Sir John Peel, one of the gynaecologists who would like the abortion law to be restricted, grudgingly admits that:

On the whole post-abortion depression is not as common a sequel as some would make out.

If we do feel depressed, however, this is not a 'punishment' that we have to put up with! The clinic we went to, or any of the referral groups mentioned in this chapter, can refer us to someone to talk with – social worker, counsellor, clergyman. Or maybe what we most need is a chance to share our feelings with friends.

As we move back into our 'real life', the life that was so drastically interrupted by the pregnancy, we can carry a lot of feelings from the experience we've had. Many of us, for instance, feel intense frustration and anger at what we've had to go through. It can take a long time for these feelings to go away.

Even though my husband was very supportive, I felt angry – not so much because he put the sperm in me as because he in no way could understand what I had experienced.

We may feel isolated, even from the people we are close to.

My boyfriend's attitude afterwards was depressingly callous. His idea was: 'Well, it's over now, why bother thinking about it.' That's when I started to have to pull away from him emotionally.

Sometimes having an abortion marks the end of a relationship, leaving us with all those mixed high and low feelings of being on our own again, in addition to the feelings from the abortion experience. Sometimes the whole episode strengthens the relationship we are in.

Some of us have negative feelings about sex for a while after the abortion.

For a good month or two I felt like sex was repulsive. We'd start to make love and I'd feel, 'I hope I don't have to pay for this.' Also, we were using a diaphragm for the first time, and I didn't trust it yet. My husband was gentle and tried to help by pulling out to ejaculate outside my vagina. But I never relaxed, and I kept asking him, 'Are you going to come soon?'

Afterwards I felt very much that my boyfriend was potentially my destroyer, or even my enemy, because he had the capacity to impregnate me again. When I used two applicators full of foam while waiting for the Pill to become effective, I used to think that I was arming myself against the act itself. This was not the most pleasant feeling to have just before making love.

On the other hand, some of us had a chance to choose a reliable method of birth control for the first time when we had the abortion, and we feel more relaxed about sex than we ever did. It can be a drag to wait two or three weeks to have intercourse – yet this is a good chance to explore ways of pleasuring each other without intercourse (see Chapter 3).

Any of the negative or confused feelings we do have after an abortion tend to pass away with time – for some of us quickly, for some of us more slowly. For a few, feelings of depression and loss can come back again in cycles around the time of year when we had the abortion or when the baby would have been born. This often depends on how good or bad we are feeling about ourselves and our lives at the time.

What's important for us to realize is that positive, negative, ambivalent feelings are all natural after an abortion. We need to accept them all as part of us, give them space in our lives, and not put ourselves down for having them – only then can we make our peace with them. For many of us a crucial part of this process has been the chance to share our feelings with supportive friends.

Fortunately all my conflicts about the abortion were resolved about a year and a half later, when I found the courage to speak of it in a women's group I was in. Because of the calmness and caring the other women shared with me, as well as some of their own experiences with abortion, I came away from that meeting feeling that this thing that had haunted me for so long was finally resolved. I no longer felt bitter about the only choice I could possibly have made in order not to totally wreck my own life and that of others.

Two Personal Experiences*

1967 (AN ILLEGAL ABORTION)

Probably the most insidious untruth about abortion concerns the so-called post-abortion guilt feelings on the part of the woman. In fact, many women have been taught to expect and, in some perverse way, may welcome the 'cleansing effect' that anticipated post-abortion guilt offers them – as though they have to atone for their crime. For as long as this society fails to recognize and refuses to sanction the right of a woman to have an abortion whenever she chooses to do so, the fear of post-abortion self-recriminations represses her as surely and as effectively as any prohibitive law is capable of doing. The problem, then, is how to get women to face the reality of post-abortion *feelings* while shaking off the shackles of superimposed guilt feelings. Ironically, guilt, the psychologists tell us, grows out of anger – anger at ourselves for feeling inadequate and unwomanly, but also anger at a society that reveres us as mothers and child-raisers but despises our rights to make the decision not to have a child. Perhaps, then, sharing my personal experience might in some way show my sisters that guilt and its attendant emotions need not follow an abortion.

'I'm sorry,' the voice said to me over the phone, 'the test was positive.' From that moment on I was a changed woman. I was going to become a mother. But was I really, in the true sense of the word? Any woman who

* Although these experiences happened in America they could as easily have happened here.

has ever conceived understands the mixed emotions I was feeling. Understand, then, the thrill I felt in knowing that life was beginning. My body is constructed to bear children, and it was fulfilling that purpose. But then I was forced to ask myself: Is that *my* purpose as a rational as well as a biological human being, and am I not reacting to a societal stimulus as well as a biological one in feeling good about being pregnant?

For me the answers to these questions resulted in the decision to abort my pregnancy. For I realized that these vague biological stirrings inside of me could never justify giving birth to a child I did not want and was not prepared to raise. Neither was I willing to subject myself to the ordeal of pregnancy and waiting, only to relinquish the child at the end of it all. It's all crystal clear to me now in telling about it. At the time, my decision was not so well thought out, but rather grew out of the conviction that I could not in my circumstances continue with an unwanted pregnancy. For me the foetus represented an undesirable growth that had to be expelled, and with it also any guilt feelings about what I intended to do. Not once did I ever think of the foetus as a human being, but rather as an entity that contained some of the properties and carried the potential for human life in much the same way that a fertilized egg contains the properties and potential for life. If, then, the destruction of a fertilized egg is within our power, why not a foetus?

Finding an illegal abortionist was not easy. The few legal avenues that are open did not even occur to me (I had my abortion in 1967), although I'm sure I would not have qualified for a so-called therapeutic abortion. Like millions of desperate women before me, I went underground. My search led to a registered nurse (I was told) who did illegal abortions. My contact was a woman who had recently undergone an abortion by this nurse, and seemingly had suffered no physical ill effects from it. The negotiating was done entirely through my intermediary, and after settling on the price, the date was fixed. All the while, I was unable to pry out of my contact many details about the procedure, which really panicked me. There was no one else to ask, so I went into the thing 'cold turkey', and all of my dreaded fears about the physical pain were realized.

The woman came to my apartment on Friday, spread me out on the kitchen table, and inserted a catheter tube up my vagina into my uterus. This, I was told, would in time start the contractions in the uterus that would lead to the expulsion of the foetus. When I questioned the abortionist further, she put me off as though I were undeserving of anything more than what she had just done for me. I had to be content with her vague instructions about what to do when the bleeding began, while trying to stifle my anxiety about complications. The entire procedure took about 15 minutes, and her attitude was one of 'do the abortion and run'. It was apparent that with the exception of two friends who remained with me (who were as ignorant of the process as I was), I was strictly on my own.

And so began a 48-hour ordeal of pain and anguished waiting for it to be over. At that point I had little regard for myself as a worthwhile human being: I was someone to be scorned and avoided – I was a walking, bleeding catheter tube. On Sunday the contractions began, and by the middle of the afternoon, it was over. The force of the uterine contractions had dislodged the catheter tube and it slipped out easily, and along with it, the foetus. Looking at the foetus was an experience I will never forget. I had been approximately two months pregnant, and at that stage the foetus had acquired some of the characteristics of a human being as we know it. It was about an inch long, and I am unable to remember its colour. I do remember staring at it in a curious, somewhat detached way; it looked so strange, and indeed it was. Its appearance did not shock or repel me, partially because of the fact that by that time I had shut myself down emotionally and was feeling only relief that it was over.

It was only much later that I was able to internalize how I felt – and continue to feel – and then to verbalize, as I have tried to do here. Even now my total emotional reaction to it escapes me, except in one vitally important way. At no time, even in the shadow of societal taboos, did I believe that I was doing something wrong or committing some offence against nature – since, in fact, it is my nature and my right to determine my destiny as a woman. Since that time my confidence in the rightness of my decision has grown, and along with it, a sense of dignity and self-determination about myself as a woman.

1972

It has become very important for me to write about my abortion, yet it is difficult to know where the beginning is. I am at a place in time where my life, by my own efforts, is beginning to change. After having two children (ages six and seven and a half) reach a point of some adjustment in school, I began to feel I needed and wanted more from life. I decided to return to college, to a plan that had been interrupted by my marriage and children. As many women who have gone or will go back to college know, that is a process of awakening within ourselves that is incredibly exciting. After one marvellous year (with at least one to go) I found myself pregnant. I couldn't believe it. It seemed somewhat like a very bad dream that I would wake up from at any time. The idea of a third pregnancy was suffocating. I just couldn't go through another five or six years of intensive child-rearing.

I couldn't – didn't want to – talk to anyone about my pregnancy, and I felt really alone. The burden of every anxiety and fear of childbirth, unwanted babies, guilt about abortion, death, life – everything I could possibly lay on myself, I did. I tried to accept the fact that I was pregnant so that I could make plans for my life that included a baby, but all the

while I kept hoping for a miscarriage. The idea of abortion — the word —
came in and out of my head but was quickly dismissed. I felt strongly that
abortion was not a choice for me. I, as a person I thought I had begun to
know, did not have the freedom to make that choice. I had believed
abortion was every woman's right, but those were hollow, liberal
thoughts for me. It's so easy to be a liberal when you're comfortable.
For me abortion was a whole life-death question that I could not bear to
settle.

I simply couldn't make a choice. I neither wanted to bear another
child nor felt I could allow myself the alternative of an abortion, which I
believe so strongly was a destructive, violent act. It's important to say
that my husband was adamantly opposed to a third child, which didn't
help me at all in making a decision. We argued bitterly — I defending
anything he was against. We really turned our backs completely on each
other, and the support we had so often given to each other was gone. The
situation was hopelessly deadening. It's so hard to describe those feelings.
I really just wished I could die.

I went to bed at night hoping to wake up to a miscarriage, and I guess
it was at this point — when I was down very low — that I realized that I
was actually considering an abortion. I saw that my problem was not so
much that I was having difficulty adjusting to the idea of a third child, but
that somewhere in the back of my mind I understood I could make a
choice — and that realization was really mind-blowing.

I tried to be really honest with myself, and it seemed that to hope for a
miscarriage was about the same as wanting a guilt-free abortion. That's
really the way I looked at it. If nature would only expel this foetus,
everything would be all right.

I began to talk to other women about myself — my feelings, my life,
everything. They were really supportive. I started thinking about myself
and what I really wanted. I tried to sort out my feelings — what was real,
what were the influences of my Catholic upbringing, society, my husband,
myself. I couldn't stop thinking of a foetus as a child — as my six- or
seven-year-old playing in the yard. I kept getting very entangled in the
sanctity of life: this foetus was growing within me whether I was awake
or asleep, all the time. When does one have the right to destroy life,
potential or real? When is life real? I wanted to just stop and search a bit
for an identity that I thought I had found but that had become confused
by the realization that I could consider aborting a foetus. Foetus — to me
a child.

I was completely muddled — and I had nowhere to go. But friends kept
helping and supporting — women supporting no decision, just me as I was.
At about the point when I felt completely spent and done in, I began to
think about the responsibility of making a decision. It became clear to
me that my confusion was a result of my unconscious desire to avoid

making a real decision. I couldn't come around to the reality of the situation. I had to take on the responsibility of saying 'I want to have this child and I will accept that' or 'I do not want another child and I must accept the responsibility for aborting this foetus'. I had to say that I was real, that my life was real and mine and important. Those feelings were very hard to come to. I don't think I believe in them fully even now, but I did begin to think of myself in a direct way, and I began to feel more sure of myself. There was a certain strength in knowing that I could make a choice that was mine alone and be entirely responsible to myself. It became very clear to me that this was not the way to have a child, that in thinking about the sanctity of life I had to think about the outcome of my pregnancy, which would be a human being/child that was not wanted. On the strength that I had begun to feel as a woman I made the decision to have an abortion. There was no decision of right or wrong or morality — it simply seemed the most responsible choice to make. It is still upsetting to me — the logic of it all — but somewhere within me it is still very clear, and I'm still very sure of that decision.

After I made my decision to have the abortion I had a great deal of support from some beautiful women who helped me over a lot of bumps. That support became very crucial to me — I'll never forget it.

My feelings the day of the abortion were in some ways very much numbed and at the same time quite clear. I was very sure of my decision that day, much more than at any other time, but my emotions were somewhat shut down. Perhaps it was in self-defence; I had questioned my decision so many times that I just had to stop. I remember thinking the next day that what had happened to me had nothing to do with my concept of the word 'abortion' and all the images that word brings into one's head. What in reality had happened was that I had become a person I control — someone who is able to say, 'This is the way my life must go.' I was fully awake during my abortion, and although it was difficult to go through, it was especially important because I felt in control of the situation. I had made my decision and was able to carry it through without losing touch with what was happening to my body. (Also, being awake and aware alleviates some of those fantasies about what has happened to you, what a foetus may look like, and so on.) I also had a woman friend with me throughout the abortion, which was a really beautiful thing. Mentioning her in one sentence can give no indication of the feelings we shared, but because of her and because of two very loving friends who accompanied me to New York, I remember that day as one of strength.

In retrospect, my feelings are very contrary and complex — some high, some low. I do not feel guilt — almost rather guilty over my astonishing (to me) lack of guilt. I have felt at many times very strong and sure in my identity as a woman — a very real person.

Bibliography

Abortion: the Evidence, A report from the Tribunal on Abortion Rights 1977 and *Abortion, Where We Stand*, 1977. (Short articles on aspects of the abortion campaign), both from the National Abortion Campaign (see below).

Ashdown-Sharp, Patricia, *The Single Woman's Guide to Pregnancy and Parenthood*, Penguin, 1975.

The Benefits of Birth Control — Aberdeen's experience 1946—1970, Birth control Campaign, 1973.

Campaigning For Better Abortion Facilities in Your Area and reading list available from A Woman's Right to Choose Campaign (see below).

Evidence to The Select Committee on The Abortion Amendment Bill, HMSO 1976.

Greenwood, Victoria, and Young, Jock, *Abortion in Demand*, Pluto Press, 1976. Historical view of abortion reform and the inherent problems of reformism.

Hardin, Garrett, *Mandatory Motherhood*, Beacon Press, 1974. Obtainable from Compendium (see p. 573).

The Lane Report: Report of the Committee on the Abortion Act, Vols. I—III, from HMSO, High Holborn, London WC1. Summary of this report available from A Woman's Right to Choose Campaign (see below).

Montreal Health Press, *Birth Control Handbook*, from Rising Free (see p. 573).

Rowbotham, Sheila, *A New World for Women: Stella Browne — Socialist Feminist*, Pluto, 1977. An important book about a feminist campaigner for birth control and abortion in the 20s and 30s.

Simms, Madeline, *Abortion Law Reformed*, Peter Owen, 1971.

Women's Abortion and Contraception Campaign: Evidence to the Lane Committee, from Rising Free (see p. 573).

CAMPAIGNING ORGANIZATIONS

The National Abortion Campaign, 374 Grays Inn Road, London WC1 (01 278 0153).

A Woman's Right to Choose Campaign, 88a Islington High Street, London N1 (01 359 5209).

The Women's Abortion and Contraception Campaign, c/o Merseyside Women's Centre, 49 Seel Street, Liverpool 1 (051 709 4141).

HELP AND ADVICE

The British Pregnancy Advisory Service (a non-profit-making referral service):

Birmingham: Guildhall Buildings, Navigation Street, Birmingham B2 4BT (021 643 1461) — head office.

Bournemouth: Pelhams Clinic, Millhams Road, Kinson, Bournemouth (020 1677720).

Brighton: 138 Dyke Road, Brighton BN1 5PA (0273 509 726).

Cardiff: 4 High Street Arcade Chambers, Cardiff (0222 372389).

Chester: 26 Queen Street, Chester (0244 27113).

Coventry: Coundon Clinic, Barker Butts Lane, Coventry CV6 1DU (0203 51663).

Glasgow: 245 North Street, Glasgow G3 (041 204 1832).

Leeds: 2nd Floor, 8 The Headrow, Leeds LS1 6PT (0532 443861).

Liverpool: 5th Floor, Harley Buildings, 11 Old Hall Street, Liverpool L2 1BB (051 227 3721).

London: 2nd Floor, 58 Petty France, Victoria, London SW1 (01 222 0985).

Manchester: Suite F, Ground Floor, 57 Hilton Street, Manchester M12 EJ (061 236 7777).

Sheffield: 160 Charles Street, Sheffield SW2 9E (0742 738 326).

BPAS clinics are in Brighton, Leamington Spa and Liverpool.

The Family Planning Association, 27 Mortimer Street, London W1 (01 636 7866).

Pregnancy Advisory Service (a non profit-making referral service), 40 Margaret Street, London W1 (01 409 0281). Uses a London clinic.

Release, 1 Elgin Avenue, London W9 (01 289 1123) – a free advice service which can sometimes refer through the NHS.

Brook Advisory Centres, head office: 233 Tottenham Court Road, London W1P 9 AE (01 323 1522/01 580 2991), for address of local clinic.

Local Women's Centres: addresses available through WIRES (see p. 570). Some women's centres do pregnancy testing, most will give advice on where to get help.

11 Considering Parenthood

Do we want to become mothers? This was not a question asked by our grandmothers. For them motherhood was the natural outcome of sex and the duty of all women. Even with the introduction of efficient contraceptive and abortion methods the choice until recently has not been whether to have children but when to have them. As women have begun to establish interests outside their homes, more of us are deciding to pursue goals other than marriage and a family. With changing attitudes encouraged by the women's movement we are beginning to realize the full potential of contraception. We no longer need to have children unless we want to; the choice of motherhood can be a positive one.

But the choice is still threatened. Fertility control is not in our hands. In some countries women are still prevented by reactionary laws from using medical technology to control this aspect of their lives. In other countries they are forced to use contraceptive methods for population control rather than for their own needs, and increasingly women are inhibited from making a free choice because of economic circumstances or fear of the taboos against illegitimacy.

Unlike most decisions, the decision to have children is irrevocable and carries deep implications for the rest of our lives. The decision not to have children also becomes irrevocable once we have gone through the span of years in which pregnancy is possible. It is difficult to know what it will be like to be a mother, what our children will be like or how we will respond to them.

We may not think about motherhood at all as young women, but for many of us there comes a point when the idea of having children takes root and grows. We do not all feel this way, but for those of us who do a decision has to be made which will affect all the people who are close to us. In the end it will be largely an emotional choice but it need not be uninformed. The aim of this chapter is to help women who are making that choice.

What Happens When We Become Parents?

'It's a boy' (somehow I expected my first baby to be a girl). All of a sudden I heard him cry. The cry was not a cry of pain but the cry of life. The baby was alive and well and they brought him to me. I was amazed that this tiny human being, fully equipped for life and very beautiful, could come out of me. I was now a mother and how exciting that was.

In a sense, having a child becomes a time both to say goodbye to our childhood and to see it from a new perspective.

My daughter loves school. When I see her doing well in reading and maths, areas in which I did well, I feel proud of my influences on her. When she is poor in athletics, as I was, I relive my own sense of inadequacy and also feel frustrated that I can't help her. Recently my daughter learned how to swim. Watching her struggle to learn something difficult for her inspired me to learn how to swim myself. So at thirty-four I took lessons and learnt myself.

As parents, we are responsible for our children in a way we had previously been responsible only for ourselves. This intensely intimate relationship is quite unlike any we've experienced before. Some people find this a burden, and being a parent does have its burdens. At the same time, parenting gives us the opportunity to grow – to learn, for instance, to love and accept another person unreservedly, and to observe first hand and help a tiny infant to grow into an adult. It is crucial to see parenting as a process and not as an end to our own growth.

CARE FOR BABIES TAKES TIME AND ENERGY

Loving care for a baby takes a lot of time and energy. The responsibility of parenthood can be overwhelming during the first year.

The first week home with my baby was both fascinating and overwhelming. I was unfamiliar with infant behaviour. I did not know how much she would want to eat, and when, what her crying meant – fatigue, discomfort, pain, exercise. I was totally obsessed by this stranger and thought about her all the time: I felt this intense physical and emotional bonding with her. It was as if I was breathing with every breath and crying with every cry.

The helpless, relentlessly needy, dynamically growing infant requires 24-hour active care and passive presence of adults. Although it is possible for us to establish a rather predictable schedule for our child, fairly soon unexpected needs are always arising.

I hear Charlie cry for what seems like the fiftieth time today. It's that dry, piercing, persistent cry of a newborn. Although I often can work out what he is saying and enjoy comforting him, this time I cannot. I find myself feeling numb and a bit resentful.

We, too, need to be cared for when we are new parents, because of all the memories of being cared for in our own childhoods and because so much of our physical energy goes into nurturing the new baby. We also need mothering because we often feel shaky as we face the responsibility of caring for a helpless infant. It's not surprising that, along with the exhilaration we feel with our new status as parents, we feel overwhelmed by an incredible sense of dependency on our partners, parents, friends and relatives.

Right after I had my baby I missed my parents intensely in ways I had not felt since I was a child. Embarrassing! Friends who were parents reassured me that they had felt the same. I wanted to crawl back to my parents' home and be taken care of.

One afternoon, sitting in John's room nursing him, I had a rush of feeling unbearably lonely. Intensely, I felt, 'I need to be mothered.' My husband, who needed reassurance himself, couldn't mother me. My own mother could not mother me. My need was profound and, except in snatches, unmeetable by any one human being.

As long as our children stay relatively healthy, parenting will never again be as intensely demanding as it is during the first few years. And some of us will have more than one small child to care for. With time, naturally, the relationship(s) between us and our children becomes more reciprocal, and what our growing children bring into our lives as lively people in their own right cannot be measured. But although older children need less physical care, we are going to be called on throughout our lives and theirs to give them emotional support, guidance, limits and affirmation.

OUR RELATIONSHIP WITH OUR PARTNER CHANGES

Having a baby often complicates and changes our relationship with our partners. It's difficult to anticipate what is involved when we add a new member to our family. In addition to feeling excited about becoming a family and proud of our baby, both partners — but especially the man — may feel jealousy at being divided or excluded, and may doubt their parenting abilities. As women, especially, we feel that we are expected to know what to do as mothers, and that we are not allowed to make any mistakes. But ease and competency in mothering is learned only over time; it is not something we are born with. We all need reassurance from our partners as we try to establish ourselves in this new role. But our partners are often anxious about their fathering abilities and need re-assurance equally as much. Our culture makes it hard for men to become fathers. They receive scant support from a society in which they are most often asked to prove themselves by performance. Fearing that they will be judged inadequate, they often cannot allow themselves to ask for help from friends or relatives.

Both of us may be so preoccupied with caring for the baby and so needy ourselves that we cannot give each other the support we need. It is important to recognize this and try to be as communicative as possible — even to set aside special time to talk about it. If each partner has not had a sense of identity and confidence independent of the other, as well as good communication and the ability to offer support and acceptance to the other, the added stress of child care and financial res-ponsibilities can magnify existing problems. A child can become a football between two people who are not supportive of one another. On the other hand, many couples have found that becoming parents is a turning point; that the act itself increases their sense of confidence in themselves and each other and that sharing in the raising of their children enriches their relationship immeasurably.

During the time a couple has a small baby it's important to set aside time to be together and this requires planning and structuring. Our sex life might become less spontaneous, but we can plan for sex if we choose to — we don't have to try to make love when we're exhausted.

SHARING PARENTHOOD WITH A PARTNER

Child care brings many practical difficulties. It may not be easy to work out an equitable arrangement which allows us time with our children and time alone. We may not know in advance what the balance should be, and it may change with time. Some of us will want, or need, to return to work fairly soon, others will prefer to concentrate on child care and others will be able to work out a balance between the two. Partners may also want to adjust work time to spend more hours with their children.

It is rare that a couple can freely make a decision about how to arrange their working time. Men are expected to go out to work to support their families and society is structured accordingly. Part-time work is hard to find and whoever does it probably experiences a drop in their rate of pay as well as an overall drop in income. If a woman decides to go out to work and support her male partner at home she is likely to be discriminated against, because despite recent equal pay and opportunity legislation, 'women's work' is still undervalued in cash terms. If she should become unemployed, her National Insurance contributions will not cover her husband and child. More often than not one partner will have to increase his or her work load in order to provide enough money for the family and may therefore be largely excluded from child care in the early months.

For many of us, two incomes are essential to keep the family afloat. A survey in 1971 showed that three times as many families would have fallen below the poverty line without the wife's income. Many families *are* living in poverty because the lack of child-care facilities forces women to care for their children at home, so they are unable to work. The situation is likely to get worse as rising unemployment so often means a squeeze on jobs for women, and cuts in public expenditure are reducing the already insufficient number of nursery places.

We must fight for changes in employment patterns, benefit laws, and child-care provision if men and women are ever to share child care in a meaningful way.

However, change is in the future. For those contemplating parenthood today the hard facts of life must be understood so that a compromise can be worked out which meets the needs of adults and children. As things stand, men often have little to do with child care, it is often difficult for them to understand that it is hard and exhausting work and that mothers need time for themselves.

PARENTING ALONE

For some of us the decision to have a child is not a joint one. We may feel unable to sustain an ongoing relationship with another adult, we may prefer to take all the responsibility for child care rather than attempt to share with someone who is unwilling to take part. Perhaps, as we see the years passing and we have not established a stable relationship or home with others, we may decide to have a child without support rather than miss the opportunity of mothering. For some of us becoming a 'single parent' is not a choice, but happens through widowhood, divorce or an unexpected pregnancy. Whatever the reason, if we are alone, we share certain problems which may be with us for many years.

The biggest problem is likely to be financial. A few of us may have a good job with paid maternity leave and a crèche at work, but most of us will not be so lucky. If we go back to work we will have to find somewhere to leave the baby.

Although single parents are supposed to have priority in council nurseries, there is such pressure on places that we cannot count on it. Few of them will take very young babies and we may feel unhappy about 'institutional' care at such an early age. There are some day nurseries run partly by women's groups but they cater for very small areas and have waiting lists. Some of us may have friends or relations who are willing to look after the child during the day and for others there is the possibility of a registered baby minder (the local Social Services office will have a list). Whichever course of action we choose, it is very important to find out enough about the person who will be caring for our children so that we can feel secure about leaving them.

The majority of single parents have to rely on Social Security to support them for at least the first few years of their children's lives. Social Security is a breadline state handout which ensures a poverty existence for as long as you need it (provided you don't break the rules). Unless you have friends close at hand, or willing to visit, this may increase your isolation — money that won't cover the heating bills won't stretch to bus fares and baby-sitters. Any attempt to supplement with other income is discouraged, because money earned is deducted from Social Security payments.

The state also keeps a beady eye on your sex life. Under the 'cohabitation rule' any woman who is suspected of cohabiting with a man is likely to lose her benefit. Cohabitation is a variable matter in the eyes of the SS snoopers; it could mean only that your boyfriend occasionally spends the night (and neighbours can be questioned and investigations made for any male clothing in your room as proof). The state believes that if a man is sleeping with you he must pay for you as well.

Lack of support through pregnancy and childbirth can be very hard and the demands of a new baby are made much greater if there is no one to share the load. However concerned friends may be at the start, it is not always easy for them to understand and respond to the continuing needs of a new mother. We may feel tempted to drop out of social activities because we are tired and pressured, but it is all the more important to keep our lives open if we are not to become isolated. Groups such as 'Gingerbread' (see p. 488) offer support to single parents, and for those of us who feel the need to have contact with others in a similar situation their group meetings and social events can be useful outlets and provide much support and advice.

In spite of the enormous difficulties that society puts in the way of single parents, many women find that the close bond which grows between them and their children is worth all the hassle in the end. If you are embarking on motherhood single-handed, talk to others doing it. If at all possible, try to arrange to live close to supportive friends even if the accommodation is of a lower standard than more distant places. However well you feel at the start of your pregnancy, make your arrangements well in advance.

Perhaps you will decide to find others to share accommodation, a solution which alleviates isolation and helps to stretch the money. Communal living brings its own problems, which we discuss below, but it is a way of life which more of us are choosing. If you already live with others it is particularly important to discuss the implications of introducing a baby into the household.

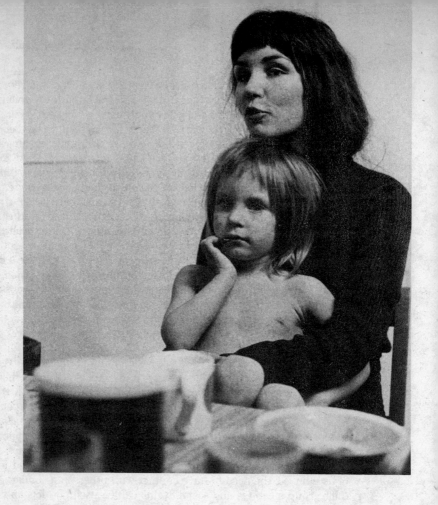

PARENTING COMMUNALLY

Communal houses are often attractive places for single or married parents to live in because child-rearing can be shared with others.

Lisa has become such a warm, open, self-sufficient girl. She doesn't cling to me as she used to. She seeks attention from other adults almost as much as from me. She has her own world with the other children here . . . And then there's me. I have more time for myself. It's a new freedom I still have trouble getting used to although we've been here over a year. I sometimes forget that I don't have to run to meet Lisa's needs; she can and will turn to others here. My time with her has been much 'better-quality' time.

Communal child-rearing challenges our ability to move out of some of the accepted restrictive ways of approaching parenthood. How do we begin to share the responsibility for raising our children? How do we trust other adults to do right by them? How do we encourage our children to turn to and respond to others? And whether or not we have children of our own, what do we risk by becoming very close to another's child? How will we and the child feel if the group breaks up and we must separate? How do we deal with deep-seated feelings about 'interfering' and begin to share in a whole new responsibility for raising a child we didn't give birth to? There are no easy answers, but some of us feel that our lives and the lives of our children will be better if we can adapt to the challenge of communal living. However, it is an important warning to keep in mind that communal living situations are often temporary and short-lived.

In this section we've tried to give you some idea of what problems and pleasures we face when we become mothers. Contrary to sentimental myths, becoming a mother, like having a relationship with a man or getting married, does not solve all one's problems.

Ideally, thinking and talking about the issues we've discussed will make us feel more informed about what is involved in parenting and more confident as we try to make our decision.

Shall I Become a Mother? — I Do Not Know

Perhaps, even after giving this issue a good deal of thought, you are deeply undecided about whether or not you want to become a mother. Again, many of us want to be parents at some point — but not now.

It feels good to be clear about my priorities. Though I have a fine relationship with a man I love very much, I know I won't choose to live with him on a long-term basis if he doesn't want to share parenthood with me. I want very much to be a parent, though I don't want to take on that responsibility alone.

I need space for myself — to work, to make music, to be alone, to be with friends — and this is pretty hard to do without sharing parental responsibilities. I also want someone else to be as important to and as involved with my children as I am — for their sake as well as my own.

I keep hearing everyone has children and loves it, wouldn't give them back and so on — but I do not comprehend it. I need a really good reason for having a child.

Others of us are not sure whether we ever want to be parents. It is important for the rest of us to offer support for this point of view. Women have been socialized so strongly to become mothers that we often feel guilty, unfeminine or a failure if we are not sure whether we want children. We have to protect our right to be undecided and help people to understand it as legitimate.

Every single month I go through a crisis. I want/don't want a child. I have period pains. I'm late again. I have to have a child before I'm too old. I don't *want to be an old mother. Why do I want a child anyway? An ego trip? Want to guarantee another me in the world? Don't want one at all practically. I'm scared stiff of being dependent and yet I'd love an excuse to drop the women's liberation image and be dependent, protected — it would save me so much effort and might force a man into looking after me. Since my father died, I've missed that safe, protected feeling. So many children in the world. I mustn't add to the numbers. Everywhere's so cram-packed with people. Buses, trains, roads, shops, houses bulging. The world just doesn't need another one. So many children uncared for, but I can't adopt or foster because the agencies are religious and moral and I'm an atheist and won't get married, even to pretend. I love kids, any age, but don't want them round my neck all the time, so I wouldn't love it any more. I love kids as equals. I don't want to become a parent. I want to learn how to feel free, not more chained down.* *

It is important to accept our feelings, understand our own point of view, and not apologize. Only then can we act with any sense of freedom.

Many of us want to do things in the near future that we could not do if we had children. We want to have children in our late twenties or early thirties, after we have had a chance to be on our own and have a variety of experiences with work, relationships and travel. Some of us want to understand ourselves better emotionally before we become parents.

Our mothering will be better if we feel comfortable with ourselves. But one danger is that cultural definitions of mothering and our own expectations of ourselves as mothers are so impossibly idealized that we may never feel ready.

When you decide to enter a contest, you do the best you can and either win or lose . . . for me motherhood looms like a big contest waiting for me to enter. But this is an event to be won. Obviously I cannot risk the motherhood game while hosting thoughts of being a losing contestant. I have to be a great, winning mother, but I have never approached any event in my life with that kind of self-assurance and/or arrogance. I am never sure of the successful outcome of my morning soft-boiled egg. Nevertheless, here I am with unfathomable control over my ova and his sperms and an outrageous inability to declare to the world that, yes, I am ready, able and strong enough to provide love, security and guidance to our creation.

But as we said, the decision to have children is irrevocable and the decision not to have them, even though that is made over a certain number of years, is, in the end, equally so. Those of us who postpone the decision to our late twenties or early thirties have a certain valuable perspective which helps us to be more realistic about parenting. But as we approach our mid-thirties, our fertility decreases and the risks to the child increase. Still, having a child and embarking on the unknown of

---

* Liz Durkin, *Peace News*, 20 February 1976.

motherhood is scary — and time and age do not change that. What we can hope for is to be honest and clear enough with ourselves that our decisions are not made by default. We are trying to develop support structures to help us consider parenthood in a balanced way. We do not want to be pressured to become parents before we are ready and comfortable, and yet we do not want to postpone the decision until it's too late.

Shall I Become a Mother? — No

More women than before are thinking seriously of not having children. Since maternity is now not our only option, we can look more critically at 'motherhood'. It's always been culturally assumed that maternity is intrinsically gratifying and is a vital step in all women's maturation. Now some women ask what maternity deprives us of. For one, it requires that we shelve or reduce our involvement in non-family interests. Some of us feel that the gratifications of maternity are not sufficient compensation.

I like kids and like my friends to have kids . . . but not me. My mother gave up a career to have us, and acted like she was in prison the whole time. Now that we're grown up, she's back to work and finally enjoys her marriage. I know a lot of women have kids and interesting work, but it's hard. My work demands most of my time and hardly pays at all — but I love it. My boyfriend is in the same situation. We just wouldn't risk it all to have a kid.

Secondly, maternity can shift the balance in our equitable marital or couple relationships. Some of us have established relationships in which both partners have satisfying careers, share many common experiences, and share equally in decision-making and household responsibilities. We want to be competent mothers, and we think this means taking on a more traditional role, which may create distance between us and our partners and slow our occupational growth.

[A woman]: *People say, 'But when you get older, you'll be sorry you didn't have children.' If they mean that I'll have no one to take care of me, I wouldn't want my children to baby-sit me in my senility. If they mean that in my old age I'll have only my children to spark up my life, then what about my friends, my interests, my work? As for immortality, I've never craved it. If some of my ideas live on in people's memories, fine. If they don't, fine.*

When I state my reasons for not having children, everything starts sounding egocentric — until I realize that my honest feelings and anxieties are going to affect the child in many ways. My relationship with my husband, my teaching career, and my plans to pursue a PhD are my most important considerations. A child simply would not get enough attention or even 'quality time' with me. Some women fulfil their personal goals while the children are being brought up by day-care centres or live-in baby-sitters. I do not trust any kind of surrogate parent to bring up my child with the atmosphere and ideals that I would want the child to have.

[Her husband]: *When my wife and I decided to marry, it was with the idea that we would not have children. We believe that it is hard enough to maintain a viable, working marriage, and in order to keep it lively, we have to have the time to work at it. With a child, our time together would probably be reduced by eighty per cent. We also want to make sure that both of us fulfil our own personal dreams, which do not include having a child. We hear so much about people who always wanted to do something but never did because they had the responsibility of caring for their children.*

Neither of us wants the sole responsibility of supporting the child and the other parent. And neither can take five years out of careers. We entered marriage intending to share everything, including the finances.

The funny thing is that people have told us that we would be great parents, but that doesn't mean that we would be. We both know that we would transfer many of our phobias and worries, and our lack of confidence to our children.

Thirdly, the additional responsibilities of maternity sometimes cause us to regress rather than mature. Social pressure to have children has been so great that it has been hard for us to assess our actual desire for children and our ability to perform as parents. Although our culture is rather resistant to the image of a non-nurturant woman, some of us feel we are not interested nor cut out to be mothers.

It's possible to incorporate children into our lives even if we choose not to have any.

It's too bad that young women think that they have to have children in order to be a 'fulfilled' woman. I'm fifty-six, never had kids, and feel as 'fulfilled' as I could possibly be. Our lives can be rich with work, friends, other people's children, and many other things. I don't think that motherhood is the right choice for every woman.

Shall I Become a Mother? — Yes

For those of us who make the decision it may be hard to keep a sense of individuality, to cope with the problems that motherhood brings, but we feel that the joys of having children can outweigh the problems.

When we become mothers our response to our child borders on the sentimental, or cliché, since it involves us in the universal experience of childbearing and child-rearing, and there is obviously little new to be said. Still, when it is our experience and our baby, it's a new miracle, and familiar words take on new meanings.

Before I had a child, although I loved being with other people's children, any time something went wrong or the child irritated me, I would think to myself, How could I ever stand the full-time responsibility of being a mother? I guess it is not for me. Somehow becoming a mother changed that. There is an intangible, indescribable bond intrinsic to the relationship, which mothers talk about, that in the long run transcends the petty, everyday irritating occurrences.

I heard a squeal of delight across the room and turned around to see my seven-month-old pulling himself up with the support of a box to a standing position for the first time. It was miraculous to see him growing before my eyes.

The dynamic relationship between ourselves and our children changes as we grow and our children grow.

I have learned to stop and watch my kids. All the energy I have put into getting in touch with the child in me I use now to stop and just listen to all the messages my children are giving me . . . I feel like it's taken me a good part of my kid's lives to enjoy them. It's as if one day I woke up and said, 'Hey, there are two people here.' I feel I don't have to be doing all the giving; they have been giving me a lot of attention all the time, but I have not been seeing that. The giving and receiving between parent and child is different from that between me and my friends.

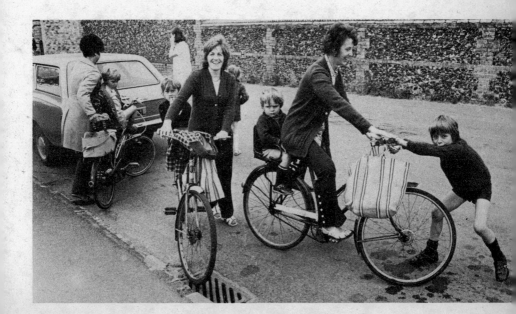

I feel a real old-fashioned possessive pride in them as MY kids — I want to say, 'Look, everybody, aren't they great?' Other times it's almost a detached kind of wonder or curiosity that the helpless little babies I cared for such a short time ago are developing into separate human beings whom I genuinely like and enjoy.

When they were little, my husband and I had total responsibility for them. We could structure their experience, teach them, select their friends, etc.

Now they are at school, which is not only freeing for me but freeing for them. They are learning things that I remember learning myself, and sometimes they come home with new ideas that they want to tell me about. I feel very excited when they want to share their new interests and their school life with me. It is a little like when a woman who has always been very home-centred goes out to a job or community work. She has new interests to share in her own work. At the same time, my kids take an interest in my work and seem to have a strong identification with our political involvements, particularly feminism.

So some of us have said and are saying, Yes, I shall become a mother — I want to know what mothering is all about.

For books and addresses concerning children and child care, see end of Chapter 14.

Introduction to Childbearing Chapters

Our preparation for childbirth is often marred by fears, misinformation and a feeling of helplessness as we cope with a medical system that can quickly dehumanize us during this most deeply human of experiences. The aim of this section is to affirm childbearing as a dignified and creative act; to educate ourselves; to discuss alternatives to orthodox medical practice; to encourage women to work for woman-controlled, woman-oriented health care and to pressure medical institutions to respond to our needs.

Rarely are we allowed to experience childbearing with dignity. Our present socioeconomic system refuses many of us the right to be well-nourished and well-educated and secure. Our present medical system, with its increasingly centralized institutions, its abuse of technological devices, and its crisis-intervention mentality, does not cope adequately with the humanness, naturalness and continuity of childbearing.

We usually give birth in an unfamiliar place for sick people and are separated at a crucial time from family and friends. We are depersonalized and lose our identity. We are expected to be passive and acquiescent and to make no trouble. We may just feel insignificant as we wait and wait to be seen by the doctor; we may feel silly for asking questions which he or she brushes aside or answers sketchily. We may even be made to feel that we are downright annoying to the doctor. Inside ourselves we may feel angry and yet powerless to do anything about what we know to be an affront to our dignity. There are many of us who have experienced these feelings of disappointment and anger, although individually we may feel isolated.

What we want from the obstetrician is thorough prenatal care, and competent technical assistance if we really need it at the time of delivery. Moreover, we would like to include the doctor as an ally who respects our entire birth process. This, however, is rarely possible. For most doctors have been taught throughout their entire medical education to see patients as a class rather than as individual people with special needs. They have learned to treat us paternally; they have been taught that we want them to take care of us, and we as patients often play into that role. The strength and anger that we may feel have no opportunity for expression in the usual doctor-patient relationship. We, as pregnant women, are expected to put ourselves in the doctor's hands, and he or she expects to take control of our birth experience.

Doctors are trained mainly to deal with complications of childbirth. 'Well,' we say, 'you never know. Something might happen. We need our doctor.' We are afraid on many levels. We have been taught to have very little confidence in ourselves, in our bodies. In fact at least 90% of our deliveries have no complications. Most of us could very easily give birth with the help of a midwife, in a hospital, a special maternity unit, or at home among family and friends. In actuality the doctor or midwife should have very little part to play in a normal delivery.

What really worries us is that, despite the whole childbirth education movement over the last twenty years, doctors intervene more and more in our birth experience. We are not ungrateful for the medical advances that have saved many lives. We simply don't want our childbirth experience *unnecessarily* mechanized and interfered with. At least 90% of us will have perfectly normal, healthy deliveries if our labours are not in some way tampered with by the doctor.

Nurses, too, can cause us distress during the childbearing experience.

As we have pointed out in the section on battered women, we think there are reasons for oppressive behaviour. It is not surprising that a nurse can be brutal to a vulnerable, defenceless woman when she herself suffers from being near the bottom of an extremely oppressive, hierarchical system. While working together to make changes in our health care system, we must remember to give our support to those people working within it who suffer from its oppressive influence.

As women, we know that childbirth is an extremely important experience in our lives. If we are prepared and unanesthetized during childbirth, we are in touch with our entire self, mind and body, and we are working intelligently along with this inevitable biological process. We are in control. The experience of childbirth can have a positive effect on all the other aspects of our being. We can feel freer sexually, having experienced such a massive physical and sexual event. We can feel more independent, having survived on our own merits this incredibly powerful experience. We can feel more in control of ourselves as whole people, having used both our mind and our body, together, to see us through labour and delivery. We can be more confident mothers, having done our best from the start to give our children a safe and satisfying birth. And finally, we can be sure that as women we are strong, competent and beautiful!

We hope that this section is a beginning in the attempt to re-own our childbearing experience.

12 Pregnancy

What You Can Do to Prepare Yourself

PROCEDURES FOR DETECTING PREGNANCY

Importance of Detection. Some women can become pregnant and not be aware of it for a few months. But if you suspect you are pregnant, you should get confirmation as soon as possible. This is so that (a) you can decide what you want to do, and (b) if you want to have the baby, you can start essential antenatal care and controlling your diet and drug intake. (For antenatal care, see p. 366; for diet and drugs, see p. 353.)

Tests. The main kind of test uses a hormone (HCG – human chorionic gonadotropin) secreted by the developing embryo and found in the urine of pregnant women. A drop of urine is mixed on a slide with a drop of serum sensitized to it and two drops of another substance; if HCG is present, the mixture won't coagulate.

This test can detect pregnancy after your period is about 2 weeks late. It is 95 to 98% accurate, but can be false if performed too early (before there's enough hormone in the urine), or if there are technical errors in handling or storing the urine. Sometimes, even if you are pregnant, your first or second tests will be negative. This is particularly true if you are approaching the menopause or taking anti-depressant drugs. It is therefore important to keep testing. Some women don't show positive signs at all in tests. There are also rare occasions when a test can be falsely positive. Usually a diagnosis of pregnancy can be made independent of these tests, for example by a bimanual examination (see p. 140).

To collect a sample of urine, drink no liquids after supper the night before and then when you wake up in the morning collect half a cupful of urine in a clean, dry, soap-free jar (if there is any trace of detergent in the jar the result may be inaccurate). Most testing agencies will provide you with a bottle (and with special envelopes if you are using their mail order service).

The sample may be sent or delivered to any of the following places for testing:

1. You can deliver it to your local hospital or your GP for a free test, but check how long it will take. They often keep you waiting for a fortnight, which is far too long. In any case, you might not wish to use your GP for fear of his not treating the result as confidential. (If your GP does ever breach confidence, you should report him to the General Medical Council, see p. 543. This applies even if you are under 16.)

2. You can take it to a chemist; chemists usually display a sign if they do pregnancy testing. The service is usually quick and accurate but they charge a fee. Some chemists sell do-it-yourself pregnancy testing kits. They are expensive and not very reliable.

3. Commercial laboratories advertise extensively in magazines and in 'Yellow Pages', often providing a mail order and while-you-wait service. They charge at least £2 and some of them offer advice on abortion as well. You do not have to take their advice.

4. The British Pregnancy Advisory Service, a charitable agency with branches in several major towns (see addresses, p. 332) will test you for £2 on the spot. They also do a mail order service; if you enclose a written request they will give you the result by telephone.

5. Family planning clinics test on the spot, or with a 24-hour delay. Charges vary from nothing (usually if you use the clinic for contraceptive purposes) to about £1·50.

6. Some women's liberation groups do pregnancy testing. They do it for free but you may be asked for a donation to go towards helping other women. If you have a choice between a commercial (as opposed to charitable) agency and a WL group, it would be best to choose the latter since WL groups are obviously committed to providing accurate results. Not all commercial agencies can be so relied on. Contact WIRES for the address of your local WL group (see p. 570).

It is now possible to detect HCG in a woman's urine 10 days after *conception*, but this new test, involving special equipment, is not yet widely available in the UK. One agency – Belmont Laboratories (see Resources, p. 479) – does provide this early test, charging an extra £2 over the cost of the usual test. They also do a mail order service. (For more details about this new test, see Jill Rakusen, *Spare Rib*, 41.)

Some doctors use two pills containing oestrogen and progestogen as a way of detecting pregnancy. The idea is that if you are not pregnant, the pills will produce withdrawal bleeding. They will not induce a period if you are already pregnant. In any case, *these pills should not be used*. They are less accurate than the urine tests (you can have withdrawal bleeding and still be pregnant), and they have also resulted in the foetus developing deformities. Even though it is well known that all drugs should be avoided during pregnancy, about 100,000 prescriptions were written for these pills in 1974.

Pelvic Examination. By means of a pelvic examination (see pp. 139–40) your uterus can be felt and your cervix examined. If you are pregnant: (1) the top of the cervix becomes softened; (2) the tip of the cervix changes from a pale pink to a bluish hue because of increased venous blood circulation; (3) the uterus feels softer; and (4) the shape of the uterus changes: where the embryo attaches itself to the inside of the uterus it makes a bulge, which can sometimes be felt on the outside of the uterus. Despite these signs, pregnancies can be misdiagnosed, and tests are advisable to be sure.

Some Women Just Know They Are Pregnant

With my first child I missed a period and my breasts hurt. With Jesse, I knew the moment I conceived him. There's no way of pinning that down, no way of explaining how I felt. I just knew.

I realized I was pregnant the same night I became pregnant. I lay there all night. I'd had a very active sex life, and it was the first time I had ever felt this way. I wasn't expecting to get pregnant, but I felt different that night.

TAKING CARE OF YOURSELF: CHOICE, COMMITMENT, PREPARATION, FEELINGS, EMOTIONAL NEEDS

If you have planned your pregnancy, when you find you are pregnant you know you have already chosen to keep your baby. If you haven't planned your pregnancy, you have to decide whether or not you will continue with it. When you decide to continue it you have made your first crucial choice — to be pregnant. Sometimes it takes a few months to make this choice. Some women let time decide.

After three months I knew my pregnancy was irrevocable, I wasn't going to end it. I felt it was taken out of my hands.

I didn't want to have another abortion, I really was amused by the idea of having a kid; I wanted a kid. I didn't feel I could ever consciously decide to have a kid, I didn't know what grounds to base that decision on.

If your pregnancy was unexpected, you might be so confused and so hassled that for a long time you drift along not being able to think clearly. It's not uncommon during pregnancy to feel often out of control. It's to your advantage that you take on/assume/choose your pregnancy as early as possible, for the more you know about the process (what's happening in and to your body) and about your feelings, the more you can be in control of what happens during pregnancy, childbirth and the postpartum time.

The first step in planning to have your first child begins with planning for a fundamental change in your life. It's not easy to experience beforehand what that change will mean. Your body and mind will change during your pregnancy; your life will change with the birth of your child. Begin to think of these changes and then take advantage of every tool and every scrap of information available. Use what used to be thought of as a time of 'waiting', of simple passivity, to prepare for the changes ahead.

For many of us it has been important to spend time with sympathetic people during our pregnancy — to be in contact, talking, sharing work, checking feelings and questions. But some of us find it can be hard to move out of isolation. Some of us marry and move away from our families and friends, often isolated in our homes. In our isolation it's hard to find other pregnant women to talk to.

It can be hard to bring up our questions and anxieties, because our bodily functions have traditionally been taboo subjects. Doctors or nurses often can't answer us satisfactorily. They might not know the things we need to know, or be aware of feelings we may be having, or have the time to talk to us. So we have to make an effort to talk among ourselves. (One thing to be a little careful about here is that some people who offer information and advice can misinform us or frighten us needlessly with stories of their own pregnancies and births, which they themselves didn't understand.)

During pregnancy we need to depend on someone.

You have to know how to ask for help. It's all right to ask, even for a cup of tea. Most of the time I had a lot of energy and was able to do things for myself, but there were times when I was really tired and I really didn't want to do physical things. The thing to aim for is instead of denying that the pregnancy makes a difference, just admit it. It made me aware of my own physical limitations.

At the beginning I felt independent. But towards the fifth month, when we came back from vacation, Dick went to work, and I felt very isolated from the 'real' world. Then I had no one. I needed to be able to talk to people, and I wasn't talking to people.

Pregnancy shatters the illusion of our separateness and reminds us of our interconnectedness with others.

You need to make a continuity for yourself. If you can, find one or more supportive women or men to share your whole experience with, to lean on at times of need and stress, to whom you can easily say, 'I need you.'

I depended on my mother and two friends. One friend had factual information that I trusted.

Often you can ask for help from the man you're close to. Sometimes you can't. He might be too busy, not able to cope too helpfully with your problems. But it's good to have him involved as much as possible as he will be living with all the joys and problems of your childbearing and he'll need preparation too.

This emphasis on preparation may begin to sound repetitious. But establishing a new human being, especially during the early weeks and months of its life, is an extremely complicated, demanding piece of work. So keeping your health and sanity is vitally important. It's also important to realize that no matter how well prepared and ready you feel at each step, something unexpected will usually happen. At least the knowledge you have will help you be more open, more flexible, more able to meet new situations with confidence. And, finally, don't knock yourself out as you learn about yourself. There will be enough time. Take it easy.

TAKING CARE OF YOUR PHYSICAL NEEDS

There are three crucial ways for you to take care of your physical needs during pregnancy. First you must obtain good antenatal care (see p. 366). Second, it is good to exercise to develop and strengthen your body. Develop your perineal muscles (see 'Pelvic Floor [Kegel] Exercises', p. 137). Strengthen your back muscles to prevent backache by (1) bending and touching your toes, (2) sit-ups, (3) bicycling exercises. Simple daily walking is always good.

Third, you must eat well throughout your pregnancy.
Nutrition. Studies made over the past forty years show that eating well is vitally important to ensure the health of your growing body during pregnancy, for pregnancy increases the body's requirements for most nutrients. But in general, doctors and obstetricians do not apply this knowledge.

There is strong evidence that if we eat well, we bear strong, large, lively babies. During the Second World War in Britain pregnant women were given priority in food-rationing programmes, and even under adverse conditions the stillbirth rate fell from 38 per 1,000 live births to 28 – a decrease of about 25%.

If women eat well during pregnancy and gain weight, there's much more chance that the baby's weight will be adequate. It should be obvious that if the baby's birth weight is adequate, the baby is less apt to die or get sick after birth.

Women and babies from poor homes are most vulnerable to disease and complications, since they are unlikely to have adequate medical care or adequate diet. Infants of low birth weight are more often born to women who don't have much money; who are under 17; who don't gain much weight during pregnancy; who are poorly nourished; who have infections and chronic disease. Good nutrition, then, helps prevent stillbirth, low birth weight and prematurity from low birth weight. It also helps prevent infections, anaemia in mothers, and brain damage and retardation in babies.

What should we eat during pregnancy? A good diet is necessary for all women all the time (see 'Nutrition' chapter). There are no 'special diets' for pregnancy and no unrefined foods (in suitable quantities) need to be avoided. Women around the world choose, or are forced, to eat completely different combinations of foods but most are still able to meet the nutrition requirements of pregnancy. A woman with a special diet due to religious beliefs, vegetarianism, etc. can still consume a diet perfectly adequate for herself and her growing foetus, but special attention is required and vitamin pills may prove particularly useful. A woman's nutritional requirements during pregnancy are also affected by personal requirements, physical exercise, general state of health, and demands of this particular pregnancy.

An Example of a Good Daily Diet During Pregnancy: (a) Milk: 3–4 glasses of either low-fat, whole or buttermilk (equivalents such as cottage cheese and yogurt are fine; skim milk is also good). If you are taking an adequate, well-balanced diet, you don't need as much milk. But milk is ideal for providing you with protein and calcium if you cannot afford much for food; (b) one or two servings of fish, liver, chicken, lean beef, lamb, pork or cheese (alternatives are dried beans, peas or nuts*); (c) one or two servings of fresh green leafy vegetables, e.g. spinach, lettuce, or cabbage, or fresh frozen vegetables as a second choice; (d) two or three slices of wholewheat bread; (e) a piece of citrus fruit or glass of lemon, lime, orange or grapefruit juice; and (f) one pat of butter or vitamin-enriched margarine. Also (a) four times a week a serving of whole-grain cereal; (b) five times a week a yellow- or orange-coloured vegetable; (c) liver once a week; and (d) a potato, preferably baked, three times a week, or half a cup of brown rice; (e) occasionally you can have an egg but preferably not more than four a week. Remember that all these foods together contain combinations of proteins, vitamins and minerals which must remain in a certain balance in order for your body to function well and provide good materials for the growth of your baby. (For more on 'Nutrition', see p. 114.) As your pregnancy progresses – and particularly if you are expecting more than one baby – it becomes even more necessary that you eat a well-balanced diet.

A Word about Calories. Pregnancy increases the body's energy (calorie) requirements, so most women will need to eat more during pregnancy than usual. However, if you are less active than usual during pregnancy, you may not need to eat more. Women under seventeen especially need a lot of calories as they are still growing.

* If these sources are depended on regularly, they may need to be combined with other grains (see Nutrition, p. 117).

A Word about Protein. Protein requirements are also increased during pregnancy. A good way of getting enough protein is to drink extra milk. Pregnant teenagers need to be especially careful to provide enough protein (and other nutrients) for their own growing bodies and the foetus.

Fluids. It is also important to drink plenty of fluids, say six to eight glasses daily. Water aids the circulation of blood and body fluids and stimulates the digestion and assimilation of foods. It also helps prevent urinary infections. But try to avoid excessive amounts of coffee or tea; caffeine crosses the placenta, but is relatively harmless in moderation.

Food and Vitamin Supplements during Pregnancy

Iron, folic acid and some vitamins (see below) are given routinely to most pregnant women, in an attempt to prevent deficiencies which might be caused by the growing foetus. For how to get them, see 'Your Rights during Pregnancy', p. 362. They tend not to be given before the 15th week of pregnancy since it is always best to avoid any drugs during the first trimester. Routine multivitamin supplementation is necessary during pregnancy if your diet is not well balanced. Do not take grossly more vitamins than the recommended amounts (see 'The Effect of Drugs, Vitamins etc.', p. 359).

The following three vitamin tablets are most usually handed out to pregnant women: *vitamin A* (found in vegetables, whole milk etc.), *vitamin C* (found in citrus fruits), and *vitamin D* (found in fish-liver oil, vitamin-D-fortified milk and sunshine; do *not* use ultra-violet sunray lamps in an attempt to absorb vitamin D). The two other most commonly-used supplements are iron and folic acid. We discuss these below.

Iron (found in liver, yeast, wheat germ, fish, meat etc.). Iron is a main component of blood haemoglobin, which carries oxygen to your baby and your cells. The baby also draws on your iron reserve to store iron in its liver to last for the duration of its milk diet after birth. However, breast-fed babies do receive iron through their mothers' milk. Also during labour you'll need a lot of oxygen (supplied by haemoglobin) for your uterus; the baby's brain cells need oxygen, too. Your own iron stores are seldom large enough to meet the requirements of pregnancy, and many young women are already iron-deficient before pregnancy. But many other dietary factors influence the absorption of iron; so, if you suffer from iron deficiency, you may need something else — for example, vitamin B or C — not iron. Not all doctors are aware of this and may hand out iron tablets routinely.

Iron tablets can cause an upset stomach. But if the tablets are not started until the 15th week of pregnancy, it is unlikely that this will happen. If symptoms do occur, the problem can often be cured by switching to another brand of tablet; failing that, you can have injections instead. Iron tablets are poisonous to children, so keep them hidden.

Calcium (found in milk, green leafy vegetables, small fish bones, stone-ground grain). Calcium is necessary for making the bones of the foetus, so extra calcium is needed during pregnancy. Supplements are commonly given to pregnant women, especially if they suffer from cramps – one of the symptoms of calcium deficiency. Other symptoms such as sleeplessness, irritability, nerve pains and uterine ligament pains can also be signs of lack of calcium.

Trace Elements, such as zinc, cobalt, copper, manganese and magnesium are also necessary – but only in minute quantities. The majority of these elements are found in the iron preparations available and in foods commonly eaten. (For more about trace elements, see Adelle Davis, *Let's Eat Right.*) Lack of them can lead to gross deficiencies. For example, too little iodine (which occurs more often in other parts of the world) can be even worse than lack of iron, leading to an abnormal baby. (Pregnant women need more magnesium than normal.)

B Vitamins (found in bread, whole grains, liver, wheat germ etc). Pregnancy increases the requirement for the B vitamins. Deficiencies are most apt to occur in folic acid (see below) and vitamin B_6, so supplements for those may be given later in pregnancy.

Folic acid, one of the B vitamins, is found in leafy green vegetables, liver, kidneys. Symptoms of folic acid deficiency are anaemia and fatigue. Excessive folic-acid deficiency can lead to nerve damage. Folic acid tablets can remedy the deficiency. They are usually given routinely, together with iron tablets (see above). Folic acid deficiency tends to affect those with repeated or multiple pregnancies; women are particularly prone during the last three months of pregnancy.

The B vitamins are said to help prevent nervousness, skin problems, lack of energy, constipation and changes of pigmentation in your skin. Pregnant women may be deficient in *vitamin B_6;* iron tablets can even make it worse. Nausea, cramps, headaches and water retention, among other things, can be helped by B_6 (Davis, *Let's Eat Right*). Good sources include whole grains, and especially brewer's yeast.

Vitamin E (found in whole grains, corn, peanuts, eggs). While most nutritionists agree that practically nothing is known about the need for vitamin E or what it does in the human, some believe strongly in its importance, for instance, that you use more oxygen than you need to if you lack vitamin E, that it promotes healing and that it influences the metabolism of vitamin A.*

---

* According to Adelle Davis in *Let's Get Well,* deficiency in vitamin E can be induced by iron supplements, and this can cause muscular weakness and hence make delivery difficult. She also believes that it can result in premature birth.

Gaining Weight. As your pregnancy advances you may feel voracious. There has been much controversy over whether or not it's okay to gain much weight beyond the weight of the uterus, placenta, foetus and amniotic fluid. Some studies show that as long as your diet is well balanced you may gain extra weight. Again, there is a positive correlation between weight gained during pregnancy by the mother and the weight of the newborn baby. The pattern of your weight gain is more important than the total amount: say one or two pounds per week. If the pattern remains fairly regular, everything is all right. A sudden large gain after the twentieth to twenty-fourth week, especially if you haven't been eating well, might mean excessive water retention (oedema) and should be checked by a doctor. Be attentive: check your own weight weekly. Weight loss or no gain should be checked by a doctor too. There are important arguments against gaining a lot of extra weight. It can put too great a strain on your circulation and your heart, and many women find it very hard to get rid of all that extra weight after the baby is born. Even if you do gain a lot of weight, keep eating a *balanced* diet (see above); do not take diet pills (see below, p. 358).

It is now thought that obese women may be able to have healthy babies without putting on very much weight during pregnancy. This, however, requires an excellent balanced diet and probably should only be tried with good medical advice or supervision. It could help prevent pregnancy from adding to the obesity problem.

Toxaemia. (See also p. 373). Many of us were cautioned by our doctors not to gain much weight during pregnancy in case we would swell up and get toxaemia. Most of us have never known exactly what toxaemia is.

During my pregnancy I thought that if my hands or ankles started to swell, something would happen — I would suddenly be in some kind of danger, a danger that I didn't understand.

[From a description of a clinic] Women . . . were threatened with frightening stories about deaths from toxaemia.

Metabolic toxaemia of late pregnancy (MTLP) is a condition that has several stages. The first stage, pre-eclampsia, is characterized by oedema (swelling due to water retention), high blood pressure, and protein in the urine. It usually occurs not before the fifth month of pregnancy, usually late in pregnancy. Pre-eclampsia may be mild or severe. In the second stage a woman might have trouble with her vision, abdominal pains, mental dullness, or severe headaches. In the most severe stage, the eclamptic stage, she might have convulsions and go into a coma. Usually women don't advance into the eclamptic stage if they are receiving medical care.

Whereas the majority of doctors are unsure of the causes of toxaemia (in one major obstetrics textbook there's a long chapter on the subject of eclampsia that contains at least eighteen theories about how the illness is caused, and a related bibliography of one hundred and eighty articles, only three of which deal with nutrition), Dr Thomas Brewer, who runs a clinic for poor women in California, is convinced after twenty years of study that toxaemia of pregnancy is caused mainly by malnutrition. When women in his clinic were placed on good diets, the incidence of toxaemia dropped radically. M. Bertha Brandt states that 'Toxaemia may be associated with undernutrition and low total serum proteins.'* Adelle Davis has found that lack of vitamin B_6 is a significant factor (*Let's Get Well*).

Certainly, the lower an area's per capita income, the higher the incidence of toxaemia and the higher the maternal mortality from toxaemia.

Whatever the answer, we cannot say too strongly that if toxaemia has already been systematically prevented by good nutrition, then it's clear that all pregnant women should be well nourished *at the very least*. Whatever symptoms and sicknesses remain, one known cause of this sickness would be eliminated. Perhaps toxaemia itself will disappear — one of those 'diseases'- that need never have been; one of the diseases of an eonomically unequal society.

Oedema. (See also 'Oedema', p. 373.) In oedema your body tissues retain water, and this retention causes face, hands, legs, or feet to swell, usually at the end of the day. Doctors in the past and present immediately connect weight gain with toxaemia. However, they must make distinctions. They must not confuse accumulation of fat with weight gained as a result of oedema. They must not confuse regular oedema with the oedema which is a manifestation of toxaemia, and which will be accompanied by other symptoms of toxaemia. Often doctors will automatically give you diuretics (water pills) if you have oedema. These can cause many undesirable side effects in mother and foetus. Their immediate effect is to cause you to urinate more. Diuretics are dehydrating. Among other things, they cause nausea, vomiting, diarrhoea, jaundice, muscle spasms, dizziness, headache and loss of appetite. These diuretics appeared in 1958 and have been pushed by the drug industry, regardless of their effects. However, when wisely used, they can be helpful.

Diet Pills (amphetamines; 'speed') are drugs. They go straight through the placenta to the foetus and can therefore harm it (see 'The Effect of Drugs, etc.' below). They are given to you to kill your appetite, but only serve to mask problems of poor nutrition. You shouldn't take them. And if you are eating adequately, you won't need them.

Salt. When you are pregnant you need a certain amount of salt. For instance, if you happen to lose some blood and you have adequate salt

* Nancy A. Lytle (ed.), *Maternal Health Nursing*. Dubuque, Iowa, William C. Brown Co., 1967.

in your system, then extra salt and water can move into your bloodstream and you don't readily go into shock. Also, if you are preparing to nurse, salt and water mean less dehydration, which is better for milk production. Women on low-salt diets can develop leg cramps; increased salt intake relieves them. So, you should not avoid salt in ordinary amounts, though it's necessary to avoid oversalted foods, since too much salt can lead to excessive fluid retention. In cases of toxaemia, salt can be harmful. It increases hypertension and blood pressure, fluid retention and oedema. If you have cardiac oedema, your salt intake might need to be restricted.

The Effect of Drugs, Vitamins, X-rays and Cigarettes during Pregnancy (for drugs during childbirth, see p. 440). In general, if you are affected by something you eat or absorb, it will get through to your baby. Your decision about whether or not to use a particular drug or procedure must therefore be a compromise between possible good effects (to you) and possible bad effects (to you, to your baby). All drugs should be avoided where possible during the first 3 months of pregnancy and if at all possible during the whole of your pregnancy.

Specific drugs to watch out for include the following.

Alcohol: a need for alcohol can be created in a baby if the mother drinks excessively, and babies born to chronic alcoholic mothers have an increased risk of congenital abnormality and death. At least one study has suggested that even a drinking level well below that termed alcoholic (e.g. the approximate equivalent of 2–3 whiskies a day) may have an effect on the foetus known as 'foetal alcohol syndrome', involving mal-formation and mental retardation.* The baby's ability to suckle may also be affected as well or instead, and some people think that nothing should be drunk while breast-feeding. We must stress that although research has only very recently begun to indicate an effect of moderate drinking on the foetus, caution does seem to be appropriate.

Aspirin, under its many brand names, if taken regularly by pregnant women, appears to increase the risk of the child being stillborn and may make the delivery more complicated, the child underweight and the mother anaemic. There also appears to be a higher risk of heavy bleeding before and after the birth (see *Lancet*, 23 August 1975). By the term 'regular aspirin-taking', the authors of the *Lancet* study mean taking the drugs as frequently as or more than once a week. However, many of the women in the study took it more often, some up to twelve times a day. It is particularly important to avoid aspirin in the last month of pregnancy, otherwise babies may be born with internal bleeding.

Drugs used for General Anaesthetics: 'Pregnant operating-room nurses

---

* 5th International Conference on Birth Defects, Montreal, Canada, 21–27 August 1977, as reported in *Excerpta Medica*, International Congress Series, No 426.

or anaesthetists who inhale over long periods low concentrations of anaesthetic drugs . . . are suspected of being at risk of abortion or of delivering a baby with congential abnormalities' (*Lancet*, 26 July 1975). Babies are also thought to be at risk if their fathers work in a similar way with these drugs. Pregnant women who undergo operations are suspected of being at risk, and until evidence to the contrary is produced, the *Lancet* recommends that operations on such women should be postponed until after the third month or, better still, until the child is born.

Commonly prescribed tranquillizers containing chlordiazepoxide (*Librium*) and meprobamate (*Equanil* or *Miltown*) may also cause birth defects in a very small proportion of babies when taken early in pregnancy. If *Valium* is taken early in pregnancy, there is an increased risk that the baby may be born with a cleft palate. If you have been on *narcotics*, especially *heroin*, your foetus will possibly become addicted before birth. Your doctor must know if you are taking narcotics (including methadone), for withdrawal symptoms in a newborn infant will be dangerous if not recognized immediately. *Large doses of vitamin C (more than 1 gm per day), and possibly vitamins A, D and K may* also harm the foetus (see *Medical Letter*, Vol. 14, p. 50, 1972).

A number of other drugs are also known occasionally to cause abnormalities and these include sex hormones (androgens, progestogens and diethylstilboestrol (see p. 182)), iodine and anti-thyroid drugs, anti-cancer drugs such as methotrexate, anticonvulsants for epilepsy, warfarin (which is used to stop blood from clotting), and the antibiotics streptomycin and tetracycline (the latter is safe up to the fifth month of pregnancy). Drugs under suspicion of causing abnormalities are antacids, iron, amphetamines and the Pill, if taken early in pregnancy. Some drugs given to the mother around the time of the birth may cause jaundice in the newborn baby, including sulphonamides, oxytocin (for induction), vitamin K and Valium.

For those of us who *have* to take drugs during pregnancy, it can be a comfort to know that drugs probably account for only a small proportion of foetal abnormalities. Even though a large number of drugs can reach the foetus, most of them are not necessarily harmful unless taken repeatedly or in large doses. It is really important to ask your chemist exactly what you've been prescribed.

Cigarettes. In the last few years we have seen a great deal of emphasis placed by doctors and government agencies on the dangers to the foetus of the mother's smoking during pregnancy. Smoking is a bad thing – particularly smoking during pregnancy – but we should put the recent campaign of the Health Education Council in perspective. The caption of one HEC poster reads: 'In just one year, in Britain alone, over 1,500 babies might not have died if their mothers had given up smoking when they were pregnant.' This is a misrepresentation of some very cautious research (Butler *et al.*, *British Medical Journal*, 1972) which called for studies to *test the hypothesis* of a causal relationship between smoking, low birth weight and higher mortality rates. Other researchers, using material from the National Child Development Study, have shown that smoking in pregnancy had less effect on the child's development (both mental and physical) than other factors, such as poverty, social class and family size (*British Medical Journal*, Vol. 4, No. 5892). While there is strong evidence that smoking affects birth weight, the guilt which this campaign will induce in those of us who can't stop smoking is clearly out of all proportion to the risks when other factors, such as living conditions, nutrition, physiological type are taken into account. We look forward to an HEC campaign against another common factor – poverty!

If you can't stop smoking we urge you to try cutting down and, if you don't eat very much, to try increasing your (nutritious) food intake: the ill effects of smoking during pregnancy tend to increase with the number of cigarettes you smoke and may be partly due to the smaller amount that smokers tend to eat (*Lancet*, 21 February 1976). It seems that it may not be good for babies to have smoking fathers either (see *Women's Report*, Vol. 2, issue 3).

X-rays can cause congenital abnormalities in a foetus, especially during the 42-day period after conception, and occasionally induce childhood cancer at any time during pregnancy. *But* these risks are not as high as they were 10 years ago since X-ray techniques have improved. However, there is still room for technical improvements and X-rays should be avoided unless they are essential. X-rays are often used to examine the foetus.* The technique of *ultrasound* (see p. 506) can sometimes be used instead, though little is yet known about its own effects on the foetus; it would seem wise, on present evidence, to avoid this technique during the first trimester.

Chemicals at work. So far, only two chemicals – lead and methyl mercury – can confidently be said to damage the human foetus, but little research has been done on other chemicals. There are, however, a number of chemicals which are known to damage the offspring of animals and to which a woman may be exposed at her place of work. Maybe more will be certain by the time you read this. To find out more, contact the Work Hazards Group at the British Society for Social Responsibility in Science (see p. 487). If you think you may be at risk from chemicals at work, you can, under the Employment Protection Act, ask to be moved to a safer area of work, without loss of pay.

---

* In some areas as many as 35% of pregnant women are exposed to X-rays. As with most technological procedures, if the machinery is available, it tends to be used. If, therefore, you are recommended for X-ray, it is worth finding out if it is really necessary. It is thought that high X-ray rates might also be due to the desire of some doctors to pinpoint the foetus's age, so that high induction rates can be maintained. There are other ways of assessing the age of the foetus: see Chapter 13, p. 431 for further discussion.

Nutrition – A Political Issue. All of us, rich and poor, have to struggle separately and together against ignorance, our own and our doctors'. Our struggle is much greater if we don't have enough money to buy needed foods; if good fresh foods aren't available; or if we have to rely too much on processed foods, many of which contain additives about whose properties little is known. For example, Red Dye No. 2, a common food additive, is now thought to be a contributory cause of miscarriages (and, incidentally, infertility). Banned in the USSR about 10 years ago, and in the US during 1977, it is in widespread use in Britain.

We must work for a social and medical system which educates its doctors to provide basic positive preventive services for pregnant women (indeed for all women and men), with an emphasis on good nutrition. We must work for a social and economic system which educates its pregnant women to expect good health and which makes good food easily available. It is clear that we can't have healthy babies unless mothers and fathers have eaten decent natural food and are healthy themselves. We must work for changes in attitudes of doctors and drug companies so that drugs are not pushed on women regardless of their harmful effects. We must be careful about what we take into our bodies when we are pregnant.

Your Rights During Pregnancy

While you are pregnant you are entitled to certain grants and services, for the benefit of both you and your baby. These rights are constantly changing with the changes in government: we still need to work together to establish a dependable and realistic support system for all pregnant women. In the meantime, you are at present entitled to the following, and should make sure you get them.

Free Prescription Charges. Medicines are free (a) to all pregnant women and (b) to women until the baby is one year old. A special certificate is needed which you obtain by filling in a form: for (a) use form FW8, obtainable from the doctor, midwife or health visitor who confirms your pregnancy. Send it to your Family Practitioner Committee (Health Board in Scotland); for (b) use form FP91/EC91, available from Post Offices, Social Security offices or Family Practitioner Committees. Prescriptions are free for children up to the age of 16.

Free Dental Treatment and Dentures, for the same period as above. You can get priority dental treatment at the local welfare clinic without having to wait. Your child can get the same up to the age of 5. It is important that you use your rights to free dental treatment at this time, for your teeth and gums can need special attention during pregnancy.

Milk and Vitamins are free in any of the following circumstances: (a) if you are pregnant and on supplementary benefit or family income supplement or if your income is below a certain level (at present roughly £38 if you have one child); (b) if you are pregnant and have two children, including foster children, under school age, regardless of your income; (c) if you have three or more children under school age, regardless of your income. To claim for supplies, your doctor, midwife or health visitor should provide you with forms FW8 and FW9. If you quality for free milk, you will be given a token book. The tokens can be used at the clinic or you can give them to your milkman. If you do the latter, you will need a receipt. Tokens are valid for 4 weeks at a time. If you qualify for free vitamins, you should be given these at your local authority clinic (e.g. maternity, child health or welfare food centre). Even if you don't qualify for free supplies, vitamins and milk can be bought at subsidized prices at the above clinics. (For details about vitamins, see under 'Nutrition', p. 355.)

Maternity Grant. This is a grant of £25 to help with the expense of having a baby; with twins you get double. You are still entitled to the grant if the baby is stillborn provided the pregnancy lasts more than 28 weeks. If you are married, you can claim this grant on your husband's National Insurance contributions. If not, claim on your own contributions. Whether or not you get the grant depends on the contributions paid. You can claim the grant any time between the 9th week before the baby is due and 3 months after the birth. Use form BM4, available from your local clinic or social security office.

Maternity Allowance. This is paid weekly for a maximum of 18 weeks and is intended to compensate you for any loss of earnings during your confinement. At present, the rate is £12·90 per week for women who have been fully employed and paying the full earnings-related national insurance contributions. If you have not paid enough contributions you may get a reduced payment or nothing at all. You should claim not later than the 11th week before the expected confinement date or you may lose some of the allowance. Use form BM4 as above. (If you get the maternity allowance you may also be entitled to an earnings related supplement. DHSS leaflet NI 155A explains how.) The government does not allow women under 16 to claim maternity benefits in their own right: it has to be done by their parents.

Maternity Leave. If you have a paid job, you may be able to have paid leave and have your job back after you have had the baby. Unfortunately, the Employment Protection Act, which is supposed to guarantee women's rights while we are pregnant, has many loopholes. For example, the Act does not apply to a large number of part-time workers who are women. The Act does, however, ensure that you cannot be dismissed simply because you are pregnant. If you want paid leave, and if you want your job back afterwards, investigate your position under the Act. *Maternity Rights* by Jean Coussins is an excellent guide.

At present there are no provisions in law for fathers who wish to spend time at home before or after the birth. We hope that something like the Sex Discrimination (Paternity Leave) Bill will eventually become law; it would go some way towards encouraging fathers to participate more fully in childrearing from the beginning. Some unions are now negotiating both longer maternity leave and paternity leave and should be encouraged to do so.

Sickness Benefit. This is available if you have to cease work for medical reasons and you cannot yet claim maternity allowance. Your doctor should sign a medical certificate and send it to your local social security office within 6 days of your having ceased work. The DHSS should then send the money to you.

If you are not eligible for any of these allowances, look into the possibility of getting Supplementary Benefit.

For more details about national insurance benefits, unemployment benefits etc., see Coote and Gill, *Women's Rights: A Practical Guide* and, if you are single, Patricia Ashdown-Sharp, *A Single Women's Guide to Pregnancy and Parenthood.* Also see Bibliography following Postpartum chapter, p. 486.

The Pregnancy Itself

INTRODUCTION

Though your pregnancy will have much in common with other women's, it is also unique. In talking to women who have been pregnant and who are pregnant at the same time you are, you will discover that there's no one, right way to be pregnant. Also realize that when we talk about experiencing changes and emotions, there are many exceptions and many combinations.

You'll all have changes to deal with. You might feel many discomforts, few, or none at all. Some minor discomforts, if neglected, can lead to major complications. And you might want to know that in every pregnancy there's a possibility of miscarriage, so that if it happens to you, you won't be totally unprepared. (See p. 500.)

As for your feelings, they will vary tremendously according to who you are; how you feel about having children; how you feel about your own childhood, your parents, or the people who reared you; whether or not you are with a man – and if you are, how you feel about your man. Sometimes you'll feel positive, sometimes negative. You'll have doubts and fears. It's important to know that these doubts and fears occur during a 'good' pregnancy too, for in a very real sense your body has been taken over by a process out of your control. You can come to terms with that takeover actively and consciously by knowing what's happening to your body, by identifying your specific feelings (especially the negative ones, because they are the most difficult to deal with), and also by learning what the foetus looks like as it grows. Its growth is dramatic and exciting.

The length of a normal pregnancy can vary from 240 to 300 days. We'll divide our discussion into trimesters (approximately three three-month periods). This division will be relevant for some of you and not for others.

FIRST TRIMESTER (FIRST 14 WEEKS)

Physical changes and how to cope with them

You might have none, some, or many of the following early signs of pregnancy. If you have had regular *periods*, you will probably miss a period (amenorrhoea). However, some women do bleed for the first 2 or 3 months even when they are pregnant, but these periods are usually short and there's scant blood. Also, about 7 days or so after conception, the *blastocyst*, the tiny group of cells to become the embryo, attaches itself to the uterine wall, and you might have slight vaginal spotting, called implantation bleeding, for new blood vessels are being formed.

You might have to *urinate* more often because of increased hormonal changes and because your growing uterus presses against your bladder. You will also be more susceptible to *urinary tract infection* (see p. 207). In the first trimester your infection should be treated with sulpha drugs.

Your *breasts* will probably swell. They might tingle, throb, or hurt. Your milk glands begin to develop. Because of an increased blood supply to your breasts, veins become more prominent. Your nipples and the area around them (areola) may darken and become broader.

You may feel *nauseated*, mildly or enough to vomit, partly because your system is changing. There are many theories about the nausea that accompanies pregnancy: that it is peculiar to Western culture; that on some deep level we are disgusted by the animal fact that we are pregnant; that nausea is a result of anxiety and tension, of the many pressures we feel. R. C. Benson for example, in *Current Diagnosis and Treatment*, says that nausea 'may indicate resentment, ambivalence and inadequacy . . .'. On the other hand, in their paper 'Alleged Psychogenic Disorders, a Possible Manifestation of Sexual Prejudice', Jean and John Lennane refute the psychological theories and show how there is a strong organic basis for the nausea that is experienced by between 75% and 88% of pregnant women. If you feel sick, eat lightly throughout the day rather than taking large meals. Don't eat too little, since it is thought that women who suffer morning sickness tend to eat far less than the recommended diet (*Women's Report*, Vol. 1, issue 3, p. 12). Munching crackers or dry toast slowly before you get up in the morning can really help. Avoid greasy, spiced food. Vitamin B$_6$ has been used to stop vomiting in pregnancy (see Davis, *Let's Get Well*). Apricot nectar also helps.*

You may feel constantly *tired*.

You may have increased *vaginal secretions*, either clear and non-irritating, or white, yellow, foamy, or itchy. The chemical makeup, as well as the amount, of your vaginal fluids is changing and because of this you will be more susceptible to thrush. If you are uncomfortable for any reason, see your doctor. (See also 'Vaginal Infections' in Chapter 7.)

The joints between your *pelvic bones* widen and become movable about the 10th or 11th week. Occasionally the separating bones come together and pinch the sciatic nerve, which runs from your buttocks down through the back of your legs.

Your *bowel movements* may become irregular, both because of the pressure of your growing uterus and again because the heightened amount of progesterone relaxes smooth muscle; therefore your bowels might not function as efficiently as they did. Also, if you are resting often, your decreased activity might cause some constipation.

During the first 10 weeks you'll feel relatively few body changes. All those above are fairly common, not too annoying.

Early pregnancy surprised me. I was expecting to feel very different and instead was feeling things I'd felt before. It was like premenstrual tension. I was a little nauseous. But it's amazing, once I realized I was pregnant the symptoms were tolerable, because they are not signs of sickness, but life-producing.

Antenatal care

You must see a doctor as early in your pregnancy as possible so that s/he can give you a complete physical check-up. The earlier and more regularly you obtain antenatal care, the greater the chance of a normal, healthy pregnancy and a live, healthy child (see Peri-Natal Mortality Survey, 1963, HMSO). There is also a greater chance that you will be able to have the baby in a place other than a consultant unit, if you wish to do so (see 'Where to Have the Baby', p. 382).

Antenatal care is free in the UK. It is available in clinics to which you

---

* For a concerned and detailed look at the treatment of nausea, see P. Rhodes in *Practitioner* (see **Bibliography**).

are referred by your G P. These are either attached to a hospital or run by the local authority. Or you can go to a G P for antenatal care (see below). Here are some guidelines for a good antenatal clinic, taken from the Maternity Care Information Sheet compiled by the Association for Improvements in the Maternity Services (the full sheet can be obtained from them):

1. The appointment system should operate so as to avoid excessive waiting.
2. The design of the clinic premises should be such that visual and aural privacy is preserved, and so that tests and consultation can take place in one room or cubicle.
3. Sufficient time should be allowed for patients to discuss their medical and social problems.
4. There should be continuity of care, so that the patient may form a relationship with the people who will attend her during her confinement.*
5. Relevant literature should be prominently displayed and made readily available.
6. Provision should be made for children who have to go with their mothers to the clinic.
7. Local transport facilities should be taken into account when the clinic timetable is being arranged.

As this guide implies, not all clinics fulfil these conditions. One woman recently took action concerning her experiences at an antenatal clinic, writing to the Secretary of State, her M P, the B M A and the administrator of the hospital. She cited among other things the lack of changing facilities and seats, heavily pregnant women being forced to queue and the refusal of doctors to tell her what they were doing to her. Often you have to wait unreasonable lengths of time at antenatal clinics.

'I always have to wait 2½ hours to see him (the consultant).' The consultant's comment: 'She should be prepared to wait 3 hours if necessary'! (*Women's Report*, 2/6)

Or hospitals and doctors' attitudes can sometimes be off-putting. Some people seem to accept this. But you don't have to. You can complain, either to the people mentioned above, and/or to your Local or Community Health Council (see p. 540). You can use the press too. Complaints might not be too successful as far as you are concerned, but they will certainly help all the women who will follow you.

In any case, you do not have to go to a clinic for antenatal care: your own G P can provide this, or if s/he does not do it, you can look up the list

---

* Continuity of care is also important from a technical point of view: it is rarely the case that two observers will reach the same conclusions when judging, say, the rate of increase in size of the uterus; lack of continuity of care can therefore lead to incorrect diagnosis of foetal gestation, and this could lead to problems if, for example, induction is recommended (see pp. 427–32).

of GPs at the Post Office and find one who is on the 'obstetric list'. S/he should then be able to provide you with antenatal care while you retain your own doctor for other purposes.

If clinics and doctors are unpleasant, it is not surprising that some women don't seek antenatal care as early as they should. There are also other reasons why women delay: 'The tragedy of Cathy Charlton, aged 21, who died alone in a bed-sitter with her newly-born baby dead beside her, for fear of making her pregnancy public, highlights the need to encourage more women to seek antenatal care. A survey carried out by the National Children's Bureau shows that in Britain less than 50% of women report to their doctors by the 16th week of pregnancy, whereas the vast majority of French women report by the 12th week. The Bureau . . . points to the 9-month antenatal allowance made available in France plus a maternity grant which encourages women to come forward . . .' (*Women's Report*, Vol. 1, issue 3).

The government inquiries into maternal deaths do not examine the psychological and social pressures which are responsible for women not obtaining antenatal care. Yet such inquiries are likely to put much of the blame for their deaths on the women themselves (see 'Death Tells No Story', *Women's Report*, Vol. 2, issue 6).

The First Antenatal Visit. The examination should consist of:

1. Medical history: menstrual history; previous babies, pregnancies, operations, abortions, illnesses (have you had German measles – rubella?), drugs taken; history of family illnesses, such as heart disease, kidney disease, diabetes,* sickle-cell anaemia.

2. General physical examination. It's important that you try to be complete in your description of what's happened to you physically. Your heart should be listened to: a large number of pregnant women have a heart murmur – often due to bodily changes during pregnancy, but many clinics refer such women to a specialist, just to make sure. Sometimes a chest X-ray for TB is performed. If it is done after 12 weeks, your abdomen should be shielded with a lead apron to protect the foetus (see 'X-rays', p. 361).

3. Examination for pregnancy, which includes: (a) examination of your breasts to see if there are changes in the glands; (b) a pelvic examination, which shows the position and consistency of the uterus, condition of ovaries and fallopian tubes, consistency and colour of the cervix; (c) taking a blood sample to determine its type and Rh factor (see p. 508) and to provide blood for a blood count, haemoglobin analysis, syphilis check-up, and a haematocrit to see if you're anaemic (wrong proportion of cells to fluid). Tests for syphilis can be false positive if you have an infection, such as a cold, so it might sometimes be necessary to have a

* For a discussion of these diseases, their relationship to pregnancy and precautions to be taken, see Gordon Bourne, *Pregnancy*.

re-test; (d) urinalysis to check for urinary infections; (e) weight and blood pressure checks; (f) a cervical smear; (g) a test to see if you have had German measles (rubella)* and a blood sugar test. Diabetics should get frequent tests of blood and urine.

You should be told of vitamin and mineral supplements and you may be given them (see 'Food and Vitamin Supplements', p. 355 and 'Your Rights', p. 362). You should also at this point be told what to take with you if you are having the baby in hospital, and whom to notify when you start labour.

It is usual at the first visit that the hospital bed or the midwife is booked for the delivery. It is therefore crucial that you have thought and discussed carefully the possible alternatives and your preferences (see 'Where to Have the Baby', p. 382). It is also important at this stage that you explain any specific wishes to the doctor and other people concerned — for example, if you wish the father or a friend to be present during labour and the birth, your feelings about pain relief etc. (see 'Companionship', p. 421 and 'Pain Relief', p. 439). In this way, if your doctor, clinic or hospital is uncooperative, you can begin to look elsewhere (see 'Choosing a Doctor', p. 555).

Subsequent Visits. These should be monthly until the 28th week and much shorter. The heartbeat and position of the foetus should be checked, as well as your urine, weight and blood pressure. You should also be able to discuss whether or not to breast-feed (see p. 457) and how to prepare your breasts for this. At 16–18 weeks you should be able to get a blood test screening for foetal abnormality which if positive will lead to further tests (see p. 506). From the 29th to the 36th week, visits will be fortnightly and then every week until the baby is born. During the weekly visits the doctor will also take internal measurements (if s/he hasn't already) to see if your pelvis is large enough for the baby to come through; and will check to see if the cervix is ripe.

If there is any doubt about the size or position of the baby or the number of babies, you will be given a 'scan'. For details of this and other tests, see 'Early Diagnosis', p. 506.

If you are attending a clinic and you need advice or treatment between visits, contact your GP even if s/he does not do antenatal care.

Cooperation Card. In some areas you are given a personal record or 'cooperation' card which you carry throughout your pregnancy and which records the details of each antenatal visit. You can learn to read

---

* If you are not immune to German measles, try to avoid exposure. When you have it, you might have a rash, tenderness of the lymph nodes in the back of your neck, and possibly mild joint pains. If you are exposed in the first trimester of pregnancy, and if you get the disease, chances are high that the foetus will be deformed. At this point you will have to make a decision about whether or not to continue your pregnancy. A blood test will tell you if you have rubella.

your card yourself (if you find the handwriting illegible, politely ask the person examining you to tell you what has been recorded. It's *your* record). Here are some common abbreviations which you may find written on your card (for an example of a card, see Bolton Women's Guide, part 1):

E or Eng	engaged: the baby's head has become fixed between the walls of the pelvic floor, ready for birth.
EDD	expected date of delivery.
Fe	you've been prescribed iron tablets.
FHH	foetal heartbeat heard (you can ask to listen).
FHNH	foetal heartbeat not heard.
FMF	foetal movement felt.
LMP	last menstrual period.
LOA	left occipito anterior ⎫
ROA	right occipito anterior ⎬ refers to the position of the baby's
LOP	left occipito posterior ⎪ head. For an explanation of what
ROP	right occipito posterior ⎭ these mean, see 'Labour', p. 399.
NAD	no abnormal deposit (in the urine). If there were abnormal deposit you could have a kidney infection or toxaemia, which would need to be treated.
T	term (40 weeks pregnant).
Vx	Vertex — the baby's head points down.

Your feelings about Yourself and Your Pregnancy

Some Positive Feelings. You might feel an increased sensuality, a kind of sexual opening out towards the world, heightened perceptions, like being in love. A lot of new energy. A feeling of being really special, fertile, potent, creative. Expectation. Great excitement. Impatience.

Being pregnant meant I was a woman. I was enthralled with my belly growing. I went out right away and got maternity clothes.

It gave me a sense that I was actually a woman. I had never felt sexy before. I went through a lot of changes. It was a very sexual thing. I felt very voluptuous.

It meant I could get pregnant finally after a lot of trying, that I could do something I wanted to do. It meant going into a new stage of life. I felt filled up.

Some Questions. What's going to happen to me? How will being pregnant change me? Will I be able to cope well? Can I physically handle birth? Will I miscarry? How long can I keep my job? Who am I? What image can I form of who I want to be? What is my baby going to be like? What about my man?

Some Negative Feelings. Shock. I'm losing my individuality. I'm not the same any more. I'm a pregnant woman; I'm in this new category, and I don't want to be. I don't want to be a vessel, a carrier. I won't matter to people now, only my baby will. I can't feel anything for this thing growing in me. I can't feel any love. I'm scared. I'm tired. I feel sick. I wish I weren't pregnant. I'm not ready. I don't understand motherhood.

Negative feelings are all relevant and natural. They should be dealt with, not avoided, or ignored. The deeper you go into these feelings, the better prepared you'll be to handle them close to the birth and afterwards.

Sometimes it seemed like I had got pregnant on a whim — and it was a hell of a responsibility to take on a whim. Sometimes I was overwhelmed by what I'd done. A lot of that came from realizing that I had chosen to have the baby without the support of a man. I was scared up until the third trimester that I wasn't going to make it.

Some of you will be too busy to think often about your pregnancy. Others will have more leisure. Some of you will be interested in your pregnancies in different degrees, your awareness switched inward at different times. You might be interested and involved in pregnancy without coming to terms with what it means to have a baby.

When I first felt her move, I knew there was life inside me. But I didn't realize I was having a baby until my doctors literally pulled her out of me upside down and she sneezed, and then she lay next to me and I felt her tiny breath on my fingers.

At the beginning of pregnancy it's sometimes a relief not to think about it, and you can even forget it if you want to. At some point during pregnancy you might want to escape from the inevitability of what is happening to you.

If pregnancy meant anything, it meant being married. I no longer felt it was easy to get out. It was like a seal on the marriage.

Growth of the foetus

This is fantastically exciting to learn about. Knowing what's going on inside our bodies at each stage makes pregnancy a much less alienating and frightening experience than it has often been in the past. We regret that we don't have enough space to describe the step-by-step development of the foetus. But there are several good books on the subject, such as Geraldine Lux Flanagan's *The First Nine Months of Life* (see Bibliography, p. 477) and Anthony Smith's *The Body*, which are available in paperback.

SECOND TRIMESTER (15TH TO 28TH WEEK)

Physical changes and how to cope with them

At about the 4th month the foetus begins its bulkier growth. Your waist becomes thicker and your *clothes* no longer fit. Clothing should be loose and comfortable. Many women modify their own slacks by inserting an elastic panel in the front. Simple smocks and men's shirts are useful and cheap since maternity clothes are often expensive. Ask your friends for any clothes they might have. Your womb starts to swell below your waist, and beginning with the 4th or 5th month you can begin to feel light movements. The foetus has been moving for months, but it's only now that you can feel it. Often you will feel it first just before you fall asleep. You are probably gaining weight now. Eat as well as you can. (See 'Nutrition,' p. 353).

Your circulatory system has been changing, your total blood volume increasing, as your bone marrow produces more blood corpuscles and you drink and retain more liquid. Because of the increase in blood production, you may need more iron. Your heart is changing position and increasing slightly in size.

The line from the navel to the pubic region gets dark, and sometimes pigment in the face becomes dark, making a kind of mask. The mask goes away after pregnancy, but usually the increased colour around your nipples and in the line of your abdomen remains.

Some women salivate more. You might sweat more, which is helpful in eliminating waste material from your body. Sometimes you'll get *cramps* in your legs and feet, perhaps because of disturbed circulation. Calcium can relieve these cramps, as can cramp bark (see *Herbs for Feminine Ailments*). Just relax — the cramps will go away. Or try pulling your foot forward with your hands, massaging afterwards and keeping your feet elevated and warm.

The weight of your uterus increases twenty times, and the greater part of this weight is gained before the 20th week. As your abdomen grows larger the *skin* over it will stretch and lines may appear, pink or reddish streaks. Your skin may become very dry; add oil to your bath and rub your skin with oil.

By mid-pregnancy, your *breasts*, stimulated by hormones, are functionally complete for nursing purposes. After about the 19th week a thin amber or yellow substance called colostrum may come out of your nipples; if it doesn't appear, there is no need to worry: you will still be able to breast-feed. Your breasts are probably larger and heavier than before. If you are planning to breast-feed some experts feel it's a good idea to begin gently massaging your nipples. If your nipples are inverted (turned in), pull them out gently several times a day by putting your thumbs on each side of your nipples, pressing down into the breasts and away from the nipple. The nipples will improve with time, but if progress is too slow, your doctor or midwife can provide you with 'woolwich shells' to help. You should wash your breasts daily with mild soap or clean water. You can support them with a good supportive bra when they begin to feel heavy. The MAVA bra, available from the National Childbirth Trust, is excellent for this purpose; it is also uniquely designed to adjust to the changing size of your breasts, and for ease during breast-feeding.*

Indigestion and *constipation* can occur. You might have *heartburn* because of too much acid in your stomach. Again, a good diet eases these situations. Eat frequent small meals if possible. Avoid greasy foods and coffee. Dried fruit helps constipation, also fresh fruits and vegetables. Drink a lot of fluids. Avoid laxatives containing sodium, such as baking soda, or Alka-Seltzer.

Also, as a result of pressure of pelvic organs, *veins* in your rectum (haemorrhoidal veins) may become dilated and sometimes painful. Lie down with your rectum high and apply ice packs. Witch hazel or some other compress will also help. Or take warm baths and apply vaseline. Proper diet, liquids, regular bowel movements and exercise are important. Varicose veins are veins in your legs that have become enlarged and can hurt. Again because of pressure, the veins and blood vessels that carry blood from your legs to your heart aren't working as smoothly as before. A tendency to varicose veins can be hereditary. Many women find it very helpful to wear support stockings a half size larger than their ordinary stockings. Exercising your feet with legs elevated, is good. And lots of rest.

Many women have *nosebleeds* because of the increased volume of blood and increased nasal congestion, or perhaps because of increased hormone levels (it's also possible to have sympathetic nosebleeds during periods). A little vaseline in each nostril will stop the bleeding.

We want to speak of *oedema* here again (we discussed it in the section on nutrition, p. 358). Oedema is swelling of the face, hands, ankles, wrists, or feet as a result of water retention. Some oedema during pregnancy is normal. Exercise helps squeeze water from the tissue spaces in your blood vessels. If you are uncomfortable, try to lie down with your feet raised several times a day. Exercising your feet while your legs are up helps circulation and to pump fluid around. Cut down on carbohydrates for a while, and get more physical rest. If oedema persists, check with your doctor.

Toxaemia (see 'Nutrition', p. 357): you might at this stage develop high blood pressure, oedema, or protein in your urine.† You might have mild

* For more on antenatal care of the breasts, see 'Care of the Breasts and Nipples' by the NCT (5p).

† Toxaemia develops mainly in very young (under 16) women, older women, and women with their first pregnancy. Women with diabetes, high blood pressure and chronic kidney disease are most susceptible, as are women who carry twins, or have too much fluid in their uteri.

pre-eclampsia, with the symptoms mentioned in the paragraph above. You should check with your doctor. Your blood pressure should be observed on at least two occasions at least 6 hours apart, and the amount of albumin (a protein) in your urine must be checked at least twice. Towards the third trimester you might have severe pre-eclampsia, indicated by very high blood pressure, a large amount of protein in your urine with a decrease in the amount of urine, blurred vision, a severe continuous headache, or swelling of your face and fingers. Severe pre-eclamptic conditions can develop in a few hours. Unless these pre-eclamptic stages are checked immediately, eclampsia – convulsions and coma – might occur. (Pre-eclamptic conditions *must* be treated in the hospital; your life and your baby's are at stake.) There is disagreement about the treatment of pre-eclampsia, with various claims made for the restriction of weight gain, curtailment of salt, hormonal treatments, and the use of diuretics. *The incidence of toxaemia of pregnancy is much lessened by constant prenatal care and supervision, and good diet.* Get as much rest as you possibly can.

Your Feelings

Many of us watch ourselves growing outward so quickly with mixed emotions. Our confusion is legitimate. During pregnancy we change from the slim wraiths we were (supposed to be) to large-bellied women. We are making a visible transition from one role to another, moving from one myth to another. Some women try to hide their pregnancies from the world and even from themselves either by continuing for a time to wear the same clothes as before, though they no longer fit, or by wearing clothes so baggy that no one can see what is happening underneath.

You've got to find yourself beyond and in spite of these myths. It's possible to feel comfortable and happy with the changes you are going through.

Whatever you are feeling, the first movements you feel your baby make can be very beautiful and moving.

I was lying on my stomach and felt – something, like someone lightly touching my deep insides. Then I just sat very still and for an alive moment felt the hugeness of having something living growing in me. Then I said, No, it's not possible, it's too early yet, and then I started to cry . . . That one moment was my first body awareness of another living thing inside me.

And after the first movement – in the fourth or fifth month – you might wait days for another sign of quickening. Then the movements will become frequent and familiar. You can feel from the outside the hard shape of your uterus.

If you are feeling angry, upset, or threatened by pregnancy, then your baby's movements serve to focus your anger. You might feel increasingly taken over.

Last night its kicking made me dizzy and gave me a terrible feeling of solitude. I wanted to tell it, Stop, stop, stop, let me alone. I want to lie still and whole and all single, catch my breath. But I have no control over this new part of my being, and this lack of control scares me. I felt as if I were rushing downhill at such a great speed that I'd never be able to stop.

Perhaps feeling the baby move for the first time will change you.

Sitting on a rock overlooking the domesite, trees growing right out of the rock. They cling and flourish on nothing. Images of the growing life inside me, also coming from nothing, getting nutrition from my body the way the tree does from the rock . . . Occasionally I give it warmth, mostly when it moves. The more it moves, the more I like it. I also resent it an awful lot; I feel big, ugly and uncomfortable, and in spite of Len's protestations, I feel alone.

Even during the most positive pregnancies there may be moments, hours and days of depression, anxiety and confusion. These depressions can be connected to underground anxieties in relation to your mother and your childhood; doubts that come from our society's ignorance about pregnancy and childbirth; doubts you have about your own identity; economic problems; having too many children already; and problems in your relationship with your man.

It seems that my feelings about my pregnancy, my body, the coming of the baby, were inextricably wound into my feelings, problems, hopes and fears for our relationship . . . It's hard to separate which feelings were a result of my unhappiness about us (a lot of the bad feelings about my body arose because Bob showed very little interest in my enlarged, changing body); which ones were my own negative feelings about having a less functional body (I wanted to keep working and active, but my body was so cumbersome that I was always worn out and tired); and which ones were just moods caused by pregnancy.

We all have general fears too. Fear of the unknown, especially if it's a first pregnancy. And by becoming pregnant we open ourselves to possible changes, complications and events that are risks in a sense. We become much more vulnerable.

I remember feeling overwhelmed by sad things I saw, and was overwhelmed by things that could happen to innocence. I'd wake in the night and think people were going to come in and take things, take the baby from me. I was beginning to be out of control. I was terribly afraid of chance. I've always been afraid of irrationality, of fate.

We fear that our babies will be deformed. Four per cent of babies are born with diseases and one per cent with severe physical malformations (see p. 505). Some of us have dreams, fantasies and nightmares about deformity. These are universal.

When I was about six months pregnant and Dick was starting school again, I was home alone, isolated for days at a time. My nightmares and daydreams started around then. Really terrible fears of the baby being deformed. All my life I've always been the good girl. I knew I wasn't really good. I knew I had bad thoughts, but I was never allowed to express them. So I thought that my baby's deformities would be the living proof of the ugliness and badness in me.

We fear our own death, the child's death.

In fact, we do have to face the fact that some women miscarry, and some babies die. (See p. 500.) While it's difficult, threatening and sad to think of, we know it happens. Though it's not usually useful, and is also very hard, to prepare ourselves for death, it helps to know what has happened to some of us in case we or our friends experience such tragedy. Knowledge is a kind of preparation. It's vitally important to be able to reach out to friends when tragic things happen, and to help break down their feelings of isolation. It also helps us to know that we can and need to ask for help if such a thing happens to us.

To deny that unpleasant things happen is to deny to ourselves and to our friends the reality and totality of our experience. Recognition of misfortune is an affirmation.

And then, we feel guilty about having fears. Don't they in some way suggest that as mothers we will be weak and inadequate? The myth is that we can't allow ourselves these depressions, because we are supposed to be strong, mature, maternal, accepting, loving all the time.

It's vital to us to realize that our feelings are legitimate. We should feel free and right in expressing them.

Men's Feelings About You and Your Pregnancy

How will the man you are involved with feel about you? That depends on how you feel about yourself; on the relationship between you; on how he feels about himself, and what he feels his part to be in your pregnancy. If he feels like getting involved, it's a very good idea to prepare with him and learn together, especially if he lives with you after your baby is born. He might feel attracted to you and close, and fascinated by your growing body. Or, for reasons having to do with his own background and upbringing, with his hang-ups, he might feel repelled, confused and threatened by all your changes and your impending motherhood (his impending fatherhood). Or he might feel positive sometimes, negative sometimes. One man says:

Sometimes I thought you were very beautiful and your belly was beautiful.

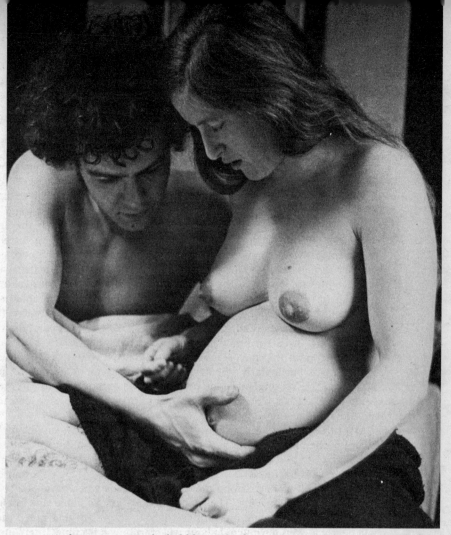

And sometimes you looked like a ridiculous pregnant insect. Your navel bulging out looked strange.

If you are having problems it's certainly best if you can talk together and realize that often your and his complex feelings are changeable. Talk can also lead to some deep, good questioning about the conventional ideas of beauty we are all brainwashed with. It's possible that he won't be able to talk about or to cope at all with the changes and responsibilities that your pregnancy implies. He might be jealous or resentful. Some men for many reasons seek out women other than the pregnant woman they are living with, whether they're married or unmarried. Some men, while not actually leaving you, may withdraw from you emotionally at this crucial time.

If you are single and get involved with men during your pregnancy, these men will all have different kinds of attitudes towards you as a person, as a pregnant women, and as a sexual being.

Intercourse

Intercourse towards the end of pregnancy is usually not dangerous, but you should not make love at any time during your pregnancy (1) if you have vaginal or abdominal pain, (2) if you have any uterine bleeding, (3) if your membranes have already ruptured (then there is danger of infection). If you have miscarried before, avoid intercourse for the first 3 months during the time your period is due. That's important for you psychologically, so that if a miscarriage should occur, you won't consider yourself responsible. And for the same reasons you shouldn't masturbate or make love to orgasm as this could bring on miscarriage.* Masters and Johnson have some evidence that the contractions of orgasm could set off labour, but the women in their study were close to term anyway. (In some cultures women ready to go into labour make love to induce labour.) If you have a threatened miscarriage or recurrent ones, it is best to cease intercourse until the doctor advises that it can be resumed (Bourne, p. 166). This is particularly important in the first 3 months and the last 10–12 weeks. Throughout your pregnancy, be aware that during oral-genital contact, air blown into your vagina may be dangerous, causing air embolism.

All these remarks refer to unusual circumstances. It's useful to be aware of them, for our main worries are that we will harm the baby in some (unknown) way. The truth is that intercourse during pregnancy is almost always harmless.

Some of you will get strong uterine contractions when you make love or when you masturbate. These contractions are valuable and useful. They strengthen the uterine muscles. If you lie quietly and relax, they will nearly always die down. Labour will start only if it's time. Intercourse can be a good exercise for the muscles of the pelvic floor. Also note how completely you can relax after making love. It's helpful to know how it feels to relax, because later, during labour contractions, that kind of complete relaxation can be useful.

Later in your pregnancy the 'traditional' position (man on top) can be uncomfortable. Pillows under your back can make you more comfortable. Sheila Kitzinger recommends that 'The first prescription for intercourse during pregnancy is to go out and buy some more pillows – more

---

* Some recent studies are finding that a substance in a man's semen, called prostaglandin, and possibly a like substance created by a woman's orgasm, can induce labour a little earlier than it might ordinarily occur.

than you think you will need. (They will come in very useful afterwards when feeding the baby on the bed.)' (From an article 'Sex in Pregnancy', available from the National Childbirth Trust.) But at no time should the man's whole weight rest on you, nor should great pressure be put upon your uterus. You can use other positions more happily; you can be on top, or he behind you. You can be side by side or sitting. Or, you might not want intercourse at all but might prefer to use hands, a tongue, or a vibrator. For more on sex during pregnancy see the above article or *The Experience of Childbirth* (Penguin), and p. 50, 'There's More than Intercourse'.

Your Feelings about Making Love. You'll each have many different feelings about making love.

I remember feeling very sexy. We were trying all these different positions. Now that we were having a baby, I felt a lot looser, a lot freer. I used to feel uptight about sex for its own sake, but when I was pregnant I felt a lot freer.

I felt very ambivalent about making love. I had miscarried several times. I wanted to make love and I was scared to make love. As a single woman it was hard to find men who found me attractive with my belly so big. I had no sexual contact at all the last two months.

Some of you might have times when you really turn inward, when you won't want or be able to 'give' to a man.

Masters and Johnson report an increase in sexual desire during the second trimester and a decrease during the third.

If You Are Living with a Group of People

It's a good idea to think about how you want them to relate to your child. Some communities exist that are themselves large extended families. But many groups are composed of people who will have very different commitments to your child. Often people don't want to have anything much to do with taking care of children. They either don't want to or don't feel ready to. Try to work out just what you are expecting of each person and whether your expectations are realistic. Talk to each person if you can and find out how s/he feels about your coming child. Do it early.

You can't assume that people will automatically help on their own and know you need help. Also, with people who don't have children you have to be explicit and tell them what to do. I don't think it's a good thing to have a lot of people take care of the baby at first, but I was glad that people helped me out. Also find out how they feel about you. Having chosen these people as your new family, you might expect to be cared for and nurtured, and you might find that people won't be able to meet your increased needs.

THIRD TRIMESTER (29TH WEEK TO TERM — 40 WEEKS)

Physical Changes

Your uterus is becoming very large.

I remember my friends' surprise when they put their hands on my belly to feel it. They expected it to be soft and somehow jellylike and were amazed at its hardness and bulk.

You can feel and see the movements of your foetus from the outside now too, as it changes position, turns somersaults, hiccups. Sometimes it puts pressure on your bladder, which makes you feel that you need to urinate even when you don't, and which can hurt a little, or sometimes a lot, for very brief periods. Sometimes, towards the end of pregnancy, it puts pressure on the nerves at the top of your legs, which can be painful too.

Your baby will be lying in a particular position, sometimes head down, back to your front, sometimes crossways. It moves around. Your doctor can help you discover which position the baby is in.

Sometimes your baby lies still. It's known that babies sleep in utero. If you don't feel movement for 48 hours in this last part of your pregnancy and you're wondering, call your doctor if you can and ask whether s/he thinks it's a good idea to check the foetal heartbeat. Usually these are periods of 'rest' for the baby and can last several days.

You will feel your uterus tighten every now and then. These are painless contractions called Braxton-Hicks contractions. They are believed to strengthen uterine muscles, preparing them for eventual labour. (See p. 399.)

It becomes increasingly uncomfortable for you to lie on your stomach. You might experience shortness of breath. There's pressure on your lungs from your uterus, and your diaphragm may be moved up as much as an inch. Even so, because your thoracic (chest) cage widens, you breathe in more air when you are pregnant than when you are not. Sometimes when you lie down you might not be able to breathe well for a moment. Prop yourself up with pillows and the pressure on your diaphragm will be lessened.

The peak load on your heart occurs in about the 30th week. After that the heart doesn't have to work so hard, usually, until delivery.

You are still gaining weight. If you have haemorrhoids or varicose veins, try to avoid standing up for long periods of time, and when you sit or lie down, be sure your feet are raised. 'Since pregnant women are notoriously deficient in vitamin B_6, a lack of this vitamin may prove to be the cause of the haemorrhoids so common during this period' (Davis, *Let's Get Well*, p. 134).

Your stomach is pushed up by your uterus and flattened. Indigestion is common. Eat small amounts. Take Gelusil or Milk of Magnesia, very mild medication. Sucking on the tablets is better than swallowing them. Don't take mineral oil — it causes you to excrete necessary vitamins. Avoid indigestion remedies that contain sodium, such as Andrews Liver Salts or Alka-Seltzer.

If you have insomnia, or trouble sleeping because of the baby moving around, take walks, hot baths, or some wine at bedtime. Avoid sleeping pills.

Your navel will probably be pushed out. Since your body has become heavier, you'll tend to walk differently for balance, often leaning back to counteract a heavier front. This can cause backaches, for which there are exercises. But the Alexander Technique (see p. 134) can enable you to prevent backaches. Your pelvic joints are also much more separated.

At about 4 to 2 weeks before birth, and sometimes as early as the 7th month, the baby's head settles into your pelvis. This is called 'lightening', or 'dropping' or 'engagement'. It takes pressure off your stomach. Some women feel much lighter. And if you have been having trouble breathing, pressure is now off your diaphragm. This 'dropping' can cause constipation; your bowels are more obstructed than they were.

As for water retention, an average pregnant woman retains from $6\frac{1}{2}$ to 13 pints of liquid, half of this in the last 10 weeks. Ankle swelling is common.

Your Feelings about Yourself and Your Pregnancy

I thought it would never end. I was enormous. I couldn't bend over and wash my feet. And it was incredibly hot.

At the end I started to feel it was too long. Dick took pictures of me during the eighth month. I saw my face as faraway and sad.

Fairly confidently and calmly awaiting the baby — quite set on a home delivery. Doctor said Thursday I was already dilated two and a half centimetres, so it must be getting close. Getting a bit anxious, listening to every Braxton-Hicks contraction, awaiting with hope and fear too, its change into the real thing.

I felt exultant and tired and rich inside. My belly is large, and last night the baby beat around inside it like a wild tempest. I thought the time had come and was panicked and nauseated, then very excited. I woke Gene up. Then at five I fell asleep. Meanwhile I move in slow motion and wait.

My kid is dancing inside under my heart.

The relationship of mother carrying child is most beautiful and simplest. I pity a baby who must come out of the womb.

13 Childbirth

Even if we haven't had a baby before, most of us have heard or read something about labour and delivery. We may be looking forward to the event with excitement and eager anticipation, or we may fear that labour will be hard for us to endure and wish we didn't have to go through with it. Much of our expectation is based on other women's stories or on our own previous experiences. By preparing ourselves for childbirth we will be giving ourselves more control over it: preparation for childbirth means finding ways to make childbirth more understandable, less frightening, and finding someone to share with and support us during the experience.

If you don't prepare for childbirth you probably won't be able to resist the hospital routine of drugs and interventions. If you have never thought about preparation before, we hope you will read this chapter as a description of a way to make an important choice in your life as a woman. If you have been considering preparation, we hope this chapter will be a useful overview.

Since, for the time being, most women in the United Kingdom are going to be having their babies in hospital, we are going to spend a good deal of this chapter talking about what that experience is like and how to handle it. However, there are growing numbers of women who don't want to have to fight the hospital and the doctors just to have a normal, untampered-with birth. Many of these women are choosing to try to have their babies at home.

Where to Have the Baby

The decision as to where to have the baby should be your decision. You may decide on hospital, you may decide on home, or you may change your mind half-way through your pregnancy.

Whichever course she chooses, a woman is likely to be better off where she feels safest, whether in hospital or at home. Often there is too much emphasis

on the 'medical' side and not enough on the woman's own attitudes and feelings.
Women should always have the choice of the kind of care and medical attention
they feel to be most suitable for them. A woman's state of mind is an important
factor for happy and straightforward childbirth. (Society to Support Home
Confinements)

In this section we try to provide as much information as possible to
enable a real choice to be made, as well as to show the factors which can
affect or limit our choice. Since the scales are so heavily weighted against
the possibility of obtaining a home birth, we have devoted a large part of
this section to this aspect of the subject. By doing so, we do not intend to
imply that women should have a home birth any more than that women
should have a hospital birth. We look forward to the time when the right
to choose where to have a baby will have become a reality.

Your decision about where to have the baby hinges on a variety of
factors, not the least of which is what the facilities and the set-up are in
your area. But another very important factor concerns the advice you
are given by your doctor(s). The majority of doctors believe that most, if
not all, babies should be born in hospital. There is, however, no scientific
evidence for this argument. The main reason doctors give for recommending a hospital birth is that they believe it is safer. The evidence cited is
that the mortality rate for mothers and babies has gone down at the same
time as hospital births have increased. But just because the death rates
have gone down does not mean to say that hospital births are the cause.
A multitude of other factors can be cited as responsible for the reduction
of deaths, e.g. higher living standards, improved general health, smaller
families, better antenatal care, etc. Indeed, a recent study in Cardiff of
all births from 1965–73 showed that virtually universal hospitilization
resulted in no significant decrease in the deaths of newborn babies at all
(Chalmers *et al., British Medical Journal,* 27 March 1976). Nor were the
risks of maternal mortality reduced either. Another study of some 170
local authorities between 1956 and 1969 shows that while in the first
part of the period authorities with the higher hospital confinement rates
tended to have lower mortality rates and vice versa, by 1968 the trend
was reversed: those with most hospital births also tended to have higher
mortality rates (Fryer and Ashford, *British Journal of Preventive and Social*
Medicine, 1972, *26,* 1). Nonetheless, the number of hospital births in
Britain has increased from 15% in 1927 to about 95% in 1976. This has
been happening gradually and has been due, to some degree at least, to the
publication of two particular government reports. The decision to achieve
100% hospital births took place in 1959 with the publication of the
Cranbrook Report. The *Peel Report,* published in 1970, added weight to
this decision. The basis of the reports' conclusions was by no means
scientific, and social and psychological aspects were not considered. No
consumers of the maternity services were represented on the committees,

which consisted entirely of doctors. The Department of Health's policy
is still based on this 'expert' opinion.

Another reason why hospital births are advocated is an 'economic'
one. This is particularly argued where there are new hospitals, which
are very expensive to run compared with old ones: unless beds are kept
full, the management starts asking questions. Since the birth rate is
declining, there is more and more pressure to keep the maternity beds
filled. In fact, if there *is* a domiciliary service available, and if it is used, as
in Holland, the figures show that it is cheaper to have the baby at home.
This is not to say that on economic grounds women should have their
babies at home. It is simply to point out that there is no economic argument for running down the domiciliary service.

One reason why hospitals are not in themselves particularly safe is
because of infection: contrary to what the BMA's booklet *You and Your
Baby* implies, infectious germs in hospital present more of a threat to a
mother and her baby than do those at home (see 'Hospital infection,
causes and prevention', Williams *et al.*, p. 480).

Are Home Births Unsafe?

The *Report on Confidential Enquiries into Maternal Deaths in England and
Wales* (1970–72) reveals that for the 10·4% of mothers delivered at home,
the maternal death rate was lower than 0·055%. *But this point is not
made by the report,* which shows a comparatively high number of deaths
(44) among women booked for home births compared with 393 deaths
among the 89·6% of women booked for confinement in other institutions.
However, these are only the figures for booking – not the *actual* materni-
ties which occurred at home! In fact, only 14 of the 44 deaths could be
linked to home confinement: for example, some had been rebooked for a
hospital birth, some had died during pregnancy, and some had been
admitted to hospital prior to delivery. As the SSHC points out, the report
is based on 'an extraordinary calculation and hardly worthy of a government publication'.

The evidence from other countries is also relevant. In Holland, for
example, where about 50% of births take place at home, the infant mortality rate per 1,000 live births is 13·1 compared with 18 in England and
Wales; the maternal mortality rate is 19·4 per 100,000 live births in
both countries. Dutch obstetricians point out that when the labour of a
normal woman is unhurried and allowed to progress normally, unexpected emergencies rarely occur. They also point out that the small
risk involved in a Dutch home delivery is more than offset by the increased
hazards resulting from the use of obstetrical medication and tampering –
both of which are more likely to occur in hospital (see Haire, *The Cultural*

Warping of Childbirth). Unfortunately now, even in Holland there is a push towards hospitalization.

Some women feel that if they desire a home birth, even if their pregnancy is normal, they may be harming the baby. Others fear that, if their baby is born handicapped, a hospital might insist on trying to keep it alive, no matter what; they may therefore prefer the idea of a home birth where they would be spared the decision of whether or not to allow the use of special machines to do this. In her new book, *The Place of Birth*, Sheila Kitzinger relates the story of one woman who experienced a stillbirth at home, yet who still felt strongly that a home birth was best. She liked being able to participate in what was happening during the half-hour fight for the baby's life: 'It was a great comfort to me that I was not lying in the formal atmosphere of the hospital, shut away with soothing words, probably given Valium, not allowed to see the baby. As it was, the fact that she was not going to live dawned on me gradually . . . it was far more bearable than it might have been.'

In conclusion, home birth is safe, for certain women in certain circumstances (see below). We can only add that the value of hospitalization has been seriously questioned in other spheres (e.g. coronary care) where home care has been shown to have slightly better results than that in 'intensive care' units in hospitals. As we go to press, *The Place of Birth* (edited by Kitzinger and Davis) uses similar criteria to question mandatory hospitalization of labouring women. Read it if you want to examine the issues in more detail.

HIGH-RISK WOMEN

Ninety per cent of all pregnancies proceed normally with few or no problems at all. Most of the problems can be predicted with good antenatal care and screening. For women with the following conditions, a hospital birth is best: toxaemia, very high blood pressure, kidney, heart or circulation trouble, epilepsy or any condition which can become critical, previous severe postpartum haemorrhage or Caesarean section, very premature labour, postmature labour of more than just a few days, multiple pregnancy, and any illness to which pregnancy is an additional problem. A previous forceps delivery does not necessarily indicate a hospital birth. Nor does the fact that a woman is small in stature (under 5 ft 2 ins), provided she is otherwise well-nourished and her pregnancy proceeds normally.

Women who are very young (16 or under) tend to have more difficult labours and more problems in general so it would be best for them to have their babies in hospital. Otherwise age should not in itself prevent you from having a home birth, unless you are over 40 or well into your 30s. But many doctors in Britain refuse a home birth to women if they are over

25: this is not a valid reason in itself for refusing a home birth. The ideal childbearing age is between 22 and 32, varying from race to race and culture to culture. Pregnant women outside this age-range should pay particularly close attention to their health and the preparation for possible complications.

In Britain, the most common reason doctors give for refusing a home birth is 'It's your first baby'. Again, this is not a valid reason for disallowing a home birth. Nor is it necessary for all fifth and subsequent babies to be born in hospital if there are no complications and the previous labour was normal.

There is a high risk if the baby is presenting abnormally (see p. 410). In many cases, the baby can be turned the right way (see p. 412), but even if it can't, it is still possible to give birth to a breech baby at home safely, provided there is an adequate back-up service. Bleeding during the third trimester could mean that a Caesarean would be necessary (because the placenta is lying over the cervix, or is becoming detached). This problem can be predicted with good antenatal care.

We cannot emphasize enough the importance of good ante-natal care for all pregnant women. However, for those contemplating a home birth, this is even more essential (if that is possible!). Only with the solid foundation of good ante-natal care can a real choice concerning place of delivery be possible (see Moore and Ashford in *The Place of Birth*, edited by Kitzinger and Davis).

Rarely, even in low-risk mothers, problems can occur which are not predictable. These include lack of progress in labour, foetal or maternal distress, abnormal bleeding before, during or after the birth, prolapsed cord (meaning that the cord is being born first). If we are aware of these possible complications they can be spotted quickly and proper action can be taken. This can only happen if there is an adequate emergency service – flying squad – in the area.

I pee into a bucket and out comes the show which is more red than I expected. This doesn't worry me very much but it was at this time that Kate (the midwife) informed the doctor. The dawn is now coming through the shutters and I'm feeling quite cheerful when he arrives. He and Kate trot out of the room. When they return he tells me he's called an ambulance to take me to Barts because I need hospital cover as I am bleeding. I look at Kate and see that she thinks so too. I am extremely lucky in knowing Kate and the doctor so well that I'm confident that they wouldn't call an ambulance unless I really needed to go to hospital. I feel calm about it. I think I had unconsciously felt that Kate was worried when she saw that I was bleeding. I can hear Ron asking Kate if she'll come too and help him stop the hospital doing anything unnecessary. [This woman went on to be delivered in hospital by Kate herself with the marvelling hospital staff looking on.]

See 'Home – The Right to Choose', for details about home confinements.

Having a Baby in Hospital

Even if we are strong and healthy some of us prefer having a baby in hospital. We may feel it is safer there both for us and the baby, and want to have rest and help after the baby is born (bear in mind, however, that some women find it easier to rest at home).

CHOOSING A HOSPITAL

Hospitals vary a lot, even between wards and consultants. Before choosing a hospital it is well worth investigating their different rules and practices and the reasons for them.* This can also help us make up our minds if we're not sure whether we want a hospital or home birth. There is no reason why we shouldn't change hospitals as long as this is done early enough. Here are some of the questions we may want to ask.

1. *General rules:* these are sometimes made for the benefit of mothers, but sometimes they appear to be arbitrary and can be distressing. The following is the experience of one mother at two different hospitals; the first was a teaching hospital in London, the other, a small maternity home in Yorkshire.

The London hospital was run on flexible and permissive lines – there were no rules that were unreasonable or unnecessary. The Yorkshire home . . . was rule-laden and authoritarian. This structure was reinforced by the whims of some of the nursing staff, who seemed to make up rules and even reverse them to suit themselves. On one occasion I was told to put a pillow under the baby on my lap whilst breast-feeding, only to be harangued by a sister for 'spoiling hospital equipment'. Patients were not allowed to lie on the bed, except at the official 'rest' periods . . . All baths had to be taken between 7 a.m. and 8 a.m. and since there was one bath to twelve people and only sufficient water for three baths at a time, the others all had cold baths. This meant that the salt tablets that are given to heal stitches would not melt and were therefore ineffective. (Sue Lees, *New Society*, 25 April 1974)

Ask about the points mentioned above, and try and talk to women who have had children in the hospital.

2. *Can your partner/friend be with you at the birth?* Early father-child contact is desirable in order for both to feel secure with each other and for both mother and father to feel able to share their child from the word 'go' (see 'Companionship', p. 421, for an example of a father's experiences

---

* It is also worth checking that stated policies are actually carried out in practice – sometimes they are not. Local NCT teachers (see p. 419) are perhaps in the best position to offer advice on this matter, since they have continuous experience of hospitals' practices via their pupils – i.e. other women.

and further discussion). Not all hospitals allow the father to be present at the birth and sometimes men are not even allowed to hold their babies. As the Patients' Association advised one father: 'It will be *your* baby . . . It belongs to you and your wife, not to the hospital. So if your baby is normal and healthy, go ahead' (*Patient Voice*, No. 2). If you want your partner or another companion to be present during labour and the birth, be sure to ask early whether this is allowed. If you're unsure early on whether you want the father there, you will at least know you have a choice.

3. *Visiting:* It is not now common for fathers to be restricted in visiting but visits from the rest of your family, particularly other children, may be curtailed. This is often explained as necessary in order to enable other mothers to have peace. But it ignores the disruption that may be caused, especially to the other siblings of the newborn baby. No hospital maternity wing should be so designed that the visiting of children has to be restricted.

Increasingly, many women may have to go to a hospital far away from home. This is because many smaller, local hospitals are being shut down in favour of district general hospitals situated in larger towns. This may make the cost of visiting prohibitively expensive for your partner. Ask the social worker at the hospital about how you can be helped with these expenses.

4. *What happens during labour?* Some hospitals insist that mothers in labour stay in bed. If a woman is allowed to walk about for as long as she wishes – at least until the membranes have ruptured – this can encourage engagement of the baby's head; it can also bring relief from the discomfort or pain of contractions.

Check that the hospital does not insist on women lying down to give birth. We discuss on p. 409 how unhelpful and even dangerous this can be. In many hospitals when you are about to give birth you have to transfer from your bed in the labour room to a trolley which takes you to the delivery room. It is worth trying to find a hospital which will enable you to stay in the same room to give birth – they are becoming more common.

5. *Pain relief:* Check what the policy is. Can you have what you want when you want it? Can you refuse treatments without a fuss? What is the hospital's attitude to natural childbirth methods? Will you be given pethidine against your will? Can you have an epidural if you want one? (See 'Pain Relief', p. 439.)

6. *Obstetrical intervention:* If you give birth in a hospital you are far more likely to come across one or more of the common obstetrical procedures such as induction or stimulation of labour, forceps or episiotomy (for more on these see p. 424). Any such procedure carries some risk –

justifiable if it is necessary but hardly so on other occasions. Check the policy of the hospital and the particular attendant in charge – though this will still not necessarily guarantee you the kind of birth you want even if there are no complications.

7. *Can you have your baby with you?* Some hospitals do not allow mothers to be with their children after delivery for hours or even days despite all the evidence about the importance of early mother-child contact and many mothers' wishes. Research shows that conventional hospital routines tend to inhibit maternal response, such as routines involving only brief contact immediately after delivery and then from 6–12 hours later, or four-hourly feeding sessions. See also 'Postnatal Depression', p. 470, which can be caused or exacerbated by separation. Even in the case of a sick baby, separation is rarely necessary so it is also worth checking on the hospital's rate of admission to Special Care Baby Units (see p. 439 for further discussion).

'Put that baby down,' the ward sister called as she strutted across the corridor towards me, indignantly: 'You know the rules of the hospital.' I glanced at the 2-day-old baby crying fiercely in my arms and wondered whom to give way to. 'Your first child, I assume?' . . . 'No,' I replied, 'I have another.' 'I suppose that's molly-coddled too.' (Lees, Hospital Confinement)

You should also find out whether the hospital has facilities for 'rooming in', whereby you can keep the baby with you in the ward, or 'modified rooming in' – part ward, part nursery (see p. 450).

8. *Attitudes to breast-feeding:* Even though national policy is now in favour of breast-feeding, not all hospitals are encouraging and some by their practices actively discourage. Check whether there is a policy of scheduled feeding or feeding on demand, and whether mothers are allowed to feed immediately after the birth. Four-hourly schedules are particularly inhuman for breast-fed babies because the quantity of a mother's milk varies throughout the day and is of such a consistency that more frequent feeding is necessary. In any case, all babies seem to thrive on frequent, moderate feeds. If we want to breast-feed we have to be well-informed and prepared (see Feeding, p. 457).

9. *How soon can you go home?* Policies vary enormously on this. You may be able to leave after 6 hours, 48 hours or you may have to stay in for at least a week. You should have a choice about what you want to do. (See also Early Discharge, p. 392.)

WHAT DOES IT FEEL LIKE GIVING BIRTH IN HOSPITAL?

The strange environment of a hospital can be disconcerting at the very least. Some hospitals have made an effort to improve the environment, lessen inflexible routines and impersonal behaviour, for example the

West Middlesex. This hospital also enables women to be supervised by the same midwife throughout the pregnancy, birth and postpartum period. Another hospital in the West Midlands is prepared to assist women to give birth in any way they wish, provided the birth is normal (AIMS newsletter, March 1976). However, bear in mind that the very nature of hospital makes it difficult to contemplate this ever being the same as giving birth at home: their hierarchical nature, and the different interests of patients and staff militate against this.

The inhumanity that many hospitals have to offer mothers has been known for some time. For example, the *Cranbrook Report* (1959) comments on 'A general complaint that there was in many hospitals too little regard for the personal dignity and emotional condition of women during pregnancy and childbirth'. (See also *Human Relations in Obstetrics* (HMSO, 1961) and *Human Relations in Obstetric Practice* (*Lancet*, 1960). But there has been no official public discussion of this subject since then.

I was accused of not telling them that my waters had already broken . . . and then they tried to break them, but got no result. Turning their backs on me they started muttering things like, 'Well, you know what this looks like, don't you,' and using abbreviations I didn't know the meaning of. Finally Sister pronounced I must be shaved completely in case I needed a Caesarean! By this time I was in tears as I felt so alone and utterly panic-stricken at the thought of a general anaesthetic which had never crossed my mind at all . . . How badly I needed a few words of comfort but I had got on the wrong side of Sister and she was being very efficient but very remote . . . a middle-aged ward orderly was the first person to say something kind to me. (Newcastle NCT newsletter, 1976)

There were three of them shouting and nagging trying to force an unwanted mask on my face . . . I hadn't even groaned and was so happy till then. One of them told me that she couldn't bear screaming; they didn't even pretend it was really for my benefit. (AIMS newsletter, 1975)

The whole experience of my second pregnancy was much better. At the Withington in Manchester one didn't have to ask for nighties or nappies whereas in St Mary's (Leeds) it was God help you if you'd changed a nighty and the baby was sick . . . My GP was very good, although of course the fact that we were 'middle-class' and Nick worked for the health service helped. He gave me a lot of confidence with this second pregnancy. The hospital was going to induce it 'because the baby isn't growing properly'; I went to the GP horrified, who told me not to listen to them and to go into hospital when I wanted to.

We had a super doctor and midwife in attendance (in hospital) who explained everything that happened, showing us the afterbirth and let us have a long cuddling session with our baby. (Newcastle NCT newsletter, 1976)

I went into hospital to have a baby, fully conscious and with joy. I was subjected to the degradation of being on a bloody production line. I was insulted, intimidated, treated like a lump of meat on a slab. I'm in the process of writing out my birth experience (after 16 months) in an attempt to purge my bitterness. I will never get over it and will fight for women's rights in pregnancy and birth as long as there is a struggle. (Peace News, February 1976)

GP UNITS

GP units are usually in a separate building close to a hospital. They are run by midwives, with a GP being in charge of each mother. Some are excellent with fewer rules and routines than in ordinary hospital maternity units; they also provide continuity of care throughout pregnancy, birth and the postpartum period. The atmosphere is less clinical and more informal so that it is easier for the human side of the staff to emerge. However, other GP units may be as bad as the worst hospitals: you will have to make enquiries, e.g. from local NCT teachers, to find out about your own local unit (if there is one − see below).

She [the midwife] had got me into the GP unit and there she stayed with me. It was lovely, just David, me, her and a pupil midwife. I had no medical treatment whatever and all went perfectly. I was given my own room and left in peace with Melanie. (from a letter to the Society to Support Home Confinements, 1975)

GP units tend to be available only for women with 'normal' pregnancies, which does reduce their advantage over a home birth. However, if home birth is precluded, e.g. because no flying squad is available, a good GP unit close to a hospital may be the answer.

To arrange for a confinement in a GP unit, find a GP who is on the 'obstetric list' (available at the Post Office). The list shows those GPs who have the necessary qualifications for delivering babies. If your own GP is not on the list, it does not matter: you can retain her or him, and use another one simply to look after your pregnancy. It is worth asking around about GP obstetricians. To be included on the list at present a GP does not need much experience. It would be wise to choose a GP who is not only experienced, but who is in close and relatively frequent involvement with childbirth (memories can fade quickly) and who does not favour unnecessary obstetrical interference (see p. 424).

Some GP units, particularly in rural areas, are threatened with closure or are already closed. The DHSS feels that it is open to question whether isolated GP units are safer than home confinement. It appears that financial reasons are also involved in order to fill up the under-used beds in the district general hospital which have resulted from the falling birth rate. We feel that DHSS policy is extremely short-sighted: those that are inadequate should be improved, and their facilities and consultant cover increased. Women *need* a personal, local service.

COMMUNITY AND MATERNITY HOSPITALS

These are small, local hospitals where care is provided by GPs and midwives – consultants visiting as needed. Based in the community, they involve little travelling and are usually far less impersonal than the large hospitals (though they are not necessarily more humane – see the above quotes from *Hospital Confinement*, see Bibliography).

Like GP units, many of these hospitals are being run down in favour of the bigger, centralized hospitals in large towns. Not surprisingly, no women as consumers have been involved in this decision. In 1974, Barbara Castle – then Secretary of State for Social Services – issued a memo to all health authorities: 'We accept the need for hospitals which can be sited nearer where people live for those patients who do not require or no longer need the specialized services and equipment which can only be economically and efficiently provided at district general hospitals.' It would seem clear that most pregnant women fitted this category but this is not so. The memo goes on to say that community hospitals 'would not normally provide maternity beds'.

As local hospitals are being closed down, people are getting together to fight for their retention. Following the closure of some of the last remaining maternity hospitals in Devon, a group of mothers in Bude threatened to take over a hotel and set up their own health group, refusing to use the hospital service (AIMS newsletter, June 1976). Unless women take such action, it is likely that in the not-too-distant future, the choice for all women will be between a district general hospital . . . or home.

EARLY DISCHARGE

If you are having your baby in hospital but want to get out quickly, it is often possible for a 48-hour or even 6-hour discharge to be arranged. Once at home you may find that you can adapt to the baby's routine very easily; breast-feeding is often easier to establish at home when one is relaxed. Often, too, home is much less noisy than hospital and you can sleep better. But being at home can be a temptation to do too much and get overtired. And visitors may think that, because you are home, you are perfectly fit. Home helps should be available to all women who need them – and there will be few who don't need a home help after an early discharge. But there is quite a shortage of home helps and maternity patients often come at the bottom of the list.

Increasingly, the promise of an early discharge is used to press mothers into having a hospital rather than a home birth. If you do not feel that adequate help is available say so — there is no reason why you should leave early.

Not all women are allowed an early discharge. You are more likely to be given one if you've already had a baby. However, you can discharge yourself from hospital on your own responsibility, although the staff will probably try very hard to dissuade you from doing so. Provided there are no complications there is no real reason why you should not return home.

Although I was pleased to have my second baby in hospital, I was rather anxious to leave the hospital before I was allowed to. This was so I could return to my first child. I had quite a normal delivery therefore I was hoping to leave after 48 hours having my mother staying to help. Apparently this was not possible due to a shortage of outside staff.

If you decide on an early discharge, a health visitor will visit you before the baby is born to explain what equipment you'll need. Once you are home, the midwife will call every day for 10 days after the baby's birth. She is there to look after you and the baby, and is on call 24 hours a day, so if you are worried you can contact her.

DOMINO SCHEMES

In the Domino scheme, a local midwife accompanies you to the local maternity unit, delivers you and returns home with you. This is an excellent way of ensuring continuity of care. However, the Society to Support Home Confinements feels it is hardly desirable to move a woman at the height of her labour when this is not necessary: she could remain at home for the birth. Not all areas run Domino schemes, one reason being that the number of community midwives is being dramatically reduced.

Home – The Right to Choose*

We have already documented the possible shortcomings of hospitals, particularly of consultant units. Given the recent and imminent closures of the few alternatives to consultant units it is crucial that at this time, more than any other, the large number of women who have normal pregnancies should have a choice between hospital or home.

However, our choice is severely limited and is becoming more and more so. This is not only because of the way doctors 'advise' us, but also because of the lack of facilities. In order to have a safe birth at home, we need (a) a willing G P, (b) a willing domiciliary (home) midwife, and (c) an obstetric flying squad service on hand in case of emergency.

* See also 'Are Home Births Unsafe?', p. 384.

(a) GPs are becoming less and less willing to do home births. This is not only because they, like many of us, have been persuaded into believing that giving birth at home is by definition unsafe. It is also because, since so few women are allowed to give birth at home (less than 5% in 1976), many GPs can have little practice in attending home births. Actually finding a GP can therefore be difficult (see 'How to get a home confinement', below). At least one Area Health Authority is making this more so by laying down that 'The midwife is not in a position to advise any patient of those GPs who would be willing to accept home confinements' (AIMS newsletter, September 1975).

(b) Midwives: the DHSS states in a press release that the total number of nursing and midwifery staff continues to increase (Health and Personal Social Services Statistics, 1975). But if we look at these statistics closely, we find that the number of domiciliary midwives is steadily decreasing. Furthermore, the number of pupils being trained as domiciliary midwives is also steadily decreasing. (The number of hospital midwives is, on the other hand, increasing, but such midwives are trained to be subservient to obstetricians and an increasing number of them can go through their training without ever seeing a birth which is allowed to progress normally. The Royal College of Midwives is understandably alarmed at this trend.) The DHSS is also planning to train fewer midwives in general, apparently because of the falling birth rate. As it is, in many areas, domiciliary midwives are not being trained.

In several areas, for example High Wycombe, domiciliary midwives are becoming increasingly concerned about their future as practitioners in their own right. They feel they are being phased out, as more births are being directed to the new large hospital in the area. In another area, the health authority has informed its Community Health Council that although it is not illegal for a midwife to accept a patient for home birth, such an arrangement is 'no longer satisfactory', and any midwife who took such action might well 'find herself in the position of having a case of malpractice to answer' (AIMS newsletter). Further depressing news concerns the fact that soon all midwives will have to be trained as nurses first. As Christine Beels points out, 'It cannot be to our advantage to have an attendant whose primary training has been with the sick rather than with the well, and who has also been trained to function as a subordinate to a doctor rather than as a professional in her own right' ('In the Beginning', *Spare Rib*, 49).

(c) Flying squads: these are emergency consultant teams who are on call, with equipment to deal with emergencies in home deliveries. Obviously, they are an essential back-up service for women giving birth at home. But not all areas have them. The Society to Support Home Confinements reports that in at least one area – Darlington – the flying squad has been withdrawn recently, thus making home delivery either impossible or dangerous. (Of the 355 maternal deaths in England and Wales in 1975, none was directly attributed to home delivery but one death was related to the failure of the hospital to provide a flying squad (*Report on Confidential Enquiries into Maternal Deaths in England and Wales,* 1975, HMSO)). And a recent paper in the *British Medical Journal* − 'Assessment of Obstetric Flying Squad in an Urban Area' − purports to show that it is economically unjustifiable to retain a flying squad in an urban area. This conclusion is based on one year's experience when less than 4% of deliveries in the area took place at home.

In spite of the continuing run-down of facilities, the DHSS insists that there is no central plan to force all women into hospital to have their babies. A former Minister responsible − David Owen − even stated in reply to a woman wishing to have a home birth that she had every right to have one. But where, for example, all the GPs in the area refuse to accept a home confinement there is nothing the DHSS *can or will* do. And draft plans for the NHS in the 1980s don't even contemplate babies being born at home.

We face a chicken and egg situation: women are discouraged from having home births, which leads to well over 90% of births taking place in hospitals, which in turn leads to the withdrawal of home birth services. Thus, in the not-too-distant future there will be no home births at all . . . unless we as women get together to do something about it.

The Society to Support Home Confinements (SSHC − see addresses) was formed by women very recently to advise, support and help women. Margaret Whyte − the founder − herself has five children: the first was a caesarean birth in hospital, and the rest she succeeded in having at home. Already (1976) the Society has activists in 30 counties and also in Wales and Scotland. The Society is not a registered body; it has no paid employees and it pays all its own expenses. Every letter is answered individually and the Society tries to offer as much personal contact and support 'to a group of women no other body is interested in nor caters for'. It receives hundreds of letters from women all over the country, many of whom have scoured the place for a willing GP and the support of a midwife. Although the Society reports that in about half the areas of the country it is still fairly straightforward to have a home delivery, in many of the others women can have extreme difficulty.

HOW TO GET A HOME CONFINEMENT*

If you wish to have a home confinement (read the section on 'High Risk Women', p. 385, before you decide), start making inquiries and arrange-

---

* Information for this section has been taken mainly from leaflets provided by the Society to Support Home Confinements.

ments as soon as you are pregnant. This is absolutely crucial since many women encounter opposition – see below.

Finding a GP: if you do not like your GP or s/he does not do maternity care, you can find another one. Only doctors on the 'obstetric list' do maternity care: the list should be available at the Post Office for you to look at. Remember that even if a GP is on the list, s/he may only do antenatal and postnatal care, sending women to hospital for the actual birth.

Finding a Midwife: the midwife usually has overall responsibility for the labour and delivery. In some 75% of all births she is the senior person present. A doctor who is cooperative will almost certainly know or work with a midwife with whom s/he can put you in touch. If you cannot find anyone to recommend a midwife, write to the Area Nursing Officer or the Area Medical Officer for the names of local midwives. Alternatively, midwives are listed in the telephone book under Nurses. Although a midwife can in principle book you for a home birth without your having a doctor booked as well, this is unlikely. If you give birth without notifying a doctor, you break the law, and if a midwife attends you without notifying a doctor, she may be guilty of malpractice.

If you are told that there is 'no domiciliary midwifery service', don't give up. We quote Margaret Whyte: 'All women, and this includes women expecting their first baby, are absolutely entitled to the services of a midwife, even if no doctor will look after them. If domiciliary facilities are inadequate the Area Health Authority is responsible for making them so and would possibly be actionable if anything happened to the mother or her baby as a result of medical neglect or wilful refusal to provide facilities . . . We have found that when approached the Area Health Authorities have in the main provided a swift and generous response to requests from women for domiciliary attention. However, there have also been threats of refusal of attendance at the birth which are an unpleasant and irresponsible bluff which should be called immediately by a formal demand in writing for midwifery care from the Area Nursing Officer.'

If you are tired of battling, or do not like the midwife provided by the area health authority, you may consider engaging a private one. The minimum fee was at the time of writing about £45 for a resident midwife for 7 days; the sessional fee (8 hours) for a private nurse (SRN) was £7.20 (according to *Which?* 'Pregnancy Month by Month').

Home Help: most women need help at home after a birth, whether it was at home or in hospital, particularly if there are other children to look after. As we have said earlier, the 'service' provided is not very good as home helps are few and far between. Women can be refused home birth on the grounds that there is no one to look after them after the birth. Thus, it is often a good idea for those (family or friends) who will be caring for you after the birth to inform the Medical Officer of Health that they are willing and able to do so. This is particularly useful if you are encountering opposition from any quarter. (Remember that the midwife will care for your medical needs for at least 10 days after the birth).

If You Encounter Opposition

At all stages of the battle for home delivery, make sure you have not been booked into hospital. If you *have* been booked into hospital, send a letter to the Area Nursing Officer stating your intention to stay at home.

The doctor came at 10.00 and said he would not do it now . as he had not realized I was booked in the Consultants Unit and it was unethical to take me out of their hands. Of course I was really shocked and upset. What a thing to tell a woman when she is in labour . . .

Although local authorities are legally required to provide facilities and personnel for home deliveries (see, for example, *Health Services and Public Health Act* 1968 Section 10(1)), we know that in many areas this is not the case. Even if services and personnel exist, you may still encounter opposition. It is worth remembering that 'Any doctor telling a patient that she is not allowed to give birth at home is deliberately misleading her and behaving unprofessionally' (SSHC, *Opting for a Home Confinement*).

One reason for denying a home birth is that the home conditions are 'unfavourable'. This decision will be based on a report from the health visitor who will look round your home and discuss family arrangements. It is worth obtaining evidence from family and friends that they will be around to support you during and after the birth.

Another reason is that there is no flying squad available. Your Community or Local Health Council and Family Practitioner Committee should support you in ensuring that there is one. If you cannot find a cooperative GP, ask the help of your Local or Community Health Council. Your local Christian Science Church can also help, since many Christian Science women have home births. Next, send a letter to the Area Medical Officer informing him of the situation and to the Secretary of the Family Practitioner's Committee asking advice. If you meet with severe difficulties, the press and local radio and television have been helpful with forcing officials to make a statement of service and policy. The SSHC has found that officials are not willing to admit to no longer operating an alternative to compulsory hospitalization.

If you still encounter opposition you could: (a) ask why precisely it would be unwise to have a home birth, though the doctor is not obliged to tell you; and (b) if you are not satisfied with the response, you could still insist on staying at home. If this is unacceptable to the doctor you can write to the doctor, the Area Medical Officer and if necessary to the domiciliary midwife, stating that you have been advised against a home birth, have been warned adequately, and are taking personal responsibility for your decision. If you are married, your husband would also have to state the same. If your doctor refuses to attend you at home and you have already signed the form EC 24 (which all pregnant women have to sign as a contract between themselves and their doctors), you should give the doctor notice that you are breaking the contract. Remember to make sure that you have not been booked into hospital against your will.

Medical personnel sometimes lie to women about their true medical condition, in order to prevent them from having a home birth. Phantom 'high' blood pressure has been quoted, even during labour, as a ruse for getting women into hospital – so it may be worth anticipating this by checking your blood pressure yourself. (Ask the SSHC for its leaflet on how to do this.) In any case, one raised blood pressure reading alone is not by itself grounds for entering hospital. Some doctors have told women they had placenta praevia where none existed; if, following this diagnosis you are not scheduled for a Caesarean birth, you could be wary of what you have been told.

If you are refused a home birth and decide to call a midwife to your house when you are in labour, you are very likely to end up in hospital, since she knows nothing about your pregnancy.

However well you think you can cope with the difficulties you have in obtaining a home birth, you would be wise to enlist support not just from friends but from local branches of the National Childbirth Trust, AIMS, SSHC, women's liberation groups, etc. If you are determined, and push long enough, you are likely to win: the authorities are not keen to demonstrate that they are willing to deny medical attention to home confinements.

I used a natural childbirth method on my first birth in hospital two years ago and had no need of anaesthetics or medical intervention . . . After the delivery and a minimal cuddle my first child was snatched away . . . I want to be free to cuddle my second infant immediately after birth as long as we both want this. When I became pregnant again, to my dismay my GP told me, 'There is no chance of your having the baby at home'. This was the policy of the local practice as it was 13 miles to the nearest hospital. I am now temporarily registered with a sympathetic doctor who will deliver my baby at home; the local midwife has agreed to deliver me . . . so one could say I have won the battle. But should one have to battle for such a basic right? (Letter to Guardian, 17 October 1975)

The birth of my third child was one of the most fantastic experiences my husband and I have ever known. Our son was born at home and it was wonderful . . . We tried to bring the baby into a quiet, gentle atmosphere as the doctor [Leboyer] suggests. In fact the cord was round the baby's neck but the *midwife was absolutely marvellous and took it as a matter of course. The baby did not breathe immediately but we stroked him gently and gradually he stirred and took a breath. The midwife was cheerful and extremely kind. She gave us both a tremendous feeling of confidence (AIMS newsletter, 1975).**

PREPARATIONS FOR A HOME BIRTH

You will need to make arrangements. The SSHC provides leaflets concerning what you will need – e.g. nightdresses suitable for nursing, sanitary towels, etc. The midwife will visit you during the 3rd or 4th month and she herself will probably make suggestions as to what you will need and about the arrangement of the furniture. It is often possible to borrow things like bowls and bedpans from either the Red Cross or the local authority. A 'confinement pack' supplied by the Area Health Authority will be delivered to you by the midwife 10 days before the baby is due. The pack should remain sealed, to be opened by the midwife when labour begins.

Labour

Delivery comes only after the *effacement* (thinning) and *dilation* (opening up) of the *cervix* (neck of the uterus). Dilation refers to the size of the round opening of the cervix, which is exposing more and more of the baby's head. It is measured in centimetres, or sometimes in finger widths. When the cervix is 10 centimetres, or 5 fingers, open, the first stage of labour is over and the baby is ready to come down the birth canal.

Many women start to dilate before they are aware that labour has begun. All through your pregnancy you'll probably feel occasional tightening of your uterus. Sometimes these preliminary contractions are strong enough to make you catch your breath, but they are rarely painful. Each of these 'Braxton-Hicks' contractions is exercising the uterus, preparing it for labour. They also start the effacement and dilation of the cervix. It is not unusual for a woman to be almost fully effaced and 1 or 2 centimetres dilated before she becomes aware of being in labour.

Which brings us to the question, when does labour really begin? There is no general answer, but you will probably have a few signs, such as the following. You may find some blood-tinged mucus on your under-clothes. This is the mucus plug that has been in the end of the cervix, whose purpose it was to keep the uterus free from germs that might have entered through the vagina. Many women never notice or never have a

* For other experiences of home birth, see *Having Your Baby* and *Peace News*, 'Perhaps it was the Raspberry Tea' (23 January 1976).

bloody show, as it's called, before labour. Others have an increasing amount of show all the way through the first stage of labour.

Some women begin labour when their membranes rupture (see p. 425). Once the bag of waters has burst there will be an increase of activity of contractions and usually, therefore, labour will be speeded up. It is important to contact your doctor or hospital if you think your membranes have ruptured, since (a) the baby may be born soon, and (b) there is a risk of infection, since there is no protective covering over the cervix. Many women have a diarrhoea-like urge for about 3 days before labour begins. This is nature's way of emptying the rectum before the birth process, so that there will be no unnecessary pressure on the vagina or the birth canal. Frequently women feel an increased number of Braxton-Hicks (see above) contractions for some time before labour actually begins, and often these contractions are confused with real labour contractions.

When labour does really get under way, you will probably feel contractions that are stronger and more regular than Braxton-Hicks contractions. They begin with a gradual tightening of the uterine muscles and slowly rise in intensity. Then a peak will be reached, and the tightening will slowly relax. It reminds some women of the rising, breaking, and falling of waves on the shore. The first contractions are usually not too uncomfortable; they last anywhere from 45 seconds to a minute. What is happening is that the lengthwise muscles of the uterus are involuntarily working to pull open the circular muscles around the cervix. Most books say that the difference between false and real contractions is that the former are erratic and the latter are regular, lasting for a specific amount of time, with a regular interval between them. But this isn't always the case.

I didn't begin to feel regularly spaced contractions until I was 4 centimetres dilated. My contractions from the beginning were anywhere from 2 to 5 minutes apart, and the spacing stayed that way throughout much of my first stage. Only the intensity of the contractions changed.

This first stage of labour may take anywhere from 2 to 24 hours, or more, depending on the size of the baby, the position in which it is lying, the size of the mother's pelvic area, and the behaviour of the uterus. The average length for first-stage labour in a mother who is having her first baby (primipara) is 12 hours. But, remember, not one of us is average. Labour is divided into four stages.

FIRST-STAGE LABOUR

First-stage labour is itself split into two categories: *early*, and *late*. Again, for each of us the experience of these stages will be very different.

But it is usually the case that early first-stage labour is easily handled, sometimes without any discomfort. Late first-stage labour occurs when the cervix is opening from 5 to 8 centimetres. This segment of labour is often shorter in duration and more intense in feeling than early first stage. For how to deal with it, see books recommended in 'How to Prepare for Childbirth', p. 416.

Probably the best sign that you are in labour is that you have to do breathing techniques to stay comfortable during a contraction. If you suspect you are beginning labour, *eat very lightly*, perhaps some clear soup and some jelly. This will give you a little extra energy, but it won't fill your stomach enough to make you nauseated as labour progresses. If you can, make sure you have some barley-sugar to suck on for added quick energy between contractions.

You will probably be given a vaginal or rectal examination to see how far your cervix has dilated. This should not be done while you are in the middle of a contraction as it can be painful then. The person doing this may be the resident doctor and not your own doctor at all. But don't let this stop you from asking questions. The doctor or nurse should check the vital signs, such as foetal heart rate and your temperature, blood pressure and pulse. If you suspect something is wrong, keep complaining until someone listens to you!

If you have been given an enema (see p. 425), the contractions may get stronger. Often they will fall into a pattern and you will be able to anticipate the intensity of the next one from that of the previous one. Relax during contractions during this stage, and make sure you are comfortable between them (see Positions during Labour, p. 409).

By the time you are 4–5 centimetres dilated, you'll probably be meeting heavier contractions of longer duration with shorter spaces between. Do whatever breathing you feel meets your needs. You may still be able to read, sing, play cards and talk to people around you if that helps you to relax between contractions. You may just want to sleep. Sleeping can be a hindrance, however, unless you are alert enough to jump into your breathing as soon as the next contraction starts. Usually if you don't ride the contraction from the start it is difficult to remain in control when it reaches its peak. If the people in your room are bothering you or keeping you from relaxing, ask them to leave. If, because of sleep or someone annoying you, you lose control in the middle of a contraction, do the following: relax, pant rapidly, and use the time after the contraction to relax completely. At this point a back rub or leg massage can help immensely to give you confidence (see 'Massage', p. 419). Massage is also very useful at the end of the first stage when our thighs and lower abdomen can ache (massage on the abdomen should be light).

By the time you are 6 centimetres dilated your contractions will in most cases be very strong, and you will probably feel a definitely uncomfortable rise of pressure and tension at the peak of the contractions, and then a gradual lessening of the tension until the contraction is completely over. Take full advantage of your time between contractions to rest, but be sure to start your breathing as soon as the next contraction begins. Many women ask for drugs at this point (see 'Pain Relief', p. 439). But a good companion will be sensitive to your needs and will remind you gently that a change of position might do some good, or perhaps a temporary switch to a deeper breathing. S/he could breathe with you throughout the contraction. That helps you to pace yourself and to keep alert. Unfortunately, you may resent any suggestion from someone else and stubbornly remain fixed to a certain position or breathing style. This irritability is very normal and probably indicates that you're entering transition.

TRANSITION

Transition is the hardest and the shortest part of labour, lasting from between one contraction to a couple of hours, although some women do not experience it at all. It is the time just before the cervix opens to a full 10 centimetres. These contractions are usually very discouraging, the part of labour that many of us felt was painful. Furthermore, the contractions are often very irregular in intensity and duration, and the intervals between them vary.

If you've come all this way without drugs, you can overcome transition on your own too. Very soon you'll be in second-stage labour, during which you will probably want to be wide awake. Transition is different for everyone, but some common signs are nausea and vomiting, leg cramps, shaking, feeling cold, severe low backache, pressure deep in the pelvis, increasing apprehension, irritability, frustration, and an inability to cope with contractions if left alone. It is during transition more than at any other time that your companion's presence is essential. S/he can help by breathing with you, massaging and comforting you, and continually reminding you that this is the most difficult and the shortest part of your labour.* Try to change your position if you remember. Try sitting almost upright, with the soles of your feet together and your legs relaxed. Prop pillows behind you to support your back. Use your most comfortable rapid breathing techniques − if you feel cold, blankets, socks and hot water bottles at your feet and between your thighs will help. A sip of water or some ice chunks to suck between contractions may be the thing to lift your spirits.

You will feel very vulnerable during transition, and you'll be very tempted to accept medication at this point. But by the time you ask for it,

---

* However, many women have found that breathing techniques are not necessary except as a distraction from a hostile hospital environment.

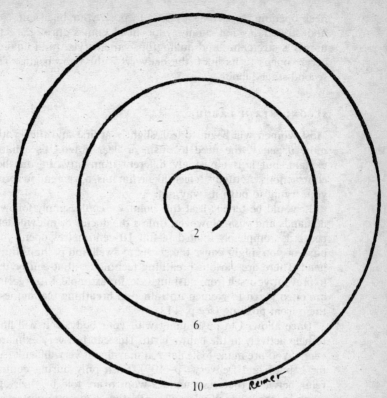

Cervical dilation in centimetres, shown actual size

and by the time it is administered and takes effect (depending on which type of analgesia you are given), you'll be very near to second-stage. And you will probably want to be awake when it's time to push. Also, the closer to delivery a drug is given, the more effect it has on the baby's responsiveness.

My legs shook all the way through transition, not just during a contraction. My husband gently held them, and that really helped. He also offered me ice chips after each contraction and wiped my forehead with a cool washcloth. I couldn't have made it without his being there every minute.

I was surprised at the strength of sensations in the transition phase and am sure that had I not been prepared I would have interpreted them as being painful.

You'll have a hard time concentrating on your breathing now unless someone is being very directive and doing it with you.

A good analogy to this first stage of labour is trying to pull on a turtle-neck sweater. At first your head fits easily. Then, as you get closer to the neck opening, it becomes harder to push your head out. You tug at it and stretch it, and finally your head comes through. Similarly, the uterus is stretching and pulling open the cervix, until finally, when the cervix opens to its limit, the delivery of the baby begins. This is called second-stage labour.

SECOND-STAGE LABOUR

Most women will begin to feel, slightly at first and then with more and more urgency, the need to push, or bear down. It's a hard feeling to explain, but it is amazingly different from anything in the preceding contractions. Actually, it feels like what it is, a tremendous pressure inside you, trying to push its way out.

It would be terrific if at this point we could simply follow our body's demands and *push*. However, unless the doctor or midwife tells you your cervix is completely dilated (a full 10 centimetres open) you must not push or you might cause the cervix to swell and perhaps hurt the baby's head. There are various breathing techniques that can be used in order to prevent yourself from pushing (see, for example, Kitzinger). Gas and air are often given to women untrained in breathing techniques, to prevent them from pushing (see p. 443).

Once allowed to push along with your body, you will finally be able to help actively in the baby's birth. This can feel very exhilarating. However, if you are made to lie flat you may find it very difficult (see 'Positions for Labour and Delivery', p. 409). Push only during contractions and relax between them. Sometimes women are told by their attendants to press in the abdominal wall onto the contracting uterus. As Sheila Kitzinger points out, this is not only unnecessary but undesirable and can cause considerable pain by preventing the full force of the contraction from being effective. Staff can, however, be very helpful during this stage – by encouraging us to get into a rhythm of pushing. Make sure you push only according to the intensity of each contraction: this may vary considerably. Research indicates that babies are born satisfactorily and with less need for forceps and episiotomies (see pp. 435 and 433) when a woman just follows her own inclinations, without being hurried and exhorted to push. If you are forced to push hard when you don't want to, it can be extremely uncomfortable as well as wasting energy. Only irresistible pushing is necessary, and only the minimum at that (see Kitzinger, *The Experience of Childbirth*). Some women don't have the urge to push: squatting can help to start more of a pushing feeling, but it is possible to give birth with minimal or no pushing.

Doctors very frequently anaesthetize women for the second stage of labour, possibly because a woman pushing during this phase looks as if she is in great pain. However, with preparation and encouragement, second-stage labour is joyful, not painful, to the overwhelming majority of women. Many women have described second-stage as 'the nice part'.

Another reason for choosing the second stage to anaesthetize a woman is that the doctor may want her desensitized so that interventions can be performed to speed up the delivery. Once again, we believe that second-stage labour should be allowed to take its normal course, usually lasting from half an hour to 2 hours, without unnecessary intervention. (Some doctors intervene if the second stage has lasted more than an hour.) If a mother is unanaesthetized and prepared, she will know when to push and how long for, without anyone telling her.

The delivery room can be a very pleasant place between contractions. If everything is going normally, there'll probably be a lot of laughing and exciting chatter during the rest intervals. There are up to 5 minutes between these second-stage contractions.

By now you're probably very tired, and perhaps you're beginning to feel a burning sensation around your perineum (the area between the anus and the vagina). This means the baby's head is about to crown and the birth is imminent. It's your body's way of saying, 'Don't push so hard; ease the baby out.' You must wait for the gradual stretching of the perineum, otherwise it will probably tear. If your perineum is tough, you may need an episiotomy (see p. 433). Try to keep your perineum relaxed by releasing those muscles. Also, keep your mouth loose; you may find this influences the relaxation of your vagina.

When the last contraction comes, the doctor will tell you to stop pushing and to use some rapid breathing to control your urge to push. Then, in the middle of the contraction, out will come your baby's head, usually facing the floor and then rotating to the side. You may be asked to give a gentle push for each shoulder and before you know it, the body will come sliding out.

Although there was no mirror, so I couldn't see my baby emerge, I could feel everything. It was the most thrilling experience I'd ever had — a perfectly formed baby slithering out of my body.

The majority of babies born in the UK are considered to be in excellent condition at birth, and this is especially true of babies born to unanaesthetized mothers. Some infants, however, will require help. Various techniques can be used to encourage the baby's respiratory functions to begin. This is vital, since lack of oxygen can cause brain damage to the infant. Also, the attendant will look for normal colour, body tone, and immediate urination.

The baby will be wet-looking, possibly covered with a milky substance called vernix, and usually not very bloody. Her/his head may look very strange at first, due to its moulding during the birth. This odd shape is temporary, and the baby's head will look normal soon.

The umbilical cord is still connecting you to your baby via the placenta,

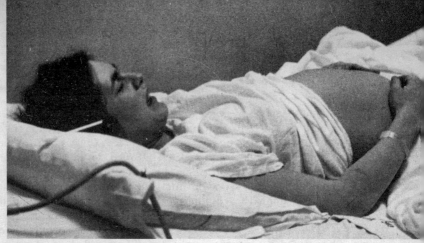

Late first stage

*In the delivery
room*

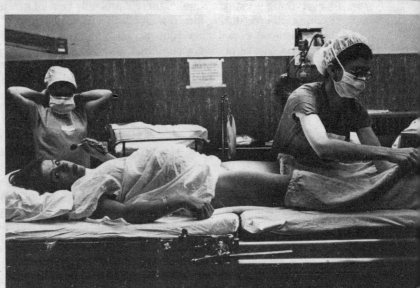

The baby's head crowning

The emergence of the pla
The tiny newborn fee
(home deliv

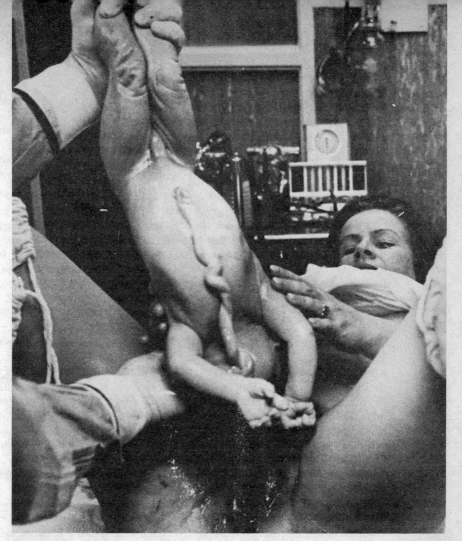

The baby is born

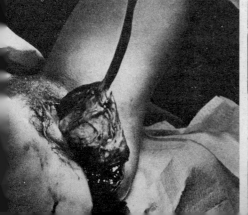
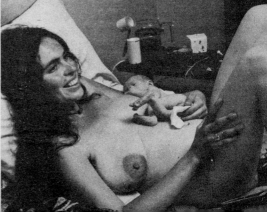

which is still inside you (except in the case of placenta praevia, see p. 413). The cord will be clamped, but this should not be done until all the blood is emptied from it, otherwise the baby will be deprived of some of its sustenance. It is worth checking with the doctors well before the birth that they will not clamp too soon. After clamping, the cord will be cut a few inches from the baby's navel. In a week or so the cord will dry out completely and fall off, leaving the baby with a normal navel.

The cord struck me as exceedingly strong and beautiful — translucent, blue, and in the shape of a telephone cord, but thicker. The doctor gave my baby to the nurse to suck out more mucus, wipe and wrap her, and only then did I get her. I was shaky, chilly, exhausted and happy. I wanted to hold and nurse my baby but had no energy left. So my husband held her close to me. I felt so close to him at that moment, and also to the woman who had been with me throughout.

THIRD-STAGE LABOUR

This is the delivery of the placenta. In Britain, women are virtually always given an injection of ergometrine or syntometrine during or after the baby's birth, whether it was in hospital or at home. This helps to contract the uterus and expel the placenta quickly which in turn prevents haemorrhage (doctors are always worried about haemorrhage after birth). In discussing the routine use of these drugs, Doris Haire points out how, together with manipulation of the uterus and other methods of speeding up the third stage, they tend to increase the incidence of retained placenta or retained tissue and maternal blood loss. 'Such obstetrical intervention is rarely found necessary when (a) the mother has received little or no medication, (b) she has been supported to a semi-sitting position for birth and (c) where placental transfusion [transference of blood to the baby via the umbilical cord] has reduced the volume of the placenta' (*The Cultural Warping of Childbirth*). In any case, suckling the baby after the birth can effectively expel the placenta but this is rarely allowed. Herbal remedies such as angelica can help with the expulsion of the placenta and thus obviate the need for injections.

Sometimes the placenta will actually follow the baby almost immediately, and sometimes it will have to be extracted manually by the doctor. With the birth of the placenta, labour is ended.

The midwife should examine the placenta to make certain it is whole. If a piece of it is left inside (retained tissue) the mother may subsequently haemorrhage due to the blood vessels being torn by the only partial removal of the placenta. If there is any doubt, she may explore inside your uterus to check. Then if you have had an episiotomy it will be sewn up.

POSITIONS FOR LABOUR AND DELIVERY

Although lying flat on your back (in the 'dorsal', 'supine' or 'lithotomy' position) is a common position for a woman to take during labour and delivery, it is neither the most efficient nor the most comfortable position, and it is quite possibly the most dangerous one. There is much evidence that the supine position not only produces more pain, but that it also leads to slower labours and more maternal and foetal distress. Foetal distress can be caused by the uterus pressing on the major sources of blood to and from the uterus, thus cutting off the oxygen supply. Furthermore, if we are lying flat, gravity cannot help us push the baby out.

It has taken a paediatrician, not an obstetrician, to raise these issues (and others) in the British medical press recently. In his paper 'Obstetric Delivery Today — For Better or for Worse?', Peter M. Dunn reminds his colleagues that less efficient uterine contractions when the woman is lying down have been a 'clinically recognized fact for hundreds of years'. He goes on to report how a study in Spain compared the effect of the supine position with the standing position, each woman alternating her posture every half hour throughout the first stage of labour. The effectiveness of contractions in dilating the cervix was *doubled* in the standing position and it was also much less uncomfortable and painful.*

The best ways of giving birth were well known long ago: 'A vast and important fund of knowledge may be derived from a study of the various positions occupied by women of different peoples in their labours . . . The recumbent position is rarely assumed among those people who live naturally . . . and have escaped the influence of civilization and modern obstetrics . . . According to their build, to the shape of their pelvis, they stand, squat, kneel, or lie on their belly [see illustrations]; so also they

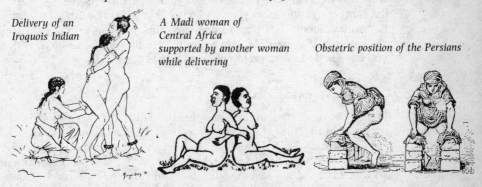

Delivery of an
Iroquois Indian

A Madi woman of
Central Africa
supported by another woman
while delivering

Obstetric position of the Persians

* You may hear quoted a recent paper by McManus and Calder which purports to show that upright posture is no better than lying down. This paper is based on the experiences of 40 women (as recounted by doctors), all of whom were induced and receiving very large amounts of drugs. It is not, therefore, surprising that they may have preferred lying down!

vary their position in various stages of labour according to the position of the child's head in the pelvis' (Prof. G. J. Engelmann, *Labour Among Primitive Peoples*, St Louis, written in *1882*). In some societies, even today, natural, logical methods of giving birth are still used. In Yucatan, for example, women may give birth in a hammock: 'The pregnant woman is suspended in space, accessible from all sides; she can be held, supported, touched, rubbed – whatever her needs are at the moment' (from an excerpt of a paper by Nancy Fuller and Brigette Jordan, published in *The Monthly Extract*, Vol. 3, issue 1).

But in the West, women are usually forced to labour and give birth lying on our backs.* A recent survey of women's views in Britain showed that 'Women wanting to get into a good position for pushing were . . . often not allowed to be propped up . . . and commented that it was a great strain to hold their legs while lying flat . . . many found themselves trying to push "up hill" ' (quoted by Peter M. Dunn, *Lancet*, 10 April 1976).

I felt I wanted to get up during labour, simply to relieve the pain, but I was not allowed to.

It is important, therefore, that women work towards a situation which enables us to give birth how we want. In the meantime, you can find out what each hospital's policy is by going to the antenatal clinic or contacting the local NCT teacher. You will probably find that you can resist pressure from doctors and nurses if you have a good companion with you, well versed in knowing your needs and wishes. Sitting up, standing, squatting, in a knee-hand position, or lying on your side are all possible. If you prefer to sit, your companion can make sure that you have a backrest and/or pillows to support your back. A large number of pillows is usually needed. S/he can also hold your legs, thus relieving you from the effort of holding them yourself and enabling you to push more easily. Remember, labour is a time to do everything you can to make yourself as comfortable as possible. Move around, change positions, do anything you have to do to keep on top of your contractions.

LESS USUAL PRESENTATIONS

In the above discussion we have assumed the baby's position in the uterus to be the most common – *left occipito anterior*. This means that the baby is head down in the uterus, lying on the left side, with the occiput, or back part of the skull, towards the mother's front. It is the most efficient way for a baby to slip past the pubic bone and into the birth canal. A baby in this position faces the floor at birth if the mother is lying flat.

---

* Things *are* changing, however: see *Spare Rib*, 18, concerning the reintroduction of the obstetrical chair in a Swedish hospital.

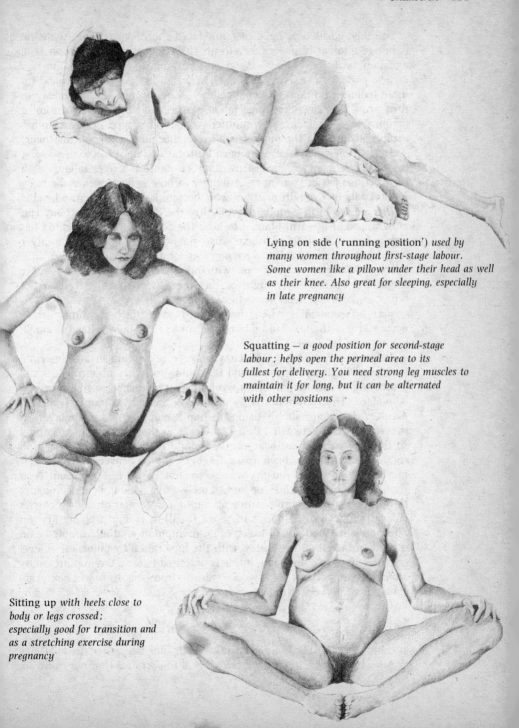

Lying on side ('running position') *used by many women throughout first-stage labour. Some women like a pillow under their head as well as their knee. Also great for sleeping, especially in late pregnancy*

Squatting – *a good position for second-stage labour; helps open the perineal area to its fullest for delivery. You need strong leg muscles to maintain it for long, but it can be alternated with other positions*

Sitting up *with heels close to body or legs crossed; especially good for transition and as a stretching exercise during pregnancy*

Another position is head first but faced the opposite way, with the baby's face towards the mother's front. This is called *posterior presentation*, and can be R.O.P. (*right occipito posterior*) or more rarely L.O.P. (*left occipito posterior*), i.e. lying on the right or the left side. It often means a more tedious and more uncomfortable labour, since the baby will try to turn around during first-stage labour in order to be born in the most favourable way, facing the mother's back. This type of presentation usually means that the mother will experience labour pains in her back.

Some babies (about 3%) are born buttocks down, or feet first, in what is called *breech presentation*. This, too, can cause a longer labour, with contractions felt in your back. A danger in breech birth is that the baby will take its first breath as soon as its bottom is born, while the head is still inside the birth canal. To avoid this, the baby's emerging body can be wrapped in a warm blanket to keep the colder air from shocking her or him into a breathful of mucus. Also, the attendant may insert a finger into the birth canal to clear a passageway for air to reach the baby's face. Forceps deliveries are common with breech births because the cervix might not be dilated enough for the head (which is bigger than the buttocks), and the head needs to be born quickly.

Face presentation is when the baby's face is the presenting part. It occurs in less than 1% of labours and, unless the baby's head is small, labour may be slower.

Before the 34th week, the baby may be presenting in an abnormal position. This is not unusual and is nothing to worry about. If it is still presenting abnormally after 34 weeks, it can be turned so that a breech is avoided. The commonest way of turning the baby (doing a 'version') involves the doctor simply using his hands placed on your abdomen. It is best to do this between 34 and 36 weeks. It should be done in hospital so that the baby's heartbeat can be monitored to check that s/he is all right. (Then if any problem arises, the baby can be delivered in safety.) It must be done while you are awake so that if you feel any pain (you shouldn't) the doctor can stop immediately. Pain could indicate damaging the placenta, for example. Since attempting a version obviously carries risks (though in good hands they are small), it is worth trying first an alternative method which involves no manipulation at all: simply lie on a hard surface for 10 minutes, with the hips raised by pillows to a level of 9–12 ins above the head. If this is practised twice a day (on an empty stomach), for at least 4–6 weeks starting from the 30th week of pregnancy it is unlikely to fail.

SOME SIGNS OF ABNORMAL LABOUR AND DELIVERY

If complications should arise during labour, our bodies will usually give us some warnings. It is, of course, of vital importance that we be aware of them and make our doctor aware of them. A woman who is awake and not medicated will have a much clearer sense of what is going on than one who is anaesthetized.

Here are a few signals that require the immediate attention of a doctor:

A continuous and severe lower abdominal pain, often accompanied by uterine tenderness. This is different from the pain of a normal labour contraction, which comes on with increasing intensity and then gradually disappears completely until the next contraction. Also, during normal contractions the uterus and entire abdomen become very hard and distended.

Cessation of good, strong contractions during first-stage labour. Labour contractions usually get more and more intense and are spaced closer and closer together as you approach second-stage. When second-stage labour is reached, however, contractions come less frequently again, though they do not cease to become effective.

Excessive vaginal bleeding. There are a number of reasons for this, such as cervical laceration, placenta abruptio (when the placenta becomes detached from the uterus), delivery before the cervix is fully dilated. It is not uncommon, however, to have a bloody mucous discharge during transition, especially if the cervix is opening up very quickly.

Abnormality in foetal heartbeat. This is a sign that the baby may be in trouble. If the mother is lying on her back, she should be turned on her left side, to take the pressure off her major blood vessels. Immediate delivery may be necessary.

Abnormally slow dilation of the cervix. If contractions are severe and still the cervix is not dilating with regularity, then the contractions may be creating undue stress on the foetus, the mother, or both.

An abnormal presentation or prolapse of cord, placenta, or a limb. If any of these occurs, an experienced obstetrician or midwife must decide if a Caesarean is required (see p. 437). Prolapsed cord and placenta praevia (placenta first instead of baby first) generally call for Caesarean section.

Any adverse change in condition of mother or baby. If the pattern of heartbeat and/or blood pressure changes; if the woman develops a fever; or if some other difficulty arises, the presence of an experienced doctor or midwife is essential to interpret the signs.

For more about complications, see, for example, Bourne, *Pregnancy*, p. 477.

PREMATURE LABOUR AND DELIVERY

A premature baby is one who is born in or before the 37th week of pregnancy. More than half the deaths of newborn babies in the United States, for example, are due to premature birth. This is a tragedy, since much prematurity can be prevented by good nutrition (see Chapter 6), good antenatal care, and adequate birth control for those who may be unable to carry a foetus to term (e.g. young teenagers whose bodies are not yet developed enough). Since the informed and better-off woman has easy access to the above, it is the poorer and ill-informed woman who is more likely to have a premature baby.

There is little known about the cause of prematurity in nearly half the cases. Poor health, inadequate nutrition, and heavy smoking all increase one's chance of having a premature delivery. Some specific causes of premature labour are infectious diseases (such as syphilis), toxaemia of pregnancy, diabetes, thyroid disturbances, foetal abnormalities (placenta praevia, placenta abruptio, etc.) and multiple pregnancies. Some of these problems can themselves be avoided through adequate health care and nutrition.

At the first sign of premature labour you should go into hospital; premature delivery may be prevented by bed rest and drugs.

Premature babies are extremely susceptible to the dangerous side effects of the drugs used during labour, so if you are prepared to handle labour without drugs you will be doing your premature baby a great service.

Most premature babies who do not live are victims of hyaline membrane disease. This is a lung disease which frequently affects premature babies and, less often, those delivered by Caesarean section. In general, the premature infant is much more susceptible to all infections.

The smaller and more feeble the baby, the more need there is for immediate care. Premature infants are placed in oxygen-, temperature-, and humidity-controlled incubators, and they must be constantly watched and carefully protected from every possible source of infection. Often parents are not even allowed to touch their own baby until his or her chances of survival are clear. This usually adds to the already high level of anxiety the parents may feel. (See Special Care Baby Units, p. 439, for further discussion.)

Feeding the premature infant may be a problem because of the baby's underdeveloped intestinal tract. One study shows that 'premature infants, fed human milk not only had the lowest incidence of major infection and mortality during the hospital stay but also proved free from infection after leaving the hospital when breast-fed at home'.* A mother can pump her own colostrum and milk with an electric or hand breast pump, and this milk can be supplied to her infant in the nursery incubator. Human colostrum, the liquid that fills the mother's breasts before her milk comes in, is so full of antibodies to fight the very infections to which the premature infant might succumb that it seems foolish not to insist that colostrum be an integral part of the premature baby's diet. In some areas, milk banks are being set up, where mothers can donate their milk

* V. Crosse, *et al.*, 'The Value of Human Milk Compared with Other Feeds for Premature Infants', as discussed in Haire and Haire, *Implementing Family-Centered Maternity Care with a Central Nursery*, pp. v. 42–3.

for premature and sick babies. Contact the National Childbirth Trust if you would like to help with this.

The birth of a premature baby may come before the mother has prepared herself psychologically for delivery and motherhood. Guilt feelings and emotional uncertainty are an almost inevitable aspect of prematurity. This anxiety is normal. Hospital staff should be aware of this and should encourage the mother and father to visit their baby, hold the baby and feed it whenever possible. If the mother feels that it is her milk that is sustaining the infant and her efforts that are helping the baby to grow stronger, then she will begin the postpartum period (see Chapter 14) with a much stronger and more confident attitude.

TWINS AND MULTIPLE PREGNANCIES

About one in 80 of all deliveries is twins. In some races they are more common (e.g. Africans) and in others they are less common (e.g. Chinese). They are not so common if you are under 20 or over 40. The predisposition to have twins can be inherited, although it is more likely to be passed through a daughter than through a son. The predisposition often skips generations, so you are more likely to have twins if your mother's mother had them, than if only your mother had them. Many people insure against having twins and many insurance companies offer policies. You have to insure before the end of the 3rd month of pregnancy. Premiums are around £3 for every £100 you want to be paid in the event of having twins. Twin pregnancies can usually be diagnosed in advance; an X-ray might be necessary for confirmation, and this is not usually performed before the 28th week. But in 5% of cases, twins are not recognized as such prior to the actual birth.

You should be particularly well cared for during a twin or multiple-birth pregnancy since there is a slightly increased risk of complications such as toxaemia. There is also an increased risk of complications during labour. More twin babies tend to die in the first few hours of life, usually due to prematurity. Twin labours can be longer (but not necessarily harder or more painful) because the uterine muscles are not so efficient due to over-distension during pregnancy. Breech births and postpartum haemorrhage are also more common. For these reasons it is unlikely that you will find a doctor prepared to do a home delivery unless in exceptional circumstances.

Multiple births usually occur as a result of the use of fertility drugs (see Infertility, p. 490). They cannot usually be diagnosed until the 24th or 28th week. The above applies to all multiple births. (For more on this subject, see, for example, 'Twins', a National Childbirth Trust pamphlet, and the chapter in *Pregnancy* by Gordon Bourne.)

How to Prepare for Childbirth

There is 'good statistical evidence in this country that adequately pre-pared mothers need less medication than unprepared mothers. Also, far more of them look back on labour as a tolerable or even enjoyable experience' ('Psychophysical Antenatal Preparation', published by the National Childbirth Trust).

I can honestly say that it was completely painless . . . There was only one time when they examined me towards the end of the first stage – when control was lost – and then I knew just how good the training was. The whole thing was a real thrill – and such a joke . . . After the terrible time with my first baby I was terrified. I had been having nightmares for days before, since I knew I had to go for induction. (Sylvia Close, The Know-How of Pregnancy and Labour)

I was never once frightened or distressed which I hadn't expected at all . . . I must confess I've always been sceptical about the 'joyful' bit of childbirth and was surprised to feel so happy and elated. (ibid.)

Well, in complete sincerity, I can say that it wasn't painless, and it wasn't easy, and (during transition) there were moments of near crisis – but it was a most marvellous and satisfying experience . . . It was so helpful for both my husband and me to have something positive to do and practise during the last weeks of pregnancy; it meant that I went into labour in a confident and eager state of mind; it meant that even at the most trying moments when otherwise I should have cracked up, I managed to keep on going; and it meant I was able to take the fullest advantage of the wonderful experience of second stage. (ibid.)

In this section we have decided, for reasons of space, to give simply an overview of the different ways in which a pregnant woman can prepare herself for childbirth. We believe that to prepare confidently and effect-ively for childbirth it is important to attend classes in these techniques. We can then be shown how to use them, we can practise them until they become second nature, our questions can be answered and we can share our fears and problems with other women and with an experienced teacher. Furthermore, since there are many different techniques, and since each teacher tends to have her own personal approach, it can be very confusing if we try to learn techniques different from those that she uses. Reading books is also useful, but nothing can replace person-to-person teaching.

The concept of preparation for labour and delivery was made popular in Europe and the United States by two obstetricians, although the idea was first introduced by three women: Kathleen Vaughan, Minnie Randall and Helen Heardman. In 1932 Dr Grantly Dick-Read, an Englishman, first introduced a method of concentrated relaxation during labour with his book *Childbirth Without Fear*. Dick-Read learned from watching his patients that fear causes tension, and tension adds to pain. His approach was to try to eliminate the fear of labour through education and the teaching of relaxation and exercise techniques. A French doctor, Fernand Lamaze, offered a different idea, which he learned in Russia, where he saw large numbers of women labouring with what appeared to be no pain at all. He called his technique 'psychoprophylaxis' (*psycho* — mind, *prophylactic* — prevention). Lamaze asked his patients to respond actively to labour contractions with a set of pre-learned breathing exercises. As the intensity of the contractions increased, so did the woman's rate of breathing. The labouring woman's whole posture and attitude changed. She was no longer flat on her back, pitied by all onlookers; now she was active, altering her positions and breathing patterns according to the progress of her labour.

In Britain, the National Childbirth Trust has pioneered what it calls 'psychophysical' antenatal preparation. It trains teachers in this method, provides books and leaflets, and runs classes in many parts of the country (see below). As their leaflets on this technique say, it is for those women 'who want a thorough preparation which goes beyond labour itself and helps them to adapt themselves to pregnancy and the puerperium'. Psychophysical preparation is based on the work of both Dick-Read and Lamaze, and that of many others such as Erna Wright and Sheila Kitzinger. Erna Wright's book *The New Childbirth* (see Bibliography) is basically a variation on Lamaze, and Sheila Kitzinger's work, such as her book *The Experience of Childbirth* (see Bibliography), is concerned with the preparation of the whole person, the whole couple, for parenthood as well as for birth. She calls her method 'psychosexual', and it involves the use of Touch Relaxation, massage and focussed concentration. The National Childbirth Trust trains teachers in all these approaches, and probably most teachers use a combination of them all.

TECHNIQUES TO USE DURING LABOUR*

By using these techniques, we cannot necessarily expect to kill all pain: most women must expect half an hour or so of pain or great discomfort at the end of the first stage, even though some women do have painfree labours. By preparing ourselves for childbirth we can become aware of our relationships with our bodies, we can learn to trust them and our instincts and we can acquire skills which enable us to remain in control of labour, answering stimuli and adapting accordingly.

Breathing: 'The way in which a woman breathes is closely connected with the rhythm to which her body adapts itself during the process of

* See also 'Pain Relief', p. 439.

labour. If she succeeds in harmonizing her breathing with the contractions of the uterus . . . she will be able to keep control of her labour, and
instead of its being a muddle of painful sensations she will find it very
exhilarating' (Kitzinger). Rhythmic breathing helps to steady you as
well: breathing affects your mind and your mind affects your body. It is
less easy to panic when concentrating on your breathing.

There are many kinds of breathing techniques. The following books
each have slightly different approaches; they are all equally valid: Sylvia
Close, *The Know-how of Pregnancy and Labour*, Sheila Kitzinger, *The
Experience of Childbirth*, and Lester Hazell, *Commonsense Childbirth*.

Whichever technique you use, it is very useful to practise breathing
with somebody else and we cannot emphasize enough how helpful classes
can be for this. But it is even more useful if you can practise with the
person who will be your companion during labour. You and s/he can
even do exercises together; Sheila Kitzinger's book has plenty of examples
of these.

Kegel Exercises (see Chapter 6, p. 137): this involves gradually
tightening the muscles around your vagina, the perineal area, and then
loosening them gradually. It can be done at any time and place throughout your pregnancy. Try to do it whenever you think of it. It's an important exercise since it teaches you how to relax the muscles of the pelvic
floor and perineum – which have to be relaxed for the baby to pass
through – and it also teaches you how to tighten those muscles so that
after the birth you can exercise to return to your naturally firm condition.

Relaxation and Dissociation Techniques: Since we have learned to use
muscles not singly but in combination, we have to learn to dissociate
the muscles from one another if we are going to be able to let the activity
of the uterus be as unhampered as possible.

The aim of these techniques is to learn what a tight muscle feels like
and how to relax it. Most of the books we recommend contain exercises
in these techniques. It is a good idea, as well as practising them in a class,
to do them with someone at home so that they can check your relaxation.
Here is an example of one exercise.

Lie comfortably relaxed, then think of one part of your body and
tense it. Make sure that all your other muscles stay loose. Then relax
and tense another part. These exercises should be done at least once a
day. Try doing them in different positions: during labour you may be on
your back very little. Also, check yourself from time to time when you're
not doing these exercises to see which parts of you tend to tense up
without knowing it. If you locate specific areas, such as your mouth or
your hands, you can concentrate especially on keeping them relaxed
during labour.

Hypnosis: this can be used to induce relaxation. Hypnotherapy for
childbirth is thus very much akin to the relaxation techniques we have

been talking about. The real difference is that with hypnosis a deeper form of relaxation tends to be possible. Hypnosis is useful, not just for relieving pain (where it can be totally eliminated, particularly if the therapist is actually with you during labour) – it also tends to result in shorter, easier labours with less tearing and little need for episiotomy (see p. 433), and it is also useful for problems experienced during pregnancy such as nausea.

To prepare for childbirth using hypnosis, it is necessary to attend sessions in the same way as with the more usual preparation techniques. Sessions can be organized either individually or in groups. After initial training in the technique, few extra sessions are necessary, except possibly an extra five minutes at the end of an antenatal check-up. It is also possible to practise the technique on your own.

The main problem with hypnosis is finding a therapist, although more and more doctors, including GPs, are learning how to use it. Another problem with hypnosis, as with other kinds of preparation, is that it cannot be used successfully without the cooperation of staff present (see Warnings, below). For example, there is very little chance of success if your brain is befuddled with drugs. As one hypnotherapist explained, the ideal situation for hypnosis in childbirth is a supportive atmosphere, preferably at home. To find a hypnotherapist, it is best to go to someone who is a member of a nationally recognized body (see p. 144).

The Alexander Technique (p. 134): By concentrating on keeping your head and neck free, and allowing your back to lengthen and widen, you should prevent yourself from unnecessary tensing of muscles and allow your body to get on with its job. If you want to try this technique – which involves very much 'not doing' as opposed to 'doing' – it is best to go to an Alexander teacher. Your teacher might even be prepared to accompany you through labour.

Massage: massage is often extremely helpful during labour, especially on your legs – usually the thighs – and back. Some women with backache labour rely on this massage to keep comfortable. Sheila Kitzinger gives a detailed account of massage in *The Experience of Childbirth* (pp. 94–5).

Make sure you discuss the techniques you wish to use with the people who will be looking after you, so that they understand and accept what you wish to do. If, when the time comes, they are uncooperative, your companion can help support you.

CHILDBIRTH CLASSES

Childbirth classes usually start 2–3 months before the expected date of delivery. Broadly speaking, classes in the UK fall into two categories: those run by the National Childbirth Trust (NCT) and those run by hospitals and local authorities.

National Childbirth Trust: the purpose of these classes is to prepare oneself not only physically but also emotionally. The classes are a mixture of teaching, group discussion and physical preparation. Most classes have at the maximum 8 couples or 12 women at a time and they take place in the teacher's own home. You can take a companion to the classes and you do not have to be married. Each teacher has herself experienced childbirth. She may be a nurse, midwife, physiotherapist, PE teacher or none of these things; but she will be a member of, and have been trained by, the NCT. She will also be expected to keep in touch with new ideas and techniques, and attend refresher seminars. Obviously the teaching will depend to some extent on the attitudes of the individual teacher.

The Trust, founded in 1956, is a registered charity with over 50 branches and about 40 smaller groups throughout Britain. Since it is not funded by any other body at all, it exists on the voluntary support of helpers, donations and subscriptions. For this reason also, it has to charge fees for its classes.

It is sad that the only body which can really prepare women for childbirth – set up, incidentally, by women – does not have access to public funds. Thus, there are many, many women who have to make do with the patchy service provided without charge by hospitals and local authorities. We hope that as more women become aware of this situation, they will join together to force the authorities to fund local NCT classes. In the meantime, teachers will charge a reduced fee or nothing at all if you are unable to pay. One branch at least has subsidized its fees for all women attending. If you are a single parent or on supplementary benefit, you should be eligible for a free class without question.

Hospitals and Local Authorities run free classes. They are often called 'relaxation' classes. The quality and standard of these classes varies widely – some being run by inexperienced people who might not have had a baby themselves nor even seen a normal birth. Sometimes the 'help' they give is simply to prepare us to accept drugs and instruments as a necessary part of childbirth. There are classes which simply urge you to relax and let your mind wander. Very few women can cope with the intensity of contractions if this is what they are expected to do. Other classes are simply concerned with leaping around. This can have very little effect apart from aiding circulation. Sometimes the information given is mystifying and even inaccurate.

At our local health centre we did breathing and relaxation. Pain was never mentioned. We were told that labour didn't mean pain, it just meant work. We were also told that 'they never let a woman suffer today; they have a lot of wonderful drugs they can give you if they think your labour needs it' (but not if you think you need it). This brainwashing exercise had a powerful effect on us. We were never given any impression that we had any control over what was to happen to us. This authoritarian behaviour persisted right through to the time I was breast-feeding. It simply produced a frightened and fearful mother. When I was discharged from the hospital, I wondered what on earth I would do with the baby, for I'd never been allowed even to assume I could make a decision before, let alone carry one out.

It [labour] was nothing like what I'd been told at the clinic would happen.

The best of these classes will probably have a teacher trained by the NCT. It is worth joining a local NCT or women's group and pushing the authorities to engage the services of a teacher trained by the NCT.

If you cannot easily get to a class, don't worry. The books, and even tapes, available (see Bibliography) provide enough information for you to work on your own if need be. In any case, NCT teachers can be flexible, particularly those working in rural areas, and it has been known for them to run marathon sessions at one go instead of short classes over a period of a few weeks.

COMPANIONSHIP

As we have already emphasized, having a reliable companion with us can be invaluable in many different ways. As yet, however, no woman has the *right* to have even her husband present during labour and birth, although as long ago as 1961 the government report 'Human Relations in Obstetrics' recognized the importance of a husband's presence. One of the most common complaints that mothers have had is being left alone in hospital during labour: this can be a frightening experience. A survey by the Scottish AIMS (1971–2) found that 50% of mothers were alone during the first stage of labour and 12% were alone during the second stage. A survey by *Which?* of 2,000 women found that eight were alone during the actual birth – a disturbingly high number. The Department of Health has in fact issued a recommendation that fathers' presence should be allowed, 'medical indications' permitting – but this recommendation has no authority. For several years now, AIMS has been lobbying the Department to make a ruling instead of a recommendation but it still declines to do this, saying that a ruling would interfere with doctors' 'clinical judgement'. (This is in spite of the fact that doctors would in any case be able to exercise their discretion according to whether they thought that 'medical indications' warranted fathers being present or not.)

If it is sometimes difficult to gain acceptance of fathers' presence, we have to expect that hospital staff will find it even harder to accept the presence of a companion other than the father.

Nonetheless, fathers *are* becoming more accepted. But while hospital staff are beginning to accept them during the first stage of labour, they might well not like them to be present later on, particularly if the birth involves an obstetrical procedure such as forceps . . . and such procedures are themselves becoming more and more common: 'Husbands were usually, but not invariably, sent out for forceps deliveries, and often found it difficult to get back to their wives again' (NCT report, 'Some Mothers' Experiences'). The report continues: 'Many husbands were 'expelled' or 'banished' for examinations, bedpans, and catheterization, and even for the taking of blood pressure readings and the recording of monitor readings, although wives would have liked them to stay.' Furthermore, there is a world of difference between actually welcoming fathers and grudgingly tolerating them:

While not actively discouraging my husband's presence while I was in labour and in the delivery room, there was certainly no enthusiasm for it. The nurses showed ingenuity in their efforts to persuade him to leave. Afterwards we were both made to feel as though we had been given some special privilege. (letter to *Sunday Times*, 20 October 1974)

In the NCT survey quoted above, some men felt discouraged from touching their wives at all and this was a source of great distress.

Even if you have arranged with the hospital beforehand that the father will be present, you might still run into difficulties, as this woman did:

They did all they could to get my husband to go home and threatened to have him removed. (*Sunday Times*, 13 October 1974)

Sometimes the hospital will tell the father to go home and get a good night's sleep, only to return to find that his partner has had a lonely, frightening and sleepless night. But, where the partnership of the man and woman is supported, the birth can be a very positive experience:

I could not possibly have managed without Mike beside me, reminding me about my breathing, relaxing, positioning and state of mind. It was wonderful to share such an incredible happening with him. We will never forget. (ibid.)

Some women may be made to feel that they *should* have the father there even if they don't want him. But if you'd rather be alone, that is your choice and it should be respected.

Sometimes both parents don't want the father to be present because they are anxious or frightened at the idea — such feelings are often expressed in the form of jokes. In a small survey of fathers, 15% said that the main thing they disliked was their impotence in not being able to help their wives; 20% disliked seeing their wives in pain (Richman *et al.* — see Bibliography). Feelings of bewilderment and uselessness are not at all uncommon. But if the father can go to classes or help the woman to practise her exercises, he may feel much more confident about the impending birth. Sometimes, men who have been adamantly against the idea of attending the birth can change their minds following attendance at a good antenatal class. (Increasingly, classes encourage fathers to go along; the NCT runs classes for couples and West London's women's hospital has just started thorough preparation for women and men.)

He didn't even want to be with me for the birth but I twisted his arm to come to classes and they converted him. (Guardian, 1 April 1976).

If you are having a baby and would like the father to be present to support you, both of you might find it useful to discuss your fears and anxieties with other women and men. Since many men tend to find it difficult to talk about their feelings and their fears — especially with other men — we have included below the story of two births as told by one man:

Time One. Lin had Josie in hospital. I wasn't there at the birth and saw Josie for the first time about five hours after she was born and then for an hour each day before she came home. When the nurse at the hospital made it plain I wasn't wanted or expected to stay with Lin for the birth I was quite relieved at avoiding the 'ordeal'. Though I'd agreed with Lin beforehand to stay with her, I was able to use the fact that the staff at the hospital didn't want me there as my excuse to go home. Why didn't I want to stay?
1. The obvious one — I was squeamish. I thought it would be an unpleasant physical experience — blood, etc.
2. I think I had a fear that it would be an anti-sexual experience. That somehow the image of a woman's sexual attractiveness built up in my mind would be spoilt by seeing the child born.
3. I thought I'd get in the way. In fact I probably would have done. I had not a clue what was going to happen, what the physical process of having a baby involved. Though I'd made sympathetic noises and 'taken an interest' in visits to the clinic and prenatal exercises, etc. — having the baby was Lin's job. It never occurred to me I might actually be able to do something useful at the birth.
4. Babies frightened me anyway. I'd never had much contact with them — having the baby was best left to Lin and the medical experts who know best. Afterwards looking after the baby — of course I'd share the work, etc. — but don't ask me to make any decisions about it — that was Lin's job — she knew best.
  Once out of hospital, I certainly didn't take an equal share in looking after Josie. Lin was in overall charge and I was an assistant who helped where he could. Lin was upset about the birth, the way it had happened and the way she'd been treated in hospital. Having missed out on the experience I couldn't understand what she was on about.

Time Two. By the time Jenny was born my feelings had changed considerably. We'd talked about it so much that all squeamishness had gone, and reading books on childbirth made me realize I could actually do something useful.
  Lin wanted to have the baby at home to avoid all the hang-ups of hospital birth . . . We were both worried that the midwives might have different ideas to us. Therefore one of my aims was to support Lin. In the event the midwives were really good, telling me when to hold Lin's legs, rub her back, and accepting that it was useful to have me there. I had Jenny in my arms two

minutes after she was born and started to take an equal share in looking after her from then onwards. There was no mystery or feeling that only Lin could do it.

Not to be at the birth now seems incredible to me. You usually try and support your friends when they need you so don't stop at childbirth, as sharing the kids means being in on everything from the word go. (Taken from *Having your baby* by Swansea Women and Health Group; this booklet also contains the experiences of two other men as well, and lots more).

Whatever companion we choose, early in our pregnancy s/he will need to read some of the same books, attend the same classes, and learn the same techniques that we do. If you have trouble finding someone to be with you, the NCT or your local women's liberation group should be able to help.

But be sure to explain to the people in charge of your birth well beforehand that you expect to have a companion with you during both labour *and* delivery. If you wish them to be there no matter what complications arise, you must explain this too. (When complications arise, that is often the time when we feel we need someone most.) If you can get the doctors and/or the hospital to agree to your request in writing this would help, as written evidence would be useful if and when some staff are uncooperative. If you have allowed yourself plenty of time and your request is not agreed to, you can then 'shop around' for more cooperative alternatives. You can help to make life easier for the women who follow you by informing groups such as AIMS, the NCT and your Community or Local Health Council of your experiences.

Obstetrical Interventions and Procedures

With all hospital procedures except those involving childbirth, the staff are obliged to obtain the person's signature before commencing. This is very unsatisfactory and gives rise to countless situations during childbirth where procedures are performed and drugs are given against a woman's wishes. It is possible that if you write a letter, stating that you will not have certain procedures unless you sign for them, you may have more chance of getting what you want. Also, if you have a supportive companion with you (see above), you have more chance of ensuring that procedures are not performed against your will. During the antenatal period, go over the procedures described in this section with your doctors and find out their opinions, practices and prejudices. If you have any preferences, make them known. Bear in mind that the value and safety of various procedures tends to be overestimated because the research on which figures are based is usually carried out by people who are particularly expert in their field.

Shaving Pubic Hair: The 'Prep'

This procedure is carried out virtually routinely in all British hospitals. Doctors say that prepping is done to decrease the risk of infection, since germs may be carried in the hair. However, Doris Haire, in *The Cultural Warping of Childbirth*, shows that the incidence of infection is in fact a little higher in mothers whose pubic area was shaved. Many of us feel that prepping is undignified; it is also uncomfortable, particularly when the hair starts growing back. In fact, as long ago as 1922, shaving was shown to be unnecessary. So much for medical logic.

Enemas

Enemas are also commonly given to women in labour. Since there is very often a natural diarrhoea for a few days before labour begins, many of us are already pretty well empty anyway. Furthermore, if we are in the middle of labour an enema can cause our contractions to become stronger and harder to control. If this happens, the attendant should be asked to stop until the contraction is over. If we are not in labour when we enter the hospital, sometimes the enema will cause our contractions to begin. Some hospitals give suppositories instead of enemas.

RUPTURING THE AMNIOTIC SAC (MEMBRANE)

The bag of amniotic fluid in which our baby has been floating throughout our pregnancy normally does not break until the very end of first-stage labour or during the second stage. Ten per cent of all amniotic sacs which are allowed to break spontaneously are still intact up to birth. Recent research shows that the amniotic membranes may be a beneficial buffer for the infant's head as it presses against the mother's pelvic floor during labour contractions.[*] About 10% of us will experience a premature rupture of the membranes before our labours begin. Once the membranes rupture there is an increased chance of infection, so mothers are usually advised to stay in bed and not to bathe at that time. You will probably know if your membranes rupture because water will trickle out of your vagina quite uncontrollably. If your membranes rupture, call your doctor. If labour has not started, you may have to have your labour induced (see 'Active Management of Labour', p. 427). Weigh your options carefully before choosing induction. Just because the membranes have ruptured, it does not mean that all the fluid will empty from the sac permanently; your body will continue to produce amniotic fluid.

[*] Roberto Caldeyro-Barcia, M.D., in his talk before the conference, 'Obstetrical Management and Infant Outcome', March 1974, New York. As reported by Margaret Worrall in the newsletter of the Boston Association for Childbirth Education, May–June 1974.

Doctors often artificially rupture the membranes. This is called an 'ARM', amniotomy or 'breaking of the waters'. It is often done to stimulate and speed up labour, although some studies disagree that rupture of the membranes has this effect.* On other occasions it is done so that an internal foetal monitor can be attached to the baby's head (see 'Foetal Monitors' below). Sometimes after the membranes are ruptured, our contractions feel so intense that we feel like taking drugs to ease the pain. It is helpful to realize that this intense part of our labour usually won't last too long, unless the entire labour process has been induced artificially. In that case we might experience strong contractions for a longer period of time.

Amniotomy can cause problems for both mother and baby, and the decision to rupture should not be taken lightly. It can displace the baby, cause prolapsed cord and infection, and 'In some cases the head of the foetus is completely deformed as a result. This 'moulding' can cause brain damage' (Caldeyro-Barcia, as reported in *Sunday Times*; see also Doris Haire). Drugs can add to the baby's stress.

Each doctor will have a particular feeling about how long labour should be allowed to go on after the membranes have ruptured. Since the risk of infection is greater without the amniotic sac, some doctors will try to accelerate labour in a woman whose membranes have ruptured if it seems to be progressing slowly. This causes some women to experience extremely intense contractions (see 'Active Management of Labour' below), which, without the protective membranes, may be harmful to the uterus and foetus, very difficult for the woman to control, and can lead to the use of further drugs and interventions to weaken the contractions.

The actual ARM procedure is described by many doctors, such as Bourne in *Pregnancy*, as free of any pain or discomfort. This is not necessarily the case. ARM can be particularly painful in women whose cervices are not 'ripe' (i.e ready to open): 'Artificial rupture of the membranes invariably proved painful to these women (several indicated that it was the worst pain they had ever had to bear), and there were many failed ARMs (in some women ARMs were attempted as many as four times) . . .' (NCT, 'Some Mothers' Experiences'). If doctors are considerate, the experience should be different. After discussion with you, they may change their minds about rupturing your membranes in the first place, or they may agree to insert a prostaglandin gel into the vagina, which can speed up the ripening process and hence reduce or eliminate pain during amniotomy. Some doctors recommend epidural anaesthesia (see p. 445) if amniotomy is to be performed and the cervix is unripe.

* Emanuel A. Friedman, M.D., *Labour: Clinical Evaluation and Management*, New York, Appleton-Century-Crofts, 1967, p. 256.

Intravenous Glucose Solution

Doctors usually advise us not to eat once labour begins. The idea is that if the stomach is empty we will be less likely to vomit during labour or during the administration of anaesthesia. Also, since our digestive systems virtually come to a standstill during labour, it is not very helpful if we have a full stomach. To substitute for light eating and to keep us from becoming dehydrated, doctors often administer an intravenous glucose (sugar) solution to a labouring woman by attaching a drip unit to a vein in her arm. Many childbirth educators feel that this drip adds to our apprehension and fear by making us feel that there is something wrong with our labour and by limiting our mobility. There is also the problem that once the 'drip' has been set up, it is all too easy for hospital staff to use it for an unnecessary induction or acceleration of labour (see below).

ACTIVE MANAGEMENT OF LABOUR

This refers to a delivery which is either induced or accelerated. The first step in induction* usually involves rupturing the membranes (see above) or 'stripping' them. 'Stripping' is often called a 'sweep'. Using a finger, the doctor separates the amnion (bag of waters) from the wall of the uterus. No one knows exactly why this causes labour to begin in some cases. It should be performed with caution, since if the placenta is lying over the cervix, the placenta could be stripped away from the uterus, with harmful and possibly catastrophic effect on the baby. Castor oil can also be given to start labour but this is usually successful only if it was about to begin soon anyway. If labour does not begin within a given amount of time (each doctor and hospital has a particular policy) then artificial oxytocin – Syntocinon – will be given to the mother to start labour as a substitute for the oxytocin present in natural labour. Artificial Syntocinon can be administered intravenously or intramuscularly. Given by mouth it is difficult to control and should not be used.†

Induction can be a positive experience. In the NCT's survey, 'Some Mothers' Experiences', out of 53 women who had already experienced a

---

* When we refer to induction, we also mean acceleration.

† Prostaglandins are sometimes used instead of, or as well as, oxytocin. Their use may become more common by the time you read this. Some people think they are better for induction than syntocinon, because they can be monitored more closely, for example, and, given orally, do not necessitate restricting drips and all that that implies. They also appear to be less 'fierce' on the uterus. Some doctors do not give prostaglandins intravenously because of side effects. Given as a pessary inside the vagina they are useful in 'ripening' the cervix and are not associated with side effects. However, even less is known about prostaglandins than is known about oxytocin.

non-induced birth, 16 said that their induced birth was better and they implied that they would choose induction again. This was particularly the case when their non-induced labours had been long and arduous:

'If I ever had a third child', remarked one woman, 'I would do everything in my power to arrange for an induced birth' . . . One woman was very happy after a 7-hour labour which she said was 'like a holiday' after a previous 36-hour labour, and another after a 12-hour labour compared with $19\frac{1}{2}$ hours with a severe backache labour . . .

But out of the 53 women, 34 felt that in spite of preparation to cope with induction, it was worse than last time and they would try to avoid an induced birth in the future. According to the NCT's survey, a positive experience of induction appears to be directly related to the quality of emotional support given. Below is one woman's experience of an unhappy induced birth:

I approached the birth in a state of happy expectancy and confidence, since the procedure [induction] had been explained to me. However, I received a severe shock. The membranes were ruptured, causing extreme pain and great mental distress. Then the oxytocin drip was set up, and about 10 minutes later contractions started, roughly 4 minutes apart at first. Later they were coming every 2 minutes and were very painful; at no time could I control the pain and 'ride it'. Injections had no effect, and I was thankful to be given gas-and-air, but the pain was so great and so regular that I could not use it without assistance. Afterwards I had a great deal of pain, and required 3 weeks to recover, compared with 11 days on the previous occasion. The whole birth was a very distressing experience and one I will not repeat.

The risks of induction

Since induction can clearly cause distress and since it also carries risks (see below), it should only be performed when necessary. There is no doubt that induction is essential in cases where there is some question about the baby's chances of survival, as in the question of toxaemia, haemolytic disease (Rh factor), diabetes, or severely prolonged pregnancy. Such cases comprise a very small proportion of all pregnancies, say, 5%. But in some hospitals, half or more of all women have been induced. The risks of induction are set out below so that we can discuss seriously with the doctor whether or not we wish to be induced.

. . . I was prepared for the induction drip without discussion. As a professional social worker in my late twenties I was not used to this approach and questioned why it was happening. The officious staff nurse told me in an off-hand manner that it was quite normal and for my own good so I was not to fuss. I did what any other intelligent woman might do and caused a scene. This quickly

*produced both the ward sister and the doctor who explained the general
principles behind induction. When I asked if it was necessary at this stage it
turned out that it wasn't so urgent – and the matter was left there. Some
hours later the doctor came and talked to my husband and myself about the
option, at which point we agreed to the induction drip being inserted. (Letter
to* Guardian, *13 December 1974).*

Induction can result in complications. Frequently the contractions do
not follow the normal wave-like course but reach intensity instantly and
remain intense for a long period. This can be very discouraging and the
mother may give up hope and rely on more drugs – with their own added
risks – to ease her pain. A mother whose labour is induced will probably
require extra support and good information on the progress of her labour.
She and the foetus must be closely monitored (see 'Foetal Monitoring',
below) to make sure that the uterus and the foetus are all right. Contractions of too great an intensity (*tumultuous labour*) can lead to decreased
blood supply to the uterus and the placenta (*uteroplacental ischemia*), and
uterine rupture. Induction can also result in high blood pressure,
prolapse of the umbilical cord, higher rates of infection, jaundice in the
newborn, higher rates of Caesareans, forceps deliveries and episiotomies
(with their own added risks) and foetal distress (see Bibliography under
'Obstetric Interventions'). The effect of hyperactive contractions can
increase pressure on the baby's head. This can be further exaggerated by
the fact that the membranes will probably have been ruptured artificially
(see above).

Many of the effects on the baby mean that it will have to be in a special
care baby unit immediately after birth. It is now reasonably well established that the resulting separation of mother and baby can lead to long-
term problems (see p. 439 for further discussion).

Little research has been done on the safety of induction – particularly
on possible long-term effects such as a far more painful labour leading to
long-term emotional problems.

Doctors who have high induction rates believe that this reduces
infant mortality, that it is convenient and that it avoids long and
unpleasant labours. The reduction of infant mortality does not appear
to result from an increased induction rate (Chalmers *et al.*, *British
Medical Journal*, 27 March 1976). Even if the mortality rate is reduced, it
could be due to the increased number of high-risk pregnancies being
terminated, for example. Furthermore, although deaths might not be
increased, complications – such as prematurity – are. It is difficult to
tell the true maturity of the foetus, especially if the woman has recently
been on the pill. 'Only about 5% of women have their babies on the day
they were expected, and the majority have them about a week late. First
babies are often late' (Kitzinger, *The Experience of Childbirth*). Conse-

quently there is a higher incidence of prematurity and resultant respiratory distress in induced babies (see Blacow *et al.*, *Lancet*). (See 'Avoiding Induction' below.)

The convenience of inductions has not been satisfactorily demonstrated. They are more labour-intensive on staff who could be better employed in a supportive role, and it has been suggested that induced births occur at least as often at inconvenient times — i.e. through the night — as do ordinary births (Cole *et al.*, *Lancet*).

Unpleasant labours can be helped by induction, but some doctors induce arbitrarily if labour has gone on for a certain number of hours — which can be as low as 12 or even 8. (The usual length of a first labour is 12–14 hours.) Some doctors think that long labours are by definition unpleasant but this is by no means always the case.

They said it would take too long without the drip. Too long for whom? I wondered.

Very little is known about the workings of oxytocin. Certainly, it does not mimic what happens naturally. It has been observed, for example, that during natural labour, women release oxytocin in spurts — not continuously as in induction — and that the maximum levels present are much below that usually given during induction (Gibbens, Blair Bell Research Society). The dosage used during induction has been described as 'monumental', and carries with it the danger of damaging the uterus (Theobald, *British Medical Journal*).

The safety of induction can certainly be increased, for example by careful selection of women and careful monitoring, and it has been argued that excessively frequent contractions 'usually reflect misuse' of oxytocin (*Lancet*, 16 November 1974). But there is little doubt that induction carries risks. Where induction is not medically essential, these risks are simply added risks to an otherwise normal labour.

Avoiding Induction

If you are told that induction is medically necessary for you, it is worth checking on the number of 'medical' inductions the particular hospital performs. You can do this in advance by asking the consultant direct, or asking your local health council to do this for you. (Bear in mind that induction rates may differ between obstetric teams within the same hospital.) If, say, 50% of births are induced you can be sure that the medical criteria used are less than stringent.

'Prolonged pregnancy' is the most common reason given for induction. Some doctors say that a pregnancy of 40 weeks is post-term, and induce accordingly. At best they may be inducing needlessly, and at worst their efforts result in a premature baby. Other doctors are far more cautious and are happy to leave a healthy pregnancy to at least 42 weeks – by which time roughly 95 per cent of women have given birth spontaneously.

If you fear you may be pushed into an unnecessary induction on the grounds of prolonged pregnancy, you could try asking the consultant to prove firstly that the baby *is* postmature. Good monitoring of a pregnant woman throughout her pregnancy, preferably by the same person, is, together with knowledge of menstrual history the best way of assessing the age of the foetus. Ultrasound readings after the first trimester and before 36 weeks are also pretty good at indicating gestational age. However, they are not to be recommended for routine use because as yet, little is known about the effects on the foetus.

In spite of your scepticism, the consultant may well keep insisting that your baby is postmature, in which case you could ask for proof that the baby is actually in danger of suffering (in fact many women know themselves when their babies are in need of help, without the aid of expert opinion). There are a variety of tests which can exclude postmaturity and can therefore spare you and your baby the risk of an unnecessary induction:

Placental function tests: oestriol tests involve collecting all your urine for at least 24 hours at a stretch, possibly even for 3 days – they can therefore be a bore! Results should be available within 24 hours, but unfortunately not all laboratories work very quickly. A blood test for placental lactogen is much simpler to do and can indicate a level below which the baby is at risk. *Amniocentesis* (see p. 506) can also be used to test for evidence of the baby's maturity, but done near to term there is a higher risk attached to this procedure. You may find that an *X ray* is suggested to detect the baby's maturity. This should be avoided if at all possible because of the risks involved (see X rays, p. 506).

One final point: if you are reasonably sure of your dates, you may well 'know' when your baby is overdue. Try not to be put off if your estimate differs from that of your doctor(s): they are notoriously prone to be wrong!

Fortunately, since the furore about non-medical inductions began in 1974, some doctors are beginning to change their practices. If there is still no clear medical reason for induction, if you have raised your objections to the procedure, and if you still suspect that the hospital is likely to induce you, you might feel like resorting to drastic action like this midwife did:

I locked myself in the ward lavatory until I was well into the second stage of labour. I didn't want them interfering with my baby. I only came out when it was too late for them to put me on a drip. It's a good job it was a short labour! (Women's Report, *Vol. 4, issue 5*)

We are not *recommending* this!

If you are induced by means of a drip in your vein, make sure that the catheter is firmly fixed, otherwise you will constantly be anxious about dislodging it. Make sure also that the tube is long enough to allow you to move around as much as you want.

Other methods of induction in use include: a *cervical vibrator*, which can quickly open the cervix, but it can be extremely painful to have anything inside you when you are in labour. *Acupuncture* has also been shown to be effective for inducing and stimulating labour. Its advantages probably extend to minimal effect on either mother or baby, but of course there has been little research with this technique in the West.

An alternative, often effective, and above all, *natural method* of activating labour is to stimulate the nipples, which enables the mother to produce her own oxytocin. This is completely safe as overdosage cannot occur and complicated monitoring is unnecessary. You can do it yourself, and the procedure can even be enjoyable! (For more about this, see Bibliography under Salzmann and Jhirad, pp. 481–2.)

FOETAL MONITORS

Foetal monitors are machines which electronically record the foetus's heart-rate during labour. The most accurate monitor involves temporarily sticking gummy electrodes onto the woman's chest. In addition, two straps are placed around the woman's abdomen. The upper belt holds the tocodynamometer, which records the intensity of the uterine contractions, and the lower strap holds an ultrasonic transducer, which monitors and records the foetal heart rate. When all three of these measuring devices are used, the external foetal monitor is about 90 to 95% accurate. Studies in Japan indicate that the ultrasonic device may be a factor in brain damage and birth defects when used early in pregnancy. There is no evidence which clearly proves that the ultrasonic transducer has no adverse long-term effect on the baby when used during labour. This is another instance of doctors' eagerness to use technology before the complete range of its effects is known. When the ultrasonic device is not used, the external monitor is only about 57% accurate.

While some women find that the straps present no problems for them at all, others find them uncomfortable and even painful. Monitoring can make it difficult to change position, and abdominal massage – which can be so helpful during contractions – becomes impossible. Recently, however, doctors in Birmingham have devised a technique with an internal monitor which enables the woman to walk around (see Flynn and Kelly, *British Medical Journal*, 1976).

Internal foetal monitors are thought to be about 90% accurate. They are electrodes connected to wires within a plastic tube, and are introduced into the woman's vagina and attached directly to the baby's presenting part (usually the head) by means of metal clips or screws. No one has bothered to find out if this causes pain to the baby. These electrodes measure the baby's heartbeat. The woman's contractions are measured either by a catheter, introduced into her uterus through her vagina, or by the external tocodynamometer strap described above. There is much more risk of infection with the internal monitor, especially when the uterine catheter is used as well, and there are of course potential risks to the baby, considering the possibility of bleeding due to the way the screw or clip is attached (John W. Scanlon, M.D., and Edward I. Walkley, M.D., *Paediatrics*, December 1972). In order for the internal elements to be applied, the mother's amniotic sac must first be ruptured. This adds to the possibility of infection and complications (see 'Rupturing the Amniotic Sac', p. 425).

With both monitors the mother's blood pressure is intermittently measured by means of a blood pressure cuff attached to one of her arms. The other arm is very frequently attached to an intravenous solution unit and/or an induction 'drip'. It is not hard to imagine that all these procedures during heavy labour can leave the mother feeling very restricted, immobile and apprehensive, although they can be reassuring.

Some people believe that monitors have decreased the newborn death rate and the number of brain-damaged children. On this basis, one study even recommends that monitoring should be introduced during all labours (Edington *et al.*, *British Medical Journal*, 1975). Others are raising questions about the value of monitors, and no one knows the side effects of monitoring itself. Perhaps one reason for the apparent obsession with foetal monitoring in some quarters is because of its very existence: in 1976 alone one British firm sold over 800 machines, with a turnover, incidentally, of two million pounds. Monitoring means money and, as we have seen with other types of technology, once the machinery has been acquired, hospital staff often feel the need to justify its existence.

There have, to our knowledge, been no studies to determine the cause of foetal stress that use as a control group women who have had no pain-relieving drugs and who have not had their membranes artificially ruptured. We feel certain that if the number of unnatural procedures described above was reduced, there would also be a decline in foetal and perinatal mortality and morbidity.

EPISIOTOMY

An episiotomy is an incision in the perineum (the area between the vagina and the anus) to enlarge the opening through which the baby will pass. It is performed just before the head is born. Although episiotomies are performed routinely in some hospitals, there is often no need for them. Often women need episiotomies because they are told to push too much.

As the NCT booklet on episiotomies says, 'Involuntary expulsive efforts by the mother combined with the uterine contractions will in most cases push the head down on the perineum without great physical effort on the mother's part . . . It is possible to manage the second stage without once using the word "push".' This removes a lot of stress on the pelvic floor and the need for an episiotomy in many cases. If the mother is not anaesthetized she will feel when to stop pushing and when to start easing the baby gently out. The doctor or midwife can direct her. The vaginal opening can stretch to very wide proportions without tearing.

They were prepared to do an episiotomy but I said I felt I could relax enough not to. By following the instructions of Sister L. when to push gently and when to pant the head was born without a cut or tear.

If you give birth in a semi-sitting position, this relieves tension on the perineum and you can avoid the need for an episiotomy (see 'Positions during Labour and Delivery', p. 409).

One justification for routine episiotomy is that it avoids tearing, particularly if forceps are used. But not all women tear and many wouldn't if they were helped to push the baby out gently. Moreover, the Cardiff study (Chalmers *et al.*) found that although the episiotomy rate had risen, there was no striking reduction in the incidence of perineal tears. Another reason given for episiotomy is that it helps a speedy delivery; this is necessary in some cases but rarely so.

A woman who can relax her pelvic floor is less likely to need an episiotomy – hence the importance of pelvic floor exercises such as the Kegel exercises (see p. 137) or those explained in various NCT publications (see address p. 488). Even if you have had an episiotomy you do *not* necessarily need one at a subsequent birth.

The effects of an episiotomy can last a long time. But they can be minimized and can even be non-existent if the cut and the stitching are done well. Everything hinges on the expertise of the person performing the procedure. It is therefore scandalous that in the UK, episiotomy repairs are commonly performed by students – for practice in stitching. If the cut and repair are done badly, they can involve intense pain – both during and after the procedures – and sexual problems which can last for months or longer. If it is obvious that an episiotomy will be needed, local anaesthetic can be given beforehand. If an episiotomy is performed during delivery, the cut should be made at the peak of a contraction when the nerve endings are numbed through stretching. If it is done in an emergency, it may not be possible to do either of these things but that should rarely happen. Although women commonly experience pain during stitching, this is unnecessary. The NCT booklet says, 'Analgesia is always necessary.' But some people assert that within, say, half an hour after the birth, no pain can be felt during stitching. In an NCT survey, half of those women who were stitched without pain relief, even within half an hour of delivery, complained of pain. One fifth commented spontaneously that the pain was severe: 'The stitching was far worse than the whole of the labour.' Sometimes a pain-relieving injection is given, but the doctor does not wait for it to take effect. Fifteen per cent of those who received pain relief had this kind of treatment. It is difficult to imagine a dentist behaving like this. In fact, as one woman pointed out in the *British Medical Journal* (5 January 1974), other wounds involving layers of muscle are stitched following an injection of drugs such as morphine or pethidine. Her own complaints of pain were ignored, sidestepped and ridiculed. And she was a doctor.

It is very difficult to repair a badly-performed episiotomy, for when the scar tissue has consolidated, restitching can make things worse. Unfortunately, the best time to repair the damage is after a subsequent birth – when it *must* be done by the most skilful person available. It is therefore essential that at all times episiotomy repairs are performed by someone who knows what they are doing.

I am not exaggerating when I say that I could hardly walk for six weeks. It had a disastrous effect on my sex life . . . In the end I was completely up the creek psychologically and felt I had to go to a psychiatrist because I couldn't face sex at all . . . When our second daughter was born I was told what a dreadful job had been made of the first episiotomy. Evidently my perineum was completely broken down and the vagina terribly lop-sided. No wonder it was agony. But they did a beautiful job sewing me up this time – used soluble cat gut for the internal stitches, which should have been used the first time but wasn't, and it's more or less back where it should be. (Nova, September 1974)

If you have had an episiotomy, the wound must be kept as clean and dry as possible – washing it every day is of extreme importance. It should be dried and covered with a pad which should be changed frequently. An anti-inflammatory drug like Chymoral taken for the first 3 days helps a lot to prevent inflammation and assist healing. Daily inspection is necessary to watch for infection. If there is any sign of this, a swab should be taken and an appropriate antibiotic prescribed. Infection can be unpleasant and it can delay discharge from hospital. For more on how to cope with an episiotomy, see the NCT publications listed on p. 481. They include many valuable suggestions, including the use of homeopathic arnica tablets and ointment.

FORCEPS

In a forceps delivery the doctor pulls the baby out with a double-bladed instrument which resembles salad tongs, except that the blades are longer and curved to fit the shape of the baby's head. Each blade is introduced into the vagina separately and placed carefully on the side of the baby's head. Then the two blades are clamped together outside the vagina. Depending on where the baby's head lies at the time of delivery, the doctor will use high or low forceps. The higher the forceps, the more dangerous the delivery, since that indicates that the baby will have to be pulled out a longer distance.

Delivery by forceps has saved the lives of many infants and mothers, but many unnecessary forceps deliveries are performed. 'The incidence of delivery by forceps and vacuum extractor (see below), combined, rarely rises above 5% in countries where mothers actively participate in the birth of babies' (Haire, p. 23). In some hospitals in Britain, the forceps rate is as high as one in every three births. Forceps deliveries can result in damage to the baby which often leads to separation from the mother, possibly leading to long-term problems (see p. 439). They are also thought to increase the risk of infection in the mother and should not be performed without good reason (see Haire).

The usual reasons for a forceps delivery are:

1. To speed up second-stage labour if there is severe foetal distress.
2. If the umbilical cord is wrapped tightly around the baby's neck or if the cord prolapses.
3. In case of unusual presentations (see p. 410).
4. If regional anaesthesia doesn't allow the mother to push out her baby.
5. To shorten a very long second-stage labour.

It is uncommon for a prepared, unanaesthetized mother to have her baby delivered by forceps, but should the occasion arise, the breathing techniques may be enough to carry you through without anaesthesia.

Normal second-stage labour can go on from half an hour to 2 hours, and unless there is some indication that the baby is having trouble getting out, there is no medical reason for introducing forceps. Women are designed to be able to give birth to babies. The survival of our species depended on it and still does.

VACUUM EXTRACTION (OR THE VENTOUSE)

This is sometimes used as an alternative to forceps. When the cervix is fully dilated and the baby is ready to be delivered, a small metal cup is placed on its head and this is connected to a vacuum which makes it stay on the scalp. Traction then results in the baby being delivered. The baby will have a swelling on its head but this will disappear. The ventouse can be used only when the head is presenting normally. Some doctors never use it: two babies died as a result of its use between 1964 and 1973, and St George's Hospital, London, stopped using it in 1968. However, its wide use in Scandinavia and Holland, where death rates for both mothers and babies are very low, does suggest that vacuum extraction may in some instances have advantages over forceps. Of course the unnecessary use of either is deplorable.

CAESAREAN SECTION

Occasionally, in the case of a very long, hard labour that seems to be accomplishing little in terms of cervical dilation, a caesarean section will be advised. The operation is also necessary if the mother's pelvic structure is too small to allow the baby to move into the birth canal, if the placenta comes loose and begins to prolapse, if the cord prolapses, if the mother or baby suddenly has an adverse change of condition, or if there is excessive bleeding.

Although this operation is not as safe as normal delivery it is almost always done to save your life or your baby's. Anaesthesia is given and you may request regional anaesthesia (see Pain Relief, p. 444) and thus be awake during the delivery. An incision is made through the abdominal wall and into the uterus. Both incisions, uterine and abdominal, are repaired by stitches.

After eighteen hours of labour the doctor told me I'd have to have a caesarean section because I wasn't big enough. I thought there was something wrong with the baby. Part of me believed it was because I hadn't laboured hard enough. Part of me believed I had failed because I hadn't been able to deliver normally (that's one thing Lamaze training doesn't prepare you for, how to deal with childbirth that doesn't work out normally).

I saw my baby being lifted from my stomach in the reflection of a lamp over me. That was very nice. I think my operation took longer, too, because I had a punctured bladder. I found out later that that was a fairly common thing to happen. They flashed my baby past me, and put him in intensive care for 24 hours in an incubator. I didn't understand why they took him away so quickly, because they kept telling me he was very healthy. They didn't tell me before the surgery that he would automatically be put in intensive care, so I didn't understand why I couldn't see him the next day. I thought something was wrong. Finally I got to see him that night, and he was put into the nursery.

Afterwards I had a lot of happy, normal birth feelings. I was very proud. I got over being ashamed. The day after he was born I had to walk, and my stomach hurt. One thing that helped me was that I was in a bed next to another woman who had had a caesarean 6 days before. Breast-feeding was a little hard, because I had to have this thing to prop him up, and for the first few days I couldn't turn on my side. After that I could put him next to me while I nursed.

Part of my easy postpartum adjustment was that I stayed in the hospital for 8 days and was well taken care of because I'd had surgery. Also, I had no episiotomy, and I was well rested. And when I got home, people took good care of me.

Two days after my due date, my waters broke and my labour was induced. After 12 hours of labour and one hour of transition, my cervix was only 7 centimetres dilated. The doctor recommended that I go on a half hour more before he would decide about an emergency delivery. I had been exhilarated by my labour and by the fact that I could control my rather strong contractions, but after he said that, my motivation started to decrease. One half hour later my doctor told me that I still wasn't dilating and that he would have to perform a caesarean. I was so physically involved in labour that this felt like an interruption and a disappointment, and I began to cry. But of course, anything that interfered with the safe delivery of my baby was unthinkable, and I agreed to the operation. I was wheeled to the operating room, given a spinal, and became numb from my upper waist down. A cloth was draped in front of me so I couldn't see anything. My husband was not allowed in the operating room. In contrast to my intense involvement with labour, I felt passive, numb, and I wished only for a healthy baby. I was surprised about how little discomfort I felt. I did feel slight strokes on my abdomen as the incisions were made, and after a half hour I felt a slight tug on my abdomen. Someone said, 'It's a boy.' I was so touched. His cry was not one of pain, but of life. They brought him to me: he was beautiful, and mine.

Caesarean section rates seem to be rising and, like forceps rates, they vary between different areas: this may well be due to the increased use of routine hospital procedures and interventions which hinder the normal course of labour. They are, however, being increasingly used for breech presentations (see p. 412), and, with doubtful reasoning, for premature labours. At least some of the Caesarean sections performed in the UK are unnecessary.

Although the risk of death from Caesareans is small they are associated with considerable post-operative discomfort, infection, and subsequent feeding difficulties. Hardly anything is known about their effects on the developing child.

Be sure to discuss the operation with your doctor before labour so that you understand all aspects of it. Hospitals are beginning to allow fathers into the operating room during a caesarean. Discuss this with your doctor, too, especially the idea of having him with you in the recovery room, when you can feel very confused, frightened and lonely. Usually a caesarean is a last-minute decision; if, however, a woman has delivered once that way, all future births may have to be conducted by caesarean.

A hysterectomy should be performed during a caesarean only in an emergency, when the uterus has become seriously infected or ruptured, and never without the fully informed consent and understanding of the mother. Routine hysterectomies during C-sections are deplorable (and even criminal without informed consent).

Special care baby units

Special care baby units are not strictly *obstetrical* interventions, but we are discussing them under this heading because their use has increased dramatically, at least in part due to high induction rates seen in recent years. The number of places in a special care baby unit can be a good guide to the interventionist policies of the nearby obstetrical unit. And bear in mind that special care baby units tend to be over-used in the same way as other technological innovations . . . to justify their existence.

As we have indicated earlier, a baby sometimes needs special care, for example, if it is premature. In this case, it needs to be looked after in a special care baby unit (SCBU) for a time. At present, almost 20% of all babies go to a SCBU; many of them are admitted with good reason. However, nearly half of these babies are perfectly healthy and need not be there; it is routine practice in some hospitals, for example, to admit to SCBU's all babies delivered by forceps. Several studies have indicated that separation of mother and baby can adversely affect the child's development (see for example, Klaus and Kennell, *Maternal-Infant Bonding*, and Richards, 'Possible effects of early separation on later development of children'). However, much can – and should – be done by hospital staff to ensure that the strain of separation is minimized. They should be sensitive to parents' very real fears and anxieties, and allow them to handle their babies, with access to the SCBU at any time. Breast feeding should be allowed if at all possible and, at the very least, a woman should be allowed to provide her own milk for her baby if she wishes. If staff are sensitive, they can prevent difficulties from arising; it is thought that one of the main reasons for these difficulties is the mother's lack of confidence, which results from her being encouraged to feel useless and inadequate in the face of 'expert' doctors and nurses. If your baby does have to be in a special unit, neither of you should be made to suffer as a result. But first of all, try and make sure that the hospital staff give adequate reasons for taking your baby away.

We hope that following the example of a few hospitals, such as the John Radcliffe in Oxford, more hospitals will recognize the importance of mothers being involved in these units. In the meantime, it is worth checking on hospital policies before you decide where to have your baby.

Pain Relief During Labour

Even if we prepare ourselves for labour (see p. 416), many of us will still experience some pain and we may well need additional help in dealing with it. But psychological support and encouragement, and good antenatal preparation, can go a long way towards dealing with pain, since fear and tension tend to increase painful sensations. In Sweden, Holland

and Japan, 'skilful psychological management of labour usually precludes the need for obstetrical medication' (Haire, *Cultural Warping of Childbirth*).

Many women who were given a second dose of pethidine or other analgesic when they found it difficult to cope with contractions would have preferred to have been given more emotional support at that point, and obviously felt that the pharmacological pain relief did not really take the place of encouragement, praise and oral guidance. ('Some Women's Experiences', NCT)

DRUGS FOR PAIN RELIEF

Drugs are the most common method doctors use for dealing with pain in childbirth. Often they are given as the 'first line of defence' or even routinely, sometimes when the mother does not want them. You are more likely to come across drugs for pain relief in hospital where staff have a lot of work and little time. Giving an injection also helps staff to feel that they are both effective and in control. It is a pity that psychological support and encouragement is not universally available. As we have shown, this can very often preclude the use of drugs – which can have an adverse effect on the baby.

Almost every drug given to the mother just before or during labour crosses the placenta and reaches the baby. If the baby is premature, smaller than average or in poor health, the consequences can be dangerous. Even a normal baby can suffer and we mothers can sometimes suffer more from the after-effects of the drugs used in labour than we might have from labour itself. The problem is compounded because along with each drug often come two or three other procedures designed to ensure, as much as possible, the safety of the drug used. Each of these procedures (see p. 424) carries its own potential risks and side effects.

Drugs intended to reduce pain during labour can be grouped under the following headings:

1. Sedatives or tranquillizers: sedatives relieve anxiety and induce a feeling of calmness or drowsiness; tranquillizers simply relieve anxiety.
2. Hypnotics: these induce sleep.
3. Analgesics: these decrease our sensation of pain; in large doses they will usually cause loss of consciousness.
4. Anaesthetics: these remove the sensation of pain altogether.

The possible psychological effects of these drugs on the child – and indirectly on the mother – are only beginning to be assessed (see Bibliography). Many drugs given just before or during labour which dampen down the mother's reactions will have the same effect on the baby. This can last for the first week of life or more, and can thus affect the baby's ability to suckle. Since the baby's sucking reflex soon after birth is important for ensuring a good milk supply, the ability of the mother to produce milk can also be affected by these drugs – and this in turn can affect the mother-child relationship.

Infants whose mothers had received analgesia and anaesthesia during labour and delivery have been shown to have retarded muscular, visual and neural development in the first four weeks of life. This doesn't mean all babies will be so affected, nor will the babies affected be permanently retarded in development, but many imprinting patterns can be set during the first few weeks of life.*

We do not yet know the true significance of all this information. Martin Richards, a Cambridge psychologist who has done some work in this area, says: 'My own guess, and it can only be a guess at present, is that drug effects in themselves are not of vital importance. If both mother and baby are healthy and they live in a supportive social situation the drug effects will be lost among all the other chance experiences of life. However, where a baby is already 'at risk' for medical or social reasons, things might be very different and in this situation a drugged baby might become the straw that breaks the camel's back' ('Obstetric Analgesics and the Development of Children', *Midwife, Health Visitor and Community Nurse*, February 1976).

What knowledge that is available very strongly suggests that these drugs should not be used routinely during labour, nor should they be used unnecessarily.

Sedatives, Tranquillizers and Hypnotics

These are commonly given in the first stage of labour 'to take the edge off your contractions'. They can have depressant effects on some newborn functions.† For example, sluggish respiration is common among babies whose mothers receive sedation, and Valium is thought to interfere with a newborn's ability to cope with cold stress. Valium may also cause jaundice in the baby if given around the time of labour. The total dose of Valium administered during labour should not exceed 30 mg. Other tranquillizers commonly used are Sparine (promazine) and Phenergan (promethazine). Sparine (which is commonly given with Nisentil, a narcotic), may cause labour to slow down or even cease altogether.

Tranquillizers may be helpful in allowing the mother to relax between contractions. However, she may find herself falling asleep until the contraction reaches its peak, and then she may panic, forget to breathe properly, and actually experience more pain than she would have without the drug. A good companion can help you by reminding you to breathe.

---

* Imprinting refers to certain bonds of a psychological nature that create patterns for future action and that either take place at a specific time or do not take place at all.

† Haire, *Cultural Warping of Childbirth*, refers to several papers on this.

Barbiturates such as Nembutal, Amytal, Soneryl and Seconal are seda-tives when given in small doses, but they induce sleep when given in larger doses and are then considered to be hypnotics. These drugs are dangerous to the baby; they reach the placenta easily and become lodged in the baby's brain. They can depress foetal respiration and responsiveness (see Ploman and Persson, 'On the Transfer of Barbiturates to the Human Foetus and Their Accumulation in Some of Its Vital Organs', *Journal of Obstetrics and Gynaecology of the British Empire*, 64, 706 (1967)).

Analgesics

Analgesics, like the above, are often given in the first stage of labour, as soon as the woman feels pain. The most commonly given analgesic is *pethidine*, a narcotic. It is usually given by injection, takes 15 minutes to take effect, and can last for 4 hours. In spite of its widespread use, it is not particularly effective and it does have side effects. A recent paper by Holdcroft and Morgan (see Bibliography) shows that three quarters of the women investigated received no relief from pain at all. All narcotics have a serious depressant effect on foetal respiration, and the newborn's behavioural responsiveness may be significantly decreased by these drugs. They should not be given within 2 hours of expected delivery because of this effect. If you are given too much pethidine, the baby may have to be given another drug – naloxone – to counteract its effects. Pethidine is commonly given in far too high a dose. 150 mg. or 200 mg. is sometimes routine instead of the 50 mg. or 100 mg. recommended in midwives' textbooks. Although some women just feel 'high' from the effects of pethidine, others experience nausea, a sense of unreality, and loss of control. Some people believe that many unpleasant experiences during labour are in fact caused by the effects of even small doses of pethidine on women not accustomed to hard drugs. Studies involving self-administration of pethidine are under way in Cardiff, and it has been found that this way, women tend to use less of the drug and have fewer side effects. If you have been on certain anti-depressants (monoamine oxidase inhibitors such as Nardil or Marplan), you will need to be watched carefully, since they can increase the effect of pethidine.

If pethidine works for you, and if you are in need of analgesia, it can well be the best drug to use, in spite of its side effects. 'In the short term, at least, it may be better to continue to use the well established drugs like Pethidine, when required, because we at least have some knowledge of their side effects . . . Where a mother of a drugged baby is having feeding difficulties it may be very helpful for her to know that the baby's reduced sucking response is the temporary result of the drug and not an indication of her "mishandling" of the baby' (Richards, 'Obstetric Anal-gesics and the Development of Children').

In some hospitals, pethidine is given routinely. You can refuse it. 'But your refusal may be met with bewilderment, contempt or disbelief. You can also ask to be given a half dose (50 mg.) . . . If you do refuse, try to be tactful. You might try saying you'd like to try it your way first, but realize that you might find, a little later, that you will need either or both gas and air (see below) or pethidine' (Bolton Women's Guide). On other occasions, narcotics can be withheld from you when you want them. They are ineffective if given too late.

The following provides a glimpse of the range of experiences women can have with pethidine. It is taken from the NCT's survey 'Some Mothers' Experiences of Induced Labour'. For a more detailed look at women's experiences of pethidine, pain relief and hospitalized childbirth in general, see this pamphlet.

Those who liked pethidine found that it took the edge off contractions without imperilling their control or that it gave them a chance to sleep and they 'woke refreshed'. Those who disliked pethidine said 'It was a great mistake. It stopped contractions', or slowed down the progress of dilatation, or made remarks such as 'I lost control and understanding'. Women who were left completely free to choose whether or not they had pethidine, and who felt they had good emotional support, were those more likely to find it helpful . . . It is clear that most women did not have a choice as to whether or not they had pethidine . . . The very ease with which pethidine can be given – 'It was shot into my thigh as I was lying down with my eyes closed' – contributes to its being used without the woman's consent, and sometimes when she has asked not to be given it.

Morphine – another narcotic with similar side effects to pethidine – is much stronger than pethidine and is particularly useful for the dull, continuing back pains of a baby in the occipito-posterior position (see p. 410) or for long labours. Some women vomit on being given morphine, so often an anti-emetic is given at the same time. *Fortral* – again similar to pethidine although it is less strong. It has little effect on the foetus's respiration, but if it does affect this, it cannot be reversed by Lethidrone as can the effects of pethidine and morphine. Fortral is a newer drug than pethidine; the possible psychological effect of this and of other newer drugs has not yet been investigated.

Inhalation Analgesia – This is pain relief that you inhale, usually by means of a face mask. (If you don't like the idea of a face mask, you could try making enquiries in advance about using a disposable mouthpiece instead.) The one most commonly used is *gas and air* (usually Entonox, which is a mixture of oxygen and nitrous oxide). It appears to be more effective than pethidine, producing satisfactory relief in almost half of those who use it. It is particularly effective if used with good teaching and support and could thus be used much more widely than pethidine.

As yet there is no evidence that Entonox has harmful effects on the baby. Like Trilene and Penthrane (see below), Entonox does not greatly depress foetal respiration. Even though nitrous oxide does reach the baby via the placenta, the use of oxygen at the same time – and its benefits to mother and baby – outweighs the possible disadvantages of nitrous oxide.

One overwhelming advantage of inhalation analgesia is that you can administer it yourself. It can also be used during the second stage of labour. Entonox takes some 15 seconds to work so you should start breathing the mixture at the beginning of a contraction, tailing off at its height.* Most hospitals explain well before labour how to use the machine, but if they don't you should ask to be shown.

Trilene is not so commonly used, mainly because of its smell which is like dry cleaning fluid. There is also evidence that it affects the baby's blood. *Penthrane* takes slightly longer to take effect than Entonox but it gives prolonged relief. Unfortunately, like Trilene, it has a smell which some people find unpleasant. Like Entonox, it helps you to become mentally and physically relaxed but a few women become very drowsy. It has little known effect on the baby.

Regional Anaesthesia

Regional anaesthesia is injected into the woman's body at a specific point, and it is expected to anaesthetize only a particular part of the body. If everything has gone normally and no drugs have been administered until this point, the actual delivery is the worst time to give the mother anaesthesia. If she has learned how to push and if her doctor or midwife is willing to coach her by telling her when to stop pushing, then she can experience the thrill of delivery fully, without an anaesthetic to cut off her sensations and make her recovery that much more annoying.

The pudendal block† anaesthetizes only the vulva, or external female organs. A painless forceps delivery (see p. 435) is then possible without recourse to general anaesthesia, although it is necessary to inject the perineum and the labia as well for complete pain relief. Even this relatively minor anaesthetic can cause 'a persistent decrease in oxygen

---

* It is very important to have a fixed concentration of the mixture: if the attendant keeps changing the concentrations, it is impossible to judge how much to inhale, and you can end up getting far too much (when you can fall asleep), or too little, which is ineffective. Beware, also, of those hospitals which encourage women to use inhalation analgesia during the 2nd stage: it can make coordination extremely difficult when you need to push.

† Pudendal block anaesthesia is named after the pudenum, or external female genitalia. Pudendum in Latin means 'that of which one ought to be ashamed'. Obviously, we can't think of a more inappropriate name!

saturation in the newborn during the first thirty minutes of postpartum observation'.†

The *paracervical block* is considered by many to be dangerous to both baby and mother. Maternal complications such as convulsions and severe hypotension (drop in blood pressure) are common. Since the injection is made into the area around the cervix, there is the possibility that the anaesthetic will accidentally be injected into the baby. Moreover, the injection site is very close to the main artery of the uterus, which increases the chance of its being absorbed rapidly by the placenta and depressing the baby.

Spinal anaesthesia is used during delivery to anaesthetize the entire birth area (from belly to thighs or knees). Spinals, or subarachnoid blocks, are injected into the subarachnoid space around the spinal column. Usually they are given only at the very end of labour, since there is some evidence that they slow down labour if given too early. However, they do require only a small dose of anaesthetic, thus minimizing any effects on the baby. Spinal anaesthesia obliterates our urge to bear down during the second stage, so instead of our pushing the baby out, the obstetrician often has to use forceps. The few remaining problems associated with spinal anaesthesia are similar to those involving lumbar epidural anaesthesia, which we discuss below.

The possible complications of spinal anaesthesia (e.g. hypotension), and the fact that it can result in severe headaches, stiff neck and backaches, mean that it is not commonly used in Britain. Other forms of anaesthesia are at least as efficient, and spinals should be avoided except when necessary for an emergency – e.g. caesarean – delivery.

Epidural anaesthesia is perhaps the most common form of anaesthesia in Britain. It can be used in the first and second stages and it results in a completely sensationless labour in 90–95% of cases. There are two kinds of epidural: the lumbar, which goes into the lumbar region of the spine, and the caudal, which enters the tip of the spine near the coccyx. Caudals have a slightly higher failure rate than lumbars. Epidurals can be given either as single or continuous injections. With the latter, a catheter is placed in the back, through which the anaesthetic can be 'topped' up when necessary. Epidurals must be given by specially trained anaesthetists, since a mistake can lead to serious consequences – in the extreme, paralysis, death or foetal injection. However, it is worth remembering that since epidurals were first used in Britain in the 1950s, there has been only one death due to an epidural – a very good record.

Apart from the above rare complications, many doctors think that epidurals are otherwise safe. For example, in *Pregnancy*, Gordon Bourne

---

† *Implementing Family-Centered Maternity with a Central Nursery*, pp. iii–13. Referring to an article by N. Cooperman *et al.*, 'Oxygen Saturation in the Newborn Infant'.

states that epidurals have 'absolutely no ill-effects whatsoever upon the baby'. This statement, made in 1975, is very misleading. Firstly, epidurals often cause maternal hypotension, and subsequent lack of oxygen to the baby is a potential problem that must be carefully guarded against by the attenants. (The supine position, which can reduce the baby's oxygen supply – see p. 409 – should never be used once an epidural has been given.) Because caudals require a significantly larger dose, they carry a greater risk to both mother and baby than lumbars. However, with the latter there is more risk of causing an unpleasant post-partum headache as a result of an accidental lumbar puncture. The direct effect of epidurals on the baby can inhibit sucking and cause 'floppiness'. Furthermore, there is a growing body of evidence to associate epidurals, as well as induction and acceleration techniques, with the following: the rising incidence of foetal distress, depressed respiration and jaundice in the newborn, caesareans, and admissions to special baby units (Richards, letter to *Observer*, 8 February 1976).

If we choose this form of anaesthesia we are also choosing a number of other hospital procedures which might be needed:

1. An intravenous hydrating solution – necessary to avoid or counteract hypotension. This will be attached to one arm.
2. Forceps delivery – and its attendant possible risks to the foetus. The incidence of forceps delivery has been said to increase two to three times with epidurals. Forceps is sometimes necessary because the epidural inhibits the woman's ability to push. But with skilful administration the woman's sensations can be restored gradually so that she can push the baby out herself, and the increased risk of forceps can be reduced.
3. Oxytocin (see 'Induction and Acceleration', p. 427). This may be necessary to counter the possible slowing down of contractions which some doctors associate with epidurals.
4. Artificial rupture of the membranes (see p. 425). This is to make sure that the baby's presenting part is firmly positioned in the birth outlet. There is some evidence that transverse arrest (the baby's getting stuck in a sideways position in the uterus) is a possible complication of epidurals, due to uterine relaxation brought on by the anaesthesia. Consequently it is very important that the baby's presenting part be engaged before the epidural is given.
5. A foetal monitor – if they are used by your hospital, (see p. 432). It is vitally important to have a continuous check on your contractions, since if they are too strong the baby may suffer distress or your uterus could rupture, and with anaesthesia you would feel nothing.

Consequently, when we choose an epidural, we choose a doctor/hospital-controlled birth as well as many of the above procedures and their possible side effects. We also choose to rely on the competence and skill of the medical staff. Epidurals are particularly useful and undoubtedly necessary in certain cases, for example, if you have pre-eclampsia or hypertension, heart, kidney or lung conditions, posterior presentation (see p. 412), or prolonged labour. They are also often welcomed by women undergoing Caesareans: this option should be open to more women than at present, although we must stress that a Caesarean is a major operation and epidural anaesthesia during this procedure should not be done except by an experienced anaesthetist.

Many women who do not have complications feel they would like to have an epidural — often because they have learned from doctors that there are no risks. If we do decide to have an epidural — and this decision is an informed one — then we should be able to have one. But epidurals are not widely available on the NHS (privately they cost over £50). While at Kingston, Surrey, over 50% of women have them on the NHS, in the country as a whole only 2% have them (AIMS, September 1974). The availability of epidurals depends (a) on the whims of consultants and administrators and (b) on the availability of trained staff (epidurals do not form a part of an anaesthetist's training, thus an anaesthetist has to make a special effort to learn this new skill). Since the job of pain relief for women in labour is usually given to the most junior anaesthetist, s/he is unlikely to have had this training. All staff involved in the use of epidurals must have specialized training.

It was a real pleasure to give birth under these conditions [under an epidural], whereas 'natural childbirth' might have given rise to complications. We enjoyed every bit of it. When our baby was born, I thought I was dreaming, it was so easy . . . Having had such a tireless labour, I recovered very quickly, producing lots of good milk for the baby and was able to enjoy him. The baby became a satisfied and easy-going child. (Letter to Peace News, *March 1976)*

I refused to have an epidural, and I was the only one in my ward not to have stitches or a hangover for the next couple of days. (Letter to Spare Rib, *22)**

General Anaesthesia

This puts you completely to sleep and should be avoided if at all possible. During the first stage of labour it slows down the process of labour, and it has a severely depressant effect on the baby. Furthermore, all general anaesthetics carry a slight risk. It is sometimes used for caesarean section, forceps delivery and other obstetrical procedures.

PAIN RELIEF — OTHER POSSIBILITIES, INCLUDING PREVENTION

Homeopathy (see p. 131)

A good homeopathic doctor can help prevent or treat all sorts of problems during pregnancy and labour. S/he will prescribe individually-

---

* For a wide range of women's experiences of epidurals, see NCT, 'Some Mothers' Experiences of Induced Labour'.

tailored doses of whatever is appropriate for you. One particular remedy — Squaw root — is very useful for pain relief. Taken during pregnancy it usually results in much easier labours; it helps expel the placenta and helps postpartum discomfort.

Herbal Remedies (see p. 133)

Raspberry leaf tea is an old, well-known remedy for relaxing the uterus and relieving the pain of labour.

Somewhat shamefacedly and surreptitiously I have encouraged my expectant mothers, who felt so inclined, to drink the infusion . . . In a good many cases in my own experience, the subsequent labour has been easy and free from muscular spasm . . . (Dr Violet Russell, writing to the Lancet *in 1941)*

Raspberry leaf tea is usually taken during the last few months of pregnancy. For more about herbs during pregnancy, see Bibliography under 'Alternative Medicine and Preventive Health Care', p. 142.

Acupuncture (see p. 132)

If used weekly for a few weeks before the birth, acupuncture can be a very effective method of pain relief. It is not often used in this country, and it would probably have to be arranged privately with an acupuncturist. According to one study in the USA, acupuncture not only reduced pain and shortened labour, but 'a majority of patients experienced a sensation of peacefulness and relaxation together with a feeling of warmth' (*World Medicine*, 4 December 1974). One British woman recently had acupuncture at hospital for her first baby — her comment: *The whole thing was marvellous.*

Other methods

For other methods of pain relief during labour, see 'Techniques to Use during Labour', p. 417.

14 After the Baby Is Born

The post (after) partum (birth) period is that time which encompasses the moments and days after our baby's birth, and the weeks and months of adjusting to our new role as mother.

Immediately After the Birth

During the first few hours after the birth, your body will already be beginning to get itself back into its normal condition. You will probably feel afterpains, which are caused by the uterus beginning to return to its usual shape and size (involution). Breast-feeding will speed up the process by releasing the hormones you need to trigger the uterine contractions and keep them working. These post-delivery contractions are often very strong, particularly if you are suckling. They are more common with second and subsequent babies than with first babies. Drugs can be prescribed to reduce any pain, but remember, if you are breast-feeding, all drugs you take will reach the baby through your milk.

In addition to these cramps, which are strongest during the first few days, you'll have a bloody discharge lasting several weeks. This is called *lochia*. It will change in colour over the first couple of weeks from red to pinkish-brown to yellowish-white. Have a good supply of sanitary towels (for the first few weeks at least do not use tampons because of the risk of infection which is high in the postpartum period). Lochia should not smell bad. If it does, that is a sign of infection so contact your doctor. Sometimes bits of placental tissue are left inside the uterine area, so if you experience persistent bloody lochia, inform your doctor, because it generally indicates that something is in the uterus that shouldn't be.

After a normal delivery the new mother is out of bed either the same day or the next day. Those of us who get up soon after delivery feel better and stronger sooner and have fewer bladder and bowel problems (which are very common after childbirth, especially if you have had a general anaesthetic).

Your baby will be given a thorough medical check-up by a paediatrician. S/he should inform you of your baby's health and answer any questions you might have concerning your baby's well-being. Your own temperature will be checked often to make sure you are not developing a puerperal (*puer*, 'child' + *parere*, 'to bear' = *puerperal*: 'pertaining to childbirth') infection. Also, your pulse will be checked, and you will be given a blood test after a day or so.

In most hospitals the baby will be taken from you very soon after birth and placed in a separate nursery room for anywhere from 6 to 24 hours. In some hospitals the mother is allowed to keep her baby with her whenever she desires and for as long as she desires. When she is too tired to be entirely responsible for the baby, the baby can be taken back to the nursery. This is called modified rooming-in. Some hospitals, however, work on an all or nothing plan, meaning that if the mother chooses rooming-in she must keep the baby with her at all times. This can prove to be a tremendous burden, especially for the new mother.

Rooming-in provides the right atmosphere for breast-feeding on demand rather than according to a rigid schedule. The baby usually cries less and gains weight faster if s/he is fed when s/he feels hungry and not when the hospital staff think s/he should be hungry.

Postnatal Visits

A *midwife* has to attend you by law for the first 10 days after you have had a baby. Within about 14 days of the birth, a *health visitor* will take over from her. She is a nurse with additional training in baby care, and again, should be able to help you with the immediate problems of looking after a baby. In addition, she can help with more non-medical matters and advise you concerning facilities provided by the local authority. You can call both the midwife and the health visitor at any time through the local health or antenatal clinic, the social services department of the local authority, or your G P. The health visitor will visit you on and off until the child is 5 years old.

Six weeks after the birth you should have a postnatal check-up to see that you are getting back to normal. An appointment should have been made by the hospital or your midwife. You can attend either the hospital or a G P who is on the obstetric list. An appointment should also be made for the baby to be seen around the same time. At these check-ups both you and the baby should be given a thorough medical examination including urine, weight, blood pressure, blood tests. An internal examination should be made and any pain or discomfort dealt with.

The midwife, health visitor and doctor are there to help you with any problem you may have. If you do have any problems, it is a good idea to write them down so that you don't forget to bring them up during your visits.

Baby clinics or child health centres can weigh the baby for you and give general advice. You can also obtain subsidized or free welfare foods and vitamins here, and see the health visitor and doctor if necessary. As is the case with all medical establishments and personnel, the quality of advice and help given in a baby clinic varies considerably.

Benefits and Allowances

Milk and Vitamins: in certain circumstances you can obtain free supplies of these (see Pregnancy chapter, p. 363, for details). Otherwise you can obtain them at subsidized prices (see below). Vitamins for mother and baby are recommended to be taken for 30 weeks after the birth.

Child Benefits: these are a tax-free cash allowance for each child in every family and paid weekly to the mother. The Child Benefit Scheme replaces both Family Allowances (which were not paid for the first child and which were also taxable) and most of the Child Tax Allowance which is being phased out. The proposed rates for November 1978 are: £3.00 for all children of two-parent families and, for one-parent families, £5.00 for the first child and £3.00 for subsequent children. These will rise to £4.00, £6.00, and £4.00 respectively in April 1979. However, the financial gain will be extremely small, as, for taxpayers, Child Benefits largely replace Child Tax Allowances, and Social Security payments have been correspondingly reduced. Many groups and organizations are campaigning for an *adequate* Child Benefit Scheme with built-in protection against inflation. The Child Poverty Action Group (see addresses, p. 487) is coordinating the campaign. To claim your Child Benefit – such as it is – pick up a claim form at your local post office.

Family Income Supplement: this is available to those in full-time work (i.e. 30 hours or more per week) with at least one dependent child where the income is less than a prescribed amount (at present £43.80 for a family with one child, going up by £4·00 for each additional child). But your income will only be supplemented to half the difference between what you earn and this prescribed amount (i.e. if you earn £35 and you have one child, you will receive £4·40 FIS). There is a maximum FIS payment (at present £9·50 for one child). Furthermore, if you are a member of a couple, you are only eligible for FIS if the *man* is in full-time work. You are, however, entitled to other benefits if you qualify for FIS. Claim forms are in leaflet FIS 1 available from your local post office.

Supplementary Benefit is paid as of right if your income is below a certain level laid down by Parliament and you are unable to work full-time (see leaflet SB 1 available at your local post office). If you qualify for SB, you can claim for extra payments for essential items – such as clothing, bedding, prams, heating etc. These are called 'exceptional needs payments' (see booklet published by DHSS, listed in Bibliography).

The benefits available to mothers and single parents are far too complex to be examined in detail in the space we have. They are also constantly changing. What we must point out is that the kind of support available in this country to mothers – especially single mothers – is derisory. The women's liberation movement's Campaign for Legal and Financial Independence is campaigning for enough support for women – particularly mothers – so that we can be totally independent. For a more detailed look at mothers' rights and for information about campaigning groups, see the Bibliography and resource list on p. 486. For more about single mothers, see Chapter 11, p. 338.

Coping After the Birth

During this period we will be faced with many adjustments: getting used to our body in its non-pregnant state, our role with our new baby, and our changed role with the baby's father, older children, housemates and others. This adjustment period can be marked by intense highs: 'I've done it' . . . 'I've given birth to this beautiful, perfect being' . . . 'it's over' . . . 'I'm thankful' . . . 'I DID IT' – and lows: 'What have I done?' . . . 'I can't take responsibility for a baby' . . . 'I'm a baby myself' . . . 'I can't be a mother, I'm not equipped, I'm not prepared' . . . 'HELP', accompanied by the realization that this utterly dependent newborn is our responsibility – for keeps. Or we may not feel any different and wonder what all the fuss is about.

We can talk about this postpartum adjustment period as having three stages, but it is well to remember this does not mean we will experience it as defined stages. More likely, we will have some of these feelings at various times and at various levels of intensity. For some women this adjustment period may be calmer and easier than for others.

The First Stage

Immediately after the birth we may feel incredibly high and tremendously relieved that there is nothing wrong with the baby. Then we come down with a crash, aching from stitches and general weariness. Some of us may not mind the achiness. You may have an urgent desire to talk about how you are feeling, or you may just want to be alone. Remember, all your needs are legitimate and you have the right to expect those needs to be met. If the hospital situation is miserable for you, ask to be released as soon as possible. If you can, try to arrange to have family or friends help you when you return home, to share both the excitement and the burden.

By the third day, most women have the by now familiar 'baby blues'. We may cry; have frightening dreams and fantasies; feel scared or worried by our lack of 'maternal feelings'. These blues last only a day or so (usually), and are accompanied by the milk letdown reflex (breast milk comes in) and may be due to the sudden hormonal changes in our bodies. They often coincide with the time most women are discharged from hospital when we are faced with responsibilities for which often we have not been prepared. We should not feel guilty at not experiencing the 'gush' of motherhood we have heard so much about. Usually as we get to know our baby our positive maternal feelings begin to grow.

Immediately after the birth of my first baby I felt high and exhilarated. But that night I got sad. I cried all night long. During the next few days I lay on my bed thinking of how I would kill myself. I looked at how the windows opened and I concentrated on figuring out times when no nurses were on duty. I couldn't sleep at all. I tried to tell them I was depressed, and all they gave me were sleeping pills. I felt like I'd never feel anything again but this incredible despair, that it would never end. I had nightmares. The one I remember best is where I would be feeding the baby. I would fall asleep and the baby would fall off the bed and be killed. I don't know why I had these dreams and impulses. I have a happy marriage and it was a wanted pregnancy.

Many women have vivid dreams and fantasies after having a baby. It is important to talk about our feelings and fears and to share our pain. We're not alone and we can support each other.

The Second Stage

This may last from 1 to 3 months and involves the actual coping with ourselves and our new baby. There is the incredible fatigue that comes from not having an uninterrupted night of sleep; the stress of incorporating this new person into our existing life. In addition to exhaustion, we may feel fragmentation, disorientation and chaos. Life seems a blur; we feel little control at this time.

There are enormous physical changes occurring in the postpartum period. Though they are popularly considered natural, 'under no other circumstances does such marked and rapid tissue breakdown (catabolism) take place without a departure from a condition of health,' says the author of a widely used textbook. Under any other circumstances the drastic reduction in blood volume (30%) that takes place during this period would be felt as exhaustion, but many women feel exhilarated instead. Most of the blood and metabolic alterations of pregnancy disappear within the first 2 weeks postpartum. Feelings, particularly of depression, are intensified and last longer if we allow ourselves to get run-down physically. Some of us have stubborn virus infections that may lead to depression, or substitute for it (in those of us who cannot acknowledge depression). If you feel unusually weak or tired during the first 2 weeks, anaemia may be the cause. It is very important to continue taking your iron pills through the first 6 weeks postpartum. Whether you are breast-feeding or not, you need good nutrition to get your strength back. If you use a lot of ready-prepared foods, be sure to supplement your diet with lots of fresh fruit and vegetables, cheese and whole grains. Good appetite may be an indication of postpartum adjustment.

Many women continue to feel tired and lethargic for 6 months or more. Housework should be shared by all family members, but if you have no help during your first week, plan on take-aways, frozen dinners and every possible short cut. It is important to get enough sleep to make up sleep lost in night feedings. Over-exertion can be dangerous. For 6 weeks — or longer if you find it helpful — time should be set aside for rest. But unless family responsibilities can be shared and/or day care can be provided for older children, telling a mother of several small children to nap during the day is little more than a sick joke.

Studies have shown that in the last weeks of pregnancy women experience a loss of REM (rapid-eye-movement) sleep. Rapid eye movements are associated with dreaming, which occurs in deepest sleep, and some scientists believe this deep sleep is needed for physical and psychological replenishment. The loss of REM sleep and the associated disturbance in dream patterns may be related to the impending crisis of childbirth. If the postpartum woman continues to lose sleep, she builds up a backlog of REM sleep loss, which can lead to emotional and physical disturbances.[*] Sleeping pills rarely allow us to get enough REM sleep.

Whether one can get enough REM sleep during the period when the baby is waking at night depends on the individual. Some women feel fine even though their usual sleep pattern is disrupted. If you are someone who sleeps most soundly in your sixth or seventh hour of sleep (you can tell if you feel sleepy during the day after interrupted sleep), the baby's father or someone else can feed the baby during the night, early in the morning, or during your afternoon nap, so that you can sleep for a longer stretch than the three or four hours between feedings. If you are breast-feeding, the baby can be given a relief bottle for one feed each day (see 'Feeding Your Baby', p. 457).

[*] Barbara Williams, 'Sleep Needs During the Maternity Cycle', *Nursing Outlook*, February 1967, pp. 53–5. For more on REM sleep, see Sharon Golub, 'Rapid Eye Movement Sleep', pp. 56–8.

As well as needing sleep, we also need exercise. Special postpartum exercises will help to get your abdomen back in shape. If these are not provided by your doctor or clinic, contact the National Childbirth Trust for information and literature (see Bibliography, p. 488). After the first 6 weeks see Chapter 6, for ideas on exercise.

As in pregnancy, some women will experience a number of discomforts, while others will hardly have any at all. Some common ones are sweating (especially at night), loss of appetite, thirst (due to loss of fluids), and constipation. You may feel great, you may have few or no discomforts, you may have many. Being aware of the range of possibilities, you are better equipped to cope with them when they occur.

Some of the signs of postpartum physical problems are: unusually heavy bleeding, heavier than your period on any day; strongly unpleasant odour of vaginal discharge; temperature 101 degrees or higher; breasts red, feeling hot or painful. If you have any of these start immediately to get more rest, and call your doctor.

FEELINGS ABOUT THE BABY

Many feelings, thoughts and fears come to mind: I am supposed to be fulfilled because now I am a mother, but I feel ambivalent; I have to be around all the time just to care for my baby's needs, so I don't have any time for my other interests – I've lost my independence; I feel scared – what if I do something wrong? I'm even afraid to bath the baby for fear I might drop her.

All these feelings are common to so many of us. We don't instinctively know how to care for children just because we're women. Experience is essential; we *learn* how to be good mothers. Talking over our ambivalent feelings and fears with other women also helps us to put those thoughts in proper perspective.

Once the baby is born, s/he is a separate being whom you have to get to know and who has to get to know you. S/he's not really as fragile as it might seem to you, and s/he has a built-in will to live. But don't let that stop you from calling your doctor or clinic any time you have a question about the baby's health or welfare.

The first month was awful. I loved my baby, but felt apprehensive about my ability to satisfy this totally dependent tiny creature. Every time she cried I could feel myself tense up and panic. After the first month I got the hang of it. Gradually my love feelings for her overcame my panic feelings, and I relaxed, stopped thinking so much about my inadequacies, and was just myself. It was pretty clear from her responses that I was doing something right.

Some babies are no problem at all: they sleep a lot, wake up for feedings, smile at you and go back to sleep again. Others are 'colicky' (a

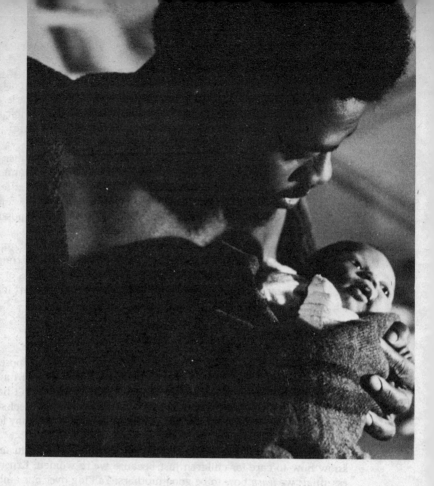

catchword to describe general discomfort, fussiness, etc.) and cry 16 hours out of 24. Then your physical and mental powers will be stretched to their limits. Much child-care literature suggests that colic is caused by parental mishandling. This is not true.* Colic can be caused by a cows' milk allergy — in which case a substitute formula might do the trick. More often, colic is due to the immature digestive system of the baby. It will grow out of it — usually by 2 months. That's little comfort while you are going through it, but there it is. No amount of preparation can really equip you to withstand this time calmly. The only advice we can offer is to try to have lots of people around to hold and walk the baby so you can get away for a period each day.

* Richards and Bernal, *New Society*, 28 February 1974, show that there is a link between the bad advice 'experts' give breast-feeding mothers and the problems their babies have (see Breast-Feeding, p. 460). The best Richards and Bernal suggest is that parents should be told that night-waking is not their fault.

When Rachel was 2–3 months old she seemed to stay awake all day and all night. She might go to sleep on your lap, but the minute we put her in her cot she woke up and started roaring till she was picked up. Three or four times she cried on and off for two whole days. The only way she would shut up was by pacing the floor with her. We felt our heads were going to burst. A friend would come round to let us have half an hour's respite when we could go to the pub to get the awful noise out of our heads. But we didn't have friends coming round on a regular basis and I'm sure this would have helped enormously. When friends did rally round, we were always left with the feeling that at the end of the day it was us who had the responsibility. A couple of times I ended up weeping because of the noise. I didn't think it would ever stop. It amazes me how any woman can put up with this sort of thing on her own. The only way I came out of it without any permanent damage to either Rachel or me was because I could share it with the man I was living with. The doctor told us it was colic; relatives told us it was because we were pandering to her. I don't think it was either of these things. Certainly, it never worked if we left her screaming – she could go on for five hours. I wonder if it was anything to do with the birth trauma: it was a long labour with foetal distress followed by a caesarean birth, and Rachel and I were separated for the first two days.

Feeding Your Baby

BREAST OR BOTTLE?

It is not surprising that most women in Britain, in the West as a whole, and increasingly in underdeveloped countries, bottle-feed their babies. We are told that our breasts are our sexiest parts, and we are whistled at and winked at until we begin to think of ourselves as little more than sex objects for men. Consequently many of us feel embarrassed or uncomfortable using our breasts to feed our babies. Then there's the problem of being a working mother. As it is there are precious few facilities for lactating mothers anywhere, but at work places? – rarely, if ever. Lastly, there's pressure from baby-milk manufacturers. Their free handouts reach 98% of expectant mothers in Britain.

Following the government report *Present Day Practice in Infant Feeding*, which concluded overwhelmingly that breast is best, if possible, even if it's only for the first week, the authorities have started producing their own propaganda in an attempt to encourage women to breast-feed. But this propaganda ignores all the pressures, conflicts and difficulties – like those mentioned above – which most of us have to face when deciding which method to choose.

The propagandists would have us believe that if we breast-feed we are good and if we bottle-feed we are bad. They do not take into account the possible disastrous effects of a mother feeding her baby in a way she does not wish or cannot do. Many of us are brought up to feel ambivalent about breast-feeding and we then feel guilty if we can't or don't want to breast-feed. There is certainly little benefit to either mother or baby if the mother feels she ought to breast-feed but doesn't really like the idea. In her article 'Breast Feeding: The Mystic Maternal Cult', Patricia Morgan points out how 'For every one woman I meet who feels that she did not get the help she wanted [to breast-feed], there are a great many more who bitterly resent being made to breast-feed or being pressured to do so.'

As a three months' pregnant mother I was made to feel even then that if I was not able to breast-feed it would be because I would not care enough for my baby to try hard enough.

We should be able to feed our babies in whichever way we feel happiest. In order to achieve such a situation the whole climate of attitudes to childbirth, sexuality, women and children will have to change, as well as the economic climate. But one of the most important things we need is information about the pros and cons of each method. And then unequivocal support for whichever one we choose.

The advantages and disadvantages of breast-feeding. Human milk is ideally suited to a baby's needs. It differs from bottled – or cows' – milk by at least 20 ingredients, containing less phosphorus, calcium, sodium, chloride and protein. The newborn's kidneys have to work that much harder to deal with the extra ingredients of cows' milk. This is particularly difficult in the case of premature babies. Furthermore, the strong urine that a bottle-fed baby has to excrete tends to produce nappy rash. This is far less common in breast-fed babies.

The colostrum which appears before the milk comes in is full of protein, minerals, vitamin A and nitrogen. The nourishment colostrum provides is very similar to that which the baby received in the womb. Colostrum has never been manufactured synthetically. Colostrum also helps protect the newborn from infections, diseases and allergies such as polio, common colds, bronchitis, pneumonia, asthma, eczema, colic and measles. Some people think that breast milk does this too. Gastroenteritis, which can be extremely dangerous to the newborn, is almost unheard of in breast-fed babies. So is constipation; although breast-fed babies might not defecate for several days, there is nothing wrong with this. It is simply because the baby absorbs breast milk so well and does not have to excrete so much.

It is possible that the tummy-ache common in newborn babies around the age of one week is caused by the common practice of hospitals of feeding them cows' milk for the first 3 nights (see Freed, *British Medical Journal*, 17 April 1976). Babies don't need extra feeding at this time: they have enough inside them to last until the mother's milk comes in.

Since breast-feeding uses up the food stores laid down in pregnancy for this purpose, it enables us to lose easily the weight we put on during pregnancy. Breast-feeding also helps the uterus to return to its previous size more quickly.

The disadvantages of breast-feeding tend to be minimized by breast-feeding supporters. Breast-fed babies require more feedings – because of the content of the milk – especially during the first 2 weeks. Sharing child care can be difficult with breast-feeding until the baby gets a little older. And if you're not careful, other members of your family may feel that you have the exclusive power to meet your baby's needs. Breast-feeding can be satisfying, sensual and fulfilling. It can be a pleasant and relaxing way for both mother and baby to enjoy feedings, and it is an affirmation of our bodies. But it cannot be delegated and it can in some cases be difficult and painful (for how to cope with breast-feeding problems, see below).

Most of us in our group who have children breast-fed our babies. We did it because we wanted that experience, and also because we were feeling proud of our bodies and glad as women that our bodies can provide nourishment for our children.

I was encouraged to breast-feed in the hospital – very ineptly, I might add; I did so and have often regretted it in the seven months since my daughter's birth. Never have I found it 'a rewarding experience' as the books claim, nor an easy one. But despite this I have come out of the experience convinced by myself – not others – that one does become particularly close to one's child, and, further, that the milk is entirely suited to the baby. (Letter to *New Society*, 25 May 1976)

The advantages and disadvantages of bottle feeding. While breast milk is more suitable for babies, particularly if they are very young, sick or premature, the dangers of bottled milk have sometimes been over-emphasized and we would like to put these in perspective.

Even very young babies can be fed by a bottle, but the milk must be of the right kind and it must be prepared properly. There are two kinds of baby-milk, 'modified' and 'unmodified'. Only modified milk is suitable for a young baby – the mineral and protein content has been made as near as possible to human milk. Many professionals have been unaware of this fact.

For the many women who are just above the breadline, modified milk can be prohibitively expensive. (Unmodified milk costs at the time of writing 20p for 20 oz, compared with 16 oz at 70p–80p for modified milks.) While breast-feeding appears to cost nothing by comparison, you must remember that it does necessitate eating well (see 'Nutrition', below).

Modified milks suitable for young or sick babies are Cow & Gate Premium Plus or V Formula; Ostermilk Complete Formula; SMA or SMA Gold

Cap. Of these, SMA Gold Cap, Ostermilk Complete Formula and Cow & Gate Premium are the nearest to breast milk. They are also the most expensive.

But at what age can a baby take unmodified milk? If you are *scrupulous* in measuring out the milk powder, and if the baby is healthy, you can probably feed it unmodified milk at 4 months. But we do not feel that any woman should have to do this, since the best milk possible should be freely available to everyone. We cannot emphasize enough that feeding overstrength milk or too much milk to a baby is harmful and even dangerous. It causes pain, discomfort, dehydration and obesity. The dehydration can be fatal; the obesity could last a lifetime.

Some people seem to think that only breast-feeding can provide the physical closeness necessary for the healthy emotional development of the baby. We do not agree with this; moreover, bottle-feeding can enable the father and other members of the family to form equally close relationships with the baby.

IF YOU DECIDE TO BREAST-FEED

About 95% of women are physically capable of breast-feeding. Indeed, it has been known for grandmothers who have not breast-fed for 20 years to lactate again if a child is put to the breast, and even if you have never had a baby and have adopted a child, breast-feeding is possible. The problem is, will social conditions and hospital practices help us to breast-feed or hinder us from doing so?

The main reason why some women are physically unable to breast-feed is because they have some serious illness or because the baby has a problem such as a cleft palate. Even if the birth was premature or by caesarean section, if the baby is shocked or drugged, if you have twins or if you are diabetic, you can still breast-feed.

The Best Conditions for Successful Breast-Feeding

1. You should prepare your nipples during pregnancy (see p. 372). This will make life a lot easier when you start breast-feeding.
2. It is best to start immediately after the birth when the sucking reflex is strongest. Each hour that sucking is delayed, the reflex becomes weaker so that suckling becomes more difficult for the baby, especially if the woman's breasts have been allowed to become full and hard. Often babies are put to the breast far too late in hospitals. Try to arrange with the staff beforehand that you would like the baby to suckle on the delivery table. Many hospitals will not allow this, but doctors and nurses have been known to change their attitudes, as in the case of this NCT teacher's experience while attending a birth:

Presently baby was whisked off to be weighed etc. while the doctor finished his embroidery (sewing up the episiotomy). After a few discreet inquiries I suggested that I might like to let the baby suckle before I had to leave to teach my class at home. Sister wanted to clean up first and put the baby to the breast later, but with a little gentle persuasion she agreed and was astonished with the baby's readiness to get on with the job. There is nothing like a strongly suckling infant to persuade the mother that the baby is alive and well and needs her! Sister remarked 'Thank you for the idea . . . I've never seen a baby get on so well.'

3. 'Demand' or 'continuous' feeding is virtually essential. Broadly this involves feeding the baby when it wants to be fed instead of when the hospital regime dictates. 3–4 hourly feeding regimes were designed for bottle-fed babies. During the early weeks, most breast-fed babies want to be fed little and often. Not all hospitals allow this, so try and choose one that does – though you may still have to insist against a disapproving member of staff.

I was the only one breast-feeding and was given no help at all, and as if that wasn't discouragement enough, I was told: 'You're not going to make it; put him on a bottle.' The baby was very large and taking a lot of fluid, vomiting and excreting a lot. He tended to wake up very hungry and scream until the next feeding time – which was religiously adhered to. The paediatrician came and I explained the situation to him; he and sister had a row over my bed, and he wrote on my notes: 'Demand feed'. At last, I thought, some sanity. But as soon as he'd gone, sister said, 'I don't care what he says, you're not demand feeding on my ward.'

Breasts are designed to produce milk according to the baby's demands. More frequent suckling increases the production of milk: hospitals that give supplementary feeds are therefore serving to prevent mothers from producing sufficient milk. Furthermore, the baby might then prefer the bottle because sucking from a bottle is easier. Even a single artificial feed can change the pH content of the baby's gut and may reduce the protective value of breast milk.

Even if the hospital states that its policy is demand feeding, they may insist on waking the baby if it hasn't fed for 4 hours or, if it wakes every 2 hours, they might say it needs an extra bottle. It is best, therefore, to make sure that all the staff know that you want to feed the baby every time it is hungry. Talking or writing to the Sister of the postnatal ward is a good idea before you've had the baby.

If the staff think that baby is not gaining weight properly, they should simply let it suckle more often instead of putting it on a bottle.

Since breast-fed babies gain far less weight in the first week than bottle-fed babies, they will always appear to be 'not getting enough'. In fact, they often lose weight in the first week: this is quite normal. Staff may also suggest that the baby is not sucking properly; this is because babies suck differently at the breast than from a bottle. Breast-feeding involves short sucking spells while bottle-feeding is more continuous.

With help and encouragement, women have been able to breast-feed their babies when otherwise the circumstances have not been ideal, for example, after the baby has already been started on the bottle or after we have been given injections to dry up our milk. It has been known for a midwife to sit with the mother through every feed, day and night, for the first few days, to make sure that feeding is successfully established.

So, in conclusion, we may have to deal with conflicting and inaccurate advice from hospital 'experts' and we may even have to do battle with them. We must make sure we are well-informed before the birth. The literature we recommend can be really helpful (see Bibliography, p. 483). If we are well-informed, we will be well-prepared to breast-feed.

Looking After Ourselves during Breast-Feeding

Wear a good, supportive bra: the MAVA bra, supplied by the NCT, is ideal (see 'Pregnancy', p. 373). Someone else can give the baby an occasional bottle once breast-feeding is established, but try not to miss two consecutive feeds. After a month or two, you can begin to share the feeding by missing one regularly. Try not to miss one feeding a day during the first 2 months. We would like to emphasize that regularity, missing the same feedings every day, is the key to successful part-time breast-feeding. You may experience some problems at first, but don't give up. Enough sleep, determination and good nutrition will see you through.

Nutrition and Drugs   We need extra calories – or energy – while breast-feeding, even more than when we are pregnant (see DHSS 'Recommended Intake of Nutrients'). We are rarely told this, in fact we are often conditioned to restrict our food intake after the baby is born, so as not to gain weight. As we have already pointed out, breast-feeding actually enables us to lose weight.

Any conscious calorie restriction to lose weight resulted in reduction of my milk supply before I noticed any reduction in my weight or waistline. With an average intake during lactation of about 3,000 calories per day, I lost 12 lb (slowly and steadily) during the nine months in which my baby gained 10 lb.

An extra pint of milk a day, together with the diet you have been following during pregnancy, would provide the extra calories you need. We also need to drink more – at least 2 pints extra. Our grandmothers used to drink 3 or 4 pints of beer or stout, which provided them with both the necessary liquid and calories. But some people believe that no alcohol

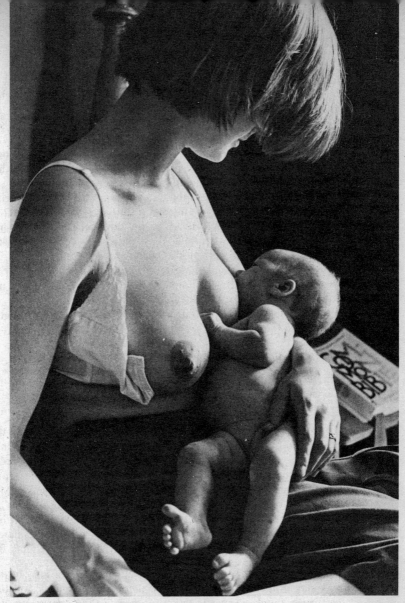

should be drunk while breast-feeding for fear of creating a need for alcohol in the baby (see *Women's Report*, Vol. 4. issue 3, p. 15). Perhaps we should stick to milk!

Other drugs may affect the baby through the milk as well. Barbiturates can pass through the milk, as can nicotine, laxatives and tranquillizers. Laxatives may cause colic or diarrhoea in babies, and tranquillizers can produce coma in babies if given to the mother in large doses. Some people believe that if you use progestogen-only contraceptive pills or injections while breast-feeding, this does not affect the baby. But although no adverse effects on lactation or on breast-feeding have been clearly and unequivocally demonstrated, little research has been done in this area. Recently, some feminist health workers have come across a surprising number of women whose breast-fed babies were 'hyperactive' and 'cranky'. One thing they all had in common was the use of the progestogen-only pill or the injectable progestogen, Depo-provera. We have also heard of difficulty with lactation in women given Depo-provera soon after birth. These examples should not be regarded as established fact, but they do indicate that more information is necessary. (Read p. 260 before considering taking Depo-provera at *any* time, and beware the increasing number of hospitals that give these injections routinely postpartum.) Even low-dose oestrogen pills appear to affect breast milk, and no-one knows about the possible long-term effects of *any* hormonal contraceptives on offspring. Thus, it might be best to choose a different method of contraception while breast-feeding. Breast-feeding in itself is not a totally reliable method of contraception, even if it is the sole method used for feeding the baby.

Difficulties during Breast-Feeding

The resources listed below can be far more helpful and encouraging than we can be in this short space. Here we look at some of the commonest problems that we can face during breast-feeding.

1. *Inability to maintain milk supply:* sometimes the blame for this is put on the mother but often the cause is that hospital staff are giving supplementary feeds. Tension can also be the cause, as well as lack of confidence. If you find that help is not forthcoming from the people around you, contact the NCT for their nearest breast-feeding counsellor. Make sure, also, that you are getting enough calories and liquids (see 'Nutrition' above). For some special hints, such as taking brewer's yeast to increase your milk supply, see Adelle Davis, *Let's Have Healthy Children*, Lester Hazell, *Commonsense Childbirth*, and the La Leche League Book, *The Womanly Art of Breastfeeding*, see Bibliography, p. 483.

2. *Engorgement:* the breasts may feel very hot, hard, heavy and tender to touch; the glands under your arms may also be swollen and you may have a temperature and a thirst. If you are allowed to suckle the baby soon after birth, engorgement will probably not occur. If you do get symptoms, immediately put cold flannels on your breasts and continue to do so until the heat subsides. This cures the problem in most women. For more details on how to deal with engorgement see, for example, *The Know-how of Breast Feeding* by Sylvia Close. The method described is unorthodox; standard hospital treatment can be very different and even painful.

3. *Cracked or sore nipples:* most experts say that this occurs because the

baby is sucking for too long. But experienced midwives have found that it usually happens because the baby is not properly 'fixed' to the breast (the whole of the nipple and the areola should be firmly in its mouth). If 'fixing' is correct, they have found that a baby can and should suck for as long as is required to get an adequate feed, and 'unlimited' sucking prevents under-production of milk. Cracking or soreness can also occur if the nipples aren't dried after feeding, or if soap is used on them. Soothing lanolin cream can be applied as a preventive. Shields can protect cracked nipples while the baby is feeding and thus assist healing. The NCT provides inexpensive nipple shields, which should be sterilized before each feed.

I stopped breast-feeding after 12 days because of sore nipples and a feeling of failure. My son was an irritable baby and never seemed to have had enough. I have now come to the conclusion that he obviously needed feeding more often than every 4 hours as insisted by the hospital . . . Sometimes my son waited 6 hours for a feed if the hospital staff were busy and was left crying in the nursery — mothers were not allowed to feed until told!

Clearly, the above three problems can be a direct result of hospital practices.

4. *Lack of weight gain.* Breast-fed babies should have regained their birth weight by the 10th day, roughly speaking. If s/he has not gained in weight after, say, 3 weeks, it might be best to check with a doctor that everything is all right. It is possible for a baby to stay the same weight for 2 months and still be perfectly healthy. Often all that is needed is for the baby to feed more often. If the baby *loses* weight after the first week, this needs to be checked on.

How Long Should We Breast-Feed?

Although the advantages of breast-feeding past the first couple of weeks have not been clearly demonstrated, there is of course much less risk of infection from contaminated milk and bottles, and breast-feeding reduces our weight gained during pregnancy. If mother and baby are happy, there are good reasons for continuing way beyond the first couple of weeks. If you are finding it difficult and/or want to stop, there is no reason to think that you are depriving your baby in any way. Up to 6 months you can supply the total nutritional needs of your baby, and up to a year you can supply three quarters of the protein needed.

RESOURCES

Many books have been written about breast-feeding. We recommend those by Sylvia Close, Mavis Gunther, Lester Hazell and Sheila Kitzinger (see Bibliography, p. 483).

Both the La Leche League and the National Childbirth Trust can help with breast-feeding difficulties and encouragement. The NCT has counsellors in many areas who have themselves experienced the problems of breast-feeding. They work on a mother-to-mother basis and are available at all times to any woman. The NCT also publishes and distributes leaflets.

The Baby Foods Action Group is concerned with the inappropriate commercial promotion and distribution of artificial baby-milks, particularly in the Third World. They are also campaigning to highlight the choices open to women, and for better maternity facilities, for example, in public places. (For addresses, see p. 487).

IF YOU DECIDE TO BOTTLE-FEED

Your milk may be suppressed with an injection of a drug such as stilboestrol (see p. 284) or bromocriptine. Most hospitals have stopped using stilboestrol because it is thought to increase the risk of thrombosis. There are other ways of drying up the milk supply, for example by binding the breasts, and drugs are probably better avoided.

In the early weeks, be sure to use modified milk and don't introduce solids or cereals before 4 months. These are not only unnecessary, they can be dangerous for the baby's immature digestive system. Don't add sugar or salt to solid foods for the same reason.

Be sure at all times that the feed is not over-concentrated. *Never* pack the powder into the scoop: loosely fill it and level it off with a knife. Remember also to sterilize the equipment as instructed.

Sex after Childbirth

Some of us may have little or no interest in sex soon after childbirth. Others of us resume sexual activity fairly quickly. We each need to set our own pace. If the vaginal area feels okay and the bleeding has stopped, there is no medical risk in having intercourse. Masters and Johnson report that many women resume sexual intercourse within 3 weeks following delivery.* The taboo period varies from culture to culture. The 6-week rule in the UK is ostensibly to prevent infection, but today it is largely for the doctor's convenience, so that the end of the celibate period coincides with the 6-week check-up. (This rule originated in the days before antibiotics.) If you sleep with one person regularly, you probably already share the same germs and have a tolerance for them.

However, some women do experience discomforts and/or low sexual interest which are physically caused and certainly legitimate reason to

---

* William H. Masters and Virginia E. Johnson, *Human Sexual Response*, p. 163.

avoid intercourse until you feel ready. Some women who are breast-feeding experience painful cramps during intercourse. In some women the stitches in the episiotomy (see p. 433) continue to be painful for several weeks. Follow your own emotions and see how you feel physically. Remember that good sex need not mean intercourse only (see Chapter 3).

Low sexual interest may be associated with lowered oestrogen levels in your body. This is fairly common and does not mean you've become 'frigid'. If you do have sexual interest but find that your vagina does not lubricate easily, this again is physical (related to low oestrogen levels) and more common in nursing mothers. Often, natural lubrication does not return for several weeks. Just use a sterile unscented lubricant such as KY Jelly or ask your doctor to prescribe oestrogen cream. Low sexual interest may also be caused by the rapid changes in your life.

You must use reliable birth control from the time you begin intercourse. Your old diaphragm will not fit, so get a new one at your 6-week check-up. Until then, you can use condoms with lots of foam or jelly. When you have started menstruating again, you can use the Pill (though preferably not if you are breast-feeding). IUDs are sometimes inserted immediately after the birth. This could mask signs of infection. It is probably better to wait at least a week. Do not rely on breast-feeding or the absence of menstruation to protect you. You can get pregnant the first time you ovulate *before* you begin to menstruate again (see Chapter 2). If you are feeding the child solely from your breast, you may well not menstruate for 4 months. But a substantial number of women do ovulate while breast-feeding.

During this time it is important to keep communications as open as possible (see Chapter 2, 'Considering Parenthood'). Talking to other couples who have recently had babies helps too. The National Childbirth Trust can often put you in touch with counsellors or postpartum groups if you feel the need for special help with sexual or emotional problems during this period.

The Third Stage

Coping with the long-term adjustments of becoming a parent may last up to a year or more. The baby may bring back our own childhood feelings of love and rejection; the experience may trigger in us feelings about death, our own, or the death of close older relatives, our parents or our grandparents. It can recall all sorts of jealous and angry feelings we may have towards our sisters and brothers. If we are single, we have the very real problem of trying to cope on our own — (see Chapter 11, p. 338). If we are in a couple relationship we may have strong feelings to work out in our relationship with our man.

Often we remain upset months after the baby's birth because we expected at some point to get our lives and feelings back to 'normal'. But once we become mothers we will never again lead altogether the same lives. For the next two decades we will have to consider the child's needs in making our own plans. If the experiences of the childbearing year are resolved in a positive way, we will have grown in strength and maturity and feel good about our new responsibilities most of the time.

It is only natural to yearn occasionally for the freedom of childlessness and to feel angry and resentful towards our kids. We have our own needs as people, and at times we need to be separate from our kids. By recognizing this need we can feel freer when away from our kids and enjoy them more when we are with them.

The first child, particularly, brings completely new experiences for the parents. For an account of the conflicts and problems see Breen, *The Birth of a First Child.*

The six or eight months after Peter was born were hard ones for me and my husband. I had wanted very much to have a baby and I enjoyed taking care of him, but I didn't seem to have any energy. My physical energy started to return when he slept through the night and more when he stopped needing a 10 p.m. feed. But my mental and emotional energy seemed to have disappeared for good. Sometimes it was all I could do to get through a day. I took long naps and I cried often. I got jealous about women my husband saw at work. I felt out of touch with the me who had been an interesting, active and humorous person. Love him as I did, in some moods I resented Peter for even existing. To most people I pretended to be a 'happy, young mother', but I was actually quite depressed. Because I didn't know about postpartum depression, I blamed what I was feeling on my own failure to be a good mother. I think I also blamed my husband, as though he could have made me feel better. He, for his part, was feeling worried about his job and resentful that I was too low to give him any comfort. He accused me of having wanted a child and now 'not wanting one'. (He didn't know about postpartum either.)

A lot of things contributed to my feeling better. I began admitting to friends how bad I was feeling; I began a cooperative play group with four other mothers. Most important, I went to a women's health course and learned that many women feel depressed for several months after childbirth. All of a sudden I knew it wasn't all my fault. I wasn't a bad person for what I was feeling. Unfortunately, even then my husband and I were not able to talk clearly about postpartum depression together. A lot of damage was done to our relationship during those months of confusion.

Contributing to our depression may be our expectations of what a good mother is or should be. Our expectations depend in part on the kind of mother we had, and in part on our fantasies of what a mother should be. The disparity between the fantasy mother within us (spotless house, floors we can eat from; serene, looking lovely when our man comes home; feeling fulfilled with full-time baby care) and the feelings we have as real mothers may cause us anxiety.* It is important at this time to get help from our own mothers, if possible, but only if they can be supportive and loving to us. We do not need to be undermined in our efforts to adjust to our new baby. We have to be strong enough to assess realistically just what kind of help we will be getting if we ask our mothers. This is not a time for us to 'prove' to ourselves or our mothers how well we can cope.

It is confusing to sort out our feelings during postpartum. There are so many of them; they sometimes change quickly and seem to come from deep within us.

I am a psychiatric nurse and therefore was aware of how angry thoughts about the baby postpartum are a normal part of the adjustment process. But I was unprepared for the enormous amount of anger I felt. I was angry about everything, it seemed. First, we had so carefully planned the conception (scientifically) of a baby girl, and I gave birth to a boy; then my sister-in-law, who had given birth six weeks before me, used the name I had reserved for my child for her baby. Then I realized how much my son resembled my father, who thirty years ago had rejected me. I also heavily identified with my oldest child about his displacement as kingpin. When I attempted to share child-care with my husband, who worked at home, I found myself at the mercy of two time-tables, the baby's and his. It wasn't until six months later that I felt my anger dissipating and it was a full two years before I felt myself again. During this time I had obsessive fantasies about hurting the baby, how fragile he was, how easily I could drop him, how maybe I would forget him and leave the house, etc. I hated myself for such thoughts, but they persisted. It wasn't until I finally accepted the fact that a 'nice woman like me' could have such anger that the fantasies abated. Postpartum for me was learning to deal with more anger than I've ever felt in my entire life. It felt like one long temper tantrum — unscreamed.

Social pressures on mothers to be with their babies constantly seem to us to be a major cause of depression. In becoming a mother for the first time, we experience an abrupt social discontinuity. We stop work. We exchange a fairly egalitarian relationship with our mate for a more traditional relationship in which the expectations for us are more stereotyped. We are deprived of adult company for six to eight hours a day or more in order to carry out full-time child-care. Yet society has no adequate built-in system of support for new mothers. We have no place to share confusing feelings. The sad fact is that parenthood is not highly valued in our society. Mothers do not get recognition for this important work.

* See Breen, *The Birth of a First Child*.

Many of us feel that sole responsibility for a newborn infant is harder than we have been prepared for. We need to have other people around right from the start to share the work, and the fun, of parenthood. We have learned that our independence and emotional well-being are as important for our children as for ourselves — we must remain people in spite of the fact that we're now mothers! Therefore, in thinking about child-care we have to talk about our own needs as well as the needs of our baby. We have to find the easiest way to share baby-care from the very beginning. Sharing, to us, means joint responsibility, not just a division of tasks. We expect the other adults who are constantly part of our children's lives to know how to take care of the baby without having to turn to us as 'the expert'. Our children need intimate, loving care from more than just one adult. If we as mothers allow ourselves to think that we are the only adults able to care for and love our children, we will almost always come to think of them as exclusively our possessions and exclusively our responsibility.

We women don't want to feel pushed out of the home, but we do want to leave the door wide open — both for ourselves and our children — to grow and develop as independent people.

Postnatal Depression

Many of us experience some form of mild or severe postnatal depression or emotional stress. In some of us, postnatal disturbance is acute. Eighty-eight thousand women a year are said to need treatment for postnatal depression. The incidence of this disturbance has not been reduced since 1915, in spite of a much lower perinatal mortality rate. In the last 10 years, 10–20,000 women have become psychotic during confinement and only about half have recovered.

We have explained above some of the obvious reasons why women experience postnatal depression. But theories as to its cause do not always take physical, emotional and practical difficulties into account. Current theories can be broken down into two schools of thought: (1) The depression is caused by physical stress — that is, hormonal imbalance and the bodily shock of labour; (2) The depression is caused by social stress.

PHYSICAL STRESS

Although it has been widely known for some time that hormone imbalance following the birth of a baby can result in postnatal depression, very little research has been done in this area. Since after successive births the recurrence of acute postpartum psychosis is high, attempts are being made to prevent this with hormone treatment and drugs. For example, tapering dosages of hormones are given over a period of about 2 months following delivery, so that hormonal changes are not so dramatic as to trigger psychosis. Tranquillizers may also be given. But the only criterion of success is if the women do not have to go into hospital.

SOCIAL AND EMOTIONAL STRESS AND PREVENTION

Social factors, including background and current environment, can be major contributors to depression in most people. Reports of depression in fathers[*] and adoptive mothers[†] indicate that the causes are not *purely* physical.

By means of a questionnaire, researchers have been able to predict the likelihood of postpartum difficulties in certain women.[**] They listed fourteen stress factors and found that the more of these stress factors the women had, the more difficulty they experienced in coping with postpartum — perhaps not surprisingly! The stress factors were as follows:

1. Primipara (woman having first baby).
2. No relatives available for help with baby-care.
3. Complications of pregnancy in family history.
4. Husband's father dead.
5. Wife's mother dead.
6. Wife ill apart from pregnancy.
7. Wife ill during pregnancy.
8. Wife's education higher than her parents'.
9. Husband's education higher than his parents'.
10. Wife's education incomplete.
11. Husband's occupation higher than his parents'.
12. Husband's occupation higher than wife's parents'.
13. Husband often away from home.
14. Wife has had no previous experience with babies.

Current environmental factors, such as lack of emotional support and assistance, husband often away, and other relatives not available for help, were significant in cases where problems persisted for longer than 6 months. It is worth remembering that 60% of the women with a high number of risk factors did not develop problems. We have included this information simply in order that it may help pregnant women to sort out

---

[*] Beatrice Liebenberg, 'Expectant Fathers', presented at annual meeting of American Orthopsychiatric Association, Washington, DC, March 1967.

[†] F. T. Melges, 'Postpartum Psychiatric Syndromes', *Psychosomatic Medicine*, 30 (January–February, 1968), pp. 95–108.

[**] Gordon, Kapostins, and Gordon, 'Factors in Postpartum Emotional Adjustment', see also Virginia Larsen, *et al.*, op. cit.

which aspects of our lives are likely to give rise to conflicting feelings and roles following childbirth. We want to suggest fruitful areas for discussion with the baby's father, the doctor, friends, antenatal classes etc., and areas where change can be made. We would also like to emphasize other factors which could equally well affect postnatal depression and which are not included in the list mentioned above.

In *Mind Out*, the magazine of the National Association for Mental Health, Jean Robinson examines the way hospitals alienate mothers. After receiving hundreds of letters from women and their husbands, she firmly believes that some cases of depression after childbirth could be caused by medical care itself. Mismanagement of labour, too many drugs, the place of delivery, the behaviour of staff, unnecessary separation of mother and baby and of mother and father, all appear to affect women's emotional adjustment after the birth.

I just felt like so much meat − a cow − a utensil − and for ages afterwards, even with a lovely little baby, I relived this bad experience over and over again. It obsessed me. I wanted to stand outside the antenatal department with a placard warning other expectant mums not to be led like lambs into this experience. (Mind Out, March/April 1977)

I was on the delivery table surrounded by nurses shouting the most unkind things, such as 'A fourteen-year-old could do better', 'Don't you want to have this baby?' and many other things − followed by a nurse losing her temper as I was 'not pushing' and it seemed to me they were literally cutting the baby out . . . Perhaps it is a natural reaction after childbirth to become upset, but, seeing the way other patients and myself were treated like imbeciles has left the most horrible impression.

A Welsh survey has come up with the fact that 65% of mothers who are delivered in hospital suffer from depression in some degree, compared with 19% confined at home.

The after-effects of artificial induction of labour with pitocin and prostaglandins have not been investigated. Ms Robinson has received around 150 letters from women who were painfully induced not for medical reasons, but to suit hospital routines. 'Many of them report long term depression, lack of feeling for their babies and sexual frigidity' (Letter to *Guardian*, 10 September 1974).

Of course, by no means all hospital births are traumatic. And as another article points out, even after a really good home birth, some women become depressed (Catherine Ballard and Hilary Hackett, *Spare Rib*, 47).

IF YOU SUFFER FROM POSTNATAL DEPRESSION

It is important for us to talk about our feelings and fears with supportive family and friends. Often, however, we do not recognize our symptoms or we are afraid of them. Feeling depressed is nothing to be ashamed of. If support from family and friends is not enough, or is not available, we can sometimes turn to the following: *Postnatal support groups*: many NCT groups are beginning to recognize the need for such groups. You can contact them through the NCT at head office or through your local branch. If no such group exists in your area, you can try setting one up yourself or through the child welfare clinic. One such group of women decided to meet once a fortnight after their babies were born. This is how one woman was helped:

I thought my life wouldn't be changed much by a baby. It took me over though — a child really brings out your deepest anxieties. I started relating differently to situations — everything became difficult, problematic; cleaning the house, washing nappies, even drinking a cup of tea. I also felt differently towards people, but my friends related to me as if I was the same and I tried to live up to their expectations. I couldn't; I freaked out, got paranoid and became a recluse with my baby and my world the size of the baby. Then I started getting together with a couple of other women with young babies. 'I just scream into my pillow at night and sometimes feel like killing myself,' one of them told me. I felt a shock of recognition. Every time we meet now we check out what we have gone through, compare, analyse, and feel a lot of mutual support. (Ballard and Hackett, op. cit.)

Your doctor: Your doctor can be extremely helpful and sympathetic, giving support for many months. However, not all GPs are helpful, and many of them do not have the time to give very much support. Far too often women are handed tranquillizers when all we need is respite from 24-hour child-care and a modicum of emotional support.

I am in a terrible state inside now. I went to my doctor and he could only examine me with one finger. I was too swollen for a proper examination ... The trouble is that I am very depressed. I told my doctor and he said 'Whatever for?'

If your doctor is unhelpful, try contacting your local *midwife* or the *health visitor* who came to see you after the birth. There may also be a branch of *Depressives Associated* in your area (see addresses p. 488).

CONCLUSION

It is clear that much research needs to be done into the cause and prevention of postnatal depression. Some exists, but it often falls down because it does not consider all the important variables. For example one

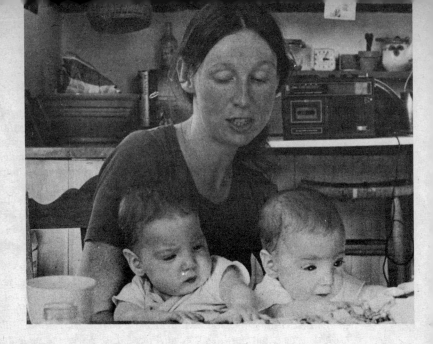

study, looking at the reasons why some women batter their children, concludes that 'Abnormal pregnancy, abnormal labour or delivery, neonatal separation, other separation in the first six months, illnesses in the first year of life, and illness in the mother in the first year of life' have been shown to be key factors in child abuse. But the study does not, for example, consider induction as abnormal. Nor does it consider the way women were treated by the medical staff. Furthermore, the study failed to emphasize two crucial factors: several of the 25 mothers examined were unsupported – and therefore had financial worries – and only four of the families were satisfactorily housed! (*Women's Report*, Vol. 3, issue 6.)

Although there are physical factors which can affect postnatal depression, there are, as we have explained, many other reasons why women become depressed after giving birth. Other factors which must not be overlooked involve the pressures society inflicts on us and the lack of help – both practical and emotional – available. If, for example, good child-care facilities were adequately available and if so many of us were not isolated in our homes, we are convinced that the incidence of postnatal depression would fall dramatically. Successful infant care is as much political as it is physical and emotional. Adequate, paid maternity and paternity leave, housing and child-care facilities are nothing more than reasonable demands which we can rightfully expect to have fulfilled. We can't hope to be 'naturally' good mothers without preparation, education, determination and help.

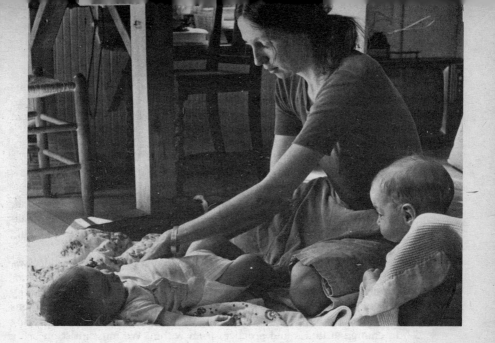

SUGGESTIONS FOR NEW PARENTS

There is little readily available instruction that prepares us emotionally and experientially for parenthood. Child-care is demanding and becomes more so if we expect ourselves to know instinctively things which are learned skills.

The responsibilities of motherhood are learned: very few books are adequate, because they rarely take into account the mother as an independent person. Talking to friends is more helpful. Dr Benjamin Spock's *Baby and Child Care* can be reassuring at times with specific information.

Get help from your mate and dependable friends and relatives. Encourage them to participate and take responsibility.

Get to know other couples who are experienced with childrearing.

Don't overload yourself with unimportant tasks.

Don't move house soon after the baby arrives.

Don't be concerned with keeping up appearances.

Time for yourself is essential — awake and asleep. When you're away from your baby, enjoy being yourself; motherhood is only one part of you.

Don't be a nurse to relatives and others during this period.

Confer and consult with family and experienced friends and discuss your plans and worries.

Don't give up outside interests, but cut down on responsibilities and rearrange schedules.

We can't emphasize enough that caring for a baby is a learned skill, and one that we are continually learning. There are no final rules to follow – our children are as different from each other as we are from our friends. The key thing is to try to relax and enjoy our children; they can be great fun as long as we don't have exclusive responsibility for them 24 hours a day.

Conclusion – What Can We Do?

As we have tried to show throughout these chapters, we as women can begin to organize ourselves to fight those aspects of our society that make childbearing and childrearing stressful rather than fulfilling experiences.

We must join with groups such as AIMS and the NCT (see addresses, p. 487). AIMS has produced several useful leaflets with ideas, for example, on how to start a local group and 'Criteria for a good maternity service'. We must work with others – such as local health councils, unions and Radical Midwives – giving support to professionals who are trying to change attitudes and practices from within. We must insist on being represented as consumers on policy-making committees; we must inform and support each other, work to deprofessionalize medicine, and persuade doctors, nurses and midwives to share their information with us. We desperately need more good, humane medical attendants, especially more women obstetricians, and we must support our sisters who embark on the long, hard and often alienating training. With more women in these fields, 'obstetric' can regain its original meaning, which is 'female who stands near'. We must work for the expansion of the midwifery services, continuity of care, community-orientated maternity homes and good child-care facilities.

We urge women who aren't in the vulnerable position of being in labour or giving birth to organize in a systematic way as consumers and evaluate the medical treatment most women receive. We urge you to investigate hospitals in your area; to assess the real needs of women in your area; to insist on whatever changes in the medical system are necessary; and to publicize your concerns throughout your community.

Doctors, hospitals and other medical institutions are powerful and unresponsive. Forcing them to become responsive to your health needs (to do in fact what they are supposed to do!) involves a difficult struggle. We need all the solidarity and sisterhood we can get. (For more discussion see Chapter 17.)

Childbearing Bibliography and Resources

GENERAL

Arms, Suzanne, *Immaculate Deception: A New Look at Women and Childbirth in America*, Houghton Mifflin, 1975. A good study of how hospitals complicate childbirth.

Association for Improvements in the Maternity Services. Various leaflets, including 'How to Set up an AIMS Group' and 'Maternity Care Information Sheet'.

Beels, Christine, *The Childbirth Book*, Turnstone Books, 1978. The first British book on childbirth written by a feminist. Highly recommended.

Bing, Elizabeth, *Six Practical Lessons for an Easier Childbirth*, Bantam Books, 1969.

Bing, Elizabeth, *Moving Through Pregnancy*, Bobbs-Merrill, 1975. Photographs of a pregnant woman exercising.

Bolton Women's Liberation Group, *Bolton Women's Guide*, available from Rising Free (p. 573). Includes good section on pregnancy.

Bourne, Gordon, *Pregnancy*, Cassell, 1972; Pan 1975. Adequate, but tends to be traditionally biased, especially when it resorts to ludicrous remarks about female sexuality.

Brazelton, T. Berry, 'Infant Outcome in Obstetric Anesthesia', *ICEA News*, November–December 1970, pp. 3–7.

Brook, Danaë, *Naturebirth*, Penguin, 1976.

Burnett, H., 'Prolonged First-stage Labour', *Nursing Mirror*, 29 July 1960.

Caldeyro-Barcia, Roberto, 'Some Consequences of Obstetrical Interference: Part 1', *Birth and the Family Journal*, March 1974. Introduction to the medical case against the use of a variety of routine medical procedures.

Close, Sylvia, *The Know-how of Pregnancy and Labour*, John Wright, 1975.

Consumers' Association, 'Pregnancy Month by Month', *Which?* booklet, 1977.

Daly, Ann, *The Birth of a Child*, Crown, 1969. Graphic photographs of a birth in Holland, with fairly good narration. Useful in helping us see how we look as we give birth.

Dick-Read, Grantly, *Childbirth Without Fear*, 2nd edn, Harper & Row, 1959. By the doctor who originated 'natural childbirth'. More stress on education and relaxation, less on activity and breathing.

Dick-Read, Grantly, *The Natural Childbirth Primer*, Harper & Row, 1956. A how-to for natural childbirth, with exercises, diet and an outstanding guide to labour and delivery.

Donnison, Jean, *Midwives and Medical Men*, Heinemann, 1977. History of childbirth in Britain, documenting the struggle between women (midwives) and men (doctors) over who should have control over childbirth.

Engelmann, *Labour among Primitive Peoples*, St Louis, 1882.

Flanagan, Geraldine L., *The First Nine Months of Life*, Heinemann, 1963. Story of conception and week-by-week progress of baby in utero. Very detailed, clear and exciting.

Garrey, M. M., *et al.*, *Obstetrics Illustrated*, Churchill Livingstone, 1974. Useful for pictures.

Gillie, Louise and Oliver, 'The Childbirth Revolution', *The Sunday Times*, 13 and 20 October 1974.

Haire, Doris, *The Cultural Warping of Childbirth*, International Childbirth Education Association, 1974 (available from National Childbirth Trust, see p. 488).

Haire, Doris and John, *Implementing Family-Centered Maternity Care with a Central Nursery*, 3rd edn, International Childbirth Education Association, 1971. Complete guide for hospitals or anyone interested in converting a conventional maternity unit into a service where prepared mothers and fathers can participate fully in labour, delivery and care of the baby afterwards. Exhaustive documentation.

Hazell, Lester D., *Commonsense Childbirth*, Putnam's, 1969. Written by a woman. Best overall book for many reasons: good to read; complete; sensible approach to childbirth. Excellent criticism of childbirth problems caused by the medical profession. Excellent section on why to have a baby at home; also good section on breast-feeding.

Heardman, Helen, *Relaxation and Exercises for Natural Childbirth* (revised by Maria Ebner), Churchill Livingstone, 1966. Cheap reprint of an old, valuable book.

Kitzinger, Sheila, *The Experience of Childbirth*, Penguin, 1970.

Leboyer, Frederick, *Birth Without Violence*, Wildwood House, 1975.

Lennane, Jean and John, *Hard Labour*, Gollancz, 1977. Very much against natural childbirth and pro epidurals etc., but provides a graphic description of what women suffer during childbirth.

McManus, T. J. and Calder, A. A., 'Upright Posture and the Efficiency of Labour', *Lancet*, 14 January 1978. Attempts, but fails, to show how lying down is the best position for labour.

Marzollo, Jean, *Nine Months, One Day, One Year*, Harper & Row, 1975. Written by parents about their experiences.

Montgomery, Eileen, *At Your Best for Birth and Later*, Wright, Bristol, 1969. Useful for exercises.

National Childbirth Trust. Numerous leaflets on pregnancy and childbirth, including breathing, exercises, sex, feeding, twins, fathers, etc. On the whole extremely useful, although some of the information is presented in a rather irritating way.

Oakley, Ann, 'Wisewoman and Medicine Man', *Rights and Wrongs of Women*, ed. Oakley and Mitchell, Penguin, 1976. Puts modern childbirth in a historical and sociological setting.

Richardson, Stephen, and Guttmacher, Alan, (eds.), *Social and Psychological Aspects of Childbearing*, Williams and Wilkins, 1967. A collection of articles that discusses many childbearing studies we wouldn't ordinarily hear about, especially on birth in other societies. Ignores the best studies of natural childbirth.

Richman, Goldthorp and Simmons, 'Fathers in Labour', *New Society*, 16 October 1975.

Swansea Women and Health Group, *Having Your Baby*, 1974 (available from Rising Free, p. 573). Great, cheap booklet.

White, Gregory, *Emergency Childbirth*, 1968 (American book reprinted by a London women's group; available from Rising Free). Indispensable for people living in remote places or for anyone who might have to deliver a baby unexpectedly. If you aren't having your baby in hospital, this is must reading.

Wright, Erna, *The New Childbirth*, Hart Pub. Co., 1968. Manual to prepare women for childbirth, written by a midwife who has had children. A woman could do all the physical preparation necessary with this book alone.

Zentner, C., *Twins*, David & Charles, 1975. Practical book.

ANTE-NATAL

Beckett, Sarah, *Herbs for Feminine Ailments*, Thorson, 1973.

Butler, *et al.*, 'Cigarette Smoking in Pregnancy: Its Influence on Birth Weight and Perinatal Mortality', *British Medical Journal*, 15 April 1972.

Davis, Adelle, *Let's Eat Right to Keep Fit*, Allen & Unwin, 1971.

Davis, Adelle, *Let's Get Well*, Allen & Unwin, 1966.

Davis, Adelle, *Let's Have Healthy Children*, Allen & Unwin, 1968.

DHSS, *Perinatal Mortality Survey*, HMSO, 1963.

DHSS, *Recommended Intake of Nutrients for the UK*, HMSO, 1969.

Lennane, Jean and John, 'Alleged Psychogenic Disorders, a Possible Manifestation of Sexual Prejudice', *New England Journal of Medicine*, Vol. 288, no. 6, p. 288, 8 February 1973.

National Childbirth Trust, 'Care of the Breasts and Nipples'.

National Childbirth Trust, 'Sex in Pregnancy'.

Rakusen, Jill, 'A New Pregnancy Test?', *Spare Rib*, 41.

Rhodes, P., Article on treatment of nausea during pregnancy, *Practitioner*, **192**, pp. 229–33, 1964.

Women's Report, 'Alcohol During Pregnancy', Vol. 4, issue 3, p. 14.

Women's Report, 'Death Tells No Story', Vol. 2, issue 6, p. 10.

Women's Report, 'Fathers' Smoking Habits', Vol. 2, issue 3.

Women's Report, 'Hormonal Pregnancy Tests', Vol. 3, issue 5, p. 6.

Women's Report, 'One Woman's Action', Vol. 3, issue 3.

Resources

Belmont Laboratories, 188 Brent Crescent, London NW10 (01 965 1477).

WHERE TO HAVE THE BABY

Anon, 'A Place to be Born', *Lancet*, 10 January 1976.

Banwell, Hamilton, *Journal of Royal College of General Practitioners*, 1970, *19*, 282, concerning 'success' of GP units.

Barnard *et al.*, *Journal of Royal College of General Practitioners*, 1970, *19*, 211, concerning 'success' of GP units.

Beels, Christine, 'In the Beginning', *Spare Rib*, 49.

Chalmers *et al.*, 'Obstetric Practice and Outcome of Pregnancy in Cardiff Residents 1965–73', *British Medical Journal*, 27 March 1976.

Crawford, J. Selwyn, 'A Critical Account of the Confidential Enquiries', *Proceedings of the Royal Society of Medicine*, Vol. 67, no. 9, September 1974: pointing out elementary statistical errors.

DHSS, *Cranbrook Report*, HMSO, 1959.

DHSS, *Health and Personal Social Services Statistics*, HMSO, 1975.

DHSS, *Health Services and Public Health Act 1968*, HMSO.

DHSS, *Human Relations in Obstetrics*, HMSO, 1961.

DHSS, *Peel Report*, HMSO, 1970.

DHSS, *Report on Confidential Enquiries into Maternal Deaths in England and Wales 1970–72*, HMSO.

Fergusson and Watson, 'Assessment of Obstetric Flying Squad in an Urban Area', *British Medical Journal*, 21 February 1976.

Fryer and Ashford, 'Study of Mortality Rates and Hospital/Home Confinement Rates', *British Journal of Preventive and Social Medicine*, 1972, 26, 1.

Garrow and Smith, paper on long-term effects of separation, *Proceedings of Royal Society of Medicine*, January 1976.

Josephine and Nicholas, 'Perhaps It Was the Raspberry Tea', *Peace News*, 23 January 1976.

Kitzinger, S. and Davis, J. A., *The Place of Birth*, Oxford University Press, 1978. Written from 'a woman's right to choose' perspective, examining the issues at far greater depth than we can. After a hasty read as we go to press, it appears relatively readable for the lay person, although a few of the articles would require help from a statistician.

Lees, Sue, 'Hospital Confinement', *New Society*, 25 April 1974.

McLachlan and Shegog (eds.), *In the Beginning – Studies of Maternity Services*, Oxford University Press, 1970.

Mehl, Lewis, 'Statistics on Low Complication and Mental Retardation Rates in Home Births', *Monthly Extract*, Vol. 5, issue 1.

Morris, N., 'Human Relations in Obstetric Practice', *Lancet*, Vol. 1, p. 913, 1960.

National Childbirth Trust, *Maternity Services in Bath*.

Oldershaw, Brudenell, 'Use by General Practitioners of Obstetric Beds in a Consultant Unit: A Further Report', *British Medical Journal*, 18 January 1975.

Oxford Consumers' Group, 'Maternity Care', *Oxford Consumer*, May 1974.

Robinson, Jean, 'How Hospitals Alienate Mothers', *Mind Out* – Journal of the National Association of Mental Health – March/April 1976.

Society to Support Home Confinements, *Maternal Deaths and Place of Confinement* (critique of DHSS 1970–72 report).

Society to Support Home Confinements, *Opting for a Home Confinement*.

Society to Support Home Confinements, *The Problem of Cross Infection in Maternity Care*.

Stacey, Margaret, 'Sociological and Psychological Implications of the New Styles of Childbirth', presented to seminar on human relations in obstetric practice, Warwick University, October 1975.

Wilkes, Dixon, and Knowelden, 'Modern Obstetrics and the General Practitioner', *British Medical Journal*, 20 December 1975.

Williams, R. E. O., *et al.*, *Hospital Infection, Causes and Prevention*, Lloyd-Luke, 1966.

Women's Report, 'A New Childbearing Centre', Vol. 4, issue 1.

Women's Report, 'More Maternity Units Threatened', Vol. 4, issue 5.

Women's Report, 'Proposals to Close Small Hospitals', Vol. 4, issue 4.

Women's Report, 'The Truth' – attitude of an area health authority to home births – Vol. 4, issue 1.

OBSTETRIC INTERVENTIONS AND PAIN RELIEF

Anon, 'Acupuncture in Obstetrics', *World Medicine*, 4 December 1974.

Anon, 'A Time to be Born', *Lancet*, 16 November 1974.

Anon, 'Induction of Labour', *British Medical Journal*, 27 March 1976: 'We as doctors must whenever possible, ensure that our patients are *made to feel* that they have taken part in decisions that affect their lives' (our italics!).

Blacow *et al.*, 'Induction of Labour', *Lancet*, 25 January 1975.

Chalmers *et al.*, 'Obstetric Practice and Outcome of Pregnancy in Cardiff Residents 1965–73, *British Medical Journal*, 27 March 1976.

Chalmers *et al.*, 'Use of Oxytocin and Incidence of Neonatal Jaundice', *British Medical Journal*, 19 April 1975.

Chard, T. and Richards, M. P. M. (eds.), *Benefits and Hazards of the New Obstetrics* SIMP with Heinemann, 1977. Gives a useful overview of the research to date, with some excellent chapters (you may need a medical dictionary for some of them).

Cole *et al.*, 'Elective Induction of Labour', *Lancet*, 5 April 1975. (See Robinson below.)

Crawford, J. Selwyn. *Principles and Practice of Obstetric Anaesthesia*, Blackwell, 1959. Attacks the 'negligence' of British anaesthetists.

Dunn, Peter M., 'Obstetric Delivery Today – for Better or for Worse?', *Lancet*, 10 April 1976, and subsequent correspondence.

Edington, P. T., *et al.*, 'Influence on Clinical Practice of Routine Intra-partum Fetal Monitoring', *British Medical Journal*, August 1975.

Froshaug, Judy, 'The Unkindest Cut of All?', *Nova*, September 1974.

Gibbens, G. D. L., 'Observations of Oxytocin Release in Human Labour', Blair Bell Research Society Meeting, 7 April 1975.

Holdcroft and Morgan, 'An Assessment of the Analgesic Effect in Labour of Pethidine and 5% Nitrous Oxide in Oxygen (Entonox)', *Journal of Obstetrics and Gynaecology of the British Commonwealth*, August 1974.

Jhirad, A., On nipple massage for induction, *Obstetrics and Gynaecology*, Vol. 41, 3, March 1973.

Liston and Campbell, 'Dangers of Oxytocin-induced Labour to Fetuses', *British Medical Journal*, 7 September 1974, and subsequent correspondence.

Melzack, Ronald, *The Puzzle of Pain*, Penguin, 1973.

Moir, Donald D., *Pain Relief in Labour*, Churchill Livingstone, 1973.

National Childbirth Trust, 'Episiotomy – Physical and Emotional Aspects' (various specialist authors, 30p).

National Childbirth Trust, 'Episiotomy' – short, cheaper leaflet.

National Childbirth Trust, *Some Mothers' Experiences of Induced Labour*, 1975.

O'Driscoll, K., 'Active Management of Labour', *British Medical Journal*, 21 July 1973: emphasizes the need for a short labour and equates long labours with pain!

O'Driscoll *et al.*, 'Selective Induction of Labour', *British Medical Journal*, 27 December, 1975.

Patient Voice, No. 1, June 1975 – 'Induced Births'.

Richards, M. P. M., 'Innovation in Medical Practice, with Special Reference to the Induction and Acceleration of Labour', presented at a study group organized by the Spastic Society, April 1975.

Richards, M. P. M., 'Obstetric Analgesics and the Development of Children', *Midwife, Health Visitor and Community Nurse*, Vol. 12, February 1976.

Richards, M. P. M., 'The One-day-old Deprived Child', *New Scientist*, 28 March 1974.

Robinson, Jean, 'Elective Induction of Labour', *Lancet*, 10 May 1975: follow-up letter and critique of the Cole study.

Salzmann, K. D., 'An Emergency Source of Oxytocin in Labour', *Journal of the Royal College of General Practitioners*, 1971, *21*, 670.

Salzmann, K. D., 'An Untapped Source of Oxytocin', *Journal of the Royal College of General Practitioners*, 1971, *21*, 282.

Scanlon and Walkley, 'Neonatal Blood Loss as a Complication of Fetal Monitoring', *Pediatrics*, December 1972.

Shearer, Madeleine, 'Fetal Monitoring: Do the Benefits Outweigh the Drawbacks?', *Birth and Family Journal*, Vol. 1, No. 1, Winter 1973–4.

Shearer, Madeleine, 'Some Deterrents to Objective Evaluation of Fetal Monitors', *Birth and Family Journal*, Spring 1975.

Standley, Kay, *et al.*, 'Local-Regional Anesthesia during Childbirth: Effect on Newborn Behaviours', *Science*, Vol. 186, 15 November 1974.

Theobald, G. W., 'Dangers of Oxytocin-induced Labour to Fetuses', letter to *British Medical Journal*, 12 October 1974.

Tipton and Lewis, 'Induction of Labour and Perinatal Mortality', *British Medical Journal*, 1, 361, 1975.

Women's Report, 'Induction', Vol. 4, issue 5.

Women's Report, 'A Ray of Light', Vol. 4, issue 4 – report of recent contributions to the induction debate.

POSTPARTUM

Ballard, Catherine, and Hackett, Hilary, 'My World Became the Size of the Baby', *Spare Rib*, 47.

Bibring, Grete L., 'Recognition of Psychological Stresses Often Neglected in OB care', *Hospital Topics*, 44, September, 1966, pp. 100–103.

Bibring, Grete L., 'Some Considerations of the Psychological Processes in Pregnancy', *The Psychoanalytic Study of the Child*, Vol. XIV, 1959, pp. 113–21.

Bibring, Grete L., *et al.*, 'A Study of the Psychological Processes in Pregnancy and of the Earliest Mother-Child Relationship', *The Psychoanalytic Study of the Child*, Vol. XVI, 1961, pp. 9–72. Excellent study of 'normal' pregnant women, with follow-up.

Breen, Dana, *The Birth of a First Child (Towards an Understanding of Femininity)*, Tavistock Publications, 1975.

Butts, Hugh F., 'Postpartum Psychiatric Problems: A Review of the Literature Dealing with Etiological Theories', *Journal of the National Medical Association*, Vol. 62, No. 2, March 1969, pp. 224–7.

Butts, Hugh F., 'Psychodynamic and Endocrine Factors in Postpartum Psychosis', *Journal of the National Medical Association*, Vol. 60, No. 3, May, 1968, pp. 224–7. Interesting case histories.

Chertok, Leon, *Motherhood and Personality*, Philadelphia, J. B. Lippincott, 1969.

Gordon, E. R., Kapostins, E. E., and Gordon, K. K., 'Factors in Postpartum Emotional Adjustment', *Obstetrics and Gynecology*, Vol. 25, No. 2, February, 1965, pp. 158–66.

Jones, Beverly, 'The Dynamics of Marriage and Motherhood', in Robin Morgan (ed.), *Sisterhood is Powerful*, New York, Random House (Vintage), 1970, pp. 57–8.

Kane, F. J., Jr, *et al.*, 'Emotional and Cognitive Disturbance in Early Puerperium', *British Journal of Psychiatry*, 1968, pp. 99–102.

Kitzinger, Sheila, 'The Fourth Trimester?', *Midwife, Health Visitor and Community Nurse*, April 1975.

Klaus, Marshal H., *et al.*, 'Maternal Attachment: Importance of the First Postpartum Days', *New England Journal of Medicine*, Vol. 286, No. 9, 2 March 1972.

Klaus, M. H. and Kennell, J., *Maternal-Infant Bonding*, St Louis, USA, C.V. Mosby, 1976.

Larsen, Virginia, *et al.*, *Attitudes and Stresses Affecting Perinatal Adjustment*. Final report, National Institute of Mental Health Grant MH-01381-01-02, 1 September 1963, to 31 August 1966. (Gordon questionnaire contained in appendices.)

Larsen, Virginia, *et al.*, *Prediction and Improvement of Postpartum Adjustment*. Final report, Children's Bureau Research Grant A-66, 1 September 1965, to 31 March 1968. Pages 95–9 have an excellent bibliography.

Liebenberg, Beatrice, 'Expectant Fathers', paper presented at annual meeting of American Orthopsychiatric Association, March 1967, Washington, DC.

Masters, William H., and Johnson, Virginia E., *Human Sexual Response*, Churchill, 1966.

Melges, F. T., 'Postpartum Psychiatric Syndromes', *Psychoanalytic Medicine*, 30, January–February, 1968, pp. 95–108.

Richards, M. P. M., 'Possible Effects of Early Separation on Later Development of Children', in Brimblecombe *et al.*, (eds.), *Early Separation and Special-Care Nurseries*, London, SIMP with Heinemann, 1978.

Richards and Bernal, *New Society*, 28 February 1974 – article concerning night waking and the bad advice parents are often given.

Robinson, Jean, 'How Hospitals Alienate Mothers', *Mind Out* – Journal of the National Association for Mental Health – March/April 1976.

Rossi, Alice, 'Transition to Parenthood', in Skolnick and Skolnick (eds), *Family in Transition*, Boston, Little, Brown and Co., 1971.

Rubin, Reva, 'Puerperal Change', in Nancy A. Lytle (ed.), *Maternal Health Nursing*, Dubuque, Iowa, William C. Brown Co., 1967.

Seashore, Marjorie, *et al.*, 'Study of Mother-Infant Separation Focusing on the Mother', *Journal of Personality and Social Psychology*, Vol. 26, No. 3, p. 369.

Stein, Rita F., 'Social Orientation to Mental Illness in Pregnancy and Childbirth', *International Journal of Social Psychiatry*, 14, Winter 1967–8, pp. 56–64.

Williams, Barbara, 'Sleep Needs During the Maternity Cycle', *Nursing Outlook*, February, 1967, pp. 53–5.

Women's Report, 'Abnormal Pregnancy . . .', Vol. 3, issue 6.

Women's Report, 'Post Partum Blues', Vol. 1, issue 5, p. 10.

FEEDING

Anon, 'Breast is Best', *Lancet*, 21 August 1976: critique of current 'evidence' that breast is best.

Barrie *et al.*, 'Milk for Babies', *Lancet*, 14 June 1975.

Close, Sylvia, *The Know-how of Breast Feeding*, John Wright & Sons, 1972: clear, simple questions and answers.

Close, Sylvia, *The Know-how of Infant Feeding*, John Wright & Sons, 3rd edn., 1973.

Gray, Anne, 'Breast Feeding – The Sociologist's Tale', *Midwife, Health Visitor and Community Nurse*, December 1975.

Gunther, Mavis, *Infant Feeding*,* Penguin, 1973: a bit medically-orientated but sensible.

HMSO, *Present-day Practice in Infant Feeding* (see also a critique of this in *Women's Report*, below).

Morgan, Patricia, 'Breast-feeding: The Mystic Maternal Cult', *New Society*, 20 May 1976.

National Childbirth Trust: various cheap leaflets including *Easy Breastfeeding, Care of Breasts and Nipples, Hand Expressing, Ante-natal Advice for Mothers Keen to Breastfeed, Analysis of Babymilks*, etc.*

Newton, M. and N., 'The Normal Course and Management of Lactation', *Clinical Obstetrics and Gynecology*, Vol. 5, 1962, p. 44. Available as a pamphlet from *Child and Family*, Box 508, Oak Park, Ill. 60303.

Raphael, Dana, *The Tender Gift*. Prentice Hall, 1973. Anthropological framework identifying new mothers' needs for support during breast-feeding.

Richards, M. P. M., 'Support for Breast Feeding', *Midwife, Health Visitor and Community Nurse*, March 1976.

Smith, B. A. M., 'Feeding Overstrength Cows' Milk to Babies', *British Medical Journal*, 28 December 1974.

The Womanly Art of Breastfeeding, Franklin Park, Ill.: La Leche League International, 1963. Vital basic information if you can get past the sickening stuff about how a woman's role is to bear and raise children. Contact La Leche League (see below).

Which?, 'Baby Milk and Food', October 1975: contains a table comparing different brands.

Whichelow, M. J., 'Breast Feeding – a Dying Art', *World Medicine*, 17 July 1974.

Women's Report, Milky, Murky Muddle (concerning confusion over artificial milk), Vol. 4, issue 3.

Women's Report, 'Present Day Practice in Infant Feeding' (critique of government document), Vol. 3, issue 1.

INFANT AND CHILD CARE

Aries, Philippe, *Centuries of Childhood*, Penguin, 1973: gives much insight into our own culture.

Barker and Skaggs, *The Mother Person*, Severn House Publishers, 1977. We haven't read it but AIMS feels it's essential reading for anyone thinking of starting a family who is not sure.

Bettelheim, Bruno, *The Children of the Dream*, Paladin, 1969: communal child-rearing.

Bettelheim, Bruno, *Love Is Not Enough*, New York, Avon Books, 1971. Although the book is not about 'normal' children, it has some important things to say about all kids. Good sections on food, inbetween times, and space.

Bowlby, John, *Child Care and the Growth of Love*, Penguin, 1953. He started the Maternal Deprivation theory; see Rutter below.

Changing Childcare: Cuba, China and the Challenging of our own values (Writers and Readers Publishing Co-operative). Three short articles aimed at nursery work trainees.

* Available from National Childbirth Trust.

Children's Community Centre, *Our Experiences of Collective Child Care* (pamphlet available from Rising Free).

Clarke, Ann and Alan (eds.), *Early Experience: Myth and Evidence*, Open Books: case studies and original research by Rutter, the Tizards and others. Very interesting.

Disabled Living Foundation, *Early Days — You and Your New Baby*, 1973 (for the disabled mother).

Edge, Patricia, *Child Care and Management from Birth to Adolescence*, Faber paperback, 1976: '. . . full of useful advice . . . Masturbation and bed-wetting are treated as a normal part of growing up, but homosexuality, contraception, working mothers, violence in the home and single parents have no place in the author's wonderland of domesticity . . .' (*Women's Report*, 4/2).

Ginott, Hima, *Between Parent and Child*, Pan: practical advice on mentally healthy communication with children.

Jarecki, Hilde, *Playgroups: A Practical approach*, Faber and Faber, 1975: perpetuates the myth that mothers should look after children and that mothers don't go out to work, but is a good guide on how to set up facilities.

Ilg, Francis L., and Ames, Louise Bates, *Gesell Institute's Child Behavior*, New York, Dell, 1955. (Get revised edition.)

Kellmer Pringle, Mia, *The Needs of Children*, Hutchinson, 1974: emphasizing psycho-social needs.

Marsden, Dennis, *Mothers Alone*, Allen Lane, 1969.

Montagu, Ashley, *Touching: The Human Significance of the Skin*, New York, Columbia University Press, 1971. Fascinating account of human needs and emotions relating to physical contact at all ages; includes some animal studies, etc. Especially shows artificiality of society in the United States.

Pre-School Playgroup Association, *At work together*: a guide for people setting up nurseries in factories, colleges and hospitals.

Pre-School Playgroup Association, *Mother and Toddler Groups — some guidelines*, from the Pre-School Playgroups Association, Playgroup House, 7 Royal Terrace, Glasgow G3 7NT.

Out of the Pumpkinshell, about a women's liberation playgroup going for over 3 years, by Birmingham women's liberation group and available from Rising Free. See p. 573.

Rayner, Claire, *You know more than you think you do* (free leaflet published by Health Education Council and Mind): on the whole, sound advice.

Rutter, Michael, *Maternal Deprivation Reassessed*. Penguin, 1972: demolishes the 'maternal deprivation' theory which grew up following Bowlby's research and which is still, alas, used as a tool for blackmailing women into being full-time mothers when they don't want to be.

Schaffer, R., *Mothering*, Fontana/Open Books, 1977. Concludes that mother love is neither inevitable nor instinctive.

Shrew magazine, Vol. 5, No. 4, 'Goodbye Dolly' — the children's books issue, available from London Women's Liberation Workshop.

Spock, Benjamin, *Baby and Child Care*, New York, Pocket Books, rev. edn., 1968. Still a classic (it's much misquoted), and the new edition is, we are assured, non-sexist. Not good on breast-feeding or socialization, but good for basic everyday troubles.

Thames Television 'Help' programme. *Information sheet on facilities for children under five*, 1977, available from 'Help' programme, Thames TV, Euston Road, London WC1. Good.

Tizard, Moss and Perry. *All Our Children*, New Society/Temple Smith, 1976: 'Fascinating information on the patterns of child care in a community, alternative forms of day care and the expressed needs of parents . . .' (Women and Education Newsletter, No. 9).

Towards Socialist Childcare by Socialist Childcare Collective. Available from Rising Free.

Woodward, W. Mary, *The Development of Behaviour*, Penguin, 1971: general book on child development.

NB: Also worthwhile, really helpful reading: books by psychiatrists such as R. D. Laing, Fritz Perls, David Cooper, Arthur Janov and other modern 'existential' psychiatrists, and books by educators John Holt, A. S. Neill, Sylvia Ashton-Warner, George Denison, Jonathan Kozol and Herbert Kohl.

Especially useful to new parents are books by family therapists. Virginia Satir's *Peoplemaking* (Palo Alto: Science & Behavior Books, Inc., 1974), has an excellent chapter on parenting.

RIGHTS, BENEFITS AND ALLOWANCES FOR MOTHERS

Ashdown-Sharp, Patricia, *The Single Woman's Guide to Pregnancy and Parenthood*, Penguin, 1975: invaluable.

Coote, Anna, and Gill, Tess, *Woman's Rights: A Practical Guide*, Penguin, 1977.

Coussins, Jean, *Maternity Rights*, National Council for Civil Liberties, 1977.

Department of Employment. *New rights for the expectant mother* (available from regional or local offices).

Equal Opportunities Commission, *Income Tax and Sex Discrimination*, available free from EOC (see address, p. 570). Useful and accessible information about the tax system.

Exceptional Needs Payments (HMSO): gives guidelines used by Social Security in exercising their discretionary powers.

Lister and Wilson, *The Unequal Breadwinner — A new perspective on women and social security*, National Council for Civil Liberties, 1976.

Lynes, Tony, *Penguin Guide to Supplementary Benefits*, Penguin, 1972.

National Welfare Benefits Handbook (published by Child Poverty Action Group): useful.

Supplementary Benefits Handbook (HMSO): useful particularly because you can quote it in your dealings with the DHSS.

Unsupported Mothers' Handbook by women in the Claimants' Union (available from Rising Free).

Women and Social Security (1975), again by the Claimants' Union, containing much useful information and advice (available from Rising Free).

FILMS AND OTHER RESOURCES

John and *Kate*, two films about the effects of separation on children. We haven't seen them, but according to AIMS they are 'essential to be seen by staff of any hospital which prohibits the visiting of children to their parents'. Available from

Concord Film Council, Nacton, Ipswich, Suffolk (tel: 0473 76012).

Birth by Julian Aston: different mothers' accounts of what it feels like to give birth, some emotional, some matter-of-fact. Also, two home births shown. 'Useful for doctors and midwives (and others) who have not experienced birth' (AIMS). Available for hire from The National Childbirth Trust.

A Child is Born (a Leboyer birth), available for hire from Guild Sound and Vision, Woodstone House, Oundle Road, Peterborough, Cambridgeshire.

Birth (with R. D. Laing) by Helen Brew. Comparison of technological and natural birth — Good, but could do without Laing. Contact NCT for details.

Journey through Birth, a series of tapes by Sheila Kitzinger; a course in preparation for couples. Very good if you can't get to good classes. Contact National Childbirth Trust.

ORGANIZATIONS

Association for Improvements in the Maternity Services (AIMS). Secretary: Christine Beels, 19 Broomfield Crescent, Leeds 6 (Leeds 751911).

Association of Radical Midwives, hon. sec.: Jenny Flintham, 17 Fairfax Road, Derby DE3 GRX.

Baby Foods Action Group, 103 Gower Street, London WC1E 6AW.

British Society for Social Responsibility in Science, 9 Poland Street, London W1 (01 437 2728).

Child Care Outside School Hours, c/o Bristol Women's Centre, 59 Union Street, Bristol BS1 2DU. Campaigns for after-school care for the children of working parents.

Child Poverty Action Group, 1 Macklin Street, London WC2 (01 242 3225). Provides information on welfare benefits and campaigns for realistic allowances for families. Also helps people to claim their benefits.

Child's Play, Action for the development of children through play: this organization, established by the charity 'Make Children Happy', keeps information and answers queries on many aspects of play provision for children aged 5 to 15. Their monthly magazine *It's Child's Play* is free to anyone who wants it. Address: Victoria Chambers, 16/20 Strutton Ground, London SW1 (01 222 0261).

Children's Rights Workshop, 73 Balfour Street, London SE17 (01 703 7217).

Cissy (Campaign for Impeding Sex Stereotyping in the Young). Contact Pam, c/o Village Books, 17 Shrubbery Road, London SW16 (01 677 2667).

Citizens' Rights Office, 1 Macklin Street, London WC2 (01 405 4517). Gives help on welfare rights and tribunal appeals and can refer you to other citizens' rights offices in the country.

Claimants' Union, East London branch at Dame Colet House, Ben Jonson Road, London E1 (01 790 3867). Helps people to claim their rights. Publishes among other things *Unsupported Mothers' Handbook* and *Women and Social Security*. Can put you in touch with other CUs.

Communes Network, c/o Laurieston Hall, Castle Douglas, Kirkcuds. Publishes a newsletter roughly every four weeks for people thinking about communal living or already engaged in it. Has contacts column for people wanting groups and groups wanting people. Network subscribers get together every six months. Send s.a.e. with all correspondence.

Conscious Birth Centre at the Community Health Foundation, 188 Old Street, London EC1 (01 251 4076) — a coordinating centre run by mothers who have had babies by the Leboyer method, to give help, advice and information to other women.

Depressives Associated, contact Ms Janet Stevenson, 19 Merley Ways, Wimborne Minster, Dorset BH21 1QN (enclose s.a.e.) (Wimborne 3957). Groups throughout the country.

Disability Alliance, 96 Portland Place, London W1. To help chronically sick and disabled mothers.

Gingerbread, head office: 35 Wellington Street, London WC2 (01 240 0953). Self-help groups throughout the country for single parents.

La Leche League, BM 3424, London WCIV 6XX. Provides information and advice on breast-feeding.

London Women's Squatters Group, contacted through WIRES (see address, p. 570).

National Campaign for Nursery Education, 33 High Street, London SW1 (01 828 2844). Campaigns against the cuts in nurseries.

National Childbirth Trust (see p. 419), head office: 9 Queensborough Terrace, London W2 3TB (01 229 9319). Addresses for hypnosis, the Alexander technique, homeopathy and acupuncture, see Further Reading to Chapter 6.

National Council for One Parent Families, 255 Kentish Town Road, London NW5 (01 267 1361).

Pre-School Playgroups' Association, Alford House, Aveline Street, London SE11 (01 582 8871). Can help you set up a playgroup.

Rights of Women (ROW) (see address, p. 571). Provides information and help with legal problems.

Single-handed Ltd, 68 Lewes Road, Haywards Heath, Sussex (Haywards Heath 4663). Commercial agency specializing in putting single parents who want to share accommodation in touch.

Society to Support Home Confinements. Organizer: Margaret Whyte, 17 Laburnum Avenue, Durham City (Durham 61325).

Women's Liberation Legal and Financial Independence Campaign, 7 Killieser Avenue, London SW2 (01 671 2779).

NON-SEXIST CHILDREN'S BOOKS: BOOK LISTS FOR ALL AGES

The Children's Rights Workshop, 73 Balfour Street, London SE17 (01 703 7217). *Sexism in Children's Books: Facts, Figures and Guidelines*, Writers and Readers Publishing Co-operative, 9–19 Rupert Street, London W1.

15 Some Exceptions in Pregnancy and Childbirth

Problems in childbirth are not uncommon, yet most of us are taken by surprise when something happens. Why are we so unprepared? One possible reason is that the *majority* of women have few serious problems. Secondly, if something goes wrong, it is often hushed up because many people are superstitious, hesitant to talk about things related to sexuality, or simply want to keep their privacy. Thirdly, many of us don't live in extended families or close communities, so we remain ignorant that certain problems are facts of life for some women. Even when we are generally healthy, things can and do go wrong.

We can learn to deal with potential problems and actual crises in two ways. First we need to have a general awareness that things can go wrong. We can tuck away such information to be used if necessary. It can't hurt us. Secondly, if we do suspect something is wrong we need specific information to answer our questions.

Often when we ask our doctors for help, either before we are pregnant or in early pregnancy, they brush aside our questions and worries. This insults our intelligence and undermines our emotional strength. We and our doctors are practising sound preventive medicine when we ask our questions as strongly as we can and they answer them respectfully to the best of their knowledge.

We can learn to develop emotional strengths to cope with what we are living through. Crisis may produce feelings of isolation, fear, anger, grief, guilt and helplessness, as well as obsessions and fantasies. During such times we need sympathetic support from our partners, friends and others who have had similar experiences. We need to be able to reach out to others.

This chapter is meant to be a first tool to help us acquire some of the information we need.

Infertility

It was a shock and a sadness to hear I'm not ovulating. That means I'm not fertile. I feel bitter towards those doctors who said 'nothing to worry about' and 'have a baby'. So now I shall undergo all kinds of tests. Today I feel optimistic, I know (I hope) my body will be set right in some way.

Every time we make love, I hope. Then, my period — blood — no child.

When we decide to have our first child, we never expect to be infertile. We know it might take a few months, that we might have some 'trouble', but we are not prepared for infertility. We're even less prepared when we already have a child or two and can't get pregnant again.

Infertility is defined by most doctors as the inability to conceive after a year or more of sexual relations without contraception. The category includes women who conceive but can't maintain a pregnancy long enough for the foetus to become viable (able to live outside the mother). You should have the right to explore whether you are infertile whenever you begin to feel concerned that you are not pregnant, although some doctors will not perform investigations unless you have been trying to conceive for 2 years. Infertility may be a temporary or permanent state, depending on your problem and on the available treatments. Many people are surprised to learn that (1) infertility is fairly common, and (2) male factors as well as female factors can be responsible. About 10 to 15% of couples are infertile. Roughly the same number of cases are caused by male factors as female factors. In about 30% of cases, combined factors are responsible.

It is clear that the man and woman must be diagnosed and treated together. If the man has the problem, treatment of the woman alone has little value and usually involves many needless and painful tests. A man, by his very anatomy, is easier to diagnose: semen analysis is one of the first tests that should be performed. Also, the temperature of the scrotal sac should be checked: the temperature could be too high simply because the man's pants or trousers are too tight (fairly ordinary jeans have been known to cause this problem).

As new research and techniques become available the cure rate for infertility is improving. Some problems respond easily to treatment, while others are incurable or respond in less than 20% of cases. Infertility appears to be increasing, possibly because little is known about the effect of prolonged use of birth control — the Pill and the IUD — on fertility, and because the higher VD rate (see Chapter 7) is causing more long-term infections that women may not be aware of.

POSSIBLE CAUSES OF INFERTILITY

A man may be infertile because of:

1. *No sperm or low sperm production.* This is probably due to an infection after puberty accompanied by high fever; unrepaired undescended testicles; taking of certain drugs; exposure to large amounts of X-ray; trauma to testicles; temperature of the scrotal sac chronically higher than it should be (see above); congenital malformation or absence of testicles.

2. *Inability of sperm to swim (low motility).* This may be due to chronic prostatitis, surgical removal of the prostate, or hormonal factors.

3. *Inability to deposit sperm in the vagina near the cervix.* This may be due to impotence; the opening of the penis being either on the underside or the top side of the penis; premature ejaculation; obesity (causing inability to penetrate); or lack of knowledge of the most effective sexual techniques.

4. *Blockage of the passageway carrying the sperm.* May be caused by untreated VD or other infection, varicocele, or vasectomy.

5. *Other factors.* Emotional stress, poor nutrition, or psychological problems.

A woman might be infertile because of:

1. *Pelvic inflammatory disease* (*PID*, see p. 205).

2. *Endometriosis.* See p. 174.

3. *Venereal disease* (gonorrhoea, see Chapter 7). If not properly treated, gonorrhoea can cause tubal blockage.

4. *Endocrine problems.* Failure to ovulate may be due to any malfunction of the glands that influence the menstrual cycle — pituitary, thyroid, or adrenals.

5. *Cervical factors.* Cervical infection; cervical mucus which repels the sperm for some reason; polyps (growths) all might keep sperm from entering the uterus.

6. *Tuberculosis* can inflame or block the fallopian tubes. Infertility clinics check for tuberculosis routinely.

7. *Other factors.* Congenital malformation; premature ageing of the ovaries; polycystic ovaries (Stein-Levinthal's syndrome); poor nutrition; obesity; emotional stress (which may occur in as many as 25% of cases).

Some shared causes of infertility are:

1. *Immunologic response.* There may be sperm antibodies present in either the man or woman which tend to destroy the sperms' action.

2. An infection called *T-mycoplasma* in either the man or the woman which can be treated by an antibiotic called doxycycline.

3. *Simple lack of knowledge.* Neither of you might know when you are fertile, how often to have intercourse during this time, or what to do during intercourse to make pregnancy more likely.

In a recent article, Masters and Johnson say that 1 out of 8 couples who have attended their infertility clinic over the past 25 years have conceived within 3 months with no treatment other than this basic information. If your menstrual cycle is regular, whether it be long or short, you will probably ovulate 14 days (give or take 24 hours either way) before the beginning of your next period. In other words, try to become pregnant the 13th, 14th and 15th days before your next period. During these 3 days, spacing your lovemaking is important. A man's sperm production decreases if he makes love too often, so you should have intercourse no more than once every 30 to 36 hours, if possible, to keep active sperm in your genital tract during that period of time. It is wise to have intercourse 2 days before this 3-day period, so that your partner's sperm production will be stimulated.

If your uterus is not tilted back the most effective position for intercourse will be with your partner above and facing you, and a folded pillow under your hips to raise them. Make love in the ways that give you pleasure, and when he penetrates you, draw your knees up to your chest and make room for him between your legs. He should penetrate as deeply as possible, and when he has an orgasm he should stop thrusting and hold quite still deep in your vagina. Approximately 60 to 70% of the sperm are contained in the first few drops of ejaculate. It's best if he withdraws immediately after ejaculation, and gently props the pillow underneath your hips if it has become flattened. Remain there for an hour, if possible, with your knees still close to your chest. This way you are more likely to retain seminal fluid until the sperm make their way up through your cervix.

Use no artificial lubricant, such as jellies or creams, and never douche afterwards.

Though these methods may at times seem too mechanical and make you tense, try to keep in your minds and hearts your good feelings for each other.

DIAGNOSIS OF INFERTILITY

British clinics vary a lot in the diagnostic tests they do. In many hospitals – particularly non-teaching hospitals – the man is not even examined. As we have already explained, this is an unacceptable way to investigate infertility. Make sure that both of you are examined and the full medical histories are taken. A disturbingly high number of hospitals are inadequate either in the tests they perform or in the way they perform them. (See survey by Sandler, in Bibliography.) Teaching hospitals are most likely to have special infertility clinics, so obviously it is best if you try to be referred to one of these. However, a hospital with even limited facilities should be able to perform a good, sound investigation. Most infertility problems should be resolved without additional facilities required for such procedures as radioimmune assays (see below). In fact, you can become pregnant before treatment has even been carried out: 13% of women become pregnant after their first consultation and a further 20% after 3 months' investigation.

Though a sequence of diagnostic studies will vary with both doctors and individuals, it should include the following:

1. *A general physical examination and medical history of both man and woman.*

2. *A pelvic examination of the woman.* Your reproductive tract, your breasts and your general development will be checked for hormone balance. Tell your doctor about your menstrual history, its onset and pattern; about any previous pregnancies, episodes of VD, or abortions; about your use of birth control; about your sexual relations (frequency, position and related feelings).

3. *A basal temperature chart* (see p. 278). From the chart you can find out if you are ovulating or not, and if you are, the date of ovulation, so that you can time your sex to coincide. If you are ovulating normally, from the time of your last period until your ovulation you'll have a fluctuating, low temperature (around 98 degrees or less). About the time of ovulation there's usually a sharp dip followed by a rise of half a degree or more. Some cycles show just a rise with no preceding dip. The higher plateau (usually around 98·4 degrees) is maintained until the day before your next period, when it drops again. NB: The rise may not happen when you expect it. Ovulatory patterns vary – don't ignore fluctuations even late in the month. You can obtain a chart from your doctor or from your local family planning clinic.

The chart, while very useful, can make us feel as if we are scheduling sex, especially if we have to use it over a long period of time.

I felt very regulated and calculating, both with my own body and in my relationship with my husband. I need not say what it did to our natural sexual impulses. But a child at all cost. That's how we felt.

You must wait at least two cycles to begin to interpret the chart.

4. *Semen analysis for the man.* Your partner will ejaculate a sample of his semen into a clean container. It must be examined as soon as possible under a microscope to find out the sperm count and motility. A count below 50 million sperm per c.c. is considered below average, but pregnancies have been known to occur with counts much lower. The sperm must be able to swim actively, and at least 80% should be normal in size and shape. A semen analysis is usually repeated, since a man's sperm can fluctuate for many reasons. If the semen analysis is abnormal, your partner will want to pursue his own diagnosis before further tests are done on you.

Any diagnosis of infertility can make things difficult for both man and woman.

My husband's sperm count was very low; we were both crushed. I don't think my husband believed it was actually happening. In fact he often talked in the third person, not truly accepting the results. I didn't know what to say. I couldn't say the typical 'Oh, it's all right' because we both knew it really wasn't all right. For some reason, I found I could handle a problem with myself but found it very difficult to handle my reaction to his problem. I was even more concerned that he couldn't handle his problem.

If all male factors are normal, study of the woman continues. You should have a *post-coital test* (*Hühner test*). This involves having intercourse just before you expect to ovulate and then seeing the doctor within several hours without having washed or douched. The doctor will take a small amount of mucus from your vagina and cervix to be studied for the number of live, active sperm. A normal test shows that sperm have the ability to penetrate cervical mucus and live in this environment. This test may be combined with another, also done at this time in your cycle, called *tubal insufflation*. It is usually done on an out-patient basis but if you find this painful, ask the doctor to arrange for it to be done under a general anaesthetic. You will then have to go into hospital for 2 or 3 days. A gas, carbon dioxide, is blown under carefully monitored pressure into your uterus, through the cervix. In a normal situation it will escape out of the tubes into the surrounding cavity, causing shoulder pain when you sit up (it is eventually absorbed into your body). If the test is abnormal, it may be repeated or confirmed by X-ray studies. It is often difficult to tell the difference between tubes that are blocked permanently and those which are only in spasm. Sometimes the insufflation solves the blockage problem, clearing the tubes of mucus or small adhesions.

If your tubes appear blocked, you can have a *hysterosalpingogram*. This is commonly done on an in-patient basis under general anaesthesia. It can be done quite safely (although sometimes painfully) on an out-patient basis with sedatives. We think that women should be able to choose the method they would be happiest with. It involves injecting a dye that shows up on X-rays into your uterus and tubes. If the tubes are open, the dye passes into the surrounding cavity to be harmlessly re-absorbed by your body.

To determine whether you are ovulating, an *endometrial biopsy* may be performed. It can be done any time from a week after ovulation is suspected to the first day of your period. A small instrument is inserted into your uterus after your cervix has been partially dilated (this will cause some unpleasant cramping). The instrument scrapes a tiny piece of tissue from the lining of the uterus (endometrium), and this is examined microscopically. Tissue formed while progesterone is being produced (after ovulation) is different from tissue formed under the influence of oestrogen (before ovulation) or under no hormonal influence. Hormonal levels in urine and blood serum can also be helpful in diagnosis of ovulation and the total hormone picture.

If no problem has been found, your doctor can do a laparoscopy (see p. 287), which allows the tubes, ovaries, exterior of uterus and surrounding cavities to be seen. A small incision is made near your navel under anaesthesia. A great deal of information can be obtained from this procedure. Even if the hysterosalpingogram showed that your tubes were all right, a laparoscopy can show up small pieces of endometriosis (see p. 174) at critical sites which might be preventing you from conceiving. Treatment for this can result in pregnancy. Sometimes a *laparotomy* (see p. 286) is performed for the same purpose as laparoscopy. This is a much more major operation and should be avoided if at all possible.

In women with few, scanty or no periods, further tests can be performed such as *serum and urinary hormone assays*, the *Metapyrone test*, the *Lysine Vasopressin test* and the *Clomiphene Pituitary Reserve test*. They involve monitoring the urine and blood over a period of time and, since they involve special techniques, can usually be performed only in the larger gynaecology units.

WHERE TO GO FOR TESTS

Ideally, ask your GP to refer you to a clinic which specializes in infertility and where the same doctor sees both you and your partner. Many family planning clinics run infertility sessions; you can refer yourself to these. You usually have to wait for an appointment at a fertility clinic – but it should not be more than 3 months.

TREATMENT

After all diagnosis has been carried out, a problem is often found and appropriate treatment can begin.

In general, male problems respond poorly to treatment. In low sperm counts which are motile, you can be artificially inseminated with your partner's sperm. Collecting and concentrating semen specimens is also being tried currently, but without much success. If the problem is a blocked passageway or a varicocele, surgery may be indicated. Some motility problems respond to steroid treatment, and male hormones may help to increase a count temporarily. Artificial insemination by donor (AID) is also possible if your partner cannot provide sperm. You can ask at your infertility clinic if there is an NHS AID service available; some doctors provide a service outside the NHS, sometimes on a charitable basis. The main problem with AID is finding suitable men willing to donate sperm. Partners of women who have been successfully treated at an infertility clinic would probably be the most willing. It is not easy to get referred for AID, although it is possible: keep trying.

For women, the highest degree of success is currently with endocrine disorders, such as failure to ovulate, short luteal (post-ovulatory) phase where the egg does not have enough time to mature before menstruation, or problems of implantation. 'Fertility pills' – such as clomiphene – can be used to stimulate the ovary. Much publicity centres on these because they sometimes cause multiple births, but if they are used carefully and the woman is properly monitored, they only increase the incidence of twins – at the most.

Cervical problems, such as cervicitis, hostile mucus, or incompetent (weak) cervix, also respond well to treatment. If uterine adhesions are found, dilatation and curettage (D & C) may be performed. Surgery on polycystic ovaries may produce normal ovulation. Tubal adhesions and blockages respond at a low rate of success to tubal surgery or medical irrigations with antibiotics and steroids. If you are found to have many adhesions due to long-term pelvic infection, you may require abdominal surgery to 'clean out' scar tissue, suspend the uterus, and improve chances of conception. Success in all treatment is highly individual.

Shared infertility problems are often treated by separate doctors. The man gets sent to a urologist while the woman is treated by a gynaecologist or infertility specialist. It is very important that your doctors communicate with each other. The potential for any couple with a shared problem to achieve a pregnancy is improved dramatically if even one member of the couple can be treated and helped. If both of you can be helped, then your chances are excellent.

In over 10% of all infertile couples no reason for infertility is found. This is called 'normal infertility'. You might be told your problems are all in your heads. This kind of attitude is not helpful at all. Often you may be victims of a condition whose cause or cure has yet to be discovered. It is a pity that commonly, people are not recalled to clinics when new discoveries have been made.

In all cases, a 5% spontaneous cure rate exists. This means a cure without any treatment whatever. Often after many years of trying pregnancy will finally occur. It may occur in our early 30s when a second 'fertile phase' may occur (the first phase being from our teens to mid-20s).

Diet can also help, and nature cure methods have been shown to be successful when all else has failed. The nature cure treatment hinges on the vaginal secretions, which can apparently be affected by diet or tension. If the secretions are too acid, sperm can be destroyed. To ensure alkaline secretions, a lot of vegetables – especially raw ones – and fruit need to be eaten. Alkaline pessaries or solutions can also be used. If you have a constant, heavy discharge – leucorrhoea – diet can also deal with this. One booklet – *Women's Ailments* (see Bibliography) – recommends a specific diet along the lines suggested above which 'should be carefully followed by any woman who appears to be infertile'. For further nature cure treatments, see this booklet.

Although a lot can be done if you are infertile, there is still much research needed. One problem is that the subject of infertility is not usually considered a priority. Those of us concerned about A Woman's Right to Choose can join together to achieve that end. For details of groups and organizations, see the end of this chapter.

THE EXPERIENCE OF INFERTILITY

The process of finding causes for infertility can be wearing and depressing. It takes a lot of strength for a woman to go through some or all of the above tests. It is crucial to have a good, supportive doctor. Relatives may not be too helpful either:

My parents and parents-in-law want grandchildren and make me feel a failure because I'm not producing them. My husband wants children very badly and sometimes reminds me that other women could provide him with them. I always feel guilty about my jealousy whenever any of my friends becomes pregnant. (Letter to *Guardian*, 5 March 1975.)

Not all people feel the pain of infertility with equal intensity. Certain feelings will appear, disappear and reappear. Hopefully, during these difficult times, we can call on help from our partners, and can both find support from close friends or an infertility support group.*

Both Jane and Ann had very similar experiences and feelings, and derived much support from each other when they discovered that they were not alone; we hope that by documenting their experiences, other women will be more able to talk about their feelings and thus derive support from each other:

Jane: *Just decided we'd like kids and thought we ought to go ahead straight away, as I was 28. As the months went by, the worry and tension mounted. I was worried anyway as I'd always taken lots of risks and nothing had ever happened, and I'd had gonorrhoea and knew this could cause infertility. The doctor wouldn't help as I wasn't married and he said my fellow would leave me, and if I had a boy it would grow up homosexual! The FPA told me I'd got to try for at least 2 years before they'd begin investigating although I was worried about my age. I kept getting ill with other things, and eventually*

---

* The National Association for the Childless and Childfree sees as one of its main functions the support of people going through tests and treatment for infertility, and of these where treatment is unsuccessful. For their address, see p. 510.

saw a partner of my doctor who was sympathetic and could see the worry was affecting my health and who referred me to the infertility clinic.

The tests were terrible and long drawn out — well over a year. Never once were the emotional problems referred to. Each new test was a major trauma.

Ann: *My tests went on for the best part of 2 years. Somewhere I've read 2 months should be possible. My overwhelming feeling was hoping something would be found — I couldn't even be treated if there was nothing wrong.*

For both Jane and Ann, sex became very difficult.

Ann: *This was one of the worst aspects, so dominated by the idea of reproduction it ceased to be an expression of anything for each other and became much more mechanical.*

Jane: *Quarrels assume enormous proportions when they mean you don't make love on the crucial day, or terrible bitterness is caused when your partner just doesn't feel like it on the crucial day.*

Ann: *The other side of it is quite as bad — if you don't feel sexy on the 'right' day — it becomes dominant enough to turn you off anyway. That causes huge problems with any other relationships too. I didn't know which came first: the totally unexpected feeling of jealousy or the idea that someone other than I might conceive by my husband. It totally squashed any ideas or practice we'd had of not being exclusive — I couldn't face using contraceptives (emotionally) at that time and couldn't do to him what I couldn't face and get pregnant by someone else. And the aftermath — it must have been nearly 2 years after the last tests before I felt really relaxed and spontaneous about sex again, which used to be good before it had to be functional.*

Jane: *All this time I'm feeling that nature has passed judgement on me that I'm not fit to be a mother. You start asking — Do I really want children anyway? You forget, because it has by now become a need to find out, to prove that you're not infertile. I never managed to work that one out — I didn't really want (deserve) children anyway because I'd be a hopeless mother. I didn't like babies and didn't know how to get on with children. I'd never had any contact with babies, nor much with children, so I couldn't say about myself — I just love kids and get on well with them. The trouble was, I couldn't remember what I'd been like with kids before I started trying to get pregnant, but after I'd started, I always imagined everyone was watching me and thinking how hopeless I was with kids and why the hell did I want any, and probably, how lucky it was I couldn't produce 'cos I'd be so hopeless with them. All this was my own fears, both in me and projected onto other people. So I had to bury all these fears just to undergo the tests: just to have the tests, pregnancy has to be a really dominant, obsessive desire.*

If you realize that you may not be able to give birth to children, you will probably feel great grief. To deny or repress this feeling of grief can prolong its resolution. You have the choice of living it as consciously and directly as you can or suppressing these very natural but painful emotions. Sometimes the pain of infertility is never completely resolved but is accepted as a familiar ache which may recur, unpredictably, throughout life.

But if we are infertile, we can still become parents — either by artificial insemination (see above) or by adoption.

Adoption

After we had stopped trying to have a baby, I baulked at the idea of adopting a child — bearing one, having the mixture of us had seemed important as well as living and changing with a child. I felt I had to really believe I would never produce children before I could even consider adopting because if I had the slightest 'perhaps' in my head, I couldn't know I would totally accept an adopted child. That took a long time. But it gradually became clear that living through growing up with a child was far more important to me than producing one.

Organizations such as *Parent to Parent Information on Adoption* in London and the *Guild of Service* in Edinburgh have originated the idea of holding group discussions for prospective adopters. It can be very helpful to talk over thoughts and feelings in an atmosphere free from the pressures of an interview with an adoption agency. We may decide, after much thought, that adoption would not be the best thing. We may feel like this because at present, adoption agencies tend to consider you only if you're 'perfect'. This puts an enormous burden on prospective adoptive parents.

I'd want 'our own' child because I feel that I can't really see myself as a mother as I am now and I see pregnancy as a process of transformation which would make me into a mother. Me, as I am now, couldn't possibly cope with a baby. To take on the commitment of bringing up 'someone else's' kid, you'd have to be really confident that you were being fair imposing yourself as a mother on the poor little thing.

If you do decide to adopt, the process *can* be long, difficult and painful, so be prepared.

The adoption process involved endless interviews and personal questions. Since there are so few babies available (the reasons for that are all good), adoption societies don't know how to choose. They make choices on narrower and narrower grounds, so your chances of adopting are very slim if your life hasn't been, at least to all external appearances, utterly conformist. We were lucky, having contacts abroad, and adopted a child born in India, because it became clear that we were unlikely to be accepted by our local adoption society.

If you wish to adopt a child, you will need to approach either your local authority (in which case, write to the Director of Social Services) or a registered voluntary adoption agency. It is now illegal to adopt through any other third party, unless you are a relative of the child or you are 'acting in pursuance of an order of the High Court' (Children Act, section 28). Although attitudes amongst agencies – particularly local authorities – are *beginning* to change, this means that unless you are extremely conformist in every aspect of your life, adopting a child may be very difficult. In theory, anyone can adopt a child provided they don't have a serious criminal record. But in practice, adoption agencies make their own rules. Thus, although in theory single people can adopt, most agencies will only place a child with a married couple. Many of these agencies set an upper age limit (which might be 40 or even 35), or stipulate that you must have been married for a certain period of time, or that you must not have been divorced. If the wife of a married couple is working, the couple may be refused a child on the grounds that children need a mother's full-time care. An agency may inform you euphemistically that 'we do not have a suitable baby at the moment' which can be their way of telling you that they will never have a suitable baby. Make sure they give you a straight answer. You may have to try a large number of agencies – and be prepared for detailed questioning about every aspect of your life. Local authorities tend to be more flexible than many other agencies. What happens may well depend on the individual social worker in charge of your case. Social workers have a lot of power. It is crucial that attitudes to adoption change, otherwise people considered in any way deviants, whether feminists, unemployed, lesbians, communards or plain cohabitees, will be unable to adopt.

(For more details about how to adopt and what is involved, see Bibliography, p. 510.)

Miscarriage (Natural Abortion)

It is a surprising statistic that in women who know they are pregnant, about 1 in 6 pregnancies ends in miscarriage. About 75% of these miscarriages occur in the first trimester of pregnancy (weeks 1 to 14). These are usually the result of a failure of the fertilized egg to undergo its first important chromosomal divisions correctly. The germ plasm dies, and in the 2nd or 3rd month your body expels this matter. Miscarriages occurring after this period are more often due to the inability of the growing foetus to maintain its placental attachment, either because of some mechanical or hormonal problem, or because a weak (incompetent) cervix dilates too early, expelling the foetus. (Any foetus delivered after the 28th week is called a premature delivery and not a miscarriage. Such a baby has a statistical chance of surviving which improves for every week in the uterus after this point.)

Miscarriage is both a physical event for a woman and a serious emotional crisis which may be shared by a partner or experienced by each of you in very different ways. Miscarriages come at a joyful time of beginning pregnancy, and thus are all the more of a shock.

Early miscarriage can feel no worse physically than a very heavy menstrual period. With late first-trimester miscarriages there can be bleeding and cramping lasting for a few days, sometimes starting and stopping irregularly, until the contents are completely expelled. If you bleed a lot, that does not necessarily mean that a miscarriage is inevitable; pain is a more reliable indication. Afterwards there is a period of bleeding until the uterine lining heals. Second trimester miscarriages are like a mini-labour, with regular strong uterine contractions.

Miscarriages are characterized by stages, each of which has an official name.

Threatened abortion. You might have bleeding or spotting, which may or may not be accompanied by minor cramps. Your cervix is closed. The process may stop by itself, or it may continue. Some doctors recommend bedrest and hormone treatment, but they are unlikely to be of any real value. Your doctor will usually advise you to stay in bed for 24 hours, to see what happens.

Inevitable abortions. The process has gone so far that miscarriage cannot be prevented. Bleeding becomes profuse; is usually brighter red as the placenta begins its separation from the uterine wall; and cramps are more intense. The foetus, amniotic sac and placenta, along with a lot of blood, may be expelled completely intact. You'll probably know when this is happening. It's very important to say here that if you are not in a hospital you must do the difficult task of collecting foetus and afterbirth, putting it in a clean container, and taking it to hospital for the laboratory to examine. This will yield important information as to why you miscarried. If tests show you have lost a 'blighted pregnancy' (where egg and sperm together have failed to divide correctly) then this has been a random event and your chances of its happening again are as random as before. If tests show genetic abnormalities or that you had an illness or infection, you can work together with your doctor on how to proceed. If the foetal tissue is normal, you might learn that your hormone levels were insufficient, or that a weak cervix was at fault. Both these conditions can be treated.

An *incomplete abortion* means that only part of the 'products of conception' has been passed. Usually a doctor will do a D&C to clean your uterus so it will heal. A *complete abortion* means that everything in your uterus has been expelled. You will continue to bleed, but less and less. If you think you are bleeding for too long, ask your doctor. (Perhaps a D&C will be necessary after all.)

Another kind of abortion is a *missed abortion*, when a foetus dies in the uterus but is not expelled. It can remain within for several months. Signs are no periods, cessation of signs of pregnancy, and sometimes occasional spotting. Treatment is either a D&C or induction of labour.

After you miscarry, you can usually resume sexual relations in 4 to 6 weeks, or after your cervix has closed (to prevent infection). You can attempt another pregnancy after one or two normal menstrual cycles. Check with your doctor.

After a miscarriage you will have to deal with your feelings.

We went home from the hospital dazed and tired. I was weak and enormously sad. I don't know that I've ever experienced such deep emotional pain. The loss was so great and so complete in the way that only death is. For the first few days I couldn't talk to anyone, but at the same time it was painful to be alone. I just would cry and cry without stopping. One of the clearest reminders that I was no longer pregnant were all the speedy changes my body went through. Within two days my breasts, which had grown quite swollen, were back to their normal size. My stomach, which had grown hard, was now soft again. My body was no longer preparing for the birth of a child. It was simple and blatant. Tiredness was replaced with weakness. And then there was the bleeding. My body would not let me forget. I knew things would improve once we could make love again and would be even better when we were full of hope. But it seemed so far away.

Almost always you will feel grief and anger. You will need the support of friends.

Most people didn't know how to give me support and perhaps I didn't really know how to ask for it. People were more comfortable talking about the physical and not the emotional side of miscarriage. I needed to talk about both. It was also difficult for my husband, because people could at least ask how my body was doing. Unfortunately he would sometimes be completely bypassed when someone called to talk with us, despite the fact that he too was in deep emotional pain.

Feelings of grief are often complicated by guilt, which can cause tension between you and your partner.

My husband said it was so hard to be supportive because he had such strong feelings: Anger: 'God damn that woman! How could she have done that!' And misery — he wanted to crawl into a corner — and self-doubts: 'Can I have any children at all?' Maybe if we could have talked about it during the days I was beginning to miscarry, we could be less tense now.

You might wonder if either of you did something 'wrong' (too much activity, too much sex, not enough good food, etc.). Such factors rarely cause miscarriage. Dispelling the tension will take a while, and longer for some than for others. It is best if your feelings are acknowledged and talked out.

Another common feeling is fear: you have lost control over your body. It could happen again.

One miscarriage does not mean you are infertile. However, if you have two or more in a row you might want to begin investigating. Try to learn why you had a miscarriage. Some of the diagnostic procedures described above for infertility will be useful here. Ask to see the pathology report, and ask that all terminology be explained fully. If you are not satisfied with the explanation, ask if there are other tests that could be done.

Arrange with your doctor to plan each detail of your next pregnancy as it progresses, including possible reasons for any spotting or cramps, definite ways to deal with contingencies, tests to be made as they become necessary, and so forth. You will need support in this project from your partner, possibly friends, or a support group. One woman, Chris Pope, wrote about her miscarriage as a means of communicating to herself and to other women. She ends her article (see Bibliography) by asking people to write to her if she can help.

The rate of miscarriage for couples who have had difficulty conceiving is much higher than for other couples. It's probably that the reasons involved in your infertility are also the ones which cause a 'high risk' pregnancy. Again, working with a competent and careful specialist will be essential for both woman and man, as hopes run high. Precautions must be taken step by step, with a great deal of consideration for the fragile feelings involved. To go from the despair of endless cycles without conception to the absolute joy of having finally conceived only to come crashing down to the reality of a miscarriage is emotionally devastating.

Feelings when the Baby Dies

Your body knows nothing about the baby's death, whether the death occurred at birth or a few days afterwards. Your breasts are filled with milk, never to be used. If the baby's death takes place before delivery, anaesthesia and delivery in the quickest and least hazardous way are desirable. Your partner should be included as long as he feels he can be supportive. The baby, once delivered, should be handled in a reverent and careful manner. If you can touch or hold the baby, this can help you, by having *someone* tangible to remember. You should be put in a room away from the nursery and hospital personnel should be told that you have lost your baby. Above all, you and your family must be allowed your grief, in privacy if you need and want it.

You might need to withdraw at first and not confront the reality which may be too much to bear. There might be a period of numbness. If you ask for help in grieving, we hope it will be intelligently and humanely extended. Platitudes such as, 'You'll have another baby before you know it,' or, 'Think of your wonderful children at home,' have no place in grief. The death of this particular child is being experienced – no other actual or potential children have any relevance to the situation. Perhaps the best help others can offer is sympathetic listening and close physical comforting.

Unfortunately, hospital staff are rarely trained to deal with death, especially the death of a baby. They may be so unable to deal with their own feelings about death that they cannot begin to help us in this situation. This is why drugs and sedatives are so often prescribed routinely in these circumstances. This practice can actively interfere with the healthy resolution of grief. Hopefully things are beginning to change. In response to an article in *The Times*, some women wrote of the very positive help they had received after stillbirth:

Some mothers described the help they were given by being asked by staff for the baby's name, some were comforted by being asked if they wanted the baby to be christened. Most striking was the help these bereaved mothers had received from other mothers who had experienced the same loss. (The Times, *3 December 1975)*

There are other changes that we must press for. Although free dental treatment is available to women who have had a baby within the previous year, free prescriptions are only available if you have a child under 1 year. This anomaly means that women who have given birth to a dead child are discriminated against at a time when they could well do without such harsh thinking. Whether or not you have given birth to a live baby, you should still receive postnatal care.

It is important to understand if possible why the baby died. Most likely whatever happened was totally beyond anyone's control, but if you suspect negligence, you should seek legal advice quickly so that the facts can be analysed. The Patients' Association could probably help you with this (see p. 571).

It can take a long time to get over the death of a child. Feelings of guilt or shame are not uncommon. Be prepared for this and if possible, make contact with people who will understand the problems you are facing. Compassionate Friends (see Bibliography, p. 511) is a national network of people who have lost a child. It is a non-religious society. By contacting them we can give and/or receive much-needed help. The Society acts as a 24-hour service for bereaved parents, however long ago the death occurred, as well as a pressure group to urge research into children's diseases.

Nobody wants to deal with death, especially when your friends are at the childbearing age themselves and can't help being afraid of you for what you stand for. I found that my friends wanted me to pretend nothing had happened. I don't think it was just my particular friends — it's natural to want to avoid those things. And so my fantastic pregnancy, in which a lot of things went on in my head and body that helped me to change and get myself together, had to be buried. Even now, after a year, I can see their pain and fear for me as I start into my eighth month of pregnancy with my second child. I have to be the one who keeps them calm, and I especially must assure everyone that this one will be okay.

Abnormal Babies

Approximately 1% of babies born suffer from severe problems such as mongolism, spasticity, blindness, deafness, absence of limbs or congenital disorders of the heart and intestine. In one out of every 250 babies born, the abnormalities are so severe that the baby cannot live. When we are pregnant it is important that we recognize the possibility of our baby being abnormal. As with miscarriage and death, this is usually a taboo subject even though most of us experience worrying dreams or fantasies about such possibilities while we are pregnant. If talking about such fears during our antenatal classes were a common practice, it would then be much easier for us to call on our teachers, advisers and friends if and when an abnormal birth becomes a reality.

It can take a long time to get over the shock of having produced a handicapped child. Many parents, particularly mothers, have feelings of great distress:

I can't help feeling guilty that I have failed being a mother having a handicapped child. (Something Wrong, see Bibliography.)

The strain can be exacerbated by other peoples' attitudes.

We have listed in the Bibliography resources which can be called upon in the event of a baby being born handicapped. Unfortunately, we live in a society where handicapped children and their parents often do not receive the kind of help — both emotional, material and practical — which is necessary. All too often the burden of a handicapped child falls for the most part on the mother. We hope that increasingly more resources will become available for those looking after handicapped children and adults. It is unlikely that this will happen without the concerted efforts of parents and of women in general.

EARLY DIAGNOSIS

Certain disorders such as Down's Syndrome ('mongolism'), muscular dystrophy, severe spina bifida and other neural tube defects can be diagnosed early in pregnancy. Diagnoses can be made (a) by a simple blood test at 16–18 weeks, followed by (b) studying the amniotic fluid (the water surrounding the foetus), where amniotic fluid is withdrawn from the uterus by a procedure called amniocentesis, and (c) by ultrasound.

Amniocentesis is safer – and more reliable – if done not before the 16th week of pregnancy. The results can take 3–4 weeks to come through, so it is best performed as soon as possible after that time. Amniocentesis is thought very rarely to trigger a miscarriage; if properly trained staff and adequate equipment are used together with ultrasound (see below) to guide the operator, this risk is minimized. The test is about 99% reliable. The few recorded errors have been human ones.

Ultrasound involves bouncing very high frequency sound waves off the mother's abdomen. Its uses include the detection of anencephaly, hydrocephaly, some cases of spina bifida and certain limb deformities, as well as the position of the baby or of the placenta and the number of babies in the uterus. Ultrasound appears to be less potentially dangerous than X-rays but it is still inadvisable at this stage of knowledge for women to have ultrasound routinely. After all, it took some 40 years before it was realized that X-rays could damage the foetus. Amniocentesis and ultrasound are still, relatively speaking, in their infancy. (For more about ultrasound and X-rays, see 'Pregnancy', p. 361).

When might you want to have these tests?
1. If you have already had a child with an abnormality.
2. If you are a carrier of serious disorders that affect males only.
3. If you are over 35, particularly if you are over 40 since the risk of having a child with an abnormality increases as you get older.

Parents who are carriers of certain hereditary diseases can be diagnosed before the woman becomes pregnant by studying a blood or skin sample.

If you find that there might be a chance of your foetus having birth defects, it should be your decision, with the advice of your doctor, whether or not you will continue your pregnancy.

Ectopic (Misplaced) Pregnancy

Whether we intend to get pregnant or not, it is always possible to develop an ectopic pregnancy. Such a pregnancy is dangerous. We should be aware of this possibility even if we are using contraceptives such as the cap, sheath, IUD or progestogen-only Pill (see Chapter 9, 'Birth Control').

Fertilization of the egg by the sperm almost always occurs in the fallopian tube. If the function of the tube is impaired in any way, for example by pelvic inflammatory disease, then it's possible that the fertilized egg might attach itself to part of the tube instead of proceeding on into the uterus. This results in an ectopic pregnancy; more rarely an ectopic pregnancy can begin to grow in the abdominal cavity, the ovary or the cervix. Early symptoms of an ectopic pregnancy can be a missed period, breast tenderness, nausea and fatigue. The uterus may also be slightly enlarged and softened. A doctor may diagnose a normal pregnancy after examining you internally and listening to your symptoms. It's difficult to discover an unruptured early tubal pregnancy.

As the pregnancy enlarges, the tube will stretch slightly. Eventually it bursts. This usually happens between the 10th to 14th week. Just before it bursts you may feel acute (sharp) stabbing pain at the site of implantation, or cramps, or a constant, dull abdominal pain, which is temporarily relieved by the rupture. But then you'll bleed inside and soon feel lower abdominal pain again. Or later you might feel aching pain in your diaphragm and sharp shoulder pain caused by blood flowing up to your diaphragm. Your breathing may be painful too. If the bleeding is greater, you might be in shock, with low blood pressure and a high pulse rate. Symptoms of shock are hot and cold flushes, nausea, dizziness, fainting. If you experience any of the symptoms of ectopic pregnancy, see your doctor. If it is at all possible that you could be pregnant, your doctor should investigate your symptoms.

Sometimes, before or after the rupture, you might have a late period with mild, menstrual-type bleeding or fragments from your uterine lining. This bleeding can be misleading, as you and your doctor might think you have had an early 'natural' abortion. If the lining of the uterus is passed, it should be examined microscopically, and if there's no evidence of trophoblastic (early foetal) tissue, ectopic pregnancy should be suspected.

A pelvic examination might show no findings at all or a number of findings: tenderness or mass in the fallopian tubes or ovaries; enlargement of the uterus; softening of the cervix; fullness behind the uterus. Blood tests might be useful. Your doctor might do a culdocentesis, inserting a needle vaginally into the space behind the uterus (pouch of Douglas). If non-clotting blood is found, ruptured ectopic pregnancy is a possibility, because the intraperitoneal blood doesn't readily clot. The doctor might recommend operative diagnostic procedures such as culdoscopy or laparoscopy.

The treatment for tubal pregnancy is usually a salpingectomy, in which the entire tube is removed. This must be done under anaesthesia. There's disagreement over whether the ovary on that side should be removed too.

It's likely that if a woman has had one tubal pregnancy due to infection, she'll conceive less readily than if she hadn't had it. (There's a 50 to 60% chance of not conceiving.) Chances of another tubal pregnancy are increased. If there was no infection and the other tube is healthy, future conception will not be much affected.

Rh Factor in Blood

The Rh factor is a substance in the blood. At least 86% of us have this substance coating our red blood cells: we are called Rh positive (Rh +). Those of us who don't have it are Rh negative (Rh −).

If someone with Rh − blood receives transfusions of blood containing Rh +, the Rh − blood gradually builds up antibodies, which defend the blood from the hostile Rh + factor, causing some red cells to be broken down, and their products spread through the body, thus exerting a poisonous effect. Some Rh − women don't produce antibodies.

When you are pregnant there's a certain amount of blood transference between you and your foetus through the placenta. Most of the exchange goes from the mother to the foetus. At birth, however, because of the separation of the placenta from the uterus, there can be a much larger spillover, and a quantity of the baby's blood can be absorbed by the mother. This does not occur often. At birth you can absorb your baby's Rh + blood, and within the next 72 hours your own blood reacts and begins developing antibodies if you are Rh −. These antibodies will be present in your blood during your next pregnancy, and can get into the blood stream of your second child as it grows, attacking and destroying some red cells. The baby could be stillborn, severely anaemic, or retarded.

Thus every woman should have her Rh factor checked early in pregnancy. If you are Rh − :
1. You should know whether you have had previous blood transfusions. Even matched blood types contain Rh − and Rh + factors, so that it's possible (though hopefully rare now that people are aware of the Rh factor) for a woman with Rh − blood type B to have received Rh + blood type B, and thus to have already developed antibodies.
2. You should have your own blood tested for Rh sensitization (the presence of antibodies).
3. A foetal amniotic fluid sample can be taken through a needle to see whether the blood cells of the foetus are being altered. This test can be done at any time in the pregnancy. If the bilirubin level in the fluid is high, it indicates that the foetus is affected, and a blood transfusion may be given to the baby in utero.
4. An injection of *Rhogam* or *Anti 'D'*, which prevents you from producing antibodies must be given within 72 hours after a miscarriage from the 2nd month on, and after every abortion or any pregnancy in which the baby's blood group is not Rh −.

What can be done if the blood of the foetus is being invaded by maternal antibodies? There are techniques now for exchanging invaded foetal blood for good blood while the foetus is still in the uterus, and for exchanging the baby's blood after it is born. Try to check up on the benefits and risks of these techniques.

Sickle-Cell Trait and Sickle-Cell Anaemia

These problems only affect black people, or those of Mediterranean descent. Sickle-cell trait means that less than half of the haemoglobin (oxygen-carrying red protein of red blood cells) in the blood has undergone a change in the composition of its protein. This change came about thousands of years ago in people who lived in Africa and in countries around the Mediterranean, and helped protect them from malaria. It's a genetic trait, meaning that it is inherited from parents. If you have sickle-cell trait, you will be healthy and probably unaware that you have it. Only under very unusual conditions, like mountain climbing at extreme heights, might you have a problem.

Sickle-cell anaemia is a disorder resulting from inheritance of the trait for sickle-cell haemoglobin from *both* parents. About 1 in 625 black people is born with sickle-cell anaemia. Symptoms are poor physical development, jaundice, weakness, abdominal pains, lowered resistance to infections, bouts of swelling and pain in muscles and joints. Red blood cells, shaped like a farmer's sickle, don't live as long as normal cells and are destroyed at a faster rate, so movement of oxygen is at a minimum. The clinical picture is variable. Some people who have severe anaemia during childhood may find the symptoms becoming milder as they grow older. For others the anaemia is tiring at times, but tolerable. It can also be extremely painful.

If you are black or if you are of Mediterranean descent, it is wise for you and possibly your partner to be tested for sickle-cell trait. The blood test is simple and you can have the results in 30 minutes. The results should be kept absolutely confidential. If you and your partner both have the trait, you may wish to ask for genetic counselling as you decide about having children, for there is a risk of your children developing the trait and, more rarely, anaemia. If you have the anaemia, the exact form should be identified as some are not as serious as others. You should be told about the problems and risks of going through a pregnancy: some of your symptoms may be intensified by pregnancy (circulatory problems might become worse, you might be more tired or depressed than usual, and more prone to miscarriage).

Bibliography and Resources

INFERTILITY

Anon, 'Artificial Insemination (Donor)', *British Medical Journal*, 4 October 1975.

Anon, 'Fertile Foils', *Guardian*, 5 March 1975. Emotional aspects of infertility and dearth of help available.

Bolton Women's Guide (available from Rising Free Bookshop) has detailed section on infertility, of general interest but with particular reference to that area.

Consumers' Association, *Infertility*, 1972. Informative.

Elstein, Max, 'Effect of Infertility on Psychosexual Function', *British Medical Journal*, 2 August 1975. Considers emotional and sexual aspects as important.

Kelso, Isa Anderson, *Women's Ailments*. Self Help series published by Thorsons.

McGarry, John, 'Artificial Insemination', *Nursing Mirror*, 29 July 1976.

March, Rosemary, 'Barren Pains', *Guardian*, 19 February 1975. Emotional aspects of infertility and dearth of help available.

Newill, Robert, *Infertile Marriage*, Penguin, 1974. Detailed discussion of infertility, diagnosis and treatment.

Sandler, Bernard, 'Infertility, an Analysis of Investigations Used in British Hospitals', *World Medicine*, 2 July 1975.

Your local women and health group – if in doubt contact WIRES, p. 570.

National Association for the Childless and Childfree, 318 Summer Lane, Birmingham: can give support, information and help. Also conscious of the insensitivity of many people who have children and who make childless people feel inadequate.

ADOPTION

Association of British Adoption Agencies, *Adopting a Child* (30p incl. postage).

Consumers' Association, *How to Adopt*. Informative discussion of the problems involved – both practical and emotional.

Seglow, J. *et al.*, *Growing up Adopted*, National Foundation for Educational Research, 1972.

Association of British Adoption Agencies, 4 Southampton Row, London WC1B 4AA. Represents both voluntary agencies and local authorities that act as agencies. Gives advice to adopters, adopted and those wishing to place children for adoption. It is not an agency but will provide a list of agencies.

Parent to Parent Information on Adoption Society, 26 Belsize Grove, London NW3 (01 722 9996). Mutual support group formed originally by a group of parents who had adopted children considered 'hard to place'. Provides information and opportunities for group discussion.

Adoption Advice Service, free and anonymous phone-in service for anyone adopted or with adopted children. Existing phone numbers:
South-east, Tuesdays, 1 p.m. to 4.30 p.m.: Woking 69229; Thursdays, 1 p.m. to 4.30 p.m.: Tunbridge Wells 33777.

Bristol, Fridays, 12.30 p.m. to 4.30 p.m.: Bristol 776715.
Mondays, 12.30 p.m. to 4.30 p.m.: Bristol 623306.
Yorkshire, Wednesdays, 1 p.m. to 5 p.m.: Horsforth 582115.
Adoption Resource Exchange, 40 Brunswick Square, London WC1N 1AZ. Links
up would-be adopters and children who are hard to place, for example because
of racial background, handicap or age.

MISCARRIAGE

Pope, Chris, 'Miscarriage', *Peace News* (8 Elm Avenue, Nottingham), 20 February
1976.
'Management of Threatened Abortion', *British Medical Journal*, 1 May 1976.

IF THE BABY DIES

Jolly, Hugh, 'The Heartache in Facing the Facts of a Stillborn Baby', *The Times*,
3 December 1975.
Kannel, John H., *et al.*, 'The Mourning Response of Parents to the Death of a
Newborn Infant', *New England Journal of Medicine*, 13 August 1970, Vol. 283,
pp. 344–9.
Lewis, Emanuel, 'The Management of Stillbirth: Coping with an Unreality', *Lancet*,
18 September 1976: a very sympathetic account of how people — both parents
and medical attendants — can best cope.
Mooney, Bel, *Guardian*, 8 January 1976: personal account which resulted in much
correspondence (16 and 23 January 1976).

The Compassionate Friends, Mrs Joan Wills, 50 Woodwaye, Watford, Herts
(Watford 24279).
Foundation for Sudden Infant Death, 23 St Peter's Square, London W6.
British Guild for Sudden Infant Death Study, 28 Ty Gwyn Crescent, Penylan,
Cardiff (Cardiff 35252) — also offers sympathy and information to newly
bereaved parents.

ABNORMALITIES

Adams, R. C., *et al.*, *Games, Sports and Exercises for the Physically Handicapped*,
Lea & Febiger 1975.
Brock, Margaret, *Christopher, a Silent Life*, Macmillan, 1975: one woman's tale
about the difficulties she encountered with the 'helping' authorities following
the birth of her deaf and partially-sighted baby.
Carlson and Ginglend, *Play Activities for the Retarded Child*, Bailliere Tindall, 1962.
Claiborne Park, Clara, *The Siege*, Penguin, 1972: a mother's account of an
autistic child.
Clarke, A. M. and A. D. B., *Practical Help for Parents of Retarded Children: some
questions and answers*, Hull Society for Mentally Handicapped Children.
Comley, J., *Behaviour Modification and the Retarded Child*, Heinemann, 1975: gives
numerous case studies.
Copeland, James, *For the Love of Anne*, Arrow, 1976: account of an autistic daughter.
Ewing, A. and C., *Teaching Deaf Children to Talk*, Manchester University Press, 1964.

512 *Our Bodies Ourselves*

Forbes, G., *Clothing for the Handicapped Child*, Disabled Living Foundation, 1972.

Freeman, P., *Understanding the Deaf/Blind Child*, Heinemann, 1975.

Hannam, Charles, *Parents and Mentally Handicapped Children*, Penguin, 1974: contains interviews around the main problem areas.

HMSO, *Services for the Disabled.*

Hunt, Nigel, *The World of Nigel Hunt*, Darwen Finlayson, 1967: a mongol boy writes about his own life.

Lagos, J., *Help for the Epileptic Child: A Handbook for Parents, Nurses and Teachers*, Macdonald & Janes, 1974.

Massie, R. and S., *Journey*, Gollancz, 1975: parents' story of life with a haemophiliac child.

Miller, M., 'Disinherited Marriage', *Midwife, Health Visitor and Community Nurse*, January 1976: about the strain of the birth of a handicapped child.

Murray, J. B. and E., *And Say What He Is: The Life of a Special Child*, M.I.T. Press, 1975: parents' account of raising their son, born with a defective nervous system. Demonstrates the problems raised when there is no clear diagnosis and prognosis.

Nicholson, J., *Autism: A Success Story*, New Society, 18 March 1976.

Pilling, D., *Child with Cerebral Palsy: social, emotional and educational adjustment*: an annotated bibliography — available from National Foundation for Educational Research.

Sheridan, M. O., *Handicapped Child and His Home*, National Children's Home, 1973.

Smith, W. W., *Judith: Teaching our Mongol Baby*, National Society for Mentally Handicapped Children, 1973, 15p.: written to give some hope to parents of new-born mongol babies and illustrates how such children can develop with careful teaching.

Solly, Kenneth, *The Different Baby*, National Society for Mentally Handicapped Children, 1972: introductory pamphlet with advice.

Something Wrong, by parents of mentally handicapped children, Arrow Books: description of problems and critique of current methods of treatment.

Stevens, Mildred, *The Educational Needs of Severely Subnormal Children*, Williams & Wilkins, 1971: a standard work; very practical.

Stevens, Mildred, 'Music and the Mentally Handicapped Child' in *Educating Mentally Handicapped Children* (ed. Alice F. Laing), Faculty of Education, University College of Swansea: guide for the non-specialist.

Stone and Taylor, *Handbook for Parents with a Handicapped Child*, Arrow, 1977: wide-ranging and practical.

Tuckwell, P., 'Ending the Isolation of Mongol Children', *New Society*, 8 April 1976. In America, mongol children can attend normal schools; in Britain they are segregated.

West, Paul, *Words to a Deaf Daughter*, Penguin, 1972.

Whetnall, E., *The Deaf Child*, Heinemann 1971.

Wilks, John and Eileen, *Bernard — Bringing up Our Mongol Son*, Routledge & Kegan Paul, 1974.

Wing, L., *Autistic Children: a Guide for Parents*, Constable, 1971.

Wing, Lorna, *Children Apart — Autistic children and their families* (MIND pamphlet).

The Association for Children with Heart Disorders, c/o John Whitehead, 536 Colne Road, Reedley, Nr Burnley, Lancs. (Burnley 27500).

Association for the Help of Parents with Handicapped Children, 42 Rugby Road, Cubbington, Leamington (0926 22537).

Association for Spina Bifida and Hydrocephalus, Tavistock House North, Tavistock Square, London WC1 9HJ (01 388 1382–5): mutual support groups, information service, publication list, etc.

Association for the Treatment of Brain Damaged Children, 21 Rowington Close, Coventry CV6 1PR (Coventry 591837): non-profit-making centre where the child is put on a home treatment course based on the Doman/Delacato method, which can stimulate the brain cells.

Break, 20 Hookshill Road, Sheringham, Norfolk (Sheringham 823170): runs holidays for unaccompanied handicapped children.

British Epilepsy Association, 3–6 Alfred Place, London WC13 7ED (01 580 2704).

Campaign for the Mentally Handicapped, 96 Portland Place, London W1N 4EK (01 636 5020).

Cystic Fibrosis Research Trust, 5 Blyth Road, Bromley, Kent BR1 3RS (01 464 7211).

Disabled Living Foundation, 346 Kensington High Street, London W14 8NS (01 602 2491): runs information service and Aids Centre.

Down's Children's Association, c/o Chairman, Quinbourne Community Centre, Ridgacre Road, Birmingham B32 2TW (Harborne 1374): any parent of a child with Down's Syndrome can be a member of the association and obtain advice and a course in sensory and motor training.

The Family Fund, PO Box 50, York: a government fund administered by the Joseph Rowntree Memorial Trust to help families with severely handicapped children.

Handicapped Adventure Playground Association, 3 Oakley Gardens, London SW3 (01 352 2321).

In Touch, 10 Norman Road, Sale, Cheshire M33 3DP: puts people caring for mentally handicapped children or adults in touch with each other for mutual support; newsletter and literature available.

Institute for Research into Mental and Multiple Handicap, 16 Fitzroy Square, London W1P 5HQ (01 387 9571): very happy to help parents; has reading lists, etc.

Invalid Children's Aid Association, 126 Buckingham Palace Road, London SW1 9SB (01 730 9891): offers friendship and help (sometimes financial).

Lady Hoare Trust for Physically Disabled Children, 7 North Street, Midhurst, W. Sussex (073081 3696).

Leukaemia Society, 45 Craigmoor Avenue, Queens Park, Bournemouth (0202 37459).

Muscular Dystrophy Group of Great Britain, Nattrass House, 35 Macauley Road, London SW4 0QP (01 720 8055).

National Association for Deaf/Blind Rubella Handicapped, 164 Cromwell Lane, Coventry (Coventry 462579).

National Association for the Welfare of Children in Hospital, Exton House, 7 Exton Street, London SE1 8VE (01 261 1783).

National Deaf Children's Society, 31 Gloucester Place, London W1H 4EA (01 486 3251).

National Elfrida Rathbone Society, 83 Mosley Street, Manchester M2 30G (061 236 5358): concerned with provision of social facilities for educationally handicapped children and their families, pre-school playgroups, mothers' groups, etc.

National Society for Autistic Children, 1a Golders Green Road, London NW11 8EA (01 458 4375).

National Society for Mentally Handicapped Children, Pembridge Hall, Pembridge Square, London W2 4EP (01 229 8941 or 727 0536).

National Society for Phenylketonuria and Allied Disorders, 6 Rawdon Close, Palace Fields, Runcorn, Cheshire (Runcorn 65081).

Royal Association for Disability and Rehabilitation, 25 Mortimer Street, London W1N 8AB (01 637 5400): for general welfare of disabled and acts as information bureau about aids, etc. Publishes a journal and holiday guide.

Scottish Council for Spastics, 22 Corstorphine Road, Edinburgh EH12 6HP (031 337 9876)

Scottish Society for Mentally Handicapped Children, 69 West Regent Street, Glasgow C2.

Spastics Society, 12 Park Crescent, London W1N 4EQ (01 636 5020).

Toy Libraries Association, Seabrook House, Wyllyotts Manor, Darkes Lane, Potters Bar, Herts. (77 44571): central contact for toy libraries all over the country, lending toys and providing advice about learning through play for handicapped children.

Wingfield Trust, 24 Station Road, Epping (Epping 3229): helps physically handicapped children, particularly through music.

16 The Menopause

I felt generally good around the time of menopause. My children were supportive and patient, particularly when I was irritable from lack of sleep. My husband, unfortunately, was quite insensitive and frequently accused me of 'inventing' my 'afflictions'. Without the help of friends and children who did try to understand what I was going through, it might have been harder for me to be with him.

Even though menopause has been a neutral or positive experience for many women, the physical and emotional changes associated with it are often misunderstood and mystifying. Since lack of knowledge may easily lead to anxiety, it's not surprising that some women have felt that the worst part about menopause was that they did not know what to expect or had no resources to refer to.

This chapter will try to help women reduce the anxiety which results from a lack of knowledge. It also seeks to encourage women to research and study menopause, a subject which has been inexcusably neglected by the male-dominated medical profession.

Our youth-oriented culture tends to present menopause as a descent into 'uncool' middle and old age. In a society which equates our sexuality with our ability to have children, menopause is wrongly thought to mean the end of our sexuality — the end of our sexual pleasure, or even the total end of our sex lives.

As women start to value themselves as more than baby machines, as we increasingly view middle age as a welcome time offering new freedom and as we make selective use of various treatments to minimize any menopausal discomforts, the menopause can be a positive experience.

I am constantly amazed and delighted to discover new things about my body, something menstruation did not allow me to do. I have new responses, desires, sensations, freed and apart from the distraction of menses [periods].

I felt physically in better shape — in my prime — unencumbered by the cycle of pain, swelling, discomfort, nuisance, etc.

I was immensely relieved that my periods were ceasing. I hated them and resented their prolongation for so many years after childbearing had ceased. It was a damn nuisance.

I felt better and freer since menopause. I love being free of possible pregnancy and birth control. It makes my sex life better.

If we feel good about ourselves and what we are doing at this time in our lives, we will cope better with whatever menopause problems we may have. It is important to be able to talk openly with those who are close to us and to ask for the support we need.

What is the Menopause?

The menopause is the time when menstruation (see p. 26) permanently ceases. As a woman approaches menopause her ovaries stop producing a monthly ovum (egg) and stop secreting the cyclic supply of oestrogen. (Well past the menopause a much smaller amount of oestrogen continues to be produced in the body.) At the same time there is a decline in the production of the hormone progesterone.

These hormonal changes mean that we will no longer be able to conceive and that we may experience some uncomfortable physical symptoms as our bodies adjust to the often rapidly diminishing supply of hormones.

The gradual decrease in the cyclic release of oestrogen and progesterone usually begins some years before the end of menstruation. Most women are aware that menopause is coming closer when the menstrual periods become scantier, shorter and farther apart. Sometimes whole months are skipped. In some women the cycles become shorter and the flow more prolonged and profuse, in other women menstruation just stops. This period can be called the 'peri-menopausal period'. Sometimes, symptoms such as heavy bleeding can be very debilitating at this time, and can last for many years if untreated. Some doctors attempt to 'solve' the bleeding problem by performing a hysterectomy. There are other, less drastic forms of treatment (see p. 519).

It is not possible to predict when a woman will begin menopause. It usually happens between 48 and 52, though it can happen as early as 35 or as late as 56. It is not true that the younger a woman starts menstruation the earlier she will go through menopause.

An early menopause can occur when a woman's ovaries are removed (oophorectomy) or as a result of ovarian disease. A hysterectomy (see p. 183) should not bring on menopausal symptoms unless both ovaries are removed as well. The removal of one ovary does not bring on menopause, since the remaining ovary continues to produce sufficient oestrogen.

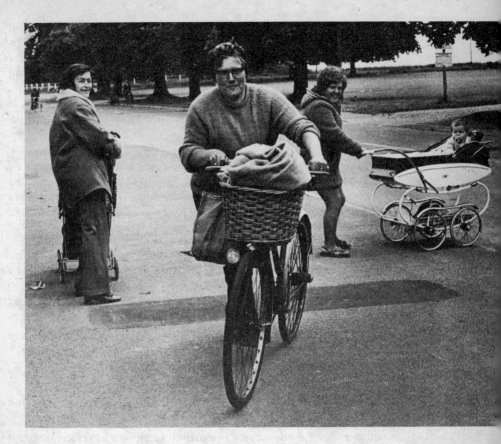

When the ovaries are removed in a younger woman who still has her uterus, HRT (see below) is usually administered afterwards to maintain menstrual periods, unless they were removed for malignancy.

Symptoms of the Menopause

The two symptoms generally accepted to be characteristic of the menopausal period are 'hot flushes' or sweats, and a decrease of moisture and elasticity in the vagina ('vaginal atrophy' is the medical term). A hot flush is a sudden sensation of heat in the upper body, sometimes accompanied by a patchy redness of skin. It usually lasts from several seconds to a minute and may involve some sweating. When it is over, a woman often feels chilly. Hot flushes may average four or five a day, most often occur at night, and may disturb sleep.

Women who have experienced them describe the hot flush as 'an all-over hot feeling with profuse perspiration'. They happen unpredictably and momentarily, 'as if I had a fleeting fever with perhaps a slight dampness on my forehead'. 'It is a feeling of heat and sweat flooding one's head without warning.'

Hot flushes are not fully understood. They may occur as a result of the body's attempt to achieve a new hormonal balance. When a woman's body has adjusted to the lower levels of oestrogen, hot flushes diminish and cease.

Even though I knew why I was having the sweats, it was a little frightening to wake up in the middle of the night with my sheets all drenched. It was hard not to feel that something was very wrong with me. And I lost a lot of sleep changing sheets and wondering how long the sweats would go on. Sometimes I felt chilled after sweating and had trouble going back to sleep. It was a good thing I could absorb myself in a book at times like that.

I also had hot flushes several times a week for almost six months. I didn't get as embarrassed as some of my friends who also had hot flushes, but I found the 'heat wave' sensation most uncomfortable.

Vaginal dryness and inelasticity results from the greatly reduced secretions of the vaginal walls. When this occurs, it is most often during the latter part of menopause (and more severe cases usually don't develop until 5 or 10 years after menstruation has ended).

The physical discomfort due to the dryness of the vagina was very sexually inhibiting. We were both concerned about the problem with intercourse. I am now using a cream to counteract the dryness. But for a long while ignorance plus poor gynaecological care were responsible for a lot of discomfort.

Often vaginal dryness can cause irritation and an increased susceptibility to vaginal infections. During intercourse, a substitute for the missing lubrication may be necessary to prevent uncomfortable friction. A water-soluble lubricant such as K Y Jelly works well. A woman who experiences painful intercourse should seek medical help, since problems other than vaginal dryness and inelasticity may be the cause (see p. 62 in Chapter 3).

So far, research has not proven that symptoms other than these two are clearly caused by menopausal changes. However, a small percentage of women do experience other troubling symptoms during menopause: palpitations, anxiety, dizziness and swollen ankles may be related in some as yet undefined way to the body's readjustment to a different level of oestrogen. Other symptoms, such as sleeplessness, less energy, headaches and fatigue, may be indirect results of distressing hot flushes.

There is not yet enough clear information about the effects of reduced oestrogen levels on our mental health. At least one study – by Mansel Aylward – appears to show that they can cause depression, but it is understandable that a night's sleep disrupted by hot flushes can result the following day in tiredness and irritability. If hot flushes occur during the day, a woman may feel anxious, or tense.

It can be embarrassing to have such an obvious and uncontrollable menopausal symptom, especially since the connotations of menopause in Western culture have been negative. As we women demystify menopause we may see that these negative connotations have been as harmful as the physical symptoms themselves.

Treatment

Since medical viewpoints differ, it is important for us to understand the present controversies as to what are and are not menopausal symptoms and how those symptoms should be treated. We do not need to accept automatically whatever our particular doctor may suggest. We should be especially wary of doctors who put every woman on medication and, equally, of those who tell us that our symptoms are 'only in the mind'.

About 1 out of every 5 women will have no (or just a few) menopausal symptoms. Although most women do experience some bothersome symptoms, many of these will not actually require treatment. We should seek help whenever symptoms significantly interfere with our normal activities, particularly because continuous and unrelieved physical distress may result in depression.

In the UK, it is still common for doctors to be less than helpful with menopausal symptoms:

My doctor told me anyone not able to cope with the menopause was just neurotic.

My doctor will only give me painkillers and Valium, and I still get the most awful headaches, flushes and night-sweats. Intercourse is now so painful my husband does not dare to come near me. (From Wendy Cooper, *If Only More Doctors Were Women*)

Women's Health Care, an agency concerned with providing information about HRT (see below), alone received 8,000 inquiries in 1975 from women who were unable to obtain either proper advice or treatment for their symptoms. We will discuss below the possible treatments for menopausal and peri-menopausal symptoms.

HORMONE REPLACEMENT THERAPY (HRT)

This involves taking oestrogen and/or progesterone (progesterone alone is more rare) in the form of pills, injections or implants.

Oestrogens

Oestrogen therapy is now in considerable vogue as a treatment for the menopause. Because of this, we are considering it in some detail. However, we must emphasize that, particularly because of recent evidence showing its association with a marked increase in the incidence of endometrial cancer (see 'Side Effects and Risks' below), we are not endorsing it as *the* answer to menopausal symptoms, nor as protection against old age. Some people believe that oestrogen replacement therapy should be every woman's right, that oestrogen given during and after the menopause will liberate us for ever. We strongly urge you to read the whole of this chapter, especially the section concerning the risks of oestrogen therapy and that relating to alternative treatments.

What Can Oestrogens Do?

Most cases of hot flushes and vaginal dryness – both of which can result from lowered levels of oestrogen in the body – are relieved by oestrogen therapy. For many cases of vaginal dryness it is sufficient to use an oestrogen cream (applied directly to the vagina) such as Dienoestrol, although it should be borne in mind that no long-term research has been done on the possible effects of oestrogen creams. These creams can also help incontinence (inability to control urination) related to dryness of vaginal and connective tissues.

Oestrogen is sometimes used to treat other symptoms thought to be related to oestrogen deficiency – such as insomnia, irritability, nervousness, depression, nausea and constipation. Though oestrogen may help these conditions, in some cases a placebo effect may be operating (i.e. a 'dummy pill' would be equally effective). In fact, placebos can be effective in relieving hot flushes as well.*

Oestrogen's effect on *osteoporosis* is controversial. Osteoporosis is a condition which affects the skeleton. Gradually, small amounts of bone mass are reabsorbed by the body. The bony mass which remains becomes fragile and susceptible to fracture. Since older women are much more prone to osteoporosis than older men, some doctors give oestrogen to women both as a prophylactic and as a cure for the problem, and they swear by its effectiveness. Others point out that as yet there is no evidence that oestrogen therapy prevents osteoporosis; they fear that the reduction in rate of bone loss brought about by oestrogen is temporary and may be followed by a more rapid progression of bone loss. No one has managed to show that oestrogen therapy decreases the incidence of bone fractures and spine curvatures. Some people believe that osteoporosis is much more related to the overall ageing process rather than to oestrogen

* See for example, Jean Coope, *British Medical Journal*, 18 October 1975.

deficiency alone, and that adequate calcium and protein intake along with exercise is best for both treatment and prevention.

Menopausal Depression and L-Tryptophan

Depression during the menopause may be linked to an insufficient oestrogen supply. Research by Dr Mansel Aylward in Merthyr Tydfil shows a link between menopausal depression and a fall in the body's free tryptophan supply at a time of hormonal imbalance, i.e. the menopause. Tryptophan is a type of protein which occurs naturally in the body and can be measured by blood test. In the menopausal state, women who are found to have an oestrogen deficiency may as a result demonstrate a low free plasma-tryptophan level because most of the plasma-tryptophan is bound to plasma albumin. Oestrogen replacement therapy can displace tryptophan from its bound state and thus enable it to reach and react upon the brain. Where there is an abnormally low tryptophan level, an additional amount can be taken orally. Thus with Dr Aylward, tryptophan treatment has been used as an extra refinement to HRT. Tryptophan treatment is new, but hopefully more doctors will have heard of it by the time you read this and will be assessing its effectiveness in clinical trials.

Side Effects and Risks

This is a very controversial area. Very little is known to date about the relative long-term risks and benefits of oestrogen therapy: it has not been in use for long enough. Some people believe that the risks (e.g. of blood clotting, heart disease, hypertension and cancer) are only associated with synthetic oestrogens. While it is true that most of the studies to date have been concerned with these oestrogens, no one has proved that 'natural' ones are in fact safer (see p. 524 below). Certainly both 'natural' and synthetic oestrogens have been implicated as involving potential risks. We list here the possible side effects and risks of oestrogen therapy that are known to date (January 1977). As more information is coming out all the time, some of this section might well be out of date by the time you read it.

Oestrogen therapy has a profound and widespread effect on the entire metabolism of the body. As with the Pill, taking oestrogen increases the risk of *blood clots, heart disease* and *hypertension*. The risks also increase with age (see p. 247 in Chapter 9 for important details). With respect to heart disease, while some studies suggest that HRT gives long-term protection against the disease (see Cooper, *No Change*), others indicate that it may contribute to an increase in triglyceride levels in the blood, which in turn are apparently related to an increased risk of heart disease.

Perhaps the most consistent worry has been the influence of oestrogen on *cancer*. A few studies suggest a dramatic decrease in the number of women on HRT with various forms of cancer (see Cooper). But they cannot be clearly interpreted, as important variables were not taken into account. Oestrogen therapy *does* appear to stimulate breast problems such as cystic mastitis, which may in itself increase the risk of a true malignancy. Furthermore, although more studies are necessary, recent research strongly suggests that oestrogen replacement therapy is associated with a marked increase in the incidence of *endometrial cancer* (see Bibliography). The risk appears to be particularly high the longer the oestrogen is taken and the higher the dose. (For women who have not had children, who are obese or diabetic, the risk of endometrial cancer is in any case greater than for women who are not in these categories.) When all the studies are taken together, they present a very persuasive argument against the use of oestrogen replacement therapy, so much so that the American Food and Drug Administration has amended its requirements for the labelling and advertising of these products to provide full warning about the endometrial cancer risk. As Mack *et al.* point out, a woman who has a uterus and who uses oestrogen replacement therapy has a risk of developing endometrial cancer that is approximately the same as for the *combined* risk from the more common cancers of the breast, cervix, lung and stomach. If the oestrogen is given together with progesterone, this stimulates the lining of the womb to shed every month; it is possible that this may ensure against too much oestrogenic stimulation of the endometrium, which may be what causes cancer to grow in some cases. (It is not known how many women, if any, in the US studies were given progesterone.) Some British specialists recommend a combined oestrogen-progesterone therapy for this reason. But the benefits of progesterone have not yet been proven, especially in its role of preventing uterine cancer. In particular, some pathologists believe that there are small immature areas of the uterine lining which do not respond to the progesterone and are not sloughed off periodically. Thus, these isolated areas would be constantly subjected to oestrogen stimulation and its possible harmful effects.

In a woman taking oestrogen, any abnormal bleeding is probably breakthrough bleeding (see p. 250). However, there is a small chance that endometrial cysts, polyps or uterine cancer could be the cause, so an endometrial biopsy, a D&C, or a suction procedure similar to menstrual extraction (see p. 28) should be performed in order to examine the endometrial tissue.

Some women on oestrogen experience gastrointestinal disturbances, fluid retention and weight gain, breast and pelvic discomfort due to tissue engorgement, headache, vaginal discharge and changes in skin pigmentation. The kinds of side effects vary with the different forms of oestrogen. Some people think that 'natural' oestrogens (see below) are the most easily tolerated, but there is as yet no clear evidence about this.

Should We Take Oestrogen Replacement Therapy?

There are at least three groups of women who should probably not take oestrogen at all: those who have a history of breast, cervical, endometrial or vaginal cancer; recurrent breast cysts; or blood clots. It is not usually prescribed for women with kidney or liver disease, certain kinds of heart disease, diabetes, high blood pressure or endometrial hyperplasia (a cell condition which could be pre-cancerous). Women who have endometriosis or fibroids (see Chapter 7) usually should not take oestrogen. However, exceptions may be made, particularly in cases of extreme menopausal symptoms. Again, some people think that 'natural' oestrogens do not affect women with these conditions. As yet, there is little evidence to support this view.

Much more research is needed in the area of HRT. Because of present uncertainties, many women are very cautious, choosing it only when symptoms are severe and when no contraindications are present. In most women, post-menopausal production of oestrogen is sufficient, and no therapy is indicated. For some women, an alternative can be found in one or other of the remedies cited below, or in carefully planned tranquillizer therapy and the strong psychological support of family and/or friends and medical personnel. We feel that the decision whether or not to take HRT should lie with each individual woman on the basis of adequate discussion with both medical personnel and other women. Those of us who do decide that any risks there may be are worth taking should not be put off by doctors who disagree with that view.

Since it is not always easy to determine which ailments are menopausal and which are simply related to ageing or other life crises, we appreciate how difficult a decision it may be to take oestrogen. But these are complexities which we women must consider while seeking help from the medical establishment.

Oestrogen is neither a fountain of youth, nor does it keep us from growing old. It does not change any of the real life crises we may be going through, but it may help some of us to adjust more easily to a possibly difficult period of our lives.

The major myth I had to overcome was the one which maintained that menopause was only a problem for neurotic women. I was taught that if a woman was physically active, busy, enjoying life and fulfilled, she would not experience any special discomfort during menopause, as these symptoms are all neurotic and psychosomatic. I am healthy, very busy and active, and was amazed to discover that certain physical menopausal symptoms did indeed occur. Night

*sweats, joint pains, dreadful nervous instability, terrible feelings of anxiety,
impending disaster — this all prompted me to talk to a gynaecologist.*

How Should Oestrogen Be Given?

If you think that oestrogen may be necessary, you should go to a doctor
who knows what s/he is doing. Bear in mind that most GPs have not
studied endocrinology (study of glands which secrete hormones), so if
at all possible it would be best to ask your GP to refer you to a menopause clinic. Women's Health Concern (see p. 534) has an up-to-
date list of clinics. Some clinics allow women to approach them direct.

If you take oestrogen, you should be screened for risk factors and
should be regularly and carefully checked, for example, for uterine cancer,
and to see that the dosages are right (they sometimes need changing).
Some doctors prescribe treatment only on the basis of a woman's
symptoms but since it is not then possible to ascertain the exact balance
of hormones in the body, this can lead to problems. See, for example,
the woman mentioned on p. 525 whose dosages of oestrogen and
progesterone needed changing. Other doctors recommend treatment on
the basis of laboratory tests. However, the equipment necessary for
sophisticated smear and blood tests to ascertain hormone balance is not
universally available; certainly no GPs have it and nor do all menopause
clinics. Hence the importance of going to a good clinic or gynaecologist.

If you have not had a hysterectomy it seems best, on theoretical
grounds, to take oestrogen cyclically, i.e. 3 weeks out of 4, so that your
uterine lining is shed every month. But it is still not clear what is the
safest way of giving oestrogen. Many doctors believe that progesterone
should be given as well, but this has not yet been fully evaluated. The
American Food and Drug Administration stresses that the lowest effective
dose should be used. Usually the goal is to prescribe as small an amount
of oestrogen as possible, to control symptoms without precipitating
side effects. Women's Health Concern reports that of 8,000 inquirers in
1975, 'many indicated that they were being given ridiculous dosages'.

As we have already pointed out, some people think that 'natural'
oestrogens such as 'Premarin' or 'Harmogen' should be used as opposed
to synthetic ones such as ethinyl-oestradiol (Climatone) or stilboestrol
(Sedestran). 'Natural' oestrogens are either extracted from mares' urine
(e.g. Premarin) or they are synthetically-produced human oestrogens,
such as Harmogen. There is no clear reason as yet why 'natural'
oestrogens might be better; it is possible that the current obsession with
these is the result of propaganda. 'Natural' oestrogens are the most
expensive. The annual sales of Premarin, perhaps the widest-selling
'natural' oestrogen, produced by Ayerst Laboratories, reportedly exceed
$70 million a year. So, while it is not possible at this stage to state

unequivocally which oestrogens are best, we *can* say that no woman should be given stilboestrol, an oestrogen which is suspect as far as cancer is concerned (see p. 182).

Some doctors believe that HRT can, or even should, be given for the rest of a woman's life; most believe that it should be given for the shortest possible time and that treatment should be stopped periodically to see if it is still needed. Whatever doctors feel, *we* should be able to make the decision about HRT, from the facts available and from our own feelings about the kinds of lives we want to lead. While it seems to us that women should be on HRT for the shortest possible time, we believe that women should have the right to be fully informed of the facts — or lack of them — and should be free to choose if, when and how to use HRT. One problem we face is sifting out the grains of truth from propaganda, 'pro-woman views' from profit-making motives, anti-HRT views from anti-woman or pro-woman views. As with all areas of health care, we will not have a choice unless (a) we have access to reliable information, (b) the medical expertise and clinics are available, and (c) we have the power to make decisions about how we wish to be treated.

Progesterone

Contrary to what is generally thought, some women — possibly one out of 250 — become deficient in progesterone, usually just before the meno-pause in the 'peri-menopausal' period. For these women, the standard oestrogen HRT can actually make their symptoms worse. This only serves to emphasize the importance of consulting a doctor who has really studied the subject of menopausal treatment. There is no one clue to progesterone deficiency. Heavy and prolonged bleeding, a common complaint at this time, can be caused by either lack of oestrogen or progesterone. Whichever treatment is found to be necessary, careful monitoring must take place to ensure maintenance of correct hormonal balance.

Apart from disabling and persistent depression (which was part menopausal and part due to a long period of extreme anxiety), my real trouble was the heavy blood loss in the peri-menopausal phase which was not only debilitating but almost impossible to cope with socially. Because I was encountering employment difficulties at the time I was inhibited from talking even to friends about the possibility of being in the menopause as I was terrified that might label me as unfit and unsuitable for employment. The doctors I finally dared to consult were quite indifferent to any suggestion of a menopausal condition. Eventually, after over five years, a new GP very reluctantly and reprovingly put me on 'Premarin' — not as a menopausal medication but because he believed it would control the bleeding by causing my blood to clot! The Pre-

marin not unexpectedly made the bleeding worse, but I went on taking it because I felt it might be even worse still if I stopped the treatment.

Finally I managed to read enough to begin to understand the menopause and I realized I needed progesterone. I then asked my doctor what he knew about (this) treatment. He was extremely rude in reply, we had a terrible row which ended by his writing out a prescription for yet another oestrogen preparation and one for a tranquillizer! I had had enough. I went straight to a Harley Street specialist who put me on progesterone at once. After the first month's treatment my periods were back to normal. But because of the distance involved my condition could not be monitored and so I gradually slipped out of balance and my periods became heavy and painful again. Also, the administration of the progesterone at that time was inexact — it can now be taken in precisely measured quantities. I was then lucky in being taken on to a local research study through which I got on to newer treatments and better monitoring. I suddenly went 'out of balance' with the other hormone — oestrogen — as the withdrawal process of that hormone had begun. In other words, the actual menopause had begun and the long, long 'run-up' to it was over. I was immediately put on to oestrogen replacement therapy with cyclical progesterone which to me means that I am having my menopause managed.

ALTERNATIVES TO HRT

1. Homeopathy (see p. 131)

One doctor we talked to never gives HRT, because she finds that her remedies are superior to hormones. However, she does believe that HRT *might* be necessary on some occasions, in which case she would prefer to use a 'natural' one. With homeopathy, the treatment has to be tailor-made to the individual. So we cannot make specific recommendations. However, it is worth bearing in mind that *sepia* is commonly effective for depression and mood changes and *pulsatilla* likewise for hot flushes. *Squid*, according to Marjorie Blackie, is often needed by most normal people at the menopause. For more details about homeopathic remedies, see her book, listed in the Bibliography.

2. Vitamin E Therapy

Little research has been done in this area, particularly latterly, and pharmacologists and nutritionists are sceptical of the value of vitamin E therapy at any time, let alone during the menopause. However, in their recent book *Women and the Crisis in Sex Hormones* (see p. 534), Barbara and Gideon Seaman unearth some extremely interesting research (ironically much of it British. In a *British Medical Journal* of 1949, Professor Hugh McLaren described Vitamin E as the 'method of choice' for treating menopausal symptoms – *British Medical Journal*, 1949, Vol. I.) which indicates that during the menopause, vitamin E can largely or totally relieve menopausal symptoms, and produce a better sense of well-being. Vitamin E requirements appear to increase during ageing. Deficiency causes FSH and LH production to increase – which is then thought to cause hot flushes. Vitamin E also prevents destruction of sex hormones, and appears to help with sleeplessness, as does *ginseng*. It appears that vitamin E treatment must be continued for 2–4 weeks before an effect can be discerned. Each woman requires tailor-made dosages, depending on her diet, if she smokes, if she has a deficiency, etc. (For natural dietary sources of vitamin E see 'Nutrition' chapter, p. 118.) The therapy seems to be especially effective when taken in conjunction with *vitamin B* or *ginseng*. Some people are sensitive to vitamin E, particularly diabetics and those with high blood pressure or a rheumatic heart condition. These people should only take it in low or moderate doses. (For more information on vitamin E, including dosages, and other alternatives to HRT, see the Seaman book.)

The reason why HRT is in vogue, and vitamin E is not, has probably more to do with the medical profession's attitude to non-prescription remedies than to any real evaluation of these respective treatments. We hope that any doctor who takes the trouble to read the research cited in the Seaman book will consider prescribing vitamin E therapy under the NHS. Otherwise it will be beyond the pockets of many, many women.

3. Other Treatments and Preventive Measures

Adequate *calcium* and *protein* intake can help enormously in keeping us healthy around the time of the menopause. Calcium deficiency can result during the menopause due to lack of ovarian hormones. Regular doses of calcium and *vitamin D*, if taken from middle age onwards, can keep our bones strong and discourage osteoporosis. Calcium tablets are also said to ease tension, hot flushes and backaches, among other things.

As we get older, we don't need so many calories, particularly if we are not taking much exercise – so we should adjust our diets accordingly. It is best to take *regular exercise* throughout our lives to keep our bodies healthy.

Nature Cure practitioners (see p. 133) believe that in a really healthy woman, the menopause produces no symptoms at all except cessation of periods. They like to concentrate on maintaining a healthy body. One school of thought suggests that when periods have stopped, poisons from the body can no longer be excreted regularly through menstruation, and therefore the body has to readjust itself, hence symptoms such as hot flushes. In her nature cure booklet, *Women's Ailments*, Isa Anderson Kelso suggests that we build up our capacities to get rid of impurities in our early thirties, so that when the menopause comes, our kidneys, bowels and lungs are prepared. We can do this by eating and drinking sensibly (too much tea, coffee and alcohol can, she says, harm the kidneys and make the symptoms of menopause more severe), not having too many hot baths, exercising our lungs and learning to breathe properly.

Certain *herbal remedies* can be very helpful. For example, Lady's Slipper is said to be excellent for women having a bad time during the menopause, and saffron is said to help with feelings of heat and headaches. Camomile tea and valerian root are useful herbal sedatives for people who find it difficult to sleep. For a detailed look at herbal treatments see *Herbs for Feminine Ailments* and *Women and the Crisis in Sex Hormones* (Bibliography, p. 533).

Clonidine, a drug used to treat raised blood pressure, can, in low doses, prevent hot flushes and sweating. But it can result in depression, and as with HRT its long-term effects are unknown.

Yoga, natural childbirth techniques (see p. 417), *hypnosis* or the *Alexander Technique* (see p. 134) can all help, for example, in dealing with hot flushes. Sheila Kitzinger is reported as saying: 'I've had a few hot flushes but I thought they were quite nice . . . As in childbirth, a sort of wave comes over you and the point is to go *with* it, instead of resisting it as something dreadful.'

It should be possible to 'turn off' hot flushes in the same way as migraines can be avoided – by means of control of the vascular system via *biofeedback*. Women working in areas like this can be contacted via *Prime Time* (see Bibliography). It would be helpful if more research were done into the role of nutrition and other preventive measures in relation to menopausal symptoms.

Feelings about the Menopause

Those of us looking ahead to menopause or just beginning to experience it can find little material that explores what most women go through during menopause.

At least one woman, the sociologist Bernice Neugarten, has done research on the menopausal experience of the average woman. One of her studies (see Bibliography) involved 100 women aged 43 to 53, from working-class and middle-class backgrounds, all in good health, all married and living with husbands, all mothers of at least one child, and none having had a hysterectomy. Women with more severe menopausal symptoms did *not* tend to view menopause more negatively than women with less severe symptoms. Only 4 out of the 100 women thought of menopause as a major source of worry. 'Losing your husband', 'just getting older' and 'fear of cancer' were much more frequent concerns.

Those women who reported more negative experiences in the areas of menstruation, first sexual experience, pregnancy and childbirth also reported more severe menopausal symptoms. There could be a variety of explanations for this correlation. Conceivably, the physical cause or causes of previous reproductive or sexual difficulties could also be the cause of menopausal problems. Or maybe negative attitudes that our culture teaches us about our bodies and about our reproductive processes continue throughout our lives to have a negative effect on all our sexual and reproductive experiences.

OUR MENOPAUSE QUESTIONNAIRE

Our Collective (in Boston), unable to find much information about menopause as most women experience it, sent out in 1974 almost 2,000 menopause questionnaires to women all over the United States. We asked women aged 25 and up (*not* just older women) to fill out the questionnaire.

In this chapter we can present only a small fraction of the information that we gathered. Those answering the questionnaire do not represent a cross section of women. However, these responses give us a better idea of what research needs to be done and also give us the privilege of hearing the voices of many women talking about this experience which society presents so negatively. In general, our questionnaires corroborate the findings of Bernice Neugarten.

The Sample

Following is a brief description of the 484 women who answered the questionnaire:

Age Range	% of Total Sample
25–40	37%
41–50	26
51–60	26
over 60	11

Most of the women who responded were living in large cities or suburbs. Three quarters had children; of these, about one half had 1 or 2 children, and half had more than 2 children. Almost all were or had been at some point in their lives, involved with full-time housework and/ or childrearing. Of the menopausal and post-menopausal women, about two thirds worked outside the home during their menopause. Including volunteer work, this figure rose to about three quarters. Post-menopausal women worked outside the home slightly more often than menopausal women.

One fifth of the women had had a hysterectomy. Slightly less than two thirds had primarily positive things to say about having had the operation.

Our Survey: Attitudes towards Menopause

The first thing we asked was, 'What comes to mind when you first see the word "menopause"?'

About half the women gave positive or neutral associations, while half referred to negative aspects. In general, younger women were more fearful and felt more negative about menopause. Older women, especially post-menopausal women, were more matter-of-fact. This suggests that younger women tend to have a distorted view of the menopausal experience, anticipating it as much worse than it usually turns out to be. Is this because of all the myths about menopause that surround us? Is it because younger women especially fear our society's attitude towards ageing women? If younger women have such fear, why don't older women answering the questionnaire express as much fear or even extreme frustration with living in a society that treats the ageing with so little respect? Possibly the older women in our sample represent a unique group of fairly active women who have managed to feel basically good about themselves despite society's generally negative attitude towards them. Another possibility is that since most (two thirds) of these older women felt that they received emotional support from family and/or friends during menopause they were more likely to have positive attitudes towards menopause. There are probably a number of likely explanations, and we would like to encourage more groups to explore these kinds of questions.

Our Survey: 'Symptoms' Experienced by Younger and Older Women Alike

We asked all women to check off any of 23 various 'symptoms' (excluding hot flushes and vaginal dryness) they might have experienced during different decades of their lives. (All of these were symptoms often associated with menopause.) The question had very interesting results. Women 25 to 40 years old checked more symptoms much more frequently than women in any other age group. And women over 60 checked by far the fewest symptoms. It is not clear what this difference might reflect: Do older women have difficulty remembering and thus recall fewer symptoms than they have actually experienced? Or do older women tend to see themselves as less 'laden' with symptoms? Or do they define a 'symptom' differently? The checklist results suggested that menopausal women *weren't* more likely than other women to report having symptoms (other than hot flushes and vaginal dryness).

Our Survey: The Experiences of Menopause

About two thirds of the menopausal and post-menopausal women reported hot flushes. Although very few women mentioned vaginal discomfort or painful intercourse, many of them may not have known that this symptom can be related to menopause. For most women menopause was reported to have lasted about 2 years or less, but for others it seemed to last as many as 4, 5, or 6 years. This is partly due to the 15% of women who resumed their periods after they had not been menstruating for a whole year. It would be interesting to know why this happens to so many women.

Following are some of the feelings and changes women reported having around the time of menopause: 'Relief' . . . 'Tearfulness' . . . 'Unexplainable periods of nervousness and irritation' . . . 'Rage at ageing' . . . 'Disorientation, crying, sense of being "over the hill", sense of failure' . . . 'Delight that childbearing years were coming to a close' . . . 'Happy to anticipate relaxed intercourse without need of contraceptive devices – disappointed because of vaginitis' . . . 'There hasn't been that much change' . . . 'I feel much better now. I had feared menopause because I was told that I would go crazy' . . . 'The lack of sex desire really bothers me' . . . 'I believe that the hot flushes I experienced were milder than most. I was always so busy with my work I didn't have time to think about them' . . . 'The changes were not drastic. I have just accepted them. They will stop one of these days' . . . 'Most of the problems at this time were due to other causes: ageing, role-stereotyping, other people's attitudes toward me' . . .

In general, about two thirds of the menopausal and post-menopausal women felt neutral or positive about the changes they experienced. One third felt clearly negative. When asked specifically about the loss of childbearing ability, 90% felt either positive or neutral. Although our culture has attached great importance to a woman's ability to reproduce, most women in our sample were not upset by the end of menstruation. Possibly this reflects the fact that, for these women, childbearing ability was only part of their self-image: after menopause they were able to value (and had the opportunity to develop) their talents and capacities beyond childbearing.

Our Survey: Sexuality and Menopause

About half of the menopausal and post-menopausal women reported no changes in their sexual desires, while the rest indicated about equally often either an increase or decrease in sexual desire. When asked if they felt differently about themselves sexually, two thirds of these women said no. (This is similar to Neugarten's finding.)

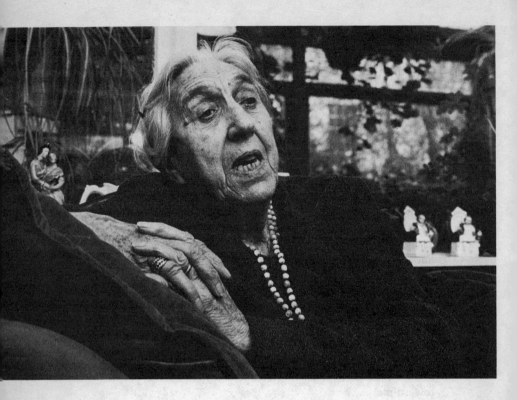

Conclusion

The responses to our questionnaire clearly indicate that many of us need much more accurate information about menopause. We don't know how meaningful the replies were. We can only hope that as women begin to respect their own experiences, further research will indicate the truth about the menopause.

If a woman has spent a large part of her life raising a family, she now has some important decisions to make about what to do with the next 30 years of her life. She may find that her options are terribly limited, since the labour market does not value her abilities and potentials. She may want to talk with other women about these problems, and women are getting together to discuss just these issues. We are all going to grow older, and we must all work to eliminate age discrimination.

We as women must work to change society's negative attitude towards ageing. We know that we can be as valuable to others and to ourselves after menopause as before — in fact more so as we grow in wisdom and experience. We must challenge the stereotypes which minimize our abilities; we must challenge social and economic forces in our culture which falsely glorify youthfulness. Let us reaffirm our potential for personal growth and contribution to society at every stage in the continuum of life.

Readings and Resources

Anon., 'Eternal Youth', *Lancet*, 7 June 1975.

Anon., 'Hormone Replacement Therapy and Endometrial Cancer', *Lancet*, 12 March 1977 (and ensuing correspondence).

Anon., 'Management of Osteoporosis', *British Medical Journal*, 8 November 1975.

Barker, Jane, and Graham, Rosie, 'Change of Life?', *Spare Rib*, 51.

Bart, P. B., 'Depression in Middle-aged Women', in *Woman in Sexist Society*, New York, Basic Books, 1971.

Beckett, Sarah, *Herbs for Feminine Ailments*, Thorsons, 1973.

Blackie, Marjorie, *The Patient, Not the Cure*, Macdonald & Janes, 1976.

Clayden, J. R. *et al.*, 'Menopause Flushing: Double-blind Trial of a Non-hormonal Medication', *British Medical Journal*, 9 March 1974.

Cooper, Wendy, 'If Only More Doctors Were Women', *Observer*, 6 February 1975.

Cooper, Wendy, *No Change: a Biological Revolution for Women*, Arrow, 1976: presents the case for HRT and its preventive and protective role.

'Drugs: Estrogen and the Menopause Patient', *Medical Letter*, 19 January 1973.

Hems, G., 'The Menopause and Breast Cancer', *Lancet*, 2 March 1974.

Hoover *et al.*, 'HRT and Breast Cancer', *New England Journal of Medicine*, 19 August 1976.

Kase, N., 'Estrogen and the Menopause', *Journal of the American Medical Association*, 21 January 1974.

Kelso, Isa Anderson, *Women's Ailments*, Thorsons, 1958.

McKinlay, S. M., *et al.*, 'Selected Studies of the Menopause', *Journal of Biosocial Science*, Vol. 5 (October, 1973).

McKinlay, S. M., and Jefferys, Margot, 'The Menopausal Syndrome', *British Journal of Preventive and Social Medicine*, 28 (1974).

Mack, T. M., *et al.*, 'Oestrogens and Endometrial Cancer in a Retirement Community', *New England Journal of Medicine*, 3 June 1976.

Masters, W., and Johnson, V., 'Human Sexual Response: The Aging Female and the Aging Male', in *Middle Age and Aging*, Chicago, University of Chicago Press, 1968.

Neugarten, B. L., *et al.*, *Personality in Middle and Late Life*, New York, Atherton Press, 1964.

Neugarten, B. L., *et al.*, 'Women's Attitudes Towards the Menopause', *Vita Humana*, Vol. 6 (1963).

Neugarten, B. L., and Kraines, R. J., 'Menopausal Symptoms in Women of Various Ages', *Psychosomatic Medicine*, Vol. 27 (1965).

Osofsky, H. J., and Seidenberg, R., 'Is Female Menopausal Depression Inevitable?' *Obstetrics and Gynecology*, Vol. 36, No. 4 (October, 1970).

Pacheco, J. C., and Kempers, R. D., 'Etiology of Postmenopausal Bleeding', *Obstetrics and Gynecology*, Vol. 32, No. 1 (July, 1968).

Poortman, H., *et al.*, 'Production of Androgens and Oestrogens in Postmenopausal Women', 8th Acta Endocrinologica Congress, Abstract No. 79, Suppl. 155 (1971).

Prescribers' Journal (a journal independent of the pharmaceutical industry published by the DHSS): Vol. 16, No. 3, June 1976. Two differing views are presented concerning treatment of menopausal symptoms.

Prime Time, an Independent Feminist Journal, available from 420 West 46th Street, New York, NY 10036.

Ryan, K., and Gibson, D. (eds.), *Menopause and Aging*, Summary Report and Selected Papers from a Research Conference, Hot Springs, Ark., May, 1971. DHEW Publication (NIH) No. 73–319, Bethesda, Md., Public Health Service, 1973.

Seaman, B. and G., *Women and the Crisis in Sex Hormones*, Rawson Co. (USA), 1977.

Smith, D., *et al.*, 'Association of Exogenous Estrogen and Endometrial Carcinoma', *New England Journal of Medicine*, 4 December 1975. See also accompanying leader article.

Symposium, 'The Management of the Menopause and Post-menopausal years' held in London, 26 November 1975 (report published by Medical & Technical Publishing Co. Ltd., Lancaster).

'Treating Menopausal Women and Climacteric Men', *Medical World News*, Vol. 15 (June 1974).

Van Keep, P. A., and Lauritzen, C. (eds.), *Frontiers of Hormone Research* (Vol. Two: *Aging and Estrogens*), Hasel, Switzerland: S. Karger, 1973.

Villadolid, L., *et al.*, 'Progress Report on Long-term Oestrogen Therapy', *Current Medical Research Opinion*, Vol. 1, No. 10 (1973).

Weideger, P., *Menstruation and Menopause: The Physiology and Psychology, the Myth and the Reality*, New York, Alfred A. Knopf, 1975.

Weiss, N. S., *et al.*, 'Increasing Incidence of Endometrial Cancer in the United States', *New England Journal of Medicine*, 3 June 1976.

White, Janet, 'Restoring the Balance in the Change', *Western Mail*, 5 March 1975.

Williams, C. W., 'Clonidine in Treatment of Menopausal Flushing', *Lancet*, 16 June 1973.

Winoker, G., 'Depression in Menopause', *American Journal of Psychiatry*, Vol. 130 (1973).

Women's Report, 'Dangers?', summary and commentary on some recent studies, Vol. 4, issue 2.

Ziel, *et al.*, 'Increased Risk of Endometrial Carcinoma among Users of Conjugated Oestrogens', *New England Journal of Medicine*, 4 December 1975.

RESOURCES

Women's Health Concern, 16 Seymour Street, London W1H 5WB (01 486 8653 or 01 788 2733): a non-profit-making agency providing information on HRT, and also on other gynaecological problems such as premenstrual tension. It supplies details of menopause clinics throughout Britain.

17 Women and Health Care

The vast majority of health workers in this country are women and the biggest users of health care facilities are women, but the role of women within the National Health Service is largely one of service.

We have not always been at the bottom of the pile. As witches, midwives and healers we were once the major source of medical care, not all of it useful but much of it learned through careful observation and knowledge of the properties of herbs. During the Middle Ages many women were forced out of medicine by witch hunts, and by the thirteenth century medicine had become a subject for study by men in universities. The training was based largely on superstition, religion and philosophy, apart from rudimentary information on herbal medicine, much of it learned from the women healers.

In the fourteenth century English doctors wrote a petition to Parliament bewailing the 'worthless and presumptuous women who usurpe the profession'* and asking for fines and long imprisonment for any woman who attempted to practise medicine. The only area in which women were left free to practise was midwifery, and by the seventeenth century even that preserve was penetrated by male 'barber surgeons' after the invention of the forceps which women were not allowed to use. During the eighteenth century doctors joined the surgeons in the lucrative trade of obstetrics. Women healers were not entirely dispensed with. Many people could not afford male doctors; the body of medical folklore was still important and midwives continued to attend the poor, delivering babies and providing virtually the only form of birth control available, which was abortion. Midwives did not believe in unnecessary interference with the natural process of childbirth and at a time when many women were dying from infections passed on by male obstetricians, with their unsterile manual examinations and forceps deliveries, the women who were attended by midwives had a higher chance of survival.

Doctors still tell us not to listen to 'old wives' tales'. To them that means the advice of our mothers and friends who have experienced our problems

* From *Witches, Midwives and Nurses*, by Barbara Ehrenreich and Deirdre English.

themselves. Doctors have tremendous power over us as the only 'reliable' source of information. Even when many of us fear and mistrust the medical profession, they have so wound us up in medical mystique that we have no one else to turn to. In taking a monopoly of medicine they have encouraged us to surrender our bodies to them.

In one survey, 250 gynaecology patients were questioned about their knowledge of their bodies and what was happening to them. Although they could describe in subjective terms what was wrong with them, 45% could not name the affected organ or describe their treatment. Of the 29% who were unable to differentiate their reproductive organs on a diagram, several made comments such as 'If I had been interested in my body I would have gone in for nursing or St John's', or 'I'm sorry I'm not a doctor or a nurse, therefore I don't understand anything medical' (Ashton General Hospital, 1975).

Many doctors realize that their patients have become unduly dependent on them. They see their surgeries filling up with patients seeking cures which they could provide for themselves. It is common to hear doctors complaining about patients who take up their time with trivial matters, but at the same time doctors have fostered this dependence by presenting themselves as experts on everything from copulation to cancer. Few doctors have the nerve to tell a patient that they don't know what is wrong or that they cannot help. Not all patients react to their lack of knowledge by constant reference to a doctor to make sure that their bodies are working. Many people conceal illness either through fear of the unknown or fear of their doctors.

When the NHS was introduced no attempt was made to change the power relationship between doctor and patient. Only the economic relationship was changed. At present doctors are not responsible to us but to the employing authority. We cannot question their clinical judgement, we cannot insist on being treated by a particular consultant, we have no right of access to information about our own case, or to insist upon a particular form of treatment, or even to have a companion with us in labour. Our only rights are negative: provided we are not incarcerated under the Mental Health Act, we can refuse treatment and we can refuse to be used as teaching material or for experiments (provided we are aware of what is happening).

Many doctors feel that our concern about our rights constitutes a lack of trust in them. They are concerned about what they see as a breakdown in the doctor-patient relationship. But many of them see the answer in a return to the cash relationship with patients either through medical insurance policies or through the disincentive of making people pay for treatment and reimbursing them later. Either of these 'solutions' would totally undermine the system of free care at the time of need. We already pay at least £60 each year for our health service through our taxes. It is *our* service and we should not be asked to pay for it twice. Certainly any system based on reimbursable payments would create a group of second-class patients carrying cards to prove their inability to pay, while the rest of us would be forced to wait months for our money to be paid back. The insurance system would be worse because it would leave out those most in need of free care. No insurance company will insure a bad risk.

These ideas ignore the real problems, the widespread ignorance about our own bodies which doctors have done nothing to tackle, combined with an emphasis on healing rather than prevention – a bias which is built into a system with a steep hierarchy topped by doctors in surgery, the most crudely curative area of medicine.

But medical staff cannot be held responsible for the current problem, which is lack of money. We spend less than 6% of our total budget on health, less even than the USA where most people pay for doctoring out of their own pockets. At present budgets are being cut back still further as a result of public spending cuts. Where a few years ago hospitals could not get the staff they needed because they didn't pay enough, now they are turning newly qualified nurses away to reduce the wages bill further, so that those who remain are more overworked than ever and waiting lists are even longer. We cannot expect adequate care from overworked, exhausted health workers. But we must look for more fundamental solutions too.

At present 60% of the health budget is spent on hospitals. Perhaps fewer people would need hospital treatment if they had the right kind of care at the start of their illness? Again, fewer people would be ill if we paid more attention to our environment, working conditions and mental health. And the NHS is paying vast amounts of money to drug firms which are still in private hands and are making vast profits from our diseases. (See *Who Needs the Drug Companies* by the Haslemere Group.)

Although our *ill-health* is in the hands of a nationalized industry, our *health* is not. Our health service spends much of its time and money patching up the victims of a profit-orientated society in which most people are isolated in their individual homes coping alone with stress and anxiety, alienated at work in dull, meaningless, or backbreaking jobs. As women become more involved in industrial work, we are facing more industrial hazards in addition to the exhaustion of doing two jobs. An industrial nurse described her job as 'keeping the workers on the lines'.

In this last section we discuss how the system works, how we can use it to advantage, and how some people are trying to change it.

The Foundation of the National Health Service

The National Health Service was set up in the teeth of fierce opposition from the medical hierarchy by the Labour Government which came to power just after the Second World War. Although Aneurin Bevan, the

1. *Secretary of State for Social Services.*
2. *Secretary of State (Health) and Parliamentary Under Secretaries of Health and Social Security.*
   The Department of Health and Social Security Scottish Home and Health Department.

3. **14 Regional Health Authorities** (England only — the Welsh Office serves this function in Wales) with responsibility for broad planning decisions, major building work, regional services, appointment of consultants and senior registrars outside teaching hospitals and allocation of funds to Area Health Authorities in the region. All members appointed by Secretary of State.

4. **Area Health Authorities** (Health Boards in Scotland). About 11 AHAs in each region. Responsibility for hospitals in the area and appointment of junior staff. Major decisions on allocation of money and cutbacks in service. Responsible for day-to-day matters and complaints about hospital or community services. 15 members appointed by the RHA, at least 4 members of local council, 2 doctors and 1 nurse.

5. *AHA full-time officials:* Medical Officer, Nursing Officer, Treasurers and administrator. Each responsible for coordinating all services in their area of responsibility.

6. *Family Practitioner Committee:* One per area, carries out duties of old executive councils; organization of GP contracts and payment, complaints and disciplinary procedures. Advise AHA on GP planning.

7. **District Management Teams.** The area breaks down into districts of 250,000—300,000 people, all of which are served by district teams. The teams are staffed by health workers but only doctors have the right to elect members to it. They comprise the District Community Physician, District Nursing Officer, District Finance Officer and District Administrator, plus 2 elected members of the District Medical Committee. The district teams assess priorities and report back to the AHA.

8. *District Medical Committees.* Special Committees for doctors to discuss medical matters and priorities from members of other specializations. No special power, but plenty of influence.

9. *Health Care Planning Teams.* Under the care of the District Community Physician. These teams focus on particular problems and are made up of representatives of particular specializations: elderly, mentally handicapped, maternity, etc.

10. *Community Health Councils* (Local Health Councils in Scotland). The consumer voice, covering the same area as a district; no real power, see p. 540.

Minister responsible for organizing the service, wanted a service which catered to everyone so that the poor would not be lumbered with a second-class service, he was unable to persuade the medical profession to drop their private practices entirely.

Changes were, however, pretty sweeping: the vast majority of people opted for NHS treatment and most doctors joined the scheme. But the obstacles to total change ensured a degree of built-in inequality which exists to this day. Working-class areas are still not as well served as middle-class areas – the availability of private patients in richer areas gives richer pickings to more mercenary doctors, and the relative poverty, bad housing conditions and more strenuous work of working-class populations put them at greater risk and give doctors more work. In practice 30% less is spent on working-class populations than on middle-class populations.*

The existence of a private sector will be a constant source of conflict in the NHS until it can be totally abolished. We have a dual system and as long as private facilities exist they provide an excuse for insufficient provision of NHS facilities (abortion services are a prime example of this). If people are desperate enough they will turn to the private sector rather than join long queues. As long as this option exists for those who can afford it there will be no improvement in the service for those who cannot. The British Medical Association which represents doctors is again battling for the preservation of privilege with their so-called Patients before Politics campaign. They have managed to convince many people that the preservation of private practice is the only way to preserve standards for patients. If doctors were not prepared to accept the bribery of the rich they would be able to give of their best to everybody. If there is a better kind of care we should all be entitled to it, not just those who can pay.

The Reorganization of the Health Service

In 1974 a sweeping reorganization of the health service, commissioned by a Conservative government, was implemented. The scheme was devised by a team of American management consultants and it pleases no one. Although doctors are represented at most levels and form a powerful interest group, much of their former control has been put into the hands of administrators. Nurses are represented at some levels and ancillary workers not at all. Patients have been given representation on the

---

* Survey by Dr Julien Le Grand, Sussex University.

Community Health Councils which have very little power and hardly any contact with, or impact on, the rest of the structure.

The changes, far from streamlining service to the public, allow the central government department (the DHSS) to make cuts in financing with greater ease and to switch funds from one area to another with little obstruction from local interest groups. This centralization of the administration means that local services are even less sensitive to the needs of the people that use them.

The Community or Local Health Councils (CHC)

These Councils were set up to represent the 'consumer' of health service facilities. They have practically no power, but they can work as a useful lobby and, in combination with local organizations, can make sure that the interests of patients are not only noted but publicized.

If CHCs are to work on behalf of the community rather than the authorities they must be composed of people who represent the community, people who are active, informed and concerned. At present each CHC has between 18 and 35 members and covers roughly the same area as a *Health District*. Half the members are appointed by the local authority, a third by those voluntary organizations selected by the Regional Health Authority, and the rest directly by the RHA.

Every CHC is funded by the Area Health Authority and has the right to find its own premises, appoint its own secretary and assistants and manage its own budget. Some have allowed themselves to be hidden away in the AHA building or in hospitals, the more go-ahead councils have separate shop front premises with easy access for local people.

All council meetings are open to the public and the press.

HOW TO GET ONTO A CHC

Members are appointed for 2 to 4 years. Half of them retire every 2 years. Any interested women's group should send an application for representation to the Regional Health Authority at least 4–6 months before the retirement date. It is likely that RHAs will be biased towards the more conservative organizations such as the FPA or the Women's Institutes. However, the Rochdale Women's group has found that just by asking questions at meetings they have been coopted onto subcommittees and offered places on the council. Attitudes vary tremendously: some CHCs use their position merely to 'rubber-stamp' cuts with the consumer seal of approval, some don't even know what their role is, or, for example that meetings are supposed to be public. In at least one area, the local authority has been persuaded to appoint members of community groups to all its seats.

THE ROLE OF THE CHC

Dealing with Complaints

Although they do not themselves investigate complaints, they should have all the necessary information, and can help individuals to formulate their complaints and give them the necessary support and assistance in making sure they are taken up. Some CHCs are monitoring complaints to make sure they are properly handled.

Fighting closures

CHCs must be consulted about new developments or closures in the locality. If they disagree with the Area Health Authority the decision must be postponed until the CHC sends alternative plans to the Secretary of State who makes the final decision. In a campaign to stop cuts, or to set up an out-patient abortion clinic, the CHC can play an important role.

Identifying priorities

The CHC should use its contact with the public to discover the real needs of the area and work for improvements. This is only possible if it is actually listening to local people. The 1975 Annual Report of the Wandsworth and East Merton CHC gives some idea of the difficulties experienced by the 'consumer voice'.

We have already seen how quickly some consultants lose their benign bedside manner when their monopoly of the 'facts' is questioned . . . Most of the Hospital Administrators with which our CHC has contact are nice and friendly but have yet to grasp the meaning of participation. Conflict has surrounded whether or not we are entitled to confidential information regarding future plans and policy and whether we can or cannot make this information more widely available, whether or not we are entitled to visit NHS establishments without an official entourage and whether or not it would be wise to fraternize with the Trade Unions. It is just an unfortunate fact that this conflict must go on over our right to proper involvement in decision making.

The Unions

Nursing and ancillary workers are represented only in a limited way in the health service administration, though together they make up the bulk of health service employees and 80% of them are women. Over the last few years increasing numbers of health workers have joined unions.

The 1973 ancillary workers' strike, followed by the nurses' action in 1974, have shown that despite the difficulties of taking industrial action in a hospital, union organization is effective.

At present most of the energy of the unions is being used in fighting cuts in staffing. Although union executives take a very cautious line over industrial action there has been an upsurge of activity at hospital level against threatened or existing staff shortages. One significant effect of this increased militancy is that the staff at the bottom of the hierarchy are for the first time challenging those at the top and taking overtly political action against them. The campaign against private practice in which ancillary and nursing staffs refused to attend private patients caused a crisis and confrontation with the consultants. Recently more unions have been taking up other types of issues: in September 1976, members of the Confederation of Health Service Employees caused real consternation in the ranks of the consultants by forcing the suspension of a consultant psychiatrist at Normansfield Hospital, Middlesex, through strike action.

Despite the large majority of women in the hospital unions, women are not well represented in the union hierarchy. In the National Union of Public Employees (NUPE), with a 59% female membership, only 1 out of 90 officials is a woman. Branch meetings are not well attended by women, partly because they tend to be held at times when women workers are home 'minding the babies' and partly because women feel alienated by the bureaucratic nature of trade union organization. It is often as hard to get women's needs properly recognized in the union as it would be through official NHS machinery. In addition, there are a number of different unions serving similar sections all with different policies and different officials and representatives. This means that when action is proposed by one union, others may not even have been informed and this leads to conflict instead of cooperation.

In one or two hospitals active women trade unionists have managed to make changes. For example, in the Charing Cross Hospital in London, meetings are now held in work time to allow more women to attend. At the same hospital a cleaners' section has been organized, which is effectively a women's section, where discussion has ranged beyond immediate economic issues and women feel more able to participate effectively.

Women have been in the forefront of the major industrial actions within the health service but they tend only to involve themselves when the action affects them directly. If we are to influence union activity we must participate on a day-to-day level, not only in times of crisis. We have the numbers, what we need is the determination and confidence to push for change both outside and inside the unions.

Trade union organization is important, but it must be broadened to look at health care and the needs of the people it serves rather than to concentrate only on the economic aspects of the service. A forum for discussion and joint action between health workers and the community is badly needed. The women's health movement is beginning to show how useful it can be to bring health workers into discussions with women's groups when the balance of power is reversed and they are doing the listening rather than the talking. Some other attempts are being made to establish links between health workers and the rest of us to form a basis for combined action on health care, and these are discussed in the last section.

Complaints Procedures

For many of us the only time we challenge the NHS monolith is when we make a complaint. But few of us know who to complain to and we are often left dissatisfied. In 1974, following a number of major hospital scandals involving treatment of 'long-stay' patients, the Davies Committee was set up to look into the complaints procedure in hospitals. The committee concluded that there was no existing procedure to study. Recommendations had been made by the DHSS, but every hospital had a different system and few of them actually informed patients of their procedures. At the time of writing, the Davies Committee proposals are under examination and some of them may be implemented, so this is a review of the present system and a preview of what could happen.

If you make a complaint it is important (under the present system) to do so in writing and to keep a copy of your letter. Send a copy to your CHC so that they can follow it up. If you run into any trouble contact your CHC or the Patients' Association for assistance (see p. 571).

COMPLAINTS ABOUT MEDICAL CARE

As things stand at present there is no NHS machinery for dealing with complaints about medical care. The doctor's 'clinical judgement' cannot be challenged by anybody unless professional negligence can be proved (i.e. they have not given the kind of care that other members of the profession would consider reasonable). Professional negligence would have to be proved in court if you want any kind of compensation, which could involve a complainant in heavy legal costs.

If you feel that a doctor is unfit to practise s/he can be reported to the employing authority (RHA for consultants, AHA for other health workers, Health Service Tribunal* for GPs). They will investigate and decide whether anything should be done. Alternatively you can report

---

* Health Service Tribunal, write c/o The H.S.T. Clerk, 86 High St., Lewes, Sussex.

the person to his/her professional body (The General Medical Council, The General Nursing Council, etc.). If the complaint is sufficiently serious the doctor could be barred from practising. These councils will only take up cases which are very serious in their eyes (they seem to be obsessed by 'improper' sexual relationships with patients) and which clearly reflect on a person's general competence to practise, i.e. drug addiction, alcoholism, assault on patients, etc.

These procedures cannot and are not intended to handle matters of mis-judgement, mental cruelty, or callousness, and even in matters of life and death it is hard to prove a case when you don't fully understand the jargon and the doctor has the full backing of his profession in his defence. The Davies Committee recommended that independent tribunals be set up to investigate matters of patient care which are not taken to court, and this is currently under discussion.

BREACH OF GP CONTRACT

GPs, because they are under contract to the NHS and are not full-time employees, are responsible for keeping to their contracts and providing a reasonable service. If, for example, they refuse to visit a sick patient who clearly cannot get to the surgery, they can be reported to the Family Practitioner Committee (see p. 538) for breach of contract. Any complaint must be made within 8 weeks of the incident. The FPC cannot award damages but can discipline the doctor concerned. However, the committee which looks into disciplinary matters is at present composed of a majority of doctors, all of whom are likely to be colleagues of the 'accused'.

HOSPITAL COMPLAINTS

Any complaint in a hospital should where possible be made immediately to the ward sister. If the complaint is made later it should be sent to the hospital secretary and if things are still not adequately cleared up they can be reported to the Area Health Authority, who should investigate. In a teaching hospital the complaint should be made to the Board of Governors.

In most cases the 'responsible body' will simply make inquiries of the person complained against and pass on their explanation; it is unlikely that the person complaining will be brought into the discussion.

The Davies Committee has proposed that a code of practice should be brought into universal use in the NHS. Under this code, every complaint whether verbal or written should be recorded in a complaints book by the most senior member of staff available at the time (usually a ward sister). The matter should be cleared up immediately if possible and if not, should be referred to the next person up the hierarchy in the relevant department. If the question is medical the matter should be referred to the consultant concerned and the complainant should have the right to discuss it. If this code is implemented it would be compulsory for admission leaflets to include information about it so that every one would know.

OTHER NHS EMPLOYEES

These complaints should be referred directly to the Area Health Authority.

FURTHER ACTION

If the complainant is not satisfied, there is another level of the bureaucracy to appeal to: the Health Services Commissioner ('Ombudsman'), who can be written to at Church House, Great Smith Street, London SW1. The HSC also has powers of investigation, but at present cannot deal with clinical matters. He has, however, been known to express concern about women being asked to wait 3 hours in an antenatal clinic!

Whatever the changes being contemplated or even implemented, it is clear that the individual use of the complaints procedure will not change the basic problems that we are confronted with. Some kind of direct action may be more effective: writing to newspapers, radio, MPs, etc. One woman we heard of got so fed up with using the machinery that she started to picket the private patients' entrance of the hospital concerned with a placard stating the treatment she had received. That did create a reaction. It affected the doctors where it hurt most – in their private-patient-purses. It is important to complain when we are badly treated, but individual action cannot be as effective as group action, so if you are contemplating a complaint read the rest of the section and particularly the section on organization, pp. 559ff.

The Hospital Hierarchy

Hospitals run on a rigid system. At the top the consultants (specialists) reign supreme. All doctors below that are junior doctors, still considered to be in training. The junior grades go down in status and pay from senior registrar to junior registrar, senior house officer, junior house officer and student. All other hospital staff are lower in status. The highest wage for the top clinical nursing grade is only fractionally above that for a newly qualified junior doctor. A 50-year-old nurse with 30 years experience is expected to take orders from a doctor even if she has to show him what to do.

Below the professional staff come the cleaners, porters and other 'ancillary' workers who keep the whole system afloat and rarely get noticed until they go on strike. Here is a cleaner's view of the hospital system.*

The snobbery is horrific, real upstairs downstairs. There was one consultant who a few years ago walked on a woman's hand as she was scrubbing the floor. He never even apologized. She got her own back though when she tripped him up with her mop. The sister and the doctors on the ward usually expect the auxiliaries (untrained nurses) to make them cups of tea or coffee, endless cups served in the middle of whatever she is doing. The consultants and most doctors walk around as though no one else exists — walking over floors we're cleaning without a murmur.

WHERE DOCTORS COME FROM

The work load and wages of doctors are unevenly distributed. Consultants and senior registrars are supposed to be available on a shift basis for urgent consultation (their actual hours will depend a lot on their field), but most of the weight of day-to-day medical care falls on the more junior doctors who may have to be on call or working for well over 80 hours a week. This means that by the time the average doctor struggles to the top of the tree he's so fed up with long hours and lack of sleep that he doesn't think to lighten the load for those below. On the contrary, he's likely to feel that if he's come through it, so can they. At the top, particularly in a popular specialization like surgery, gynaecology or general medicine, the rewards are sizeable. Consultants are powerful, the hospital revolves around them and they are responsible to no one other than their employing Regional Authority. In addition they can earn thousands of pounds a year above their NHS salary through private work.

Needless to say, few of those at the top are women (only 1% of surgeons and 12% of gynaecologists). Women are a minority in any branch of the profession: a little over 30% of medical students are women now that the quota system limiting female entry to the profession has been lifted, and 22% of practising doctors. Women do not get promoted easily and they have a struggle getting into the popular specializations. The reason given is that they will not devote their lives to medicine and their training will be lost. However, those women doctors who do have children do seven-eighths as much work over 40 years as their colleagues who are not burdened with such responsibility,† and they do it in spite of the fact that practically no consideration is given to the needs of doctors with families; there are few child-care facilities, part-time work is less

---

* From Big Flame, *Women's Struggle Notes*, No. 6.
† Violet Johnson, *Sunday Telegraph*, 25 January 1976.

available than it should be (except in clinics) and of lower status than full-time work. Most women therefore go into general practice where they can structure their time more easily.

The struggle to the top is not in itself conducive to a caring and sympathetic attitude to patients, a creative attitude to health care organization or a thoughtful attitude towards other members of staff. It is a rare man or woman who escapes the stereotyping (though they certainly exist) and does not emerge like the conservative, unquestioning, complacent consultant who trained them. Two female medical students have written about their experiences. Here are extracts from those articles.

I went to St Thomas's Hospital medical school to do First MB. The bar in the students' union looked like an Edwardian club for the aristocracy, there were deep scratchy armchairs that 21-year-old men would sink into in order to talk about cricket and recall catastrophe in the operating theatre. They camped it up in short white coats and bought drinks for you. I felt foolish if I talked about the emerging women's movement. I wanted to connect my political ideas to the medical education I had embarked on but it was hard because the students were mostly upper-class and their minds were complacent. I was upset when they talked of how good it was going to be when they were big earners and big spenders. They seemed to look on life processes and illness processes as things which enabled you to earn £4,000 a year [in 1974!] and screw a few nurses.

Things became clearer when I went to Cambridge to do Second MB, two years of anatomy, physiology, and biochemistry. For a long while I had considered myself neither male nor female, human rather. Now I was sitting in lecture rooms whose words told me outright it was no accident women's brains were smaller than men's. The implicit orthodoxy of the medical faculty allowed them (women) two possibilities only. Either you could be an easy lay and preferably dumb, or you could be miraculously hard-working and reticent. If you were neither you felt lost.

Medicine was only rarely Elizabeth Garrett Anderson, mainly it was Doctor in the House and lascivious mnemonics. A lot of the teachers were men in their fifties and sixties who had gone into academic medicine because they weren't prepared to work in the National Health Service when it was introduced in 1948. They tended to restrain their sexism until very drunk, then it came out in venomous laughter. 'But of course women are incapable of being doctors.'

Doing anatomy taught me a lot about the extent to which the human body has been defined as male. Women are described only when their anatomy differs from men's. I suggested this to one of the men on the course when we came to study sex organs. His eyes went cold with impatience: 'I suppose you think it's sexist that the instruction sheet for the dissection starts with male genitals.' (Anne Scott, Spare Rib, *22)*

The fact that patients come to see us with problems other than simply of diagnosis was recognized in our training, but not solved. It was somehow implied that our expertise in physical diagnosis (and perhaps our innate and god-given superiority?) should equip us to advise and make decisions for our patients. The presence of moral issues was recognized and often discussed but with no critical framework. The personal beliefs and prejudices of the particular practitioner concerned were decisive. The fact that this involved power relationships between doctor and patient was never discussed.

I saw the way nurses were treated (ordered around and condescended to), the way ward aides would melt away from the gaze of doctors as they entered the wards, the slapping of physiotherapists' bottoms. The contradictions were reinforced by my discovery that my identification with nurses was not welcome (they were suspicious of women playing at doctors, just as they felt disgust at the thought of male nurses doing work normally considered fit only for females). The supposedly benevolent nature of medicine was belied daily on the wards as patients were not listened to, talked down to, made the subject of long irrelevant discussions (usually just within earshot), and sometimes used as research material without their full understanding. (Barbara Jacobs, Spare Rib, 26)

A glance at Jeffcoate's standard textbook of gynaecology* gives us some idea of where doctors get their attitude to women from. Apparently 'girls' experience period pains because 'their outlook on sex, health and menstruation is faulty', and pre-menstrual tension is the result of 'The underlay of over-anxiety and emotional instability . . . [which] makes it necessary to regard the condition as a psychosomatic disorder . . . there is nearly always a fundamental constitutional weakness which makes the individual fail to cope with the ordinary day-to-day stresses of life.' Is it any wonder if we sometimes feel we are banging our heads against a brick wall when we try to explain how we feel to our doctors?

Nursing – The Lady and the Lamp?

In the last few years an increasing number of men have entered nursing and (inevitably?) many of them have risen to the administrative grades. As a result titles like 'sister' and 'matron' are being phased out in favour of 'charge nurse' and 'nursing officer'. The same logic has not been applied to the case of women rising to the top of the medical profession and becoming 'fellows' or 'masters' of the Royal Colleges. However, in spite of this concern for male nurses, women still make up 89% of the profession. It is traditionally a 'woman's job' and the romantic side of it emerged

---

* 1975 edition of *Principles of Gynaecology* by Sir Norman Jeffcoate, Butterworths.

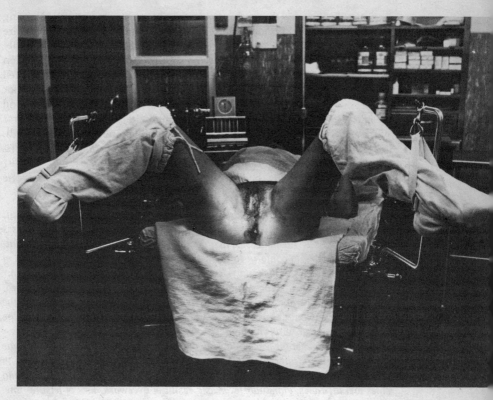

The obstetrician-gynaecologist's view of women

from fiction into reality when Enoch Powell, as Health Minister, suggested that their low wages were justified by their marriage prospects.

Up until the Crimean War nursing as a profession did not exist and what nursing there was could not have been described as romantic. The war created a surplus of well-bred young ladies who, with no chance of a husband, were looking for respectable independence. It was those women, organized by Florence Nightingale, who created nursing as it is today. Until they arrived on the scene and licked the filthy hospitals of the day into something more resembling the Victorian middle-class home, nursing had been the job of down-and-outs, acting as cleaners in the hospitals. The gentry had always been attended by their servants at home. The Victorian influence didn't only affect the hygiene, it imbued nursing with a high-flown moral tone which it still attempts to keep up today.

Under the present system there are three grades of nurses: untrained Auxiliaries, semi-trained State Enrolled Nurses, and fully-trained State

Registered Nurses (the only grade eligible for promotion). Nursing auxiliaries are paid more than student nurses, so women who are interested in nursing but cannot afford to train because of family commitments are attracted to the job and then find that they are often expected to do the work of trained staff. Lower qualifications are accepted for SEN training than for the SRN course but there is no channel for advancement. The SEN qualification is not accepted outside Britain, and foreign women coming here to train are often channelled into this course without being aware that they will not get qualifications to go home with. They become instead the NHS's source of low paid labour, easily dispensed with in times of unemployment.

The SRN training is the first step on the promotion ladder. Here is one woman's experience of training at a London hospital:

Long hours, extra duties, tiredness, night duty — lots of it, bedpans, vomit, sputum, blood, a rigid class system from maids and porters through nurses and technicians to medical students, doctors and God himself, the Consultant. One was expected to conform to the stereotyped image of the ideal nurse full of meekness and self-sacrifice, naivety, lack of individuality and awareness of our position as a mere nurse, a smiling slave. At one of the first lectures I attended, we were told that one doesn't discuss politics, sex, or religion, on or off the ward. We spent only three weeks a year in the lecture room. The rest of the year was practical with an emphasis on bedpans.

We lived in constant fear of nursing officers and sisters, trying to bring some status into their 'inferior' profession and status by using male methods to control and keep so-called order. The result was injustice, strict and inhuman rules and attitudes, glandular fever as a result of overwork, lack of leisure time, short holidays, and bad diet from hospital canteens. We were encouraged to join that right-wing watchdog of the nursing hierarchy, the Royal College of Nursing.

A possible reward for taking all this shit was marriage to a nice young doctor. 'Nice' meaning a right-wing, pompous, rugger-playing, sexist (unpleasantly so) consumer of large quantities of alcohol. If you resisted the stereotyping, punishment ranged from being ostracized or picked on incessantly, to constant fear of expulsion or exam failure.

At present midwifery is a specialization on its own. It can be studied as a postgraduate course for nurses or as a subject on its own without other training. It is likely, however, that in the future all midwives will have to train as nurses first.

From Where We Lie

How do we, as patients, experience the hospital system? Obviously our experiences vary according to what we are suffering from, where we live, our class and colour, our knowledge and ability to express what we feel. There are times when we are very ill or very frightened when we may find the rigid atmosphere reassuring; at those times the total abdication of responsibility for our bodies may seem welcome. The health service is at its best when dealing with crises; it is when we are feeling well enough to care that the system appears at its most oppressive. When we are having babies, or being examined for infection, we do not want to be taken over and managed by an efficient army of people trained to do a certain job a certain way and not to take our needs into account.

Here is a comment from a woman who had a baby at Hackney Hospital a few years ago (Hackney Women's Paper).

I asked for the father of my baby to be with me at the time of confinement. A sister told me, 'We do not allow the father of the child to be there or just in special cases. Besides you are unmarried and foreign and think of how many English wives would like to have their husbands with them.'

And here is another experience of hospital from a woman who was suffering from a severe drug reaction:

Group gathers at end of bed — consultant surrounded by registrars, students, ward sisters, etc. I am not consulted. 'How old is she?' — to sister — 'Get that thing off her' (my nightie) 'What does she want to wear those for?' (Cotton briefs under my short nightie protecting their blasted sheets from possible menstrual leakage) — 'no wonder she's got a rash', and so on. The group then continued to waffle on a few feet away unaware that my rising blood pressure left my hearing unaffected, each airing their pet theories — including the psychosomatic bit from the registrar and the consultant's assumption that I had been self-medicating — Why not ask me? — I've repressed most of it except the feeling of fury and frustration at being treated like an insentient slab of flesh, spotty to boot. I knew what caused the reaction and my subsequent refusal of the suspect drug and consequent improvement justified my conviction.

Although the quotes we have used in this book do not necessarily reflect the opinion of a balanced sample of health service employees and users, they do reflect the same concern about the entrenched conservatism and elitism of the medical profession and show how these attitudes, far from being the harmless eccentricities of otherwise compassionate and efficient health workers, affect staff morale and patient care. We have not described in detail the good experiences that some of us have had in hospitals because we feel that good care should be the rule and not, as it is fast becoming, the exception. We realize too that only a small proportion of people complain about their treatment but we feel that this reflects our expectations of medical treatment. It is only when we come together to talk about our experiences that we begin to realize that the individual bad experiences are not exceptions, that we are not merely 'complainers' and that we are not unreasonable in our demands.

We cannot simply dispense with trained medical personnel. Those years of detailed study in any field of medicine are important to us, but we can demand that health workers (particularly doctors) use their information responsibly and put their technical skills at our disposal rather than using them to enhance their own status.

Patients' Rights in Hospital

We have only three 'rights' and two of them are negative.

1. We may refuse treatment.
2. We may refuse to be used for teaching.
3. We have a right to competent treatment – as defined by the doctors themselves.

Here is an adaptation of a model bill of rights for hospital patients. It was originally compiled by George Annas for the American Civil Liberties union. We feel it is something to work towards. Its language is precise. Where it refers to a 'legal right', it is a right recognized by law. Where it states 'right' it would probably be recognized under clause 3 above, in a court of law. Where it says 'we recognize the right', it refers to what ought to be. Those rights marked with an asterisk exist in law in the USA but not in Britain.

The model bill is set out as it would apply to a patient in his or her chronological relations with the hospital: sections 1–4 for a person not hospitalized but a *potential* patient; 5 for emergency admission; 6–15 for in-patients; 16–19 for discharge and after discharge; and 20 relating back to all 20 rights.

1. We recognize the patient's right to informed participation in all decisions involving his/her health care.
2. We recognize the right of all potential patients to know what research and experiments are being used in the hospital and what alternatives are available elsewhere.
3. We recognize the right of a potential patient to complete and accurate information concerning medical care and procedures.
4. The patient has a right to prompt attention, especially in an emergency situation.*
5. We recognize the right to a clear, concise explanation in layperson's terms of all proposed procedures, including the possibilities of any risk of mortality or

serious side effects, problems related to recuperation, and probability of success.*

6. The patient has a legal right not to be subjected to any procedure without his/her voluntary, competent and understanding consent. The specifics of such consent shall be set out in a written consent form, signed by the patient.

(This is of particular importance to us. We are under no obligation to sign consent-forms until we have *read* them, *understood* them and *freely consented* to what is in them. We may insist on amending them if we so wish.)

7. The patient has a right to a clear, complete, and accurate evaluation of his/her condition and prognosis without treatment before being asked to consent to any test or procedure.*

8. We recognize the right of the patient to know the identity and professional status of all those providing service. All personnel have been instructed to introduce themselves, state their status, and explain their role in the health care of the patient. Part of this right is the right of the patient to know the identity of the physician responsible for his/her care.

9. We recognize the right of any patient who does not speak English to have access to an interpreter.

10. We recognize the right of the patient to all the information contained in his/her medical record while in the hospital, and to examine the record on request.

We recognize the right of a patient to discuss his/her condition with a consultant specialist, at the patient's request.

11. The patient has a legal right not to have any test or procedure, designed for educational purposes rather than his/her direct personal benefit, performed on him/her.

12. The patient has a legal right to refuse any particular drug, test, procedure, or treatment.

13. We recognize the right to privacy of both person and information with respect to: the hospital staff, other doctors, residents, interns and medical students, researchers, nurses, other hospital personnel, and other patients.*

14. We recognize the patient's right of access to people outside the hospital by means of visitors and the telephone. Parents may stay with their children and relatives with terminally ill patients 24 hours a day.

15. The patient has a legal right to leave the hospital.

16. The patient has a legal right to leave the hospital regardless of his/her physical condition, although the patient may be requested to sign a release stating that he/she is leaving against the medical judgement of his/her doctor or the hospital.

17. We recognize the right of the patient not to be transferred to another hospital unless he/she has received a complete explanation of the desirability and need for the transfer, the other hospital has accepted the patient for transfer, and the patient has agreed to transfer. If the patient does not agree to transfer, the patient has the right to a consultant's opinion on the desirability of transfer.

18. We recognize the right of the patient to be notified of his/her impending discharge at least one day before it is accomplished, to insist on a consultation by an expert on the desirability of discharge, and to have a person of the patient's choice notified in advance.

19. At the termination of his/her stay at the hospital we recognize the right of a patient to a complete copy of the information contained in his/her medical record.

20. We recognize the right of all patients to have 24-hour-a-day access to a patient's rights advocate who may act on behalf of the patient to assert or protect the rights set out in this document. (George Annas believes, and we agree, that 'a statement of rights alone is insufficient. What is needed in addition is someone, whom I term an advocate, to assist patients in asserting their rights. As indicated previously, this advocate is necessary because a sick person's first concern is to regain health, and in pursuit of health patients are willing to give up rights that they otherwise would vigorously assert'.)

Even the few rights we have are often ignored. It is common to hear of patients being examined by students without being asked for their permission. Most patients are too embarrassed and overawed to complain. Many people are given treatments they would rather not have, by default; either they are not told what they are being given or they sign a consent form without being given the time or help to read and understand it. Our right to competent treatment is so hard to define that few people complain unless 'incompetence' is of proportions that cannot be ignored.

For many of us the hospital atmosphere combined with our own illness renders us incapable of defending ourselves. Some women's groups have taken up the idea of 'patient advocacy' by accompanying each other to doctors and confronting the system with support. This idea could be extended if community advocacy groups could be organized locally around hospitals.

General Practitioners (Family Doctors)

General practitioners are doctors who, having completed their basic medical training in a hospital, have been registered by the General Medical Council and set up in practice to provide 'general medical services'. Most GPs will have done 1 year's traineeship with a practising GP before starting practice (this will soon be compulsory) and some will have done 2 years extra in a hospital. Once they are registered, GPs may either start up their own practice, or join an existing group practice or partnership or a health centre.

HOW THEY ARE PAID (figures for November 1977)

A basic salary of £2,595 plus capitation fees per patient per year: £2.45 for patients under 65, £3.35 for those between 65 and 75 and £4.00 for patients above that age. In addition the BMA fought and won an extra allowance for giving family planning advice on the grounds that it is non-medical! That means an extra £3.50 usually for writing a prescription for the Pill; for fitting an IUD, £10. Then there are certain extra sums, for example: for night visits (£4.60), for every patient above the first 1,000 (47p), maternity work (£35.75 with obstetrical training and £20.85 without), cervical smears in specified cases (£2.30). There is an inducement of £420 for working in a group practice and added allowances for working in undesirable areas. The DHSS considers that £8,818 per annum should be the average net income (after overheads) that a GP should earn (in 1977). Allowances for expenses such as receptionists' salaries and equipment are paid on top – as long as the services of receptionist are not provided by the doctor's wife who is not considered an employee and is therefore expected to work for free (it is not clear whether the reverse would be true if the wife was a doctor and the husband a receptionist). In an urban area most doctors earn more than the minimum and many of them do extra work in clinics or hospitals for which they are paid sessional fees.

It is clear from the structure of GPs' pay that male patients are considered the norm: almost all the regular health work for women comes under a special category with extra pay. It seems absurd that a doctor can be paid more for work such as contraception advice than for the total care of the rest of our bodies, and this added inducement has meant that a large number of doctors are now giving contraceptive 'advice' without the necessary training. It is common for GPs to write Pill prescriptions year after year without even a blood pressure check.

CHOOSING A DOCTOR

Everyone, whether living temporarily or permanently in this country, is entitled to free medical care and to register with a general practitioner. Visitors to Britain are entitled to the same treatment for any diseases, accidents, etc. which occur while in this country (e.g. you cannot get an NHS abortion if you became pregnant before entering this country).

In order to sign on to a doctor's list he must first accept you, and sign your medical card. If you do not have a card the doctor will give you a form to fill in after which a card will be sent to you. If you have lost your card, write to the Family Practitioner Committee for a new one (address and phone number in the phone book).

It is important to register with a doctor before you actually need one so that you can make sure you do not end up registering in an emergency with someone you dislike. You can change your doctor (see p. 557) but it is a hassle worth avoiding. Lists of doctors should be available from the Community Health Council, Library, Citizens' Advice Bureau, Post Office or Family Practitioner Committee. The names on the list should have coded letters after them to tell you a little about their qualifications.

'M' means maternity – the doctor is trained in obstetrics. 'MSO' means maternity only, not general practice. 'C' means contraception and that the doctor will prescribe for women other than those on his normal list. 'C*' means contraceptives may be prescribed for those women on his list only. 'CSO' means contraceptive work only, and 'X' means limited list, the doctor will only take a certain number of patients so the list may be full. There may also be other letters indicating that the doctor has taken specialist examinations. If you want to know more consult the Medical Directory in the library – this has pocket histories of each doctor in it. However, the best way of finding a good doctor is usually by word of mouth.

Contact the doctors in your immediate area. Make sure they are convenient to get to. If a doctor has room on the list ask for an appointment *before* registering. If you live in a rural area you may not have a choice but it is still worth visiting your doctor before you become ill. Here is a list of questions to ask at your initial visit.

1. Is there an appointment or open surgery system? Appointments often cut down on waiting time but are inconvenient if you don't have a phone.
2. If an appointment system, do they allow exceptions? Some surgeries will try to fit you in if you turn up. How long must you wait for an appointment? (3–5 days in some group practices.)
3. How long is the average waiting time at the surgery?
4. What is the attitude to home visits? Some doctors expect you to come to the surgery unless you are virtually unable to move.
5. Are there any surgeries after working hours or at weekends?
6. Is the doctor easily available in emergencies and what kind of locum cover will there be?
7. If it is a group practice can you always see the same doctor?
8. What is the doctor's attitude to babies and small children (if relevant)? Some doctors cannot cope with them and wise ones will say so.
9. What is the doctor's attitude to (a) birth control – will s/he prescribe, and is s/he trained in contraceptive work? (b) abortion – does s/he consider the choice to be yours? (c) how does s/he feel about home births? is s/he trained in obstetrics and could s/he arrange delivery in a GP unit?
10. Does s/he have private patients? This could mean that they will be getting a better service in which case you won't be getting the best care.
11. Is s/he a member of any health service committees? If so, s/he is likely to have good hospital contacts which can be useful.

Not all these questions will be relevant to you and there may be other ones which you consider more so, but one of the most important considerations is how the doctor deals with your questioning. If he is impatient or irritable it is likely that you will find the same attitude to medical questions at a later date.

GROUP OR SOLO PRACTICE

There is a tendency for younger doctors to join up with others in group practices, health centres or partnerships. There is a financial advantage to them in doing this because the cost of overheads is shared, and government grants are available. Doctors on their own are paying for everything out of their own pockets. A financial advantage to them should be passed on to you in better facilities. They can afford to buy more expensive diagnostic equipment which saves time waiting for samples to be sent away. Often they will have a district nurse, midwife or health visitor attached to the practice. The doctors often share night and weekend duty so you are likely to see someone you know. On the other hand, you may get impersonal, conveyor-belt treatment from a different doctor at each visit. A doctor in a solo practice may develop a more personal relationship with you and therefore a better understanding of your needs. On the other hand s/he may be very overworked, get little time off, and employ emergency locums who don't know you. Probably the best solution is a group practice where you can always see the same doctor.

CHANGING YOUR DOCTOR

Your GP need not be yours for life. If you move you can automatically change to a new doctor nearer your home. If you decide to part company for other reasons there are mechanisms for that too.

1. If you are merely moving to a new address (it doesn't have to be outside your present doctor's area) you sign part A on your medical card and then give it to your new doctor who should sign part A as well. The new doctor then sends the card to the Family Practitioner Committee who will send you a new one.
2. If you want to change for any other reason there are two methods of doing it.
(a) You can ask your doctor to release you by signing part B of your card which you must complete. Then take the card to the new doctor who must sign part A and send it to the FPC.
(b) If you would rather not ask your doctor to sign the card, you can yourself send it to the FPC. They will return it with a slip which allows you to transfer not sooner than 2 weeks and not more than 6 weeks after they received it. You then complete part 1 of the slip and take it to your new doctor who must sign and send your card to the FPC for replacement. If you've lost your card, you will have to ask for an application form which you will send with your letter of transfer.

Doctors are often unhappy about taking another doctor's patients. According to the Patients' Association, doctors in some areas are operating a 'gentleman's agreement' not to take patients from their colleagues.

The PA's advice is: 'Write to the FPC and tell them you no longer wish to be on the list of Dr X. Then go to the new doctor of your choice and say you don't have a GP.' If you cannot find any doctor to accept you, you must send your card to the FPC listing the doctors who have refused you. You will then be allocated a doctor.

MANAGING YOUR DOCTOR

More than any other person, your GP should be a partner in your health care. The function of this 'primary' level of the Health Service is to help you deal with general health problems which do not require hospitalization or a great deal of specialist knowledge for diagnosis. The advantage of having one doctor who keeps your records and acts as a funnel to other areas of the health service is that he or she should be able to treat your body as a whole, not just a back, or a womb or an area of skin. Many of our health problems are interconnected and the increasing specialization of medicine can prevent you or your doctors from making the right connections. Your GP should be keeping track of your whole body health to prevent this compartmentalization. Unfortunately many doctors are not prepared to listen to their patients for long enough to help them make those connections. Mistaken diagnosis and inappropriate prescription may be a direct result of a doctor's inability to listen and to explain. If doctors are to be brought into a health *partnership* with us, the impetus has to come from us. Here are some ideas which may help you to help your doctor.

1. When you meet your doctor for the first time introduce yourself and shake him by the hand. Even if you are not a natural hand-shaker the gesture will probably bring him to his feet and to eye level. It is better to meet eyeball to eyeball rather than as a supplicant when he wearily raises his eyes from writing his notes to give you the once-over.
2. Go through the list of questions on p. 556 if this is your first appointment.
3. For subsequent appointments, make a list of *all* symptoms whether they appear to be related or not. Don't allow yourself to be dismissed, or any conclusions to be drawn until you've got through the list. Don't feel guilty about the others in the waiting-room. One thorough discussion at this stage may cut out future ones. It might help you to write down symptoms as they appear. It isn't always easy to remember when a pain or discharge etc. actually started.
4. If you are given a prescription ask what it is, how to use it, and how long to take it for. Doctors can instruct the chemist to leave the label and instructions in the pack by ticking a box on the prescription form with the letters NP in it. They should be encouraged to do so.
5. If you don't understand what your doctor is saying, never be ashamed to ask him to repeat it more slowly and simply.
6. If you are worried or anxious you may forget what a doctor has said, take a note pad with you and write it down.

7. If you don't feel confident you might like to have someone with you to ask the questions you feel too confused to ask.

8. Finally, we should remember that doctors are human too and they respond better to friendly familiarity than hostility.

OVER-PRESCRIBING

There are more people in this country taking tranquillizers regularly than in any other country in the world. Twelve per cent of British women take tranquillizers daily for a month or more every year. The result, according to one psychiatrist, is often no more than converting 'an anxious but clear-headed person into an anxious but woozy-headed person'.

It isn't only tranquillizers that are ladled out with apparent abandon. Antibiotics are also over-used; they are often prescribed for minor infections which would cure themselves and for viral infections which they do not cure. They are not always given in the appropriate dose with clear instructions that the course must be completed, and doctors are often lazy about getting culture tests done to make sure that the appropriate antibiotic is being prescribed. If these drugs are misused the bacteria will quickly adapt and become resistant to them and far more difficult to budge. The wrong medication may actually lower resistance to infection by disturbing the natural balance of bacteria in the body, and many women instantly develop a fungal infection if they are given antibiotics. So they shouldn't be prescribed unnecessarily.

But over-prescribing is not only the doctor's fault. Sometimes we demand concrete evidence of our doctors' concern or expect them to deal with our social problems, and doctors respond by providing signed evidence of illness. If we are to be participants in, rather than victims of, health care, we must learn to question our doctors, find out if medication is really necessary and try to avoid swallowing drugs which are unnecessary or bad for us.

Organizing for Change

Women have long recognized that the control of our health and fertility is central to the control of our lives and that while it is in the hands of male-identified lawmakers and doctors our freedom even to work for change will be severely curtailed. In many countries over recent years — America, Canada, Belgium, Italy, Chile, France etc. — women and men have faced prison sentences for their courageous work in opposing restrictive laws and organizing illegal abortion clinics and referral centres. In

America the success of the abortion campaign brought together women who are now fighting for broader changes. Self-help groups and health clinics have been started so that women can learn more about their bodies and get treatment from sympathetic people at low prices. Fighting for possession of our own bodies is a very radicalizing experience.

So what about Britain? The health movement here is gradually beginning to gather force. The abortion debate has re-emerged with greater intensity, and cuts in health service spending have made us aware that our free health system is under threat. These two issues have brought many women into the broad health movement through local groups to defend and extend the Abortion Act, and campaigns against hospital closures and cuts in public health expenditure.

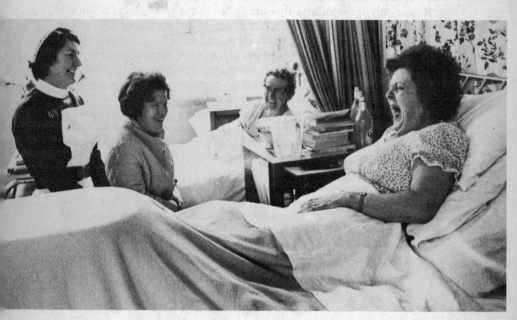

Elizabeth Garrett Anderson hospital, the only hospital in the UK run for and by women — recently saved from closure after a year's campaign

This rekindling of concern about health is encouraging, but there is a danger that those important principles about the quality of care which are at the heart of the women's health movement will get swamped in an attempt to keep the health service intact. Women are suffering from inhumane treatment in some of those very hospitals we are trying to defend, and at the hands — or tongues — of some of those health workers whose jobs we are fighting to protect. The contradictions get sharper as money becomes more scarce. We must avoid neglecting the content of the NHS while trying to preserve the form.

Everywhere health workers are being politicized by struggles against redundancies and worsening working conditions. The situation is ripe for radical changes. In every hospital, particularly where defence committees are organized, feminists could try to set up (or join), patients' committees and insist on discussing the kind of service we are protecting and how it can be changed. We must have the courage to join those organizations which have sprung up to defend the rights of health workers and fight there for our own rights and the rights of all patients to the care we need.

EDUCATING OURSELVES

One of the underlying principles of the women's liberation movement is that we should educate ourselves to understand our oppression before we can change it. Health groups are run on the same principles and these small local groups are the core of the movement. We teach ourselves and help others to learn through self-help.

Self-Help

Self-help is women sharing experiences, knowledge, and feelings — women supporting each other and learning together. Self-help begins by working from a practical base, starting with learning from physical self-examination (see p. 135), finding out what we *do* know, what we do *not* know, what we *want* to know and exploring from there.

Self-help groups are action-oriented. One self-help group might investigate menopause, another human sexuality, another lesbian health issues, another might train as paramedics and health counsellors. The possibilities are endless, depending only on our own creativity and needs.

Self-help is women relating to ourselves in order to demystify health care, the professionals and our own bodies; it involves being able to make personal choices based on our own very valid experiences and knowledge. Self-help is a positive action by which we can change our own lives and those of our sisters.

Self-help is a political act. It is deeply challenging to the existing health care system. Through sharing our knowledge collectively we have developed skills — we, not only the 'professionals', will know what is done to us medically and why it is done. We do not take the place of the doctor, but we *do* reverse the patriarchal-authority-doctor-over-'patient' roles.

Self-help represents a wide range of activities. Here are a few examples:

● A group of teenage women getting together for the first time to discuss many of the issues in this book.
● A group of women committed over a period of time to trying to change medical and health care practices at a local hospital.
● A group of women doing original research in areas vital to better health care for women.
● A group of new mothers getting together weekly to help one another cope with postpartum problems and experiences.

As we learn more about our own bodies and minds through self-examination and consciousness-raising we can pass our information on to others in a number of ways: we can help other women to start groups like our own; we can write pamphlets out of our joint experience of health care combined with a guide to local facilities and conditions; we can organize courses on self-help through the Workers' Education Association or by linking up with teachers in local schools or colleges; we can rent cheap short-life property from the council to start a women's centre where we can do pregnancy testing, provide information on local facilities and hold discussions on all aspects of our health; we can use our centres to spread information on self-help, and as campaign headquarters.

Women's Publications

Many women's groups have produced material from their own discussion and research. It covers a wide range and more is being printed all the time, so we can only produce a very selective list in the Bibliography. When work is produced by our sisters we spend less time trying to read between the lines wondering what the researchers have overlooked. Three regular publications are particularly useful – they are: *WIRES*, a bi-weekly newsletter for the women's liberation movement; *Women's Report*, a bi-monthly round up of women's news with two or three pages on the latest health information from a critical feminist perspective in every issue: and *Spare Rib*, a monthly magazine with regular, longer articles on health issues (see p. 570).

Conference reports and campaign pamphlets are also packed with useful information, and some groups have published area guides on health issues.

Information Services, Helping Organizations and Pressure Groups

Almost all the organizations which advise or refer people on health or related problems have their own educational branch and often full-time press officers to disseminate information. A need for help is usually accompanied by a need for change, and organizations which provide help such as Release (abortion referrals and help to drug addicts etc.), MIND (help and campaigning for mental patients' rights), and all the rest usually produce information about the work they do to encourage that change.

Pressure groups have been started on every conceivable subject. They collect and collate information which is used to impress government bureaucrats and MPs. Many of them also take up individual cases. One of the most important organizations for us is the Patients' Association, which has an unrivalled knowledge of complaints procedures and the red tape of the Department of Health. It is well worth joining the Association if only for the informative newsletter. Other groups which can provide information are: The Child Poverty Action Group (information on women and children on low incomes), The Consumer Association (produces reports some of which are on medicines or aspects of medical care); The Birth Control Trust produces statistics on birth control.

Pressure groups have their limitations as campaigning bodies, which we will discuss later.

ORGANIZING WOMEN'S GROUPS

Groups within the women's movement have tried to avoid building structures with leaders at the top, which is why self-education is important to us. But organizing loose structures so that everyone moves together is harder and more demanding than using the old authoritarian chains of command. The women's movement is still trying to find ways of coordinating on a national scale. Regular conferences are our most important link. They are held locally, regionally, nationally and on specialist issues.

It doesn't take much to start a new group. Just a few women meeting regularly in someone's house is all you need, and many women in the health movement will be happy to help you get off the ground (contact WIRES for addresses). It is important also to keep in contact with other groups in your area, through occasional meetings, a newsletter if there are enough of you and the invaluable method of the telephone circle. This last method requires careful organization but if it works, any person receiving information should be able to pass it on very quickly by contacting those immediately before and after her in the circle, who will in turn pass the message on. If every group subscribes to WIRES and sends in their own information as well as using others we will be better able to communicate nationally.

Mutual Help Organizations

There are a number of organizations which have set up local groups to provide mutual support for people in similar situations. They vary in the degree to which they are organized from above and the amount of political pressure they seek to exert on the authorities. These organizations are an important departure from the old 'do-gooding' organizations which strip people of the responsibility for their own lives. Although many of them are 'apolitical' and most of them would differ ideologically and structurally from women's liberation groups, there is a degree of overlap in some areas. Organizations of particular interest to us are: Association for Improvements in the Maternity Services (AIMS, see p. 487), which organizes local groups to change NHS practice all over the country; and Gingerbread, which is a network of groups for single parents. Others organize around alcoholism, obesity, hospitalized children, multiple sclerosis, etc. More and more people are recognizing the value of organizing in groups to analyse our own experience in order to counteract bureaucratic oppression and give each other comfort and support.

Pressure Groups

Some of these groups are extraordinarily successful in fighting for limited reform. However, they are limited as campaigning bodies because they operate through changing the minds of the people in power, rather than spreading ideas through the mass of people who can then take them up and if necessary defend them. They tend also to work *for* minority groups rather than helping those people to work for themselves, and they are therefore often responsible for reinforcing rather than dispelling misinformation about the fringe nature or abnormality of the people they are fighting for.

Two examples of campaigns in which limited reforms have actually hampered more radical progress are the 1967 abortion campaign and the campaign for homosexual equality. The debate on homosexuality presented homosexuals as abnormal people in need of compassion. It did not assert their right to equal treatment and they are therefore still oppressed by restrictive laws. It was not until the start of the Gay Liberation Front and the women's movement that homosexuality was presented in a positive light. Similarly, the abortion law, by putting the abortion decision into the hands of doctors rather than women, has reinforced the idea of women as mindless creatures who are unable to make their own decisions and need to be *protected* by a restrictive law. It did not activate the mass of women and as a result we were not ready to defend the law in 1975 when anti-abortionists attacked it under the pretence of *'protecting us'*.

In both these cases, limited reforms have, in the short term, alleviated much distress. While it is possible that mass campaigns would have been impossible to launch at the time the reforms were achieved, we must learn by the results of such campaigns that only changes which are demanded by all of us can be defended by all of us.

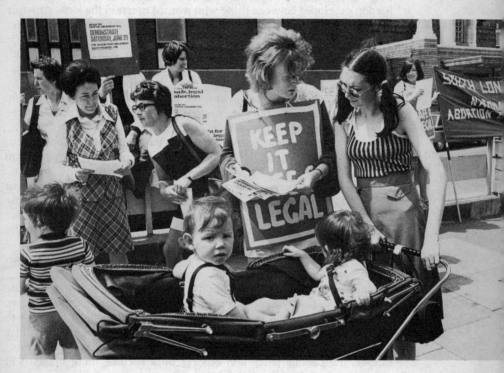

Campaigning for abortion rights

Campaigning

The most important national campaign to be fought on a health issue was started in March 1975 when women from a number of organizations realized that even the liberalization given us by the 1967 Abortion Act was threatened. The organization and history of this campaign serves as an important example to us.

The *National Abortion Campaign* which was quickly formed to fight the Abortion (Amendment) Bill (see p. 296) is worked out on lines as close as possible to the structural principles of the women's movement. Based on NAC groups which bring together people from different organizations at local level, the campaign is then coordinated through national planning meetings, which are open to all members of the campaign, and organized on a day-to-day basis by one or two full-time workers and a steering committee of volunteers which is itself open to new members.

In the first few months the overriding urgency of the situation brought people from different political backgrounds together, but as time wore on friction developed between those who wanted to retain the loose structure and others from some more traditional organizations who argued for their own hierarchical structures and tactics. Feminists in local groups as well as on the steering committee had to learn very fast to deal with the confrontal tactics of other organizations, a far cry from the cooperation with which the women's movement has always tried to organize. Many feminists felt unable to continue working in this atmosphere, and feeling angry and frustrated they withdrew. Several groups disintegrated under the strain of conflicting strategies.

Other feminists stayed on to argue for their own politics, and in some areas feminist NAC groups were formed. The Abortion Law Reform Association, which had become 'A Woman's Right to Choose Campaign', attracted some women who wanted to remain in the campaign but felt unhappy working in their NAC group. Fortunately, the loose structure of NAC allowed women to cope with these problems. The fact that local groups do not have to adhere to any 'line' and can organize independently has kept the campaign going. However, the experience of NAC has taught many of us the importance of formulating our own policies and fighting for them rather than giving up.

Many feminists avoid trade unions and socialist organizations because they see them simply as organs of male power in a slightly different guise. There are, however, a large and growing number of us who want to inject feminist principles into socialist politics. This will have particular relevance for those of us in the health movement, as the public sector unions, the Labour party and other groups become more involved in campaigns to defend the NHS. It is hard to intervene in these organizations without getting swamped, and most of us prefer to organize through the support of our own groups, joining with others where necessary. For those of us who have not ventured into the world of organized politics, here are some suggestions.

1. Never go to a meeting alone. It is easier to speak in public if you have support.
2. Find out the agenda of the meeting in advance so that you can discuss it in your group and get your thoughts straight. Other organizations do it all the time, that's why they always seem to present solutions before the rest of us have digested the questions.
3. Once you have found your feet, argue for de-formalizing meetings; rotate the chairperson every week; rotate minute-taking (make sure that the men do not always leave this to the women); get everyone to introduce themselves and say who (if anyone) they represent, if the meeting is small enough to make this convenient.

In-groups, hierarchies, and paternalism thrive on structure and organization. If you take the rules away you may not have pulled the rug out from under their feet, but you will have tweaked it at least.

4. Try and work out early on who comes from what organization. That way you can discover if you are participating in a discussion or a head-on clash between opposing party 'lines' in which case, don't expect to have an instant effect on decision-making: it will take perseverance.

5. Don't get sucked into trying to beat them at their own game. Do your damndest to change the rules. Feminist ideas depend not only on the outcome but on the mode of organization.

Alternatives to the Existing Services

While working to change the existing system, we can think about setting up alternatives. Since NHS services are free, most of us would be loath to set up a service for which women have to pay. But we can start looking for ways to set up alternatives within the NHS.

Some people feel that we should not use our energy to set up isolated clinics where only a few women can be treated rather than pressurizing the DHSS to set up a network of clinics. But isolated clinics would provide models. It is, after all, not only the content of the service which we would like to change, but the whole structure. We want to examine the relationship of medical personnel to us and to each other. We know that our minds and our bodies are indivisible. We want a medical service that recognizes this and provides support groups and counselling for us to talk about our health, particularly if we are making a decision which could affect our whole lives: whether or not to have an abortion, a hysterectomy, a breast operation, etc. We want clinics which focus on prevention rather than cure and therefore actively encourage people to examine their own bodies, discuss their health and participate in their own care.

A clinic which provides the whole range of diagnostic facilities but does not question the relationship of trained to untrained people would merely be a well-equipped clinic and nothing else. The Well Woman Centre at Marie Stopes House, London, was started to provide the sort of alternative we describe, unfortunately outside the NHS. Many women who have had bad treatment from their GPs have found the clinic helpful and friendly by comparison and have been willing to pay for their treatment. However, the clinic has not lived up to its original plans. The hierarchical structure is still very much in evidence and any improvement in relationship between medical staff and patient comes more from the attitudes of individuals working there than an attempt to change old patterns.

One way in which, theoretically at least, we could set up alternatives within the NHS is through general practice. As GPs are not employed by the NHS but are under contract, they can provide any kind of service as long as the people on their list are adequately cared for. Feminist GPs could divide up their practice allowance and the allowance for ancillary workers to pay a group of counsellors and paramedics on a sessional basis. The doctor would still have to be responsible for all the prescribing and for providing a full service for all patients of either sex, but it would be possible to run a few sessions a week for women, with group discussions, counselling and self-help as optional extras for all.

This model is by no means ideal, as it is based on the willingness of doctors to change their patterns of work. They would in the end have total financial control. It might, however, serve as an intermediate step and demonstrate that a different approach to medical care is not only possible but desirable.

There are many possibilities for the future and one way or another, medical care is going to have to change to put the emphasis on the causes of disease rather than the symptoms, prevention rather than cure. For us those changes will not be enough unless the power of the medical profession over our lives can be challenged and the relationship between people, health workers and doctors can be re-examined and re-structured. In the meantime we will have to cope with doctors and medicine as they are now. We hope that this book will have helped you to do that.

For organizations and addresses see below.

Women's Centres, Newsletters, General Resources

Some of these addresses may have changed by the time you read this, others may have disappeared completely. At the time of writing they are our most important sources of information.

HOW TO KEEP IN TOUCH

Health groups, e.g. self help or campaigning groups: address lists are available from WIRES (see below).

HealthRight (American feminist women's health magazine), 175 Fifth Avenue, New York, NY 10010, USA.

The Monthly Extract: An Irregular Periodical (Communications Network for gynaecological self-help clinics), Box 3488, Ridgeway Station, Stamford, Connecticut 06905, USA.

Scarlet Women, Socialist feminist magazine. From 5 Washington Terrace, North Shields, Tyne and Weir.

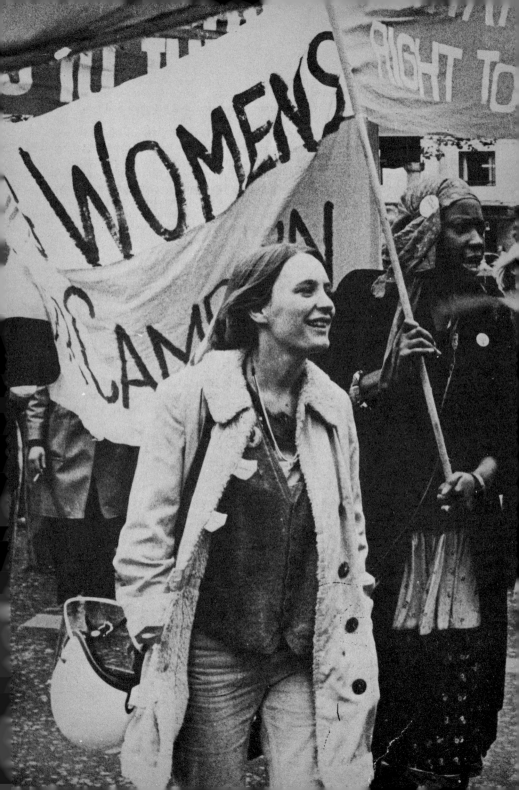

Spare Rib, a monthly women's liberation magazine. Available from bookshops and by subscription from Linda Phillips, 114 George Street, Berkhamsted, Herts. Interesting articles from a feminist viewpoint, lists activities and information on campaigns, arts, etc.

WIRES, 32a Parliament Street, York (York 35471). This produces the national newsletter of the women's liberation movement; it is also a phone-in information centre giving details of local women's groups, centres, etc.

Women's Report, a bi-monthly feminist magazine which includes a regularly up-dated health information section. Available from some bookshops and on sub-scription from Box 48, Rising Free, 182 Upper Street, London N1.

Women's Research and Resources Centre, 27 Clerkenwell Close, London EC1 (01 253 7568). Library, index of research on women, organizes talks.

ORGANIZATIONS*

Big Flame, 217 Wavertree Road, Liverpool 7 (051 263 1350). A revolutionary organization which is very active in the health service.

The Birth Control Campaign, Margaret Pyke House, 27/35 Mortimer Street, London W1A 4QW (01 580 9360).

The Consumer Association, 14 Buckingham Street, London WC1 (01 839 1222). Information on various socio/medical surveys, and tests of over-the-counter preparations.

Counter Information Services, 9 Poland Street, London WC1 (01 439 3764). Produces regular reports on various matters some of which are extremely useful to us, e.g. *Cutting the Welfare State, Unilever's World, Women and the Crisis.*

The Department of Health and Social Security, Press and PR, Alexander Fleming House, Elephant and Castle, London SE1 (01 407 5522).

Equal Opportunities Commission, Overseas House, Quay Street, Manchester 3 (061 933 9244); London office: 01 629 8233.

The King's Fund Centre, 126 Albert Street, London NW1 (01 267 6111). Charitable organization which aims to provide a forum for discussion and study of health issues and to help accelerate the introduction of 'good new ideas'. Has a library, runs conferences.

MIND (National Association for Mental Health), 22 Harley Street, London W1N 2ED (01 637 0741).

The National Council for Civil Liberties, 186 Kings Cross Road, London WC1 (01 278 4575). The NCCL women's rights officer deals with cases of sex dis-crimination. The women's committee produces useful pamphlets on current issues affecting women, analysing them from a legal and civil rights point of view.

The Patients' Association, 11 Dartmouth Street, London SW1H 9BN (01 222 4992).

Rights of Women (ROW), 374 Grays Inn Road, London WC1 (01 278 6349). Women legal workers' group, help women to understand law, help women's organizations campaigning against laws, help individuals with legal problems.

Socialist Medical Association, 9 Poland Street, London W1V 3OG (01 439 3395).

* For organizations working in specific areas, see the relevant chapters.

Women's Liberation Legal and Financial Independence Campaign, 214 Stapleton Road, London N4. Campaigns for the legal and financial independence of women.
Working Women's Charter Campaign, c/o 1a Camberwell Grove, London SE5. Set up to make links between the women's movement and the trade union movement through local groups.

FURTHER READINGS

Guides

Coote, A., and Gill, T., *Women's Rights – A Practical Guide*, Penguin, new edition, 1977. An excellent guide to our legal and economic rights (or lack of them).

Faulder, Jackson and Lewis, *The Women's Directory*, Virago, 1976. A directory of organizations and publications produced for and by women. Unfortunately dates fast and most of the listings are too short to be of lasting value. However, it is useful.

Grimstad, Kirsten, and Rennie, Susan (eds.), *The New Women's Survival Catalogue*, Knopf, 1975. An American book on everything – plenty of UK information, though obviously, some of it dated.

General Political Readings

Allen, Pamela, *Free Space: a perspective on the small group in women's liberation*, Times Change Press, 1970.

Bengis, Ingrid, *Combat in the Erogenous Zone – Writings on Love, Hate and Sex*, Wildwood House, 1973.

Chesler, Phyllis, *Women and Madness*, Allen Lane, 1974.

Comer, Lee, *The Myth of Motherhood*, B. Russell Peace Foundation, 1971.

Comer, Lee, *Wedlocked Women*, Feminist Books, 1974.

Conditions of Illusion, Feminist Books, 1976. Second Anthology of writings from the British women's movement.

Davis, Angela, *If They Come in the Morning*, Orbach and Chambers, 1971. Essays by black liberationists in the 1960s.

De Beauvoir, Simone, *The Second Sex*, Penguin, 1972. A classic which pre-dates the current women's movement. Many of us have learned from it.

Donnison, Jean, *Midwives and Medical Men, A History of Inter-Professional Rivalries and Women's Rights*. Heinemann, 1977. Careful documentation.

Engels, F., *Origin of the Family, Private Property and the State*, Pathfinder Press, 1972.

Firestone, Shulamith, *The Dialectic of Sex: the Case for Feminist Revolution*, Paladin, 1972.

Frankfort, Ellen, *Vaginal Politics*, Bantam Books, 1973. Obviously somewhat out of date, but a good read.

Friedan, Betty, *The Feminine Mystique*, Penguin 1965. An American classic on the condition of women in society.

Greer, Germaine, *The Female Eunuch*, Paladin, 1971. Heralded by the press as *the book on women's liberation*. It isn't, but it did have a big impact on women at the start of the British women's movement.

Heller, T., *Restructuring The Health Service*, Croom Helm, 1978. A useful book documenting the need for change in the NHS but limited by its omissions in relation to women.

Kollontai, Alexandra, *Sexual Relations and the Class Struggle*, Falling Wall Press, 1972.

Kollontai, Alexandra, *Selected Writings*, translated with an introduction and commentaries by Alix Holt, Allison & Busby, London, 1977.

Lerner, Gerda, *Black Women in White America*, Vintage, 1973. Anthology of essays.

Millett, Kate, *Sexual Politics*, Virago, 1977.

Millett, Kate, *The Prostitution Papers*, Paladin, 1975.

Mitchell, Juliet, *Woman's Estate*, Penguin, 1971.

Mitchell, Juliet, *Psychoanalysis and Feminism*, Penguin, 1974.

Mitchell, Juliet, and Oakley, Ann, *The Rights and Wrongs of Women*, Penguin, 1976. Collection of well-researched papers including an excellent one by Oakley on 'Wisewoman and Medical Man'.

Morgan, Robin (ed.), *Sisterhood is Powerful: an anthology of writings from the women's liberation movement*, Vintage Books, 1970.

Oakley, Ann, *Sex, Gender and Society*, Temple-Smith, 1972.

Reid, Willie May, *Black Women's Struggle for Equality*, Pathfinder Press pamphlet.

Rowbotham, Sheila, *Women's Liberation and the New Politics*, B. Russell Peace Foundation, 1971.

Rowbotham, Sheila, *Women, Resistance and Revolution*, Penguin, 1974.

Rowbotham, Sheila, *Woman's Consciousness, Man's World*, Penguin, 1973.

Rowbotham, Sheila, *Hidden From History*, Pluto, 1973.

Unbecoming Men: a men's consciousness-raising group writes on oppression and themselves. Times Change Press, 1971.

Wandor, Michelene (ed.), *The Body Politic*, Stage 1, 1972, The first anthology of writings from the British women's movement. Useful as an introduction.

Williams, Maxine, and Newman, Pamela, *Black Women's Liberation*, Pathfinder Press pamphlet.

Wilson, Elizabeth, *Women and the Welfare State*, Tavistock, 1977.

Medical

The British Medical Journal, BMA House, Tavistock Square, London WC1. Expensive and highly technical, can be ordered through a library.

Ehrenreich, Barbara, and English, Deirdre, *Complaints and Disorders: The Sexual Politics of Sickness*, Writers and Readers Publishing Co-operative.

Ehrenreich, Barbara and English, Deirdre, *Witches, Midwives and Nurses: A History of Women Healers*, Writers and Readers Publishing Co-operative. Both these available from Compendium.

First Aid Manual, published by British Red Cross, 1973.

The Haslemere Group, *Who Needs the Drug Companies*, available from Rising Free. Excellent booklet.

Klass, A., *There's Gold in Them Thar Pills*, Penguin, 1975. Useful for information, but the author seems to think, unlike the Haslemere Group (above), that the problem can best be combatted by doctors behaving more responsibly. Not surprisingly, he's a doctor.

Klein, R., *Complaints Against Doctors: A Study in Professional Accountability*, Knight, 1973.

The Lancet, 7 Adam Street, London W C2. Also highly technical.

Lanson, Lucienne, *From Woman to Woman*, Penguin, 1976. About gynaecological matters in question and answer form. Useful, but not feminist; written by a doctor.

Leach, Gerald, *The Biocrats*, Penguin, 1972.

McKeith, Nancy (ed.), *The New Women's Health Handbook*, Virago, 1978.

The Medical Letter, 56 Harrison Street, New Rochelle, NY 10801. A newsletter produced by concerned doctors.

M.I.M.S. Journal (Monthly Index of Medical Specialities): index of drugs compiled monthly from details supplied by the drug companies, and provided free to doctors. Gives up-to-date information on side effects and uses. 'For use only by registered medical practitioners', but there is nothing to stop you getting hold of a copy from a friendly doctor. Haymarket Press.

M.I.M.S. Colour Index (published annually by Haymarket Press). Contains colour charts and details of chemical constituents of all drugs.

Parish, Peter, *Medicines – A Guide for Everybody*, Penguin, 1976.

Samuels, Mike, and Bennett, Hal, *The Well Body Book*, Wildwood House, 1974.

BOOKSHOPS AND MAIL ORDER

Places where you should be able to get/order most of the books we have listed. Those marked with an asterisk put out book lists on sexual politics.

* **Compendium**, 240 Camden High Street, London NW1 (01 485 8944). Extremely good commercial bookshop.

* **Rising Free**, 182 Upper Street, London N1 (01 359 3785). Specializes in pamphlets and periodicals and material which is unlikely to be distributed commercially.

Pathfinder Book Centre, 93 Goldsmith Street, Nottingham.

Shirlee's Stall, Greyfriars Market, 14 Forrest Road, Edinburgh.

* **Grassroots**, 109 Oxford Road, Manchester.

* **Publications Distribution Co-op**, 27 Clerkenwell Close, London EC1.

* **Sisterwrite**, 190 Upper Street, London N1 (01 226 9782).

INDEX

584